Harald Kittler, Cliff Rosendahl, Alan Cameron, Philipp Tschandl · **Dermatoscopy**

Harald Kittler
Cliff Rosendahl, Alan Cameron, Philipp Tschandl

Dermatoscopy

Pattern analysis of pigmented and non-pigmented lesions

2nd edition

facultas

Harald Kittler MD, Philipp Tschandl MD
Department of Dermatology, Medical University of Vienna, Austria

Cliff Rosendahl MBBS PhD FSCCA, Alan Cameron MBBS FSCCA
School of Medicine, The University of Queensland, Australia

2nd edition 2016
© 2011 Facultas Verlags- und Buchhandels AG
facultas Universitätsverlag, Vienna, Austria
www.facultas.at/verlag

ISBN 978-3-7089-1385-8

Typeset by Norbert Novak & Florian Spielauer, Vienna, Austria, www.media-n.at

The first edition has been translated into seven languages.
We owe great thanks to the international team who made each of these translations possible.
We dedicate the 2nd edition to them.

Agata Bulinska (Polish, Russian)

Teona Shulaia, Natalia Kiladze, Dmitry Michajlowski (Russian)

Hélène Roche Plaine, Jean-Yves Gourhant, Adriana Bulinska (French)

Gabriel Salerni, Magdalena Bulinska (Spanish)

Andrea Giuseppe Di Stefano (Italian)

Bengü Nisa Akay, Cengizhan Erdem (Turkish)

Renata Hübner Frainer (Portuguese)

Preface

Dermatoscopy is a simple method that anyone can learn. However, many doctors still doubt that they can gain sufficient skill in dermatoscopy for it to be useful in their everyday clinical practice. One of the main reasons for this attitude is the discrepancy between the simplicity of the method and the difficulty of the jargon used by experts, which may be quite incomprehensible to the uninitiated. Such jargon rarely adds significant information to one's observation but it does create an irksome barrier which makes dermatoscopy unnecessarily difficult to learn. One of the main concerns of this book is to remove this barrier from the path of learning.

The reason for writing this book was the clear need for a single source of concise, easily comprehensible, and consistent learning materials to teach the method of pattern analysis. Pattern analysis is a comprehensive and powerful diagnostic tool and has proved to be the method with the greatest diagnostic accuracy in the majority of studies. The method presented here is not a new invention, or even another new algorithm, but plain and simple pattern analysis. Its novelty is merely that inaccuracies and ambiguities have been consistently avoided, and prime importance has been given to clarity, logic, and consistency in both the language used to describe lesions and the method of using these descriptions to reach a diagnosis. I would not have undertaken this project without the encouragement and support of Dr. Elisabeth Riedl and Dr. A. Bernard Ackerman, who contributed to the development of the method by providing a large number of valuable ideas and concepts. Regrettably, Dr. Ackerman passed away suddenly in December 2008. He has left a void that cannot be filled. He was a magnificent teacher, full of spirit and verve, and possessed unique originality.

I also wish to thank those who generously provided the visual material and thus made it possible to write this book at all. As the majority of clinical photographs have been derived from the archives of the Department of Dermatology in Vienna, I am most grateful to the current Head of the Department, Univ. Prof. Dr. Hubert Pehamberger who, with no hesitation and with the greatest willingness, gave permission to use these images. I also thank his retired predecessors Univ. Prof. Dr. Klaus Wolff and Univ. Prof. Dr. Herbert Hönigsmann. Most of the clinical pictures were taken by Andreas Ebner, who is an extremely talented and patient photographer at the Department of Dermatology in Vienna. I thank Univ. Prof. Dr. Michael Binder; he was my first teacher of dermatoscopy and generously provided his camera for taking many of the dermatoscopic pictures in this book. However, the photographs in this book are not derived from Vienna alone. Colleagues from all corners of the globe generously and selflessly provided photographs, include Giuseppe Argenziano, Ralph Braun, Ian McColl, Jean-Yves Gourhant, Maggie Oliviero, Harold Rabinovitz, Isil Kilinc Karaarslan, Iris Zalaudek, and of course the two co-authors Cliff Rosendahl and Alan Cameron. The English edition of this book could not have been produced without their help. Philipp Tschandl helped us to inspect and prepare the photographs, select references, and especially write the chapter on Inflammatory Skin Diseases. The excellent English draft of the German edition was produced by Sujata Wagner. I am indebted to her for her patience and accuracy. Finally, I wish to thank the staff of Facultas Verlag (publisher) for their support and cooperation. Specifically, Hani Aghakhani and Norbert Novak worked extensively in designing the book. Finally I must thank Dr. Sigrid Neulinger for her extreme patience in dealing with innumerable missed deadlines.

Vienna, October 2011   *Harald Kittler*

Preface to 2nd edition

The success of the first edition took us by surprise. It has been translated into seven languages. The second edition is not merely a reprint of the first. All chapters have been updated and new material added, incorporating suggestions of readers and correcting the (inevitable!) mistakes that were brought to our attention. Some chapters have been completely rewritten. We thank Jean-Yves Gourhant, Pedro Zaballos, Iris Zalaudek, Giuseppe Argenziano, Bengü Nisa Akay, and Bianca Carlos for providing us their images. We have worked hard on the 2nd edition and we hope that we exceeded your expectations.

Harald Kittler, Alan Cameron,
Cliff Rosendahl, Philipp Tschandl

Vienna, Austria and Brisbane, Australia,
September 2016

Contents

1 **General Principles** **9**
  1.2 Indication and Benefits of Dermatoscopy 10
  1.3 Diagnostic Accuracy 14
  1.4 Training 15
  1.5 Development of the Method 16
      1.5.1 Pattern Analysis 16
      1.5.2 Evolution of a diagnostic algorithm 17
      1.5.3 Scoring Systems for Melanocytic Lesions 17
      1.5.4 What happened to pattern analysis? 18
      1.5.5 Standardization and Consensus 19
      1.5.6 Critique of diagnostic methods and metaphoric terminology 20
2 **Principal pigmented skin lesions relevant to dermatoscopy** **27**
  2.1 Melanocytic lesions 27
      2.1.1 Melanocytic nevi 27
      2.1.2 Melanoma 42
  2.2 Non-melanocytic pigmented lesions 42
      2.2.1 Vascular proliferations, vascular malformations and hemorrhage 42
      2.2.2 Melanotic macules 45
      2.2.3 Benign epithelial neoplasms 49
      2.2.4 Malignant epithelial neoplasms ("keratinocyte cancer") 50
      2.2.5 Adnexal neoplasms 50
      2.2.6 Dermatofibroma 51
      2.2.7 Other pigmented lesions relevant to dermatoscopy 51
3 **Pattern Analysis – Basic Principles** **53**
  3.1 Basic elements 53
  3.2 Basic patterns 53
      3.2.1 Pattern of lines 53
      3.2.2 Pattern of dots 55
      3.2.3 Pattern of clods 55
      3.2.4 Pattern of circles 55
      3.2.5 Pattern of pseudopods 55
      3.2.6 Structureless pattern 55
      3.2.7 Combinations of patterns 62
  3.3 Colors 62
      3.3.1 Melanin 62
      3.3.2 Other pigments 64
      3.3.3 Color combinations 65
  3.4 Descriptions of pigmented lesions on the basis of patterns and colors 65
  3.5 Clues 66
  3.6 Characteristic features of pigmented non-melanocytic lesions 74
      3.6.1 Proliferation of vessels 74
      3.6.2 Intracorneal hemorrhage 77
      3.6.3 Solar lentigo, seborrheic keratosis and lichen planus-like keratosis 77
      3.6.4 Dermatofibroma 81

      3.6.5 Melanotic macules...81
      3.6.6 Pigmented basal cell carcinoma 89
      3.6.7 Squamous cell carcinoma 89
  3.7 Characteristic features of melanocytic lesions 97
      3.7.1 Melanocytic nevi 97
      3.7.2 Melanoma...113
      3.7.3 Metastases of melanoma 121
4 **Metaphoric dermatoscopic terms and what they mean** **125**
5 **An algorithmic method for the diagnosis of pigmented lesions** **147**
  5.1 One pattern 147
      5.1.1 Lines 147
      5.1.2 Pseudopods 156
      5.1.3 Circles 156
      5.1.4 Clods 158
      5.1.5 Dots 167
      5.1.6 Structureless 169
  5.2 More than one pattern 171
      5.2.1 Lines 173
      5.2.2 Pseudopods 184
      5.2.3 Circles 185
      5.2.4 Clods 186
      5.2.5 Dots 187
  5.3 Applying pattern analysis to clinical practice 190
  5.4 Chaos and Clues 190
6 **Non-pigmented (amelanotic) lesions**..**203**
  6.1 Clues used in the diagnosis of non-pigmented (amelanotic) lesions..........203
  6.2 Vascular patterns 211
  6.3 Differential diagnosis of non-pigmented lesions 212
7 **Clues and Clichés** **235**
  7.1 Clues 235
  7.2 Common Clichés 243
8 **Special situations** **253**
  8.1 Nails 253
  8.2 Acral lesions...260
  8.3 The face...269
  8.4 Mucosal lesions 280
  8.5 Recurrent melanocytic lesions 280
  8.6 Difficult lesions 280
  8.7 Inflammatory skin diseases 286
9 **Digital Dermatoscopic Monitoring** **297**
  9.1 Choice of lesions to monitor 298
  9.2 Interpretation of changes 302
  9.3 Growing nevus or melanoma? 302
  9.4 Benefits and Risks...306
10 **Cases** **309**
11 **Dermatoscopic-dermatopathologic correlation**...............................**373**

  Supplement **387**
  Index..**389**

1 General Principles

1.1 The Investigation Technique

Dermatoscopy is a simple and non-invasive investigation technique that enhances one's naked eye perception of skin lesions by revealing significant additional morphological features, and thus facilitating, or making possible, the establishment of a diagnosis. The first use of an instrument with an inbuilt light source and the first use of the word 'dermatoscopy' to describe the technique appears to be in 1920, by the German dermatologist Johann Saphier (1) *(1.1)*.

Saphier based his approach on previous reports published by Unna and Kromayer (1893), who described a technique of viewing skin lesions through a glass plate coupled to the skin by immersion oil (under the name 'diascopy'). Like Unna and Kromayer, Saphier's investigations were mainly focused on inflammatory skin diseases. At the time, the diagnosis of pigmented skin lesions was considered to be of little importance. The benefits of dermatoscopy for the diagnosis of pigmented lesions became recognized in the last third of the 20th century – specifically for the diagnosis of melanoma. During this renaissance dermatoscopy was given several other names such as *epiluminescence microscopy*. A more recent term frequently used in the Anglo-American literature is *dermoscopy*. However, these neologisms have contributed to the type of confusion that arises when different terms are used for one and the same entity. Saphier, who was first to describe an instrument with all the components of modern instruments, named it dermatoscopy. Therefore, this is the only term that will be used in this book.

From Saphier's time through until the 1980s, dermatoscopy was performed using cumbersome stereomicroscopes. Today one uses a simple hand-held instrument consisting of a focusable magnifying lens, LED illumination, a transparent contact plate and possibly polarizing filters *(1.2)*.

The use of a contact plate coupled to the skin with a transparent fluid is crucial to the function of the dermatoscope. When one examines lesions clinically (or with a dermatoscope without fluid), the majority of the light remitted to the observer's eye is reflected back from the most superficial layer of the epidermis, the stratum corneum. This largely obscures details of

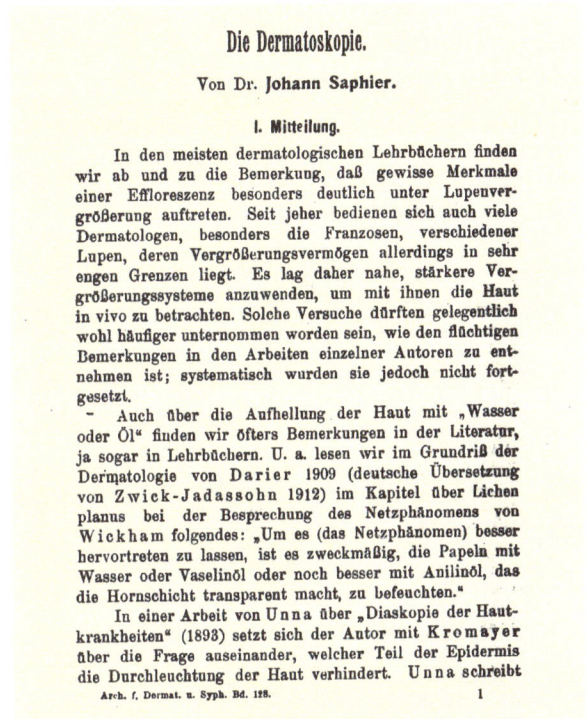

Figure 1.1a: *Extract from Johann Saphier's original paper titled "Dermatoskopie", published in 1920 in the Journal "Archiv für Dermatologie und Syphilis" (Archive for Dermatology and Syphilis).*

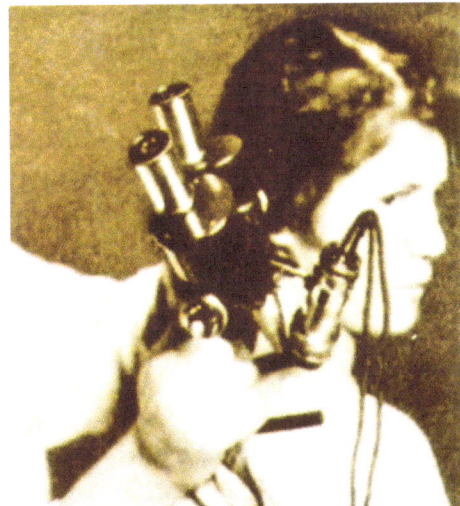

Figure 1.1b: *Binocular dermatoscope from Saphier's times (around 1920).*

Figure 1.3: *Procedure for dermatoscopy: First a contact fluid – in this case ultrasound gel – is applied on the skin lesion to be investigated. The transparent contact plate of the hand-held dermatoscope is then pressed onto the pigmented lesion covered with gel (the contact fluid smoothens the surface and reduces reflection), and the lesion can then be viewed through the magnifying lens.*

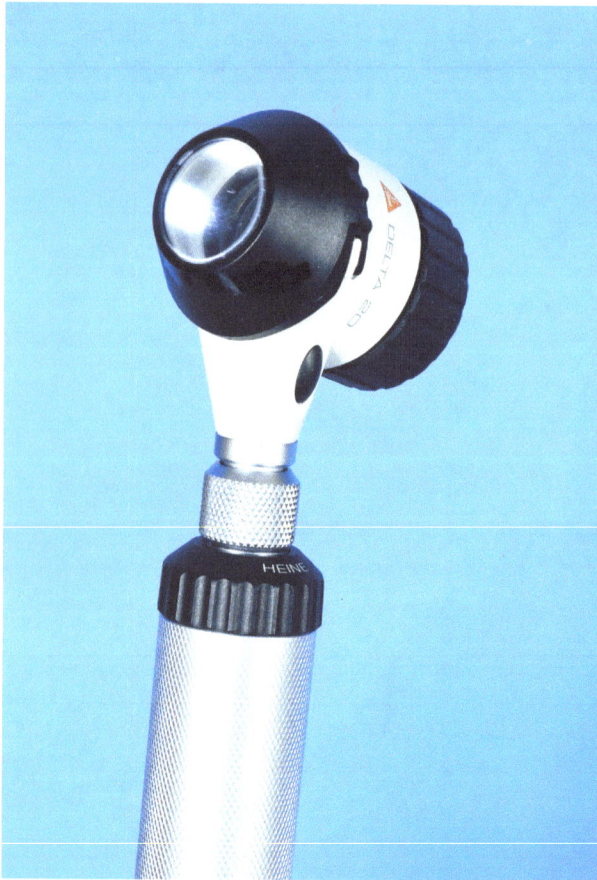

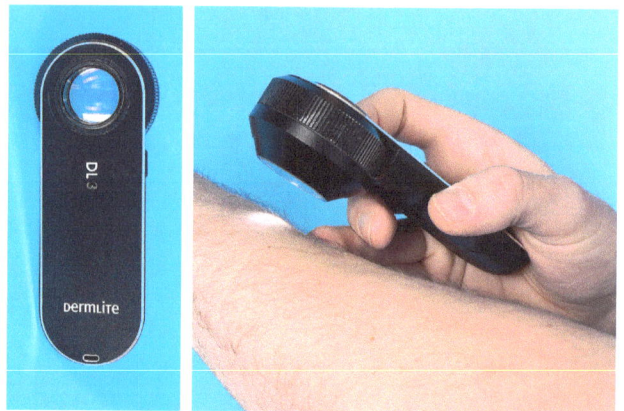

Figure 1.2: *Commonly used handheld dermatoscope of Heine Company. When using this simple hand-held device one needs a contact fluid such as paraffin oil or ultrasound gel.*

Figure 1.4: *Dermatoscope with polarized light, which dispenses with the need for a contact fluid or direct contact with the skin.*

lesion pigmentation and vascularity, as these features are located in deeper layers of the epidermis, and the dermis. Light remitted from deeper structures is irregularly refracted by the unevenness of the superficial keratin layer, further degrading the perceived image. These phenomena are largely eliminated by using a contact fluid (such as alcohol, paraffin oil or ultrasound gel) to couple the baseplate of the dermatoscope to the skin. *(1.3 and 1.5)*. Replacing the air between the skin and faceplate glass with a fluid smoothens the skin surface and creates a far better match of refractive indices, which greatly reduces reflection from the skin surface. More recently, dermatoscopes have been developed which eliminate surface reflection by the use of polarizing filters *(1.4)*. These instruments do not require a contact fluid, or even direct contact with the skin. Although the images seen using polarizing instruments are very similar to those seen using contact dermatoscopy, a few significant differences exist (2). For example, perpendicular white lines ("shiny white lines") are only

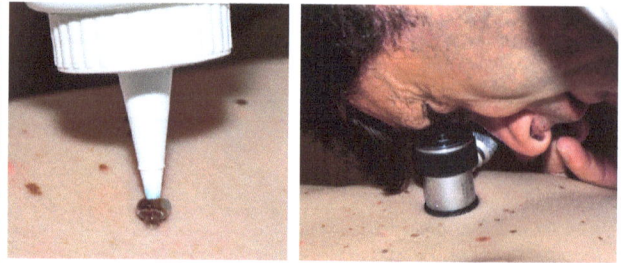

visible with polarized dermatoscopy *(1.6, bottom row)*, while the white dots and clods of seborrheic keratosis are best viewed with non-polarized dermatoscopy *(1.6, top row)* Polarized and non-polarized dermatoscopy are therefore best considered complementary. Most new handheld dermatoscopes can switch between polarized and non-polarized mode.

1.2 Indication and Benefits of Dermatoscopy
In short, dermatoscopy is indicated when better resolution of pigment or vascular structures in the epidermis or upper dermis will help resolve a differential diagnosis. Immediately after the introduction of handheld instruments, dermatoscopy was promoted as being particularly useful in differentiating nevi from melanomas by assessment of pigment patterns. While this is important, the vast majority of cutaneous malignancies are not pigmented. Furthermore, even skin neoplasms which are most commonly pigmented have lightly pigmented

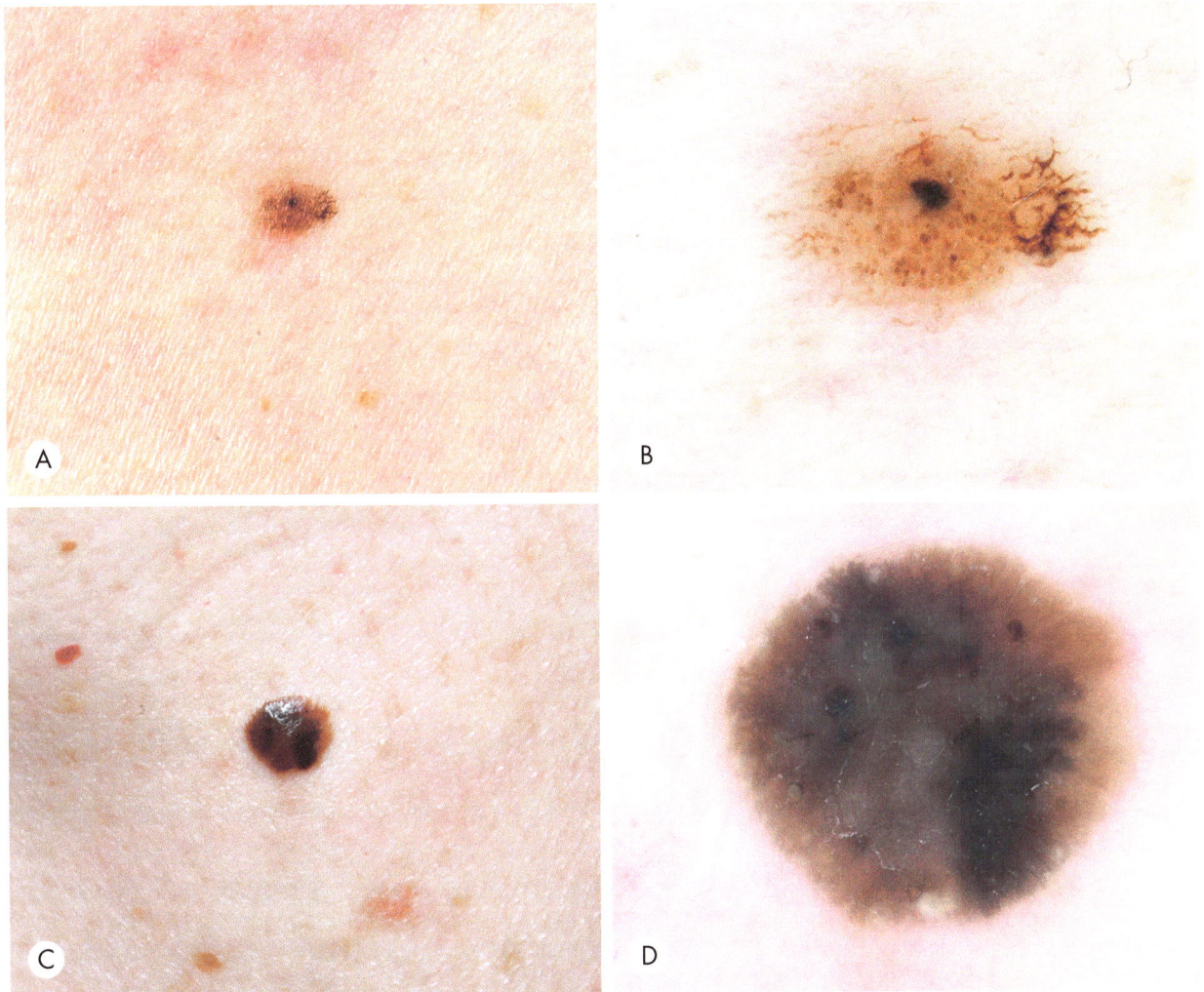

Figure 1.5: Two pigment lesions: A and B represent a melanocytic nevus while C and D show a seborrheic keratosis. The pictures in the left column (A, C) show what is seen with the naked eye while the right column (B, D) shows the image seen through the dermatoscope. In the dermatoscopic image one finds additional structural details that escape detection by the naked eye. This enhancement of detail is partly attributable to magnification, but more to the reduction of reflection on the surface of the skin.

or entirely non-pigmented variants. This includes a significant minority of melanomas.

While patterns formed by blood vessels and keratin are less diagnostically specific than patterns formed by melanin pigment, they still provide significant additional diagnostic information when pigment is absent, over and above naked eye clinical examination (3, 4).

Diagnosis of Melanoma

Despite strong evidence to the contrary, the belief that dermatoscopy adds nothing to the diagnosis of melanoma compared to naked eye examination persists into the 21st century.

In a trivial sense, this is true in that dermatoscopy does not add anything to the diagnosis of melanomas which

can confidently be diagnosed clinically, but this is a misunderstanding as to the role of dermatoscopy. The foremost role of dermatoscopy is not confirmation of a diagnosis established clearly with the naked eye but the unveiling of morphological criteria that revise the diagnosis established with the naked eye. Dermatoscopy can shift the point of diagnosis closer to the initial emergence of the neoplasm, but only if lesions with no naked eye evidence of malignancy are routinely examined.

We consider it self-evident that every melanoma goes through a stage in its evolution when it lacks the criteria required to allow diagnosis. This is the reason the clinical ABCD rule (1.7) contains a size criterion — not because melanomas are never less than 6 mm diameter,

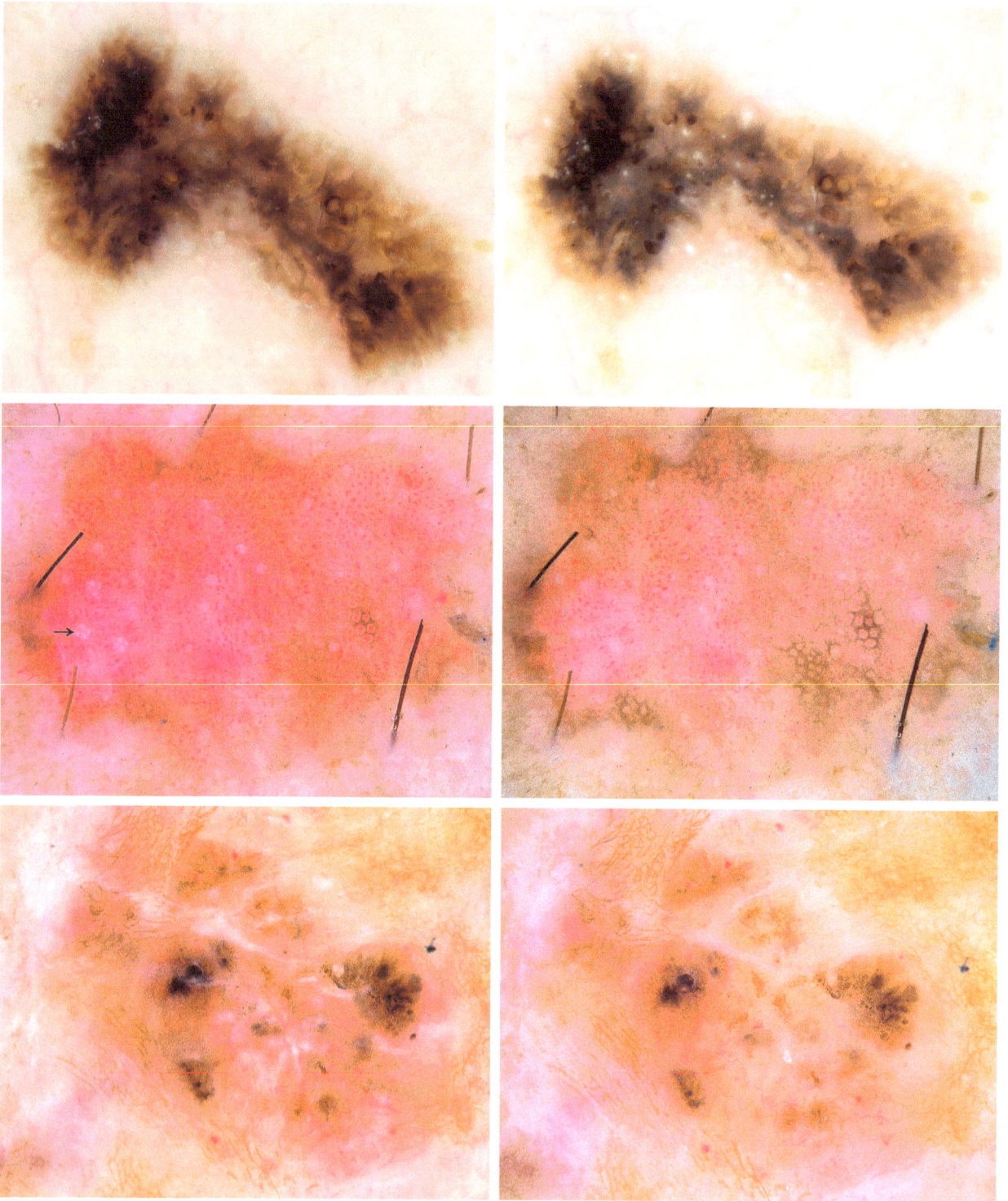

Figure 1.6: Dermatoscopy with and without polarization.
The pigmented lesions were photographed with (left column) and without (right column) polarization. **Top row:** The typical white dots and clods ("milia-like cysts") of a seborrheic keratosis are better seen with classic contact dermatoscopy without polarization (right) and are invisible with polarization (left). **Middle row:** The coiled vessels of pigmented intraepithelial carcinoma (pigmented Bowen disease) are visible with and without polarization but with polarization (left) they appear more prominent. In the left image there are also some specific structures that consist of four white dots arranged in a square (arrow). These structures are only visible with polarized dermatoscopy. **Bottom row:** A basal cell carcinoma with white lines (left), which are nearly invisible without polarization.

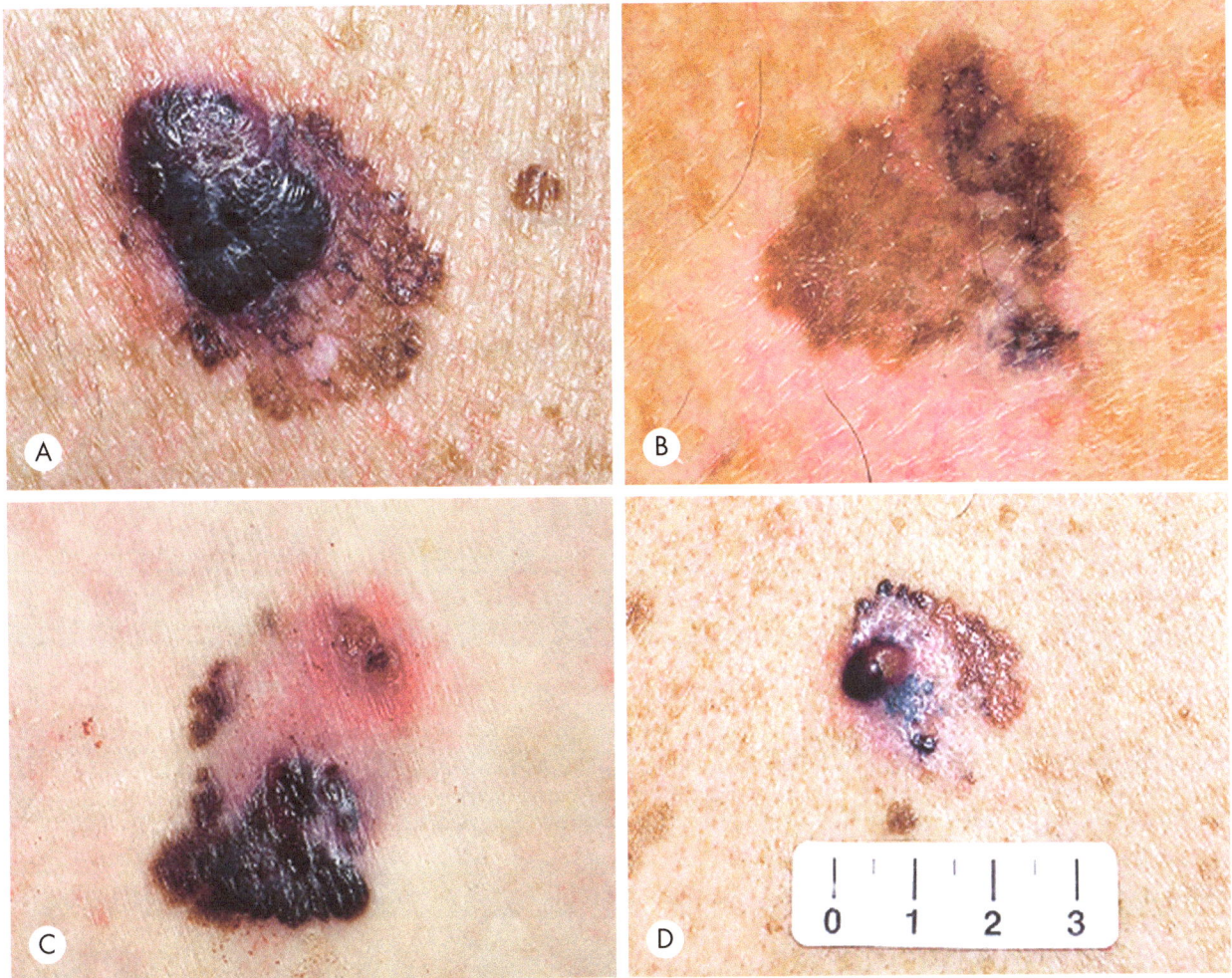

Figure 1.7: The concept of the clinical ABCD rule is illustrated by four melanomas. The ABCD criteria are applied when the melanoma has achieved a certain size and has been present for a longer period of time (usually a few years). All of these melanomas are already invasive. In other words, they are not confined to the epidermis (in situ), but have invaded the underlying dermis. The chances of cure are reduced in proportion to the increasing depth of invasion.

but because the accuracy of clinical diagnosis is only acceptable for larger lesions. Melanomas less than 6 mm diameter are routinely diagnosable by dermatoscopy. Indeed, dermatoscopic monitoring over time allows diagnosis of melanomas even before the emergence of specific dermatoscopic features.

Figure 1.8 shows a melanoma just a few millimeters in size, which shows no melanoma-specific criteria on naked-eye inspection. It is neither asymmetrical nor has irregular margins, is not multicolored, and is not larger than 6 mm in size. However, dermatoscopic investigation shows that the criteria of a melanoma are clearly fulfilled. The diagnosis was confirmed by histology showing an *in situ melanoma (1.9)*. In other words, neoplastic melanocytes are confined to the

epidermis. After excision of this melanoma, the patient may be deemed to be cured of the disease.

Like every morphological method, dermatoscopy has limitations. Dermatoscopy cannot entirely replace histopathology; in some cases histopathology is the only way to establish an unequivocal diagnosis. Rarely, dermatoscopy may be misleading; the naked eye criteria point in the right direction and dermatoscopic criteria erroneously point to a different diagnosis. However, these exceptions are only that, exceptions, and a large body of evidence demonstrates that the addition of dermatoscopy improves overall diagnostic accuracy. Histopathology is also a purely morphological method with its own limitations. Correlation of histopathologic with dermatoscopic findings may allow a diagnosis even when histopathology alone is not diagnostic.

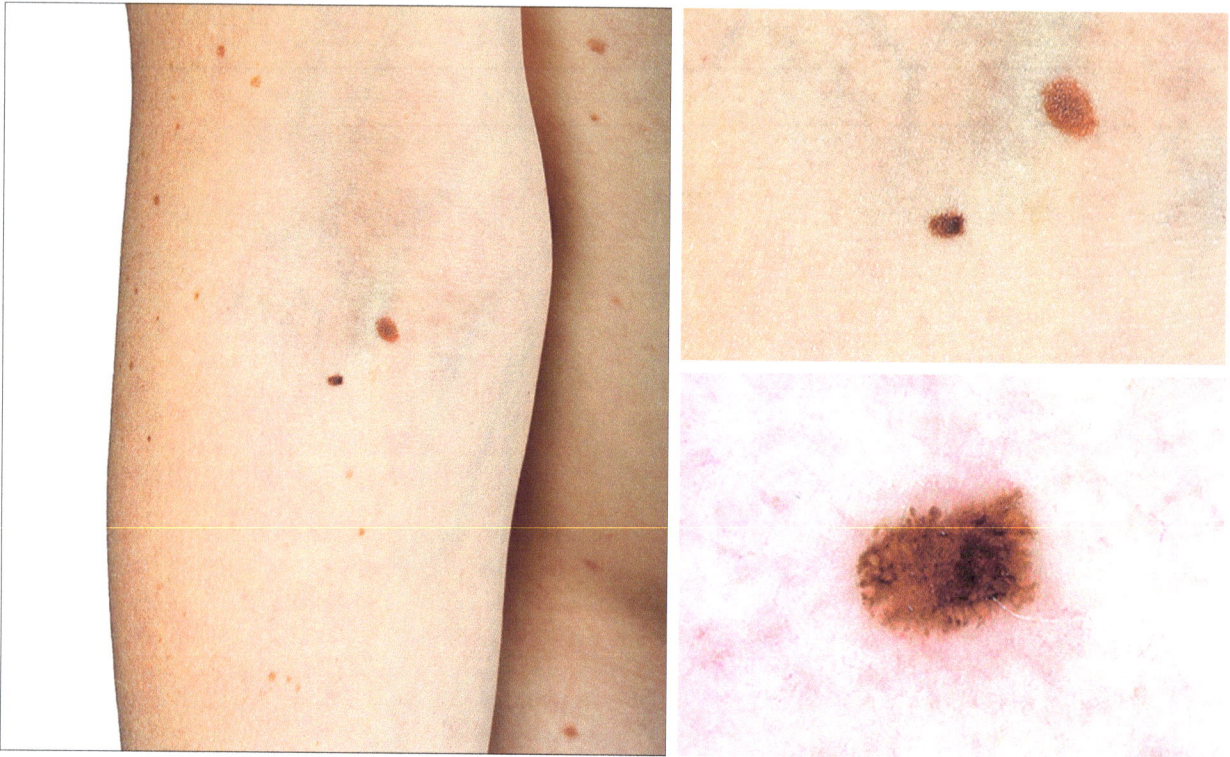

Figure 1.8: A melanoma on the forearm, just a few millimeters in size. The condition may be clearly diagnosed as a melanoma on the basis of dermatoscopy because of the presence of so-called pseudopods, whereas the application of the ABCD rule and naked-eye assessment are both unreliable. The histological image clearly shows an in situ melanoma (Figure 1.9).

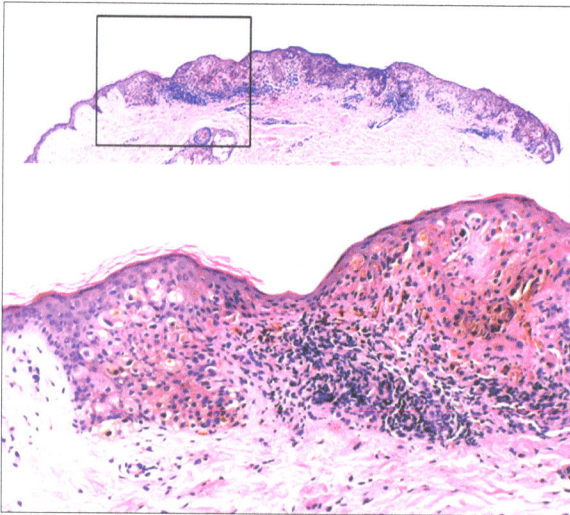

Figure 1.9: Histopathological view of the melanoma shown in Figure 1.8. Although the lesion is small, a melanoma can be diagnosed with absolute certainty. The melanocytic lesion is asymmetrical. The melanocytes in the epidermis are mainly arranged as single cells, melanocytes vary in size and shape, possess a hyperchromatic nucleus, an eosinophilic cytoplasm, and contain dusty melanin pigment. One finds several individual melanocytes in higher layers of the epidermis (pagetoid spread). The diagnosis is in situ melanoma.

1.3 Diagnostic Accuracy

The benefits of dermatoscopy as compared to examination with the naked eye alone are measurable and have been examined in multiple studies. Most of the published studies do not consider differentiating melanoma from all other skin lesions, but are limited to the distinction between melanocytic nevi and melanoma. In this simple case, the diagnostic accuracy can be expressed by two indices. Sensitivity is defined as the proportion of correctly diagnosed melanomas in relation to the total number of melanomas in the investigated sample. For instance, if 70 of 100 melanomas are diagnosed correctly as melanomas, the sensitivity of the examination is 70%. Specificity is defined as the proportion of correctly diagnosed nevi in the investigated sample. For instance, if 80 of 100 nevi are diagnosed correctly, the specificity of the examination is 80%. Table 1.1 lists the results of 13 studies in which the diagnostic accuracy of dermatoscopy was directly compared with naked-eye inspection. The given values of sensitivity and specificity refer exclusively to the distinction between melanomas and nevi. The different values found in the various studies are more a reflection of study design than any "real" differences; differences in the selection of samples,

Table 1.1

First author and year of publication	Sample size (n)	Sensitivity		Specificity	
		Unaided eye	Dermatoscopy	Unaided eye	Dermatoscopy
Benelli 1999	401	67%	80%	79%	89%
Binder 1995	240	58%	68%	91%	91%
Binder 1997	100	73%	73%	70%	78%
Carli 1998	15	42%	75%	78%	89%
Cristofolini 1994	220	85%	88%	75%	79%
Dummer 1993	824	65%	96%	93%	98%
Krähn 1998	80	79%	90%	78%	93%
Lorentzen 1999	232	77%	82%	89%	94%
Nachbar 1994	172	84%	93%	84%	91%
Soyer 1995	159	94%	94%	82%	82%
Stanganelli 1998	20	55%	73%	79%	73%
Stanganelli 2000	3.329	67%	93%	99%	100%
Westerhoff 2000	100	63%	76%	54%	58%

the manner of presenting dermatoscopic images, and the subjects' level of training, to name a few. Still, the majority of studies show the diagnostic accuracy of dermatoscopy to be higher than that of the naked-eye investigation. In 2002 and in 2008 the results of the studies were confirmed by two meta-analyses (5, 6). In 2011 Rosendahl et al. confirmed that dermatoscopy also improves the diagnostic accuracy for non-melanocytic lesions (7).

1.4 Training

Specific training in dermatoscopy is essential. Elementary training in the use of the method requires no more than a few days for beginners with a basic knowledge of pigmented skin lesions. Not only physicians but also nurses, medical students and even lay persons can be successfully trained to use dermatoscopy (8). However, as is true for all morphological methods, continuous practice and regular use of the method are absolute prerequisites for the achievement of real expertise. Without basic training, adding dermatoscopy to clinical examination has been shown to worsen diagnostic accuracy (9). The subjects in this study were physicians who had some experience in clinical diagnosis of pigmented lesions, but no formal training in dermatoscopy. The subjects were confronted with two photographs — clinical close-up and dermatoscopy — of a series of pigmented lesions. The sensitivity (the percentage of correctly diagnosed melanomas) dropped significantly after presentation of dermatoscopic photographs. It has

been speculated that the unfamiliar structures revealed by dermatoscopy only served to confuse clinicians who are trained in naked eye assessment. The trivial but important conclusion drawn from this study was that dermatoscopy serves only those who know how to use the procedure. A similarly structured study showed that a short and intensive phase of training – of just a few days' duration – is sufficient to learn the basic principles of the method and markedly improve diagnostic accuracy (10).

The best way to teach dermatoscopy to novices is still a matter of debate. Tschandl et al. tested the two common strategies used to teach dermatoscopy (11). One group of students received a more verbal-based training with detailed explanations of diagnostic criteria, the other group received a more visual-based training involving the presentation of a large number of images representative for each diagnosis without pointing out specific criteria. The first method may be called the explanatory, the second the demonstrative method. The diagnostic accuracy was similar in both groups although there were some differences with regard to certain diagnoses. The group receiving demonstrative training had a higher sensitivity for basal cell carcinoma whereas the group receiving explanatory training had a higher sensitivity for seborrheic keratosis and a higher specificity for nevi. We consider these to be complementary strategies. One needs to learn the "alphabet" of dermatoscopy, which is best explained verbally, but one also needs to see the different patterns and their subtle variations, which is best demonstrated visually.

1.5 Development of the Method

It is instructive to follow the evolution of dermatoscopy as a tool for the assessment of pigmented skin lesions – on the one hand to understand the origins of common methods, and on the other hand to comprehend and classify the diverse terms in use (the *ad hoc* proliferation of terms is a major source of confusion). Pioneers in the field of dermatoscopy such as Saphier largely confined themselves to the description of inflammatory skin lesions like lichen planus, lupus erythematosus, or scabies. At this time dermatoscopy was apparently of no importance for the diagnosis of pigmented skin lesions or melanoma. The first serious report about the value of dermatoscopy for the diagnosis of melanoma was published by Rona MacKie in 1971 (12). Ten years later the Austrians Fritsch and Pechlaner published "Differentiation of benign from malignant melanocytic lesions using incident light microscopy". In addition to other criteria, the authors describe in detail the basic anatomical features of the pigment network, which is one of the principal structures in dermatoscopy (13). This report mentions dermatoscopic differences between nevi and melanomas, but a general method for the diagnosis of pigmented skin lesions is just briefly outlined.

1.5.1 Pattern Analysis

In 1987 Pehamberger, Steiner, and Wolff described pattern analysis, the first analytical method to distinguish between the primary types of pigmented skin lesions (at the time, the rather cumbersome term *epiluminescence microscopy* was used instead of *dermatoscopy*) (14, 15). Pattern analysis is based on recognition of a number of dermatoscopic structures which constitute reproducible patterns characteristic of the more common pigmented lesions. As the first studies on pattern analysis were published in English-language journals, the Austrians Pehamberger, Steiner, and Wolff used only English terms for the structures they described, such as *radial streaming, blue-whitish veil or the milky way*. These neologisms were poorly defined or not defined at all. This artificial metaphoric language created a barrier even to those willing to learn. Furthermore, the diagnosis was based not only on the presence or absence of a dermatoscopic structure, but also on qualitative aspects. For instance, the German term "Schollen" (clods) which was given the English designation of "globules" was assessed according to whether they were distributed regularly or irregularly, and whether they were of the same size or different sizes. Qualitative aspects of the pigment network described a few years earlier by Fritsch and Pechlaner included, according to Pehamberger, Steiner, and Wolff, paired terms such as

Table 1.2: List of dermatoscopic criteria established at the consensus conference in Hamburg in 1989
Pigment network
discrete
prominent
regular
irregular
wide
narrow
broad
delicate
Irregular extensions, pseudopods
Radial streaming
Brown globules
Black dots
Whitish veil, milky way
White scar-like depigmented areas
Grayish-blue areas
Hypopigmentation
Reticular depigmentation
Milia-like cysts
Comedo-like openings
Telangiectasia
Reddish-blue areas
Maple leaf-like areas

regular/irregular, or delicate/prominent, and narrow/broad. Unfortunately (though inevitably) these poorly defined qualitative properties were subject to a wide range of inter-individual differences in interpretation, and were poorly reproducible. Despite justified criticisms, however, the studies of Pehamberger, Steiner, and Wolff were the first systematic approaches in this field and the starting point for further developments that followed in subsequent years.

Shortly afterwards, other research groups in Europe also showed interest in dermatoscopy, which soon led to a variety of approaches. The consequences were an uncontrolled growth of terms on the one hand, and the absence of consensus about fundamental aspects on the other. The first attempt to counteract this evolution and standardize dermatoscopy was made as early as in 1989 at a consensus conference in Hamburg (16). The results of this consensus conference were published in 1990. The participants established a list of diagnostic criteria that is shown in *table 1.2*. One outcome of the consensus conference was speculation about the histopathological correlates of dermatoscopic criteria, but there was no attempt to define the listed criteria. Today this list is mainly of historical value.

1.5.2 Evolution of a diagnostic algorithm

The pattern analysis published by Pehamberger, Steiner and Wolff in 1987 was mainly confined to a description of the frequencies of dermatoscopic structures for the most important pigmented skin lesions. A formal method that can be used for melanocytic as well as non-melanocytic skin lesions and which guides the investigator in a structured manner to a specific diagnosis was not provided. This was developed in the following years. In this regard, the studies of Jürgen Kreusch (17) and Wilhelm Stolz (18) are worthy of mention. They proposed a 2-step algorithm. The first step classified pigmented skin lesions as either melanocytic or non-melanocytic, and specifically diagnosed several common non-melanocytic tumors. The second step was applied to melanocytic lesions only, with the goal of distinguishing melanoma from melanocytic nevi. This method of investigation gained acceptance, although in slightly modified form and despite a few weaknesses (which will be addressed later).

1.5.3 Scoring Systems for Melanocytic Lesions

The subsequent evolution of the technique saw attempts to simplify the method and schematize it further. Attention was mainly focused on differentiating melanomas from nevi. In pattern analysis, evaluation of the identified dermatoscopic structures in the individual case was left to the investigator's judgment. However, this requires considerable experience, so simple scoring systems were developed. Their purpose is to lead the investigator to the correct diagnosis by the aid of structured algorithms. These systems include Stolz' ABCD rule (19), Argenziano's 7-point check list (20), Menzies' method (21), the 3-point checklist (22) the CASH algorithm (23), and the chaos and clues algorithm (24). All of the above mentioned algorithms are confined to a few structural characteristics and vary with respect to their inclusion of symmetry and color *(1.10)*.

Stolz' ABCD rule

The ABCD rule of dermatoscopy was published by Stolz in 1991. The fact that it followed the clinical ABCD rule was not a coincidence. The criteria of asymmetry, border and color are very important here. However, the letter D stands for dermatoscopic structures and not for diameter, as it does in the clinical ABCD rule. Since a size limit does not apply, the dermatoscopic ABCD rule is applicable to small melanomas as well.

In the dermatoscopic ABCD rule, scores are assigned to the four criteria of asymmetry, border, color and dermatoscopic structures, each of which are multiplied by a fixed factor (the latter is determined by the use of statistical methods and a large random sample). Dermatoscopic structures scored in the method of Stolz are pigment network, dots, clods ("globules"), "branched streaks", and structureless areas. These 4 scores are summed to determine a total dermatoscopy score. This score categorizes the lesion as either benign, suspicious or malignant. The ABCD rule only applies to melanocytic lesions.

Argenziano's 7-point check-list

When using Argenziano's 7-point check-list lesions are assessed for the presence of seven criteria; 3 major which score 2 each, and 4 minor which score 1 each. A total score of three or more is indicative of melanoma. The major criteria are an atypical pigment network, a blue-whitish veil, and an atypical vascular pattern. The minor criteria are irregular streaks, irregular dots/globules, irregular blotches, and regression structures. Like the ABCD rule, the 7-point check-list is only suitable for melanocytic lesions.

Menzies' Method

Menzies' method proceeds in a stepwise manner. First, symmetry and color are assessed. All lesions which are symmetrical or one color are regarded as benign and excluded from further analysis. All other pigmented lesions are assessed for the following dermatoscopic features: blue-white veil, multiple brown dots, pseudopods, radial streaming, scar-like depigmentation, peripheral black dots or globules, five or six colors, multiple blue-gray dots, and a broadened network. Melanoma is diagnosed when at least one of these features is present. According to the author, the sensitivity of this method is 92% and its specificity, 71%.

Three-point checklist

The 3-point checklist is a simple approach with a relatively high sensitivity and moderate to fair specificity. It takes into account only 3 criteria: Asymmetry, atypical network, and blue white structures. A pigmented lesion that has any 2 of these 3 criteria should be biopsied.

CASH algorithm

The acronym CASH stands for color, architecture, symmetry, and homogeneity. CASH is similar to Stolz' ABCD rule for dermatoscopy. The CASH score ranges from 2–17 and was reported to reach a sensitivity of 98% and a specificity of 68% at a cut point of 8.

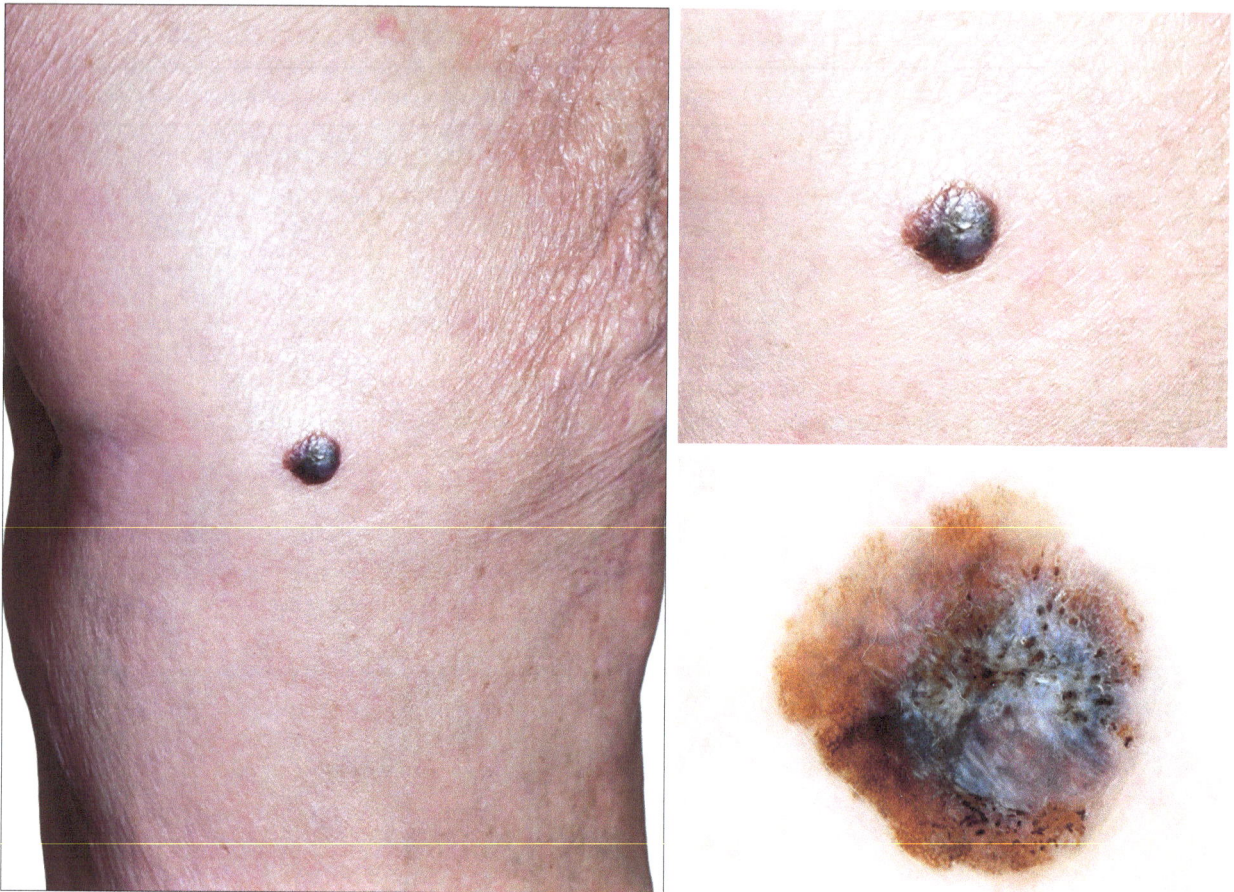

Figure 1.10: This pigmented lesion can be clearly diagnosed as a melanoma with any dermatoscopic method.

Stolz's dermatoscopic ABCD rule: A (asymmetrical in both axes; 2.6 points), B (sharp interruption of pigment in four segments; 0.4 points), C (4 different colors: light brown, dark brown, blue-gray, black; 2 points), D (4 different dermatoscopic structures: reticular lines, dots, clods, and a structureless area; 2 points) – yield 7 points in all and thus confirm the diagnosis of melanoma (if the total sum is > 4.75 points, the diagnosis is melanoma).

Argenziano's 7-point check-list: Two major criteria (asymmetry and blue-whitish veil) and a minor criterion (irregular dots/globules) yield 5 points and thus confirm the presence of a melanoma (a melanoma is presumed to exist from a score of 3 points onward).

Menzies' method: Asymmetry and more than one color and the simultaneous presence of positive criteria, such as peripheral black dots/globules or a blue-whitish veil lead to the diagnosis of melanoma.

Chaos and clues: A chaotic lesion with multiple clues to malignancy (gray/blue structures, eccentric structureless zone, peripheral black dots) should be excised to exclude malignancy.

Pattern analysis: A clearly asymmetrical pattern (reticular lines, dots, structureless area), more than one color with melanin being predominant (brown, blue, black), also arranged asymmetrically, and several specific criteria confirming the presence of a melanoma (black dots in the periphery and a structureless eccentric blue area) clearly indicate the presence of melanoma.

Chaos and clues

Like the Menzies' algorithm the chaos and clues algorithm is a stepwise procedure. First one scans for chaos (defined as asymmetry of structure or color) and only when chaos is discovered one has to search for one of nine clues to malignancy. If there are both chaos and at least one clue to malignancy then biopsy or excision is recommended. The chaos and clues algorithm does not involve any calculations. It works for melanocytic and non-melanocytic lesions.

1.5.4 What happened to pattern analysis?

In addition to these "simplified" systems, pattern analysis still exists as a comprehensive diagnostic method and it has been adapted in the last few years by the inclusion of new criteria. In this regard the work of Alfred Kopf and Ashfaq Marghoob, who defined benign and malignant patterns and included new criteria, deserves special mention (25). Also worthy of mention are the assessment of dermatoscopic criteria for pigmented basal cell carcinoma by Menzies (26), the analysis of progression patterns of facial melanoma by Stolz (27), the description of the patterns of Clark nevi by Hofmann-Wellenhof (28), the evaluation of dermatoscopic criteria of pigmented seborrheic keratosis by Braun (29), the categorization of the protean dermatoscopic patterns of dermatofibroma by Zaballos (30), the classification of patterns of acral melanocytic lesions by Saida and Tanaka (31, 32), the analysis of pigmented mucosal lesions and recurrent nevi and melanoma by Blum (33), the discovery of dermatoscopic clues for pigmented Bowen's disease by Cameron (34), and finally the dermatoscopic classification of nevi in different age groups by Zalaudek (35). All the above mentioned achievements have been accomplished by the application of pattern analysis.

In fact, it has been shown that pattern analysis is superior to other investigation techniques in many respects. Beginners find it easier to cope with the simple algorithms, but they are soon confronted with barriers which can be resolved only by a comprehensive method such as pattern analysis.

What is one talking about when one refers to pattern analysis? In actual fact, it is still not clear what a person does when he/she uses pattern analysis. Due to the large number of criteria to be considered, pattern analysis is more difficult and demanding than simple scoring systems, but it is also more powerful and flexible. How the investigator combines these criteria to reach a diagnosis remained a mystery for a long time because the rules of this skill were never clearly formulated. Thus, pattern analysis appeared to be mysteriously dependent on the user's ingenuity. Teaching this technique was a somewhat mystifying subject. The greatest challenge of this book is to render pattern analysis – this powerful methodological tool – communicable and comprehensible.

1.5.5 Standardization and Consensus

After the previously mentioned first consensus conference held in 1989 in Hamburg, nothing happened for a long time. Dermatoscopy remained split into various schools. A uniform method, homogeneous criteria, and congruent definitions were absent. It was not until the founding of the International Dermoscopy Society (IDS) in 2001, under co-founder and first president Peter Soyer, a dermatologist from Graz, that a forum was formed. This forum declared that it was responsible for answering questions relating to the consensus. As it combined all important research groups, it appeared to be legitimized to perform the task. This development culminated in a consensus conference held via the Internet and the organization of the First World Congress

of Dermatoscopy in 2002 in Rome. The results of the consensus conference were summarized in a consensus paper which was presented a year later in the Journal of the American Academy of Dermatology (JAAD) (36). The consensus included the first step of the diagnostic algorithm, namely the distinction between melanocytic and non-melanocytic lesions, as well as the previously mentioned scoring systems for melanocytic lesions and the definitions of the most commonly used terms in dermatoscopy *(1.11 to 1.13)*. Regrettably, this unique opportunity to simplify the language of dermatoscopy was missed. Instead, metaphoric terms were adhered to and incomplete or contradictory definitions were formulated.

After the results of the second consensus were published in 2003 the vocabulary of dermatoscopy expanded significantly. Even experts struggled with the multitude of terms. The main driving forces for the creation of new terms were the expansion of dermatoscopy to new realms such as inflammatory skin diseases and the introduction and dissemination of polarized dermatoscopes that allowed observations of structures previously invisible with classic contact dermatoscopy. Many new terms, especially those that were published in case reports, were ill-defined metaphors with dubious diagnostic significance.

In 2007 Harald Kittler introduced a simple descriptive terminology that avoids metaphoric terms and is based on five geometrically defined basic elements, namely lines, pseudopods, circles, clods and dots (37). The advantages of this terminology are its simplicity, its logical structure, and the lack of need for definitions beyond those of basic elements. In the following years the descriptive terminology became increasingly popular. The growing controversy between descriptive and metaphoric terminology and the growing number of new terms demanded the need for a new consensus.

In 2013 Alan Halpern initiated the International Skin Imaging collaboration (ISIC) and appointed Harald Kittler to lead a selected group of experts charged with creating a standardized dictionary of dermatoscopy. This process led to the 3rd consensus conference which was finalized during the 4th World Congress of Dermatoscopy in Vienna in April 2015. After two years of extensive discussions the expert group succeeded in creating a dictionary of standardized terms that takes into account descriptive and metaphoric terminology. This dictionary, which was published along with the consensus paper in 2016 (38), is now the standard reference for all issues related to terminology. We will deal with the dictionary in detail in chapter 4. For reasons that we will explain below the authors of this

Dermoscopic criterion	Definition
Pigment network-pseudonetwork	Network of brownish interconnected lines over a background of tan diffuse pigmentation. In facial skin a peculiar pigment network, also called pseudonetwork, is typified by round, equally sized network holes corresponding to the pre-existing follicular ostia.
Aggregated globules	Numerous, variously sized, more or less clustered, round to oval structures with various shades of brown and gray-black. They should be differentiated from multiple blue-gray globules.
Streaks	These have been previously described separately as pseudopods and radial streaming, but are now combined into the one term. They are bulbous and often kinked or finger-like projections seen at the edge of a lesion. They may arise from network structures but more commonly do not. They range in color from tan to black.
Homogeneous blue pigmentation	Structureless blue pigmentation in the absence of pigment network or other distinctive local features
Parallel pattern	Seen in melanocytic lesions of palms/soles and mucosal areas. On palms/soles the pigmentation may follow the sulci or the cristae (ie, furrows or ridges) of the dermatoglyphics. Occasionally arranged at right angles to these structures.
Multiple milia-like cysts	Numerous, variously sized, white or yellowish, roundish structures
Comedo-like openings	Brown-yellowish to brown-black, round to oval, sharply circumscribed keratotic plugs in the ostia of hair follicles. When irregularly shaped, comedo-like openings are also called irregular crypts.
Light-brown fingerprint-like structures	Light-brown, delicate, network-like structures with the pattern of a fingerprint
Cerebriform pattern	Dark-brown furrows between ridges typifying a brain-like appearance
Arborizing vessels	Tree-like branching telangiectases
Leaf-like structures	Brown to gray/blue discrete bulbous structures forming leaf-like patterns. They are discrete pigmented nests (islands) never arising from a pigment network and usually not arising from adjacent confluent pigmented areas.
Large blue-gray ovoid nests	Well-circumscribed, confluent or near confluent pigmented ovoid or elongated areas, larger than globules, and not intimately connected to a pigmented tumor body
Multiple blue-gray globules	Multiple globules (not dots) that should be differentiated from multiple blue-gray dots (melanophages)
Spoke-wheel areas	Well-circumscribed radial projections, usually tan but sometimes blue or gray, meeting at an often darker (dark brown, black or blue) central axis
Ulceration[ǁ]	Absence of the epidermis often associated with congealed blood, not due to a well-described recent history of trauma
Red-blue lacunas	More or less sharply demarcated, roundish or oval areas with a reddish, red-bluish, or dark-red to black coloration
Red-bluish to reddish-black homogeneous areas	Structureless homogeneous areas of red-bluish to red-black coloration
None of the listed criteria	Absence of the above-mentioned criteria

Dermoscopic criterion	Definition
Global features	
Reticular pattern	Pigment network covering most parts of the lesion
Globular pattern	Numerous, variously sized, round to oval structures with various shades of brown and gray-black
Cobblestone pattern	Large, closely aggregated, somehow angulated globule-like structures resembling a cobblestone
Homogeneous pattern	Diffuse, brown, gray-blue to gray-black pigmentation in the absence of other distinctive local features
Starburst pattern	Pigmented streaks in a radial arrangement at the edge of the lesion
Parallel pattern	Pigmentation on palms/soles that follows the sulci or the cristae (furrows or ridges), occasionally arranged at right angles to these structures
Multicomponent pattern	Combination of three or more above patterns
Nonspecific pattern	Pigmented lesion lacking above patterns
Local features	
Pigment network	Typical pigment network: light- to dark-brown network with small, uniformly spaced network holes and thin network lines distributed more or less regularly throughout the lesion and usually thinning out at the periphery. Atypical pigment network: black, brown or gray network with irregular holes and thick lines
Dots/globules	Black, brown, round to oval, variously sized structures regularly or irregularly distributed within the lesion
Streaks	These have been previously described separately as pseudopods and radial streaming. Streaks are bulbous and often kinked or finger-like projections seen at the edge of a lesion. They may arise from network structures but more commonly do not. They range in color from tan to black.
Blue-whitish veil	Irregular, structureless area of confluent blue pigmentation with an overlying white "ground-glass" film. The pigmentation cannot occupy the entire lesion and usually corresponds to a clinically elevated part of the lesion
Regression structures	White scar-like depigmentation and/or blue pepper-like granules usually corresponding to a clinically flat part of the lesion
Hypopigmentation	Areas with less pigmentation than the overall pigmentation of the lesion
Blotches	Black, brown, and/or gray structureless areas with symmetrical or asymmetrical distribution within the lesion

book prefer descriptive terminology, which will be the terminology of choice throughout the book. We think, however, that teachers of dermatoscopy should be familiar with both terminologies. For those who are only familiar with metaphoric terminology we have dedicated Chapter 4 to the definition and explanation of metaphoric terms, and their translation into descriptive terminology. According to a recent survey among more than 1000 IDS members 23.5 % prefer to use descriptive terminology while 20.1 % prefer metaphoric terminology. Most participants, however, use both terminologies (56.5 %), which underlines the importance of harmonizing them.

1.5.6 Critique of diagnostic methods and metaphoric terminology

On the one hand dermatoscopy appears to be mysterious and complex to the beginner because of its ambiguous terms; on the other hand it is trivialized by its scoring systems. Such trivialization is a reaction to the impermeable mist that has emanated from the dubious, metaphoric artificial language conceived by experts in dermatoscopy.

Metaphoric terms
Rather like the names of the constellations of the night sky, many dermatoscopic terms require considerable imagination before they can be related to the morphological structures they are supposed to describe. These include spoke-wheel-areas, blue-whitish veil, radial streaming, fat fingers, or moth-eaten border, to name just a few *(also see figures 1.11 and 1.12)*. In the collective memory of the dermatoscopic community, most of these terms are linked to the inventor and are certified as such. This, possibly, is the reason why new terms are being constantly created. The strength of this vivid and gripping terminology undoubtedly lies in its ability to stimulate associative thinking and therefore memory. However, this advantage is offset by the fact that most of the terms are the outcome of individual associations by their inventors. Only in ideal cases does any real similarity exist between the terms and actual structures they are intended to represent.

Figures 1.11 and 1.12: Modified original tables with the criteria and definitions worked out at the consensus conference. From: Argenziano G, Soyer HP, Chimenti S, et al. Dermoscopy of pigmented skin lesions: results of a consensus meeting via the Internet. J Am Acad Dermatol 2003; 48: 679–93. The inconsistent definitions of aggregated globules, blue-gray globules and dots and globules are highlighted.

Most observers, particularly those who focus briefly on dermatoscopy, will be unable to follow this creative act of free association. This approach is reminiscent of interpreting a Rorschach test. However, the test was developed to assess the subject's personality and not to generate consistent descriptions of structure and color. In this sense metaphoric terms act as barriers for teaching and learning – especially if they are poorly defined or not defined at all. This renders their use arbitrary because undefined terms end up mean different things to different people. This, in turn, leads to difficulties in communication and comprehension. Despite this, we do not want to condemn metaphoric terms completely.
A definite disadvantage of the descriptive terminology is that long and cumbersome descriptions are required for complex structures.
An apt metaphor to replace such descriptions has value. Some clinicians, especially those who have been trained in metaphoric terminology, still prefer metaphors to descriptive terms. We accept this and we will discuss all relevant metaphoric terms in chapter 4. This book is intended to serve everyone, including those who prefer metaphoric terminology. The use of descriptive terminology alone does not make one a better dermatoscopist. Finally, it is worth noting that the results of the 3rd consensus conference and the introduction of a dictionary of standardized terms put an end to the unlimited creation of new metaphoric terms.

Missing or inconsistent definitions

What is the difference between dots and globules? Why is the same shape a globule when it is brown, a nest when it is grey, a lacune when it is red, and a comedo-like opening when it is orange? What is the difference between streaks and pseudopods? How is fingerprinting defined? What exactly is a blue-whitish veil? Does the cobblestone pattern consist of cobblestones? Are cobblestones globules, i.e. clods? All successful formal systems have a similar structure; a few simple basic terms are defined and more complex ideas are then derived from these terms. A famous example is Euclid's "Elements", which constitutes the foundation of geometry. In this work Euclid defines a few basic terms such as a point, a straight line, a circle, etc., and from these basic terms derives a formally verifiable axiomatic system that proved very useful to describe the world. As Euclid has done for geometry, Aristotle established the foundations of logic more than 2000 years ago. In his famous syllogisms he describes the truth of linked statements. A morphological diagnostic method like dermatoscopy can also be viewed as a formal system. Proceeding from well-defined basic terms,

Second-step algorithm: pattern analysis criteria for the dermoscopic differentiation between benign melanocytic lesions and melanoma

Dermoscopic criterion	Definition	Diagnostic significance
Vascular structures	Comma-like vessels	Dermal nevus
	Hairpin vessels	If uniformly distributed, seborrheic keratosis. If irregularly distributed, consider melanoma
	Dotted vessels	Melanoma
	Linear irregular vessels	Melanoma
	Vessels and/or erythema within regression structures	Melanoma

Figure 1.13: Modified original table with the "definitions" for vascular structures worked out at the consensus conference. From: Argenziano G, Soyer HP, Chimenti S, et al. Dermoscopy of pigmented skin lesions: results of a consensus meeting via the Internet. J Am Acad Dermatol 2003; 48: 679–93. In actual fact, the definitions are not definitions at all.

one can derive verifiable and reproducible statements that follow the laws of logic.
According to the consensus paper of the IDS (International Dermoscopy Society) published in 2001, no definition exists for the term "globules". On the other hand, a term like aggregated globules is defined as a collection of round or oval structures of different sizes, arranged more or less in a grouped fashion, and may be light brown to dark brown or gray-black in color *(figure 1.11)*. Aggregated globules are thus defined on the basis of their form, design and color. Immediately thereafter, one is told that aggregated globules should not be confused with blue-gray globules. However, "aggregated" and "blue-gray" are not properties that one can compare with each other because they are not mutually exclusive. One describes a specific arrangement, whereas the other describes color.
Furthermore, it is stated that "blue-gray globules" must be distinguished from "blue-gray dots". Thus, one rightly concludes that the distinction between dots and globules is relevant *(figure 1.11)*. However, subsequently one is told that no distinction is made between dots and globules because both are defined as "black, brown, round to oval, variously sized structures" *(figure 1.12)*.
The diverse terms used for similarly shaped solid objects of different colors is a further instance of the inconsistent and illogical language of dermatoscopy. Calling these objects globules when brown, ovoid nests when blue-grey, lacunes when red, can only lead to confusion and make learning unnecessarily difficult *(1.14)*.
The section on vascular patterns also lacks definitions – the column named *Definitions* actually contains no definitions, but terms like hairpin and comma-like vessels, or even linear, irregular vessels, as if these terms were self-explanatory. Obviously, these terms are meaningless and incomprehensible without definitions *(1.13)*.
All these points of critique were addressed in the 3rd consensus paper published in 2016. The experts agreed

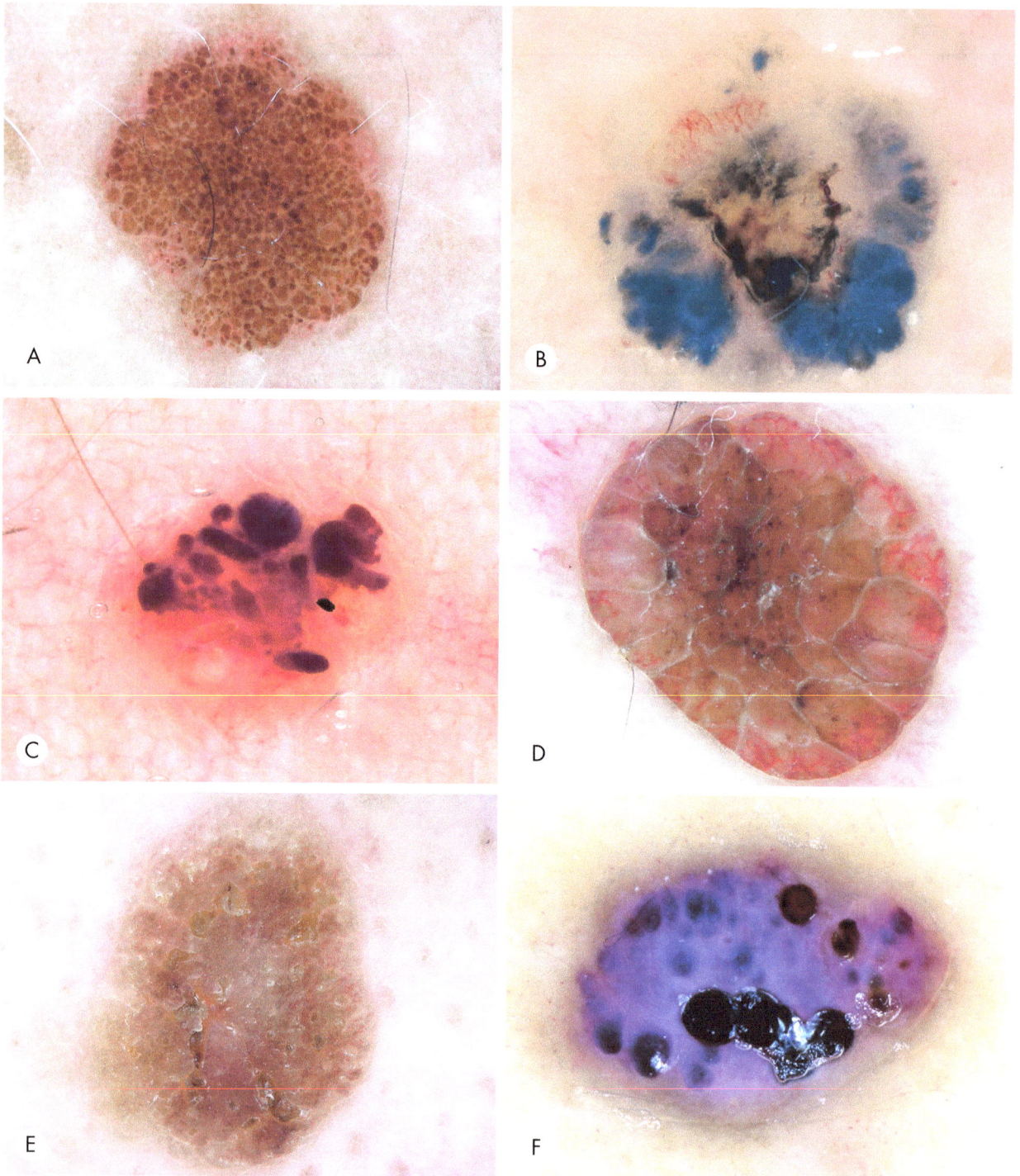

Figure 1.14: *Small brown clods of the same size and shape* **(A)**, *blue clods of different sizes and dissimilar form* **(B)**, *red clods* **(C)**, *large polygonal skin-colored and light-brown clods* **(D)**, *yellow and orange clods* **(E)**, *violet and black clods* **(F)**. *Translated into the language of classical dermatoscopy this means: globules* **(A)**, *blue ovoid nests* **(B)**, *red lacunae* **(C)**, *cobblestone pattern* **(D)**, *orange and yellow clods are not criteria in classical dermatoscopy and therefore bear no names although they are very specific for seborrheic keratoses* **(E)**, *purple and black clods are also termed lacunae* **(F)**. *Thus, the same structures, namely clods, are named differently, depending on their color.*

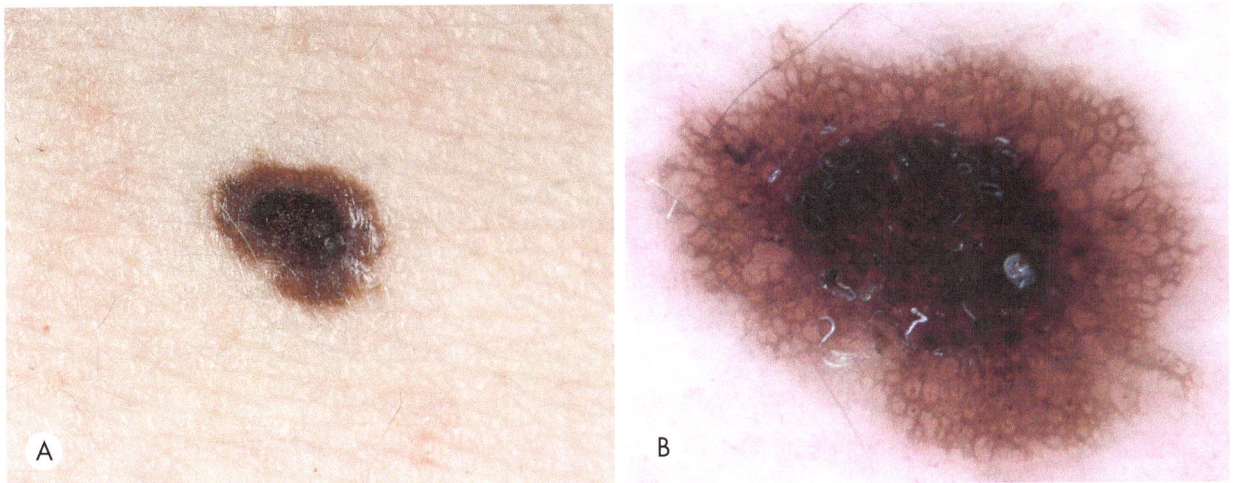

Figure 1.15: Non-melanocytic lesions with a pigmented network. **(A)** Clinical appearance; **(B)** Appearance on dermatoscopy: At the periphery one finds obvious reticular lines (pigment network). Histopathological diagnosis: seborrheic keratosis.

on consistent definitions for all suitable metaphoric terms and reached a consensus for definitions of vascular patterns. We will deal with the consensus definitions of metaphoric terms of pigmented lesions in chapter 4. The vascular patterns and their definitions will be addressed in chapter 6.

Scoring systems

The basic intention behind the so-called scoring systems was to make dermatoscopy more accessible to beginners. Like a raffle, one threw all dermatoscopy criteria ever described into a large drum, mixed them thoroughly, and selected, on the basis of statistical procedures, a few that were considered relevant to the diagnosis. All others were ignored. Then one invented complicated procedures (every author invented a different one) as to how one distinguishes between melanomas and nevi on the basis of the chosen criteria. For all scoring systems, the final diagnosis is always "benign" or "malignant", as if the world of melanocytic lesions could be reduced to these two terms. The scoring systems trivialized dermatoscopy without simplifying it.

Scoring systems have a strong framework (usually one sums up a few parameters and when the total sum exceeds a certain value it is a melanoma). The user is degraded to a robot.

A method of this type does not encourage reflection. Without reflection, one does not achieve a deeper understanding of a subject. If one wishes to achieve a more profound comprehension of a morphological method like dermatoscopy, it will not be sufficient to add one and one, or say B after one has said A. That would be tantamount to only using proverbs to guide crucial life decisions ("Slow and steady wins the race"). These proverbs may be justified as rules of thumb but are too rigid, simplified and limited to guide all (or even most) of our actions.

With the exception of the chaos and clues algorithm all scoring systems are restricted to distinguishing nevi from melanomas, and so can only be applied after one has decided whether the lesion is melanocytic or non-melanocytic ("the first step"). Furthermore, scoring systems are of limited use at some specific locations such as the face, mucosa, or the palms and soles, where different criteria apply.

Having said this, and despite any criticism one may level against scoring systems, one must acknowledge that they do perform reasonably well under many circumstances. Beginners will be able to achieve a moderate degree of diagnostic accuracy fairly rapidly by using a scoring system. In this sense, the different scoring systems have been thoroughly tested, and all found to be useful. We also acknowledge that not everybody has the time to learn a comprehensive method like pattern analysis. For those who want to achieve quick and fairly accurate results we recommend the chaos and clues algorithm (see chapter 5) because it is fast and simple and circumvents the cumbersome and problematic first step.

The first step

Established dogma is that one must distinguish between melanocytic and non-melanocytic lesions as the first step in assessing a pigmented lesion (39). In principle there is nothing wrong with this approach as it provides structure to the procedure of investigation. However, it is not self-evident that this is the best possible first step,

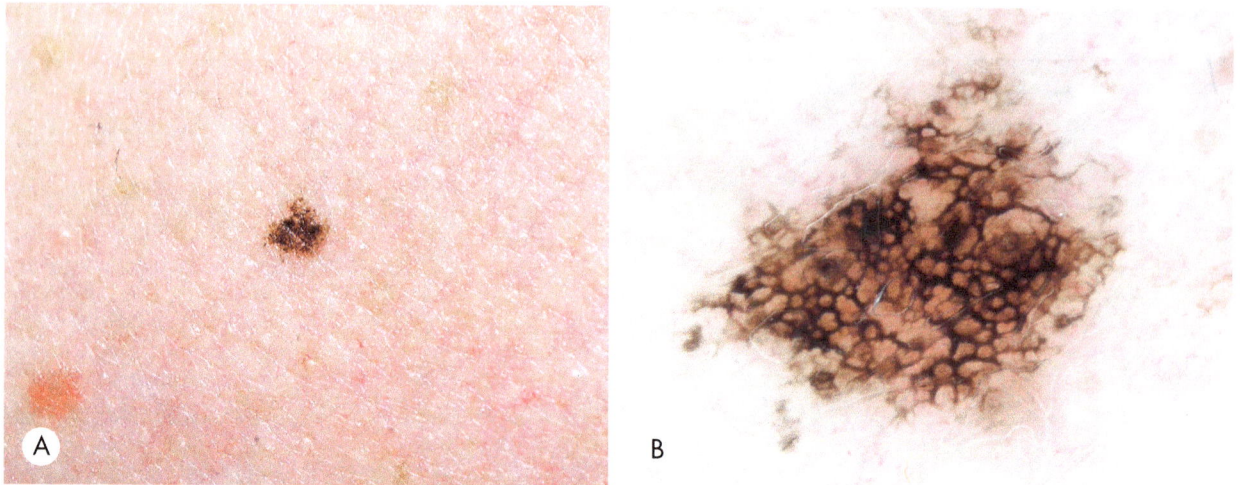

Figure 1.16: Non-melanocytic lesions with a pigment network. **(A)** Clinical appearance; **(B)** Appearance on dermatoscopy: dark brown and black reticular lines (pigment network). Histopathological diagnosis: "Ink-spot" Lentigo.

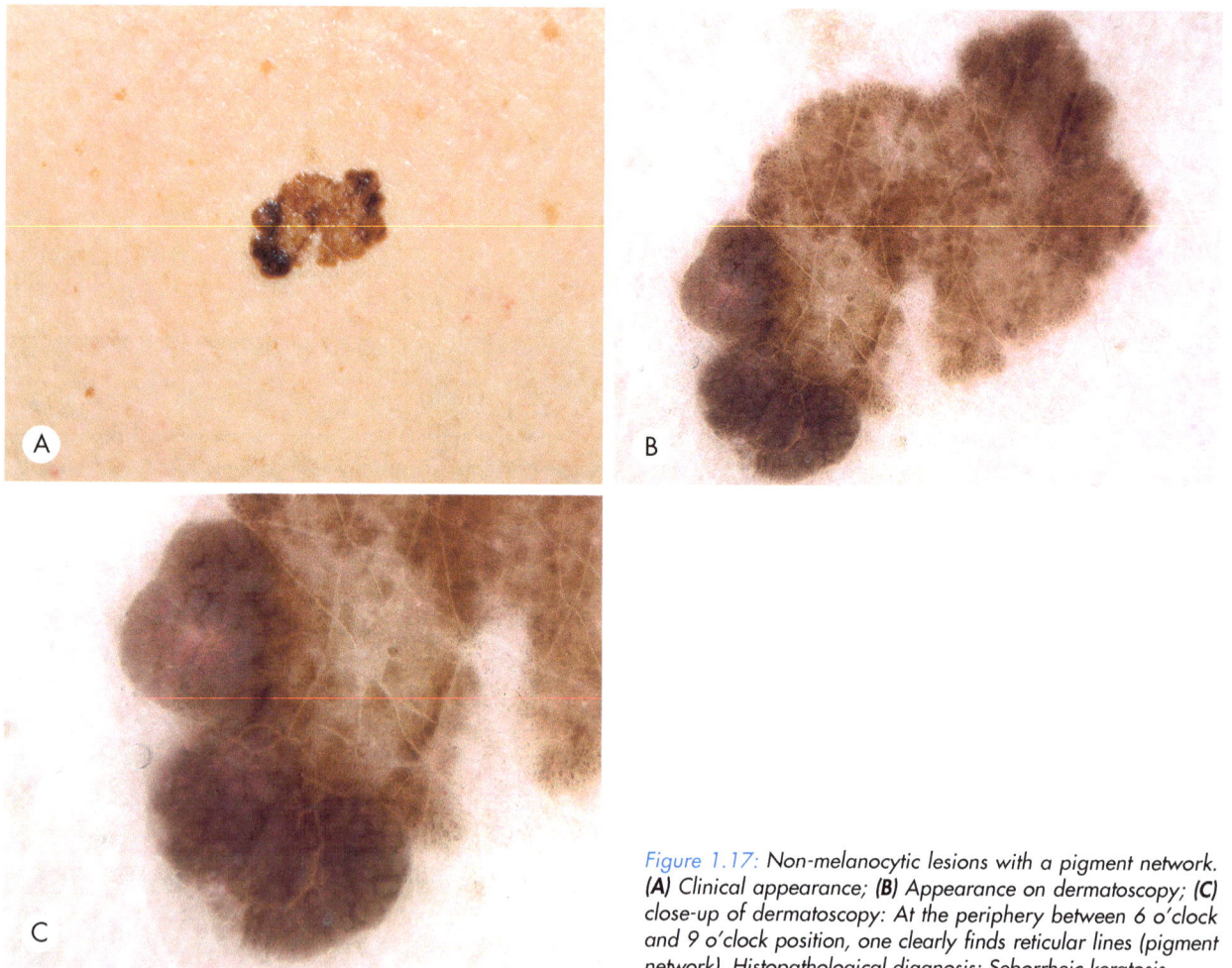

Figure 1.17: Non-melanocytic lesions with a pigment network. **(A)** Clinical appearance; **(B)** Appearance on dermatoscopy; **(C)** close-up of dermatoscopy: At the periphery between 6 o'clock and 9 o'clock position, one clearly finds reticular lines (pigment network). Histopathological diagnosis: Seborrheic keratosis.

and remarkably little evidence has been presented to support this method.

In fact, the criteria this method uses to distinguish between melanocytic and non-melanocytic lesions are not very reliable (40). For instance, in "the first step", the presence of a pigment network (reticular lines) indicates that the lesion is melanocytic. However, several non-melanocytic pigmented skin lesions may also have a pigment network. Examples are solar lentigo, some seborrheic keratoses, dermatofibroma, "ink-spot" lentigo (reticular melanotic macule), urticaria pigmentosa or the accessory mammilla *(1.15, 1.16, and 1.17)*. In all of these cases, strict application of the rules would mislead the investigator. One has entered a blind alley because one has to make a diagnostic decision before the lesion has been fully described. We contend that one should make a full description of the lesion, and only then consider the diagnosis when all morphological details can be taken into account.

Following from a full description, one could reasonably consider a wide range of "first steps" instead of the distinction between melanocytic and non-melanocytic lesions. For example one might differentiate between symmetrical and asymmetrical lesions, raised or flat lesions, or lesions that should be excised or biopsied on the one hand and ones that should not be biopsied on the other.

These methodological weaknesses are the principal reason why we propose a new approach. The method we present is pattern analysis, but presented in a form that is consistent, comprehensive, and logical. By virtue of this simple and consistent language, pattern analysis can be accessible to one and all and not just to experts. We wish you all the best on this journey.

References

1 Saphier J. Die Dermatoskopie. I. Mitteilung. Arch Dermatol Syph 1920; 128:1–19.

2 Benvenuto-Andrade C, Dusza SW, Agero AL, Scope A, Rajadhyaksha M, Halpern AC et al. Differences between polarized light dermoscopy and immersion contact dermoscopy for the evaluation of skin lesions. Arch Dermatol 2007; 143:329–38.

3 Rosendahl C, Cameron A, Argenziano G, Zalaudek I, Tschandl P, Kittler H. Dermoscopy of squamous cell carcinoma and keratoacanthoma. Arch Dermatol 2012; 148:1386–92.

4 Rosendahl C, Cameron A, Tschandl P, Bulinska A, Zalaudek I, Kittler H. Prediction without Pigment: a decision algorithm for non-pigmented skin malignancy. Dermatol Pract Concept 2014; 4: 59–66.

5 Kittler H, Pehamberger H, Wolff K, Binder M. Diagnostic accuracy of dermoscopy. Lancet Oncol 2002; 3: 159–65.

6 Vestergaard ME, Macaskill P, Holt PE, Menzies SW. Dermoscopy compared with naked eye examination for the diagnosis of primary melanoma: a meta-analysis of studies performed in a clinical setting. Br J Dermatol 2008; 159: 669–76.

7 Rosendahl C, Tschandl P, Cameron A, Kittler H. Diagnostic accuracy of dermatoscopy for melanocytic and nonmelanocytic pigmented lesions. J Am Acad Dermatol 2011; 64: 1068–73.

8 Luttrell MJ, McClenahan P, Hofmann-Wellenhof R, Fink-Puches R, Soyer HP. Laypersons' sensitivity for melanoma identification is higher with dermoscopy images than clinical photographs. Br J Dermatol 2012; 167: 1037–41.

9 Binder M, Schwarz M, Winkler A, Steiner A, Kaider A, Wolff K et al. Epiluminescence microscopy. A useful tool for the diagnosis of pigmented skin lesions for formally trained dermatologists. Arch Dermatol 1995; 131: 286–91.

10. Binder M, Puespoeck-Schwarz M, Steiner A, Kittler H, Muellner M, Wolff K et al. Epiluminescence microscopy of small pigmented skin lesions: short-term formal training improves the diagnostic performance of dermatologists. J Am Acad Dermatol 1997; 36: 197–202.

11 Tschandl P, Kittler H, Schmid K, Zalaudek I, Argenziano G. Teaching dermatoscopy of pigmented skin tumours to novices: comparison of analytic vs. heuristic approach. J Eur Acad Dermatol Venereol 2015; 29: 1198–204.

12 MacKie RM. An aid to the preoperative assessment of pigmented lesions of the skin. Br J Dermatol 1971; 85: 232–8.

13 Fritsch P, Pechlaner R. Differentiation of benign from malignant melanocytic lesions using incident light microscopy. In: A. Ackerman editor. Pathology of Malignant Melanoma. New York: Masson; 1981. p. 301–12.

14 Pehamberger H, Steiner A, Wolff K. In vivo epiluminescence microscopy of pigmented skin lesions. I. Pattern analysis of pigmented skin lesions. J Am Acad Dermatol 1987; 17: 571–83.

15 Steiner A, Pehamberger H, Wolff K. In vivo epiluminescence microscopy of pigmented skin lesions. II. Diagnosis of small pigmented skin lesions and early detection of malignant melanoma. J Am Acad Dermatol 1987; 17: 584–91.

16 Bahmer FA, Fritsch P, Kreusch J, Pehamberger H, Rohrer C, Schindera I et al. [Diagnostic criteria in epiluminescence microscopy. Consensus meeting of the professional committee of analytic morphology of the Society of Dermatologic Research, 17 November 1989 in Hamburg]. Hautarzt 1990; 41: 513–4.

17 Kreusch J, Rassner G. Auflichtmikroskopie pigmentierter Hauttumoren. Stuttgart: Thieme; 1991.

18 Stolz W, Braun-Falco O, Bilek P. Color Atlas of Dermatoscopy: Blackwell Wissenschafts-Verlag; 2002.

19 Nachbar F, Stolz W, Merkle T, Cognetta AB, Vogt T, Landthaler M et al. The ABCD rule of dermatoscopy. High prospective value in the diagnosis of doubtful melanocytic skin lesions. J Am Acad Dermatol 1994; 30: 551–9.

20 Argenziano G, Fabbrocini G, Carli P, De Giorgi V, Sammarco E, Delfino M. Epiluminescence microscopy for the diagnosis of doubtful melanocytic skin lesions. Comparison of the ABCD rule of dermatoscopy and a new 7-point checklist based on pattern analysis. Arch Dermatol 1998; 134: 1563–70.

21 Menzies SW, Crotty KA, Ingvar C, McCarthy W. Dermoscopy: An Atlas: Mcgraw-Hill Education Ltd; 2009.

22 Soyer HP, Argenziano G, Zalaudek I, Corona R, Sera F, Talamini R et al. Three-point checklist of dermoscopy. A new screening method for early detection of melanoma. Dermatology 2004; 208: 27–31.

23 Henning JS, Dusza SW, Wang SQ, Marghoob AA, Rabinovitz HS, Polsky D et al. The CASH (color, architecture, symmetry, and homogeneity) algorithm for dermoscopy. J Am Acad Dermatol 2007; 56: 45–52.

24 Rosendahl C, Cameron A, McColl I, Wilkinson D. Dermatoscopy in routine practice – 'chaos and clues'. Aust Fam Physician 2012; 41: 482–7.

25 Marghoob AA, Braun R, Kopf AW. An Atlas of Dermoscopy: Informa Healthcare; 2004.

26 Menzies SW, Westerhoff K, Rabinovitz H, Kopf AW, McCarthy WH, Katz B. Surface microscopy of pigmented basal cell carcinoma. Arch Dermatol 2000; 136: 1012–6.

27 Stolz W, Schiffner R, Burgdorf WH. Dermatoscopy for facial pigmented skin lesions. Clin Dermatol 2002; 20: 276–8.

28 Hofmann-Wellenhof R, Blum A, Wolf IH, Piccolo D, Kerl H, Garbe C et al. Dermoscopic classification of atypical melanocytic nevi (Clark nevi). Arch Dermatol 2001; 137: 1575–80.

29 Braun RP, Rabinovitz HS, Krischer J, Kreusch J, Oliviero M, Naldi L et al. Dermoscopy of pigmented seborrheic keratosis: a morphological study. Arch Dermatol 2002; 138: 1556–60.

30 Zaballos P, Puig S, Llambrich A, Malvehy J. Dermoscopy of dermatofibromas: a prospective morphological study of 412 cases. Arch Dermatol 2008; 144: 75–83.

31 Saida T, Oguchi S, Ishihara Y. In vivo observation of magnified features of pigmented lesions on volar skin using video macroscope. Usefulness of epiluminescence techniques in clinical diagnosis. Arch Dermatol 1995; 131: 298–304.

32 Saida T, Koga H, Yamazaki Y, Tanaka M. Acral Melanoma. In: H. P. Soyer editor. Color Atlas of Melanocytic Lesions of the Skin. New York: Springer; 2007. p. 196–203.

33 Blum A, Simionescu O, Argenziano G, Braun R, Cabo H, Eichhorn A et al. Dermoscopy of pigmented lesions of the mucosa and the mucocutaneous junction: results of a multicenter study by the International Dermoscopy Society (IDS). Arch Dermatol 2011; 147: 1181–7.

34 Cameron A, Rosendahl C, Tschandl P, Riedl E, Kittler H. Dermatoscopy of pigmented Bowen's disease. J Am Acad Dermatol 2010; 62: 597–604.

35 Zalaudek I, Schmid K, Marghoob AA, Scope A, Manzo M, Moscarella E et al. Frequency of dermoscopic nevus subtypes by age and body site: a cross-sectional study. Arch Dermatol 2011; 147: 663–70.

36 Argenziano G, Soyer HP, Chimenti S, Talamini R, Corona R, Sera F et al. Dermoscopy of pigmented skin lesions: results of a consensus meeting via the Internet. J Am Acad Dermatol 2003; 48: 679–93.

37 Kittler H. Introduction of a new algorithmic method based on pattern analysis for diagnosis of pigmented skin lesions. Dermatopathol: Pract & Conc 2007; 13: 3.

38 Kittler H, Marghoob AA, Argenziano G, Carrera G, Curiel-Lewandrowski C, Hofmann-Wellenhof R et al. Standardization of Terminology In Dermoscopy/Dermatoscopy: Results of the 3rd Consensus Conference of the International Society of Dermoscopy. J Am Acad Dermatol 2016; 74: 1093–106.

39 Marghoob AA, Braun R. Proposal for a revised 2-step algorithm for the classification of lesions of the skin using dermoscopy. Arch Dermatol 2010;146:426–8.

40 Tschandl P, Rosendahl C, Kittler H. Accuracy of the first step of the dermatoscopic 2-step algorithm for pigmented skin lesions. Dermatol Pract Concept 2012; 2: 203a08.

2 Principal pigmented skin lesions relevant to dermatoscopy

In this chapter we present, in the form of a glossary, a list of pigmented skin lesions for which dermatoscopic assessment is likely to be helpful. We do this to clarify terminology and to prevent misunderstanding. The usefulness of dermatoscopy is not limited to assessing the lesions mentioned in this chapter, which is restricted to conditions that are usually or commonly pigmented (never forgetting that all pigmented neoplasms also have non-pigmented variants). The universe of lesions which are (nearly) always non-pigmented, which also includes inflammatory conditions, is more complex and very large. A lexicon that includes all conditions that can usefully be examined by dermatoscopy is beyond the scope of this chapter. We strongly recommend that you read this chapter even though it does not directly address the subject of dermatoscopy. The photographs shown here are all clinical images of what would be seen when viewing these lesions with the naked eye. One purpose of doing this is to show how difficult it can be to make a diagnosis without dermatoscopy. Dermatoscopic views are shown in chapter 3 after presentation of the method.

Clinicians, "dermatoscopists" and pathologists speak languages which partly overlap, but have significant areas of difference. This is particularly confusing when the same terms are used, but with different meanings. Adding to the confusion, several competing schools of dermatopathology propagate different concepts and use different terminology. As a clinician one must therefore expect diverse histopathological reports. The definitions that now follow may not resolve the widely prevalent confusion, but they will at least not intensify it. Needless to say, we use a consistent form of terminology in this book.

2.1 Melanocytic lesions

Dermatoscopy is commonly used to confirm or exclude the diagnosis of melanoma. Melanocytic nevi and melanomas — the benign and malignant neoplasms arising from melanocytes — together form the group of lesions classified as "melanocytic". All other skin lesions are often lumped together and classified as "non-melanocytic" but this is problematic because it includes diverse conditions which are entirely unrelated, for example dermatofibroma and seborrheic keratosis. We prefer to classify conditions by what they are and not by what they are not and so whenever possible will avoid the term "non-melanocytic" by using more specific terms.

2.1.1 Melanocytic nevi

A melanocytic nevus is a benign proliferation of melanocytes, either in the form of a congenital malformation (hamartoma) or an acquired neoplasia. Melanocytes are not merely increased in number but are also (at least partly) arranged in nests, chords or strands. An increased number of melanocytes (melanocytic hyperplasia) without the formation of nests, chords or strands is not sufficient to justify calling a lesion a nevus. One may also observe an increase in the number of melanocytes in "non-melanocytic" lesions, for example solar lentigines, but nests never develop in these cases.

In this book we use a modified version of Ackerman's (1) classification for melanocytic nevi, which is based on histopathological criteria. The disadvantage of this classification is that only the pathologist can see the features required to make a definitive diagnosis; clinicians and "dermatoscopists" merely try, on the basis of their description, to predict the pathologist's diagnosis. Ideally, a classification system would incorporate clinical and dermatoscopic as well as histopathological findings. Several grave historical errors such as the interpretation of the Spitz nevus as a "juvenile melanoma" are attributable to the fact that pathologists did not look beyond the objective of their microscope. Clinicians and "dermatoscopists" who are not familiar with dermatopathology are also at risk of this type of error.

In Ackerman's modified classification of nevi, a distinction is made between the following entities: Clark nevus, Spitz nevus, Reed nevus, congenital nevus (with the sub-types "superficial" and "superficial and deep"), combined congenital nevus, blue nevus (with subtypes), Unna nevus and Miescher nevus. It should be noted that

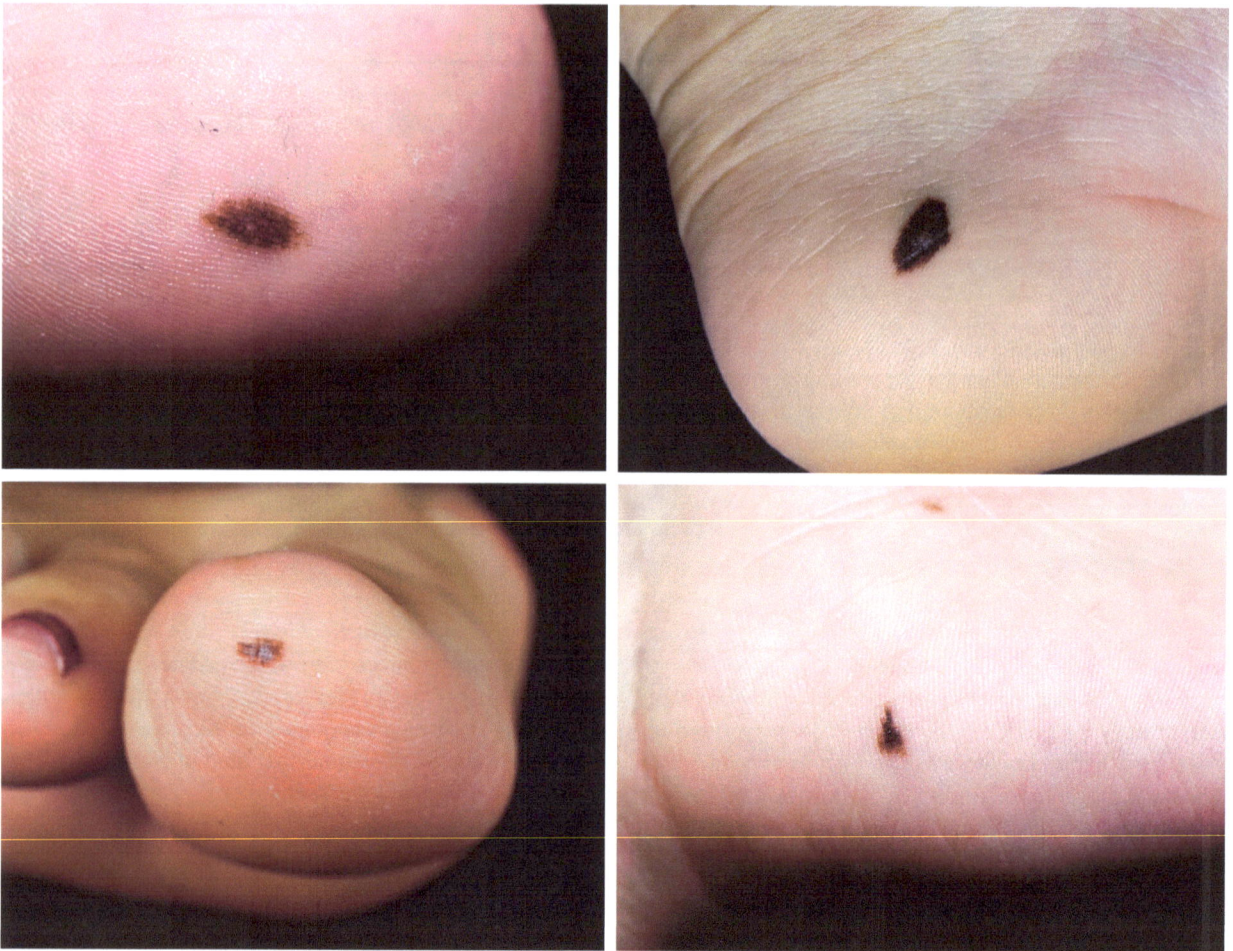

Figure 2.1: Acral nevi.
Top left: Acral nevus (histopathology: "superficial" congenital nevus). **Top right:** Acral nevus (histopathology: "superficial and deep" congenital nevus). **Bottom left:** Acral nevus (histology: classical acral nevus). **Bottom right:** Acral nevus (no histology because not excised).

the term "congenital" does not necessarily mean that the nevus was visible at birth. Many so-called congenital nevi appear after birth and some even appear as late as early adulthood (2, 3). In addition, we use the term "acral nevus" acknowledging that the designation is not consistent; location is not a histopathologic feature and is otherwise irrelevant to the classification of nevi. Contrary to common practice, the terms "dysplastic nevus" and "atypical nevus" are not used here.

The terms used in this book and their definitions are given below in alphabetical order:

Acral nevus
Acral skin is that found on the palms and soles. Anatomically the acral skin is marked by its specific arrangement of rete ridges, which are represented on the surface of the skin by characteristic papillary ridges and furrows.

In a rare example of unanimity, both clinicians and dermatopathologists use "acral nevus" as a general term for nevi at acral sites; the location determines the name. In fact, most types of nevi, such as Spitz nevi, Reed nevi and "superficial" or "superficial and deep" congenital nevi, may occur on acral skin. Whenever possible the specific diagnosis should be preferred to the general term "acral nevus". We name the special type of nevus that has no equivalent at other locations and occurs only on acral skin a "classical acral nevus". This type of nevus is small and flat, and its pigmentation is uniformly brown. In terms of histopathology it consists of small nests of melanocytes exclusively at the dermo-epidermal junction. In this book, while we have no term to replace the ambiguous "acral nevus", the specific histopathological diagnosis is additionally given when possible. Only when no histology is available and the clinical or dermatoscopic diagnosis is equivocal do

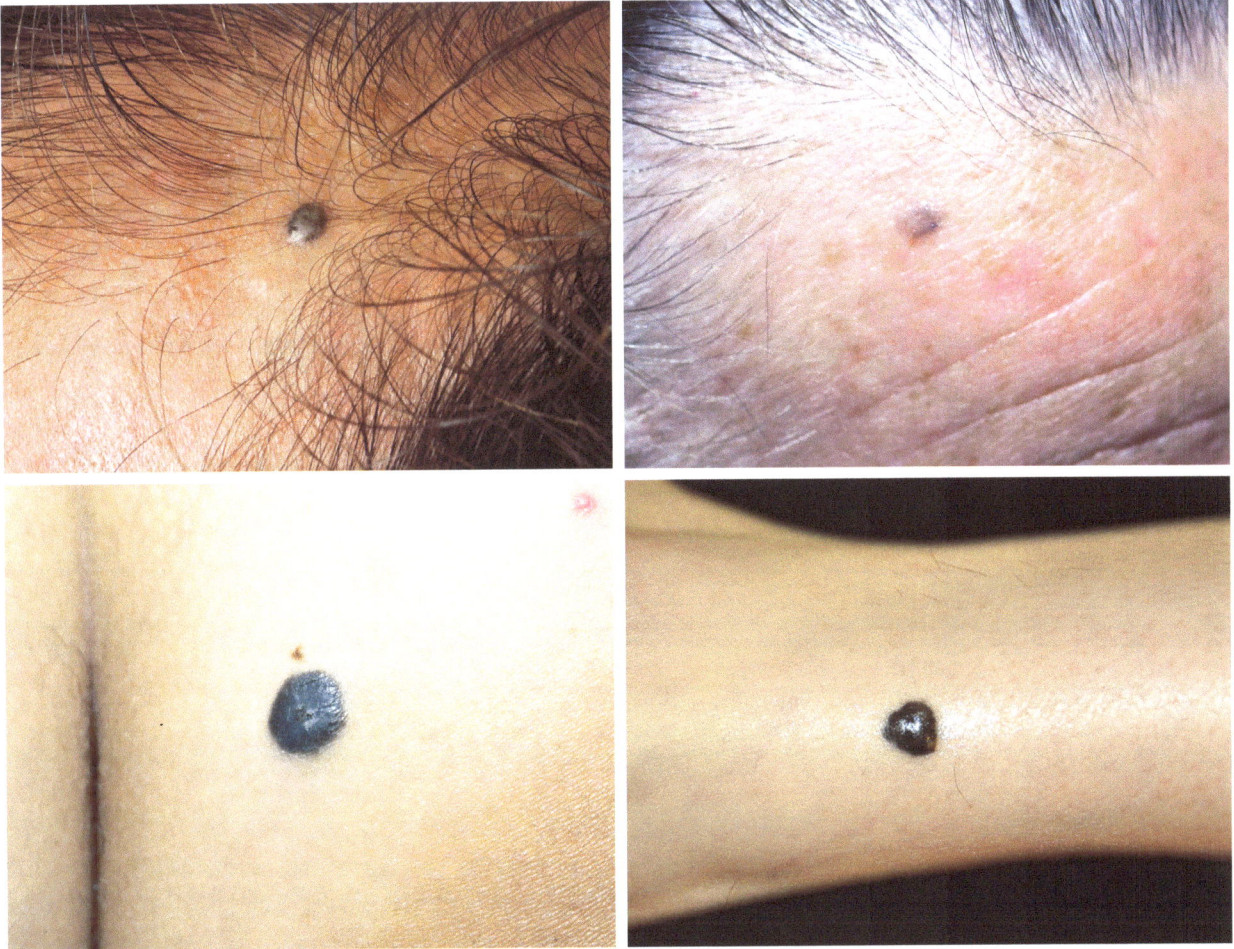

Figure 2.2: Blue nevi.
Not all "blue nevi" are uniformly blue; some are gray or brown. **Top left:** *Blue nevus (histopathology: "common blue nevus").* **Top right:** *Blue nevus (histopathology: "common blue nevus").* **Bottom left:** *Blue nevus (histopathology: "Masson's neuronevus").* **Bottom right:** *Blue nevus (histopathology: "common blue nevus").*

we use the collective term "acral nevus" with no further specification *(2.1)*.

Blue nevus

This is a collective term for several types of nevi whose principal common pathological criterion is the proliferation of spindle-shaped and dendritic melanocytes in the dermis. As a rule these dermal melanocytes contain abundant melanin. This gives rise to the characteristic eponymous blue color on clinical *(2.2)* as well as dermatoscopic examination. Dermatopathologists distinguish between several sub-types of blue nevi. The most important of these are the so-called common blue nevus and the cellular blue nevus. Because these dermatopathological sub-groups cannot be identified clinically or by dermatoscopy, when we only show the clinical or dermatoscopic appearance, we use the collective term "blue nevus". If the nevus was excised and

subjected to histological investigation (which occurred in most cases), the dermatopathological sub-classification is also given.

Not all "blue nevi" are blue on clinical examination or dermatoscopy. Some may be gray or skin-colored while others may be partly brown. There are also non-pigmented varieties which are white. Conversely, of course, not all blue melanocytic lesions are "blue nevi". The term "malignant blue nevus" is not used in this book. The entity known as a malignant blue nevus is, in our opinion, a melanoma (4).

Clark nevus

The Clark nevus is the most common type of acquired melanocytic neoplasm. They are usually macular, ranging in size from a few millimeters up to about 1 cm. Colour is usually brown and may be variegate. Occasionally, but more commonly in persons with a

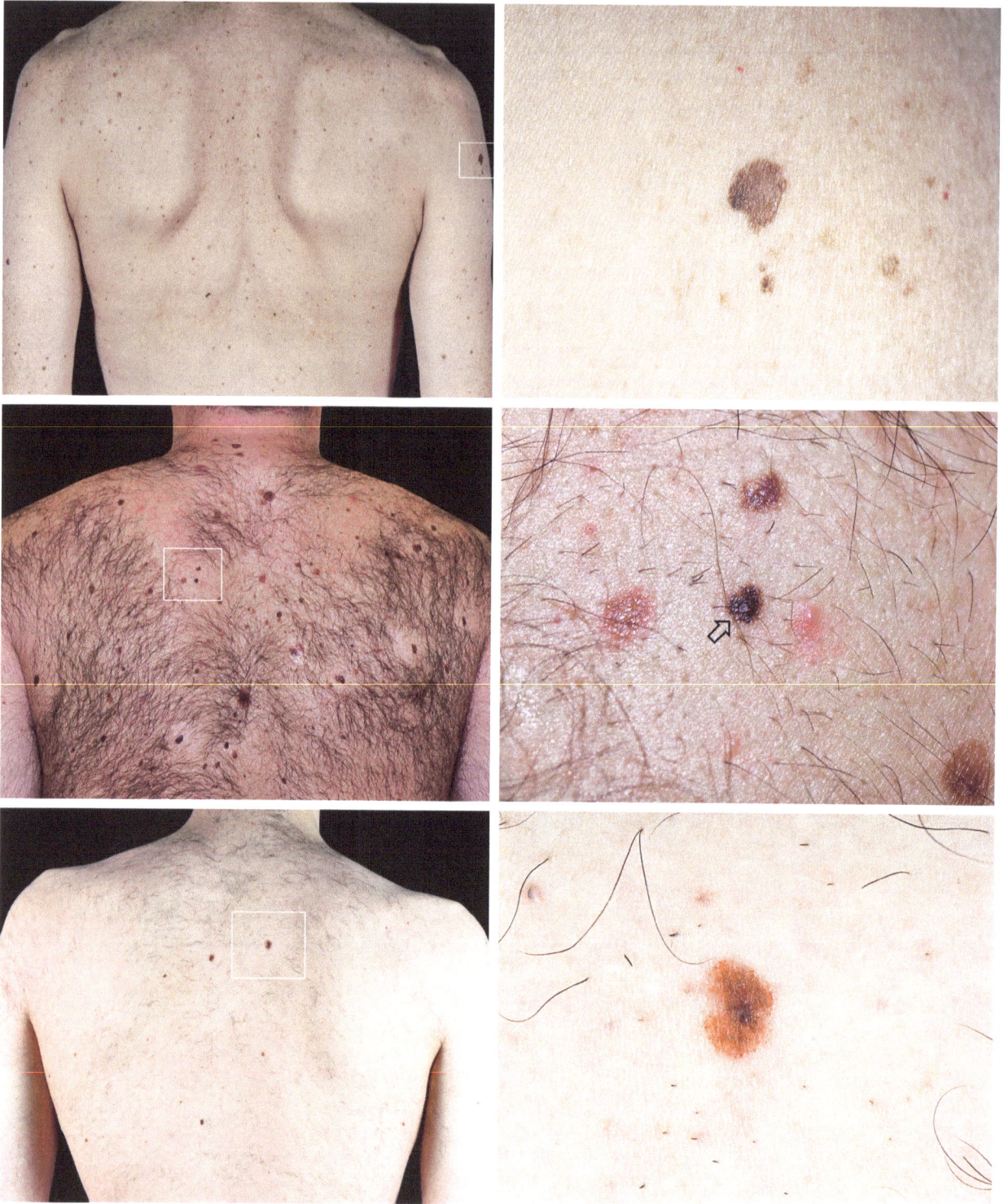

Figure 2.3: Clark nevi.

Clark nevi are typically flat and light-brown or dark-brown. Most Clark nevi are much smaller than 1 cm in size. **Top left:** A patient with several Clark nevi. The largest of them is on the right upper arm **(Top, right). Middle row, left:** This patient has several Clark nevi as well as numerous "small" congenital nevi, of which the majority are larger than the Clark nevi. In some cases it may not be possible to distinguish between a Clark nevus and a congenital nevus with the naked eye. **Middle row, right:** A typical Clark nevus (arrow), surrounded by other nevi which cannot be definitely classified on clinical investigation (Clark nevus or "superficial" congenital nevus). **Bottom left:** Several Clark nevi of different sizes. **Bottom right:** Close-up of a relatively large Clark nevus.

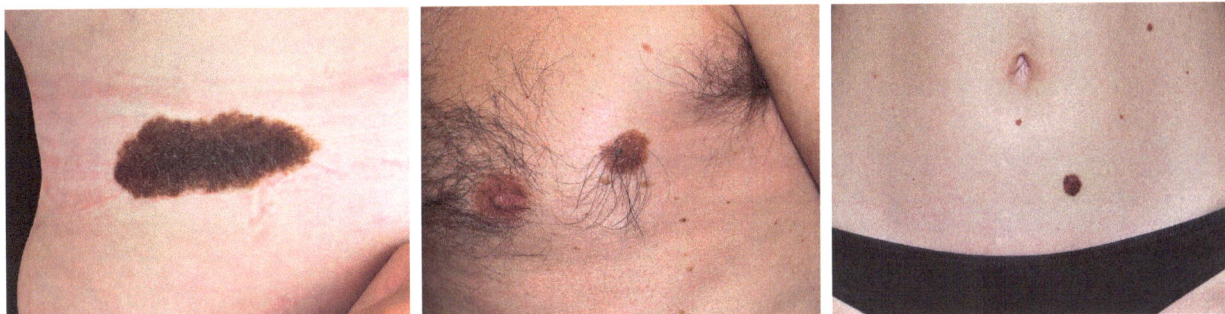

Figure 2.4: Congenital nevi of different sizes

very light skin, one finds lightly pigmented or non-pigmented varieties. Clark nevi usually occur on the trunk and the proximal portion of the extremities, but not on facial or acral skin. Clark nevi are very common. On average, people with lighter skin phototypes have ten to twenty, but it is not unusual to see people with hundreds of Clark nevi.

In terms of dermatopathology Clark nevi have a characteristic appearance: the silhouette is symmetrical and flat, and the melanocytes are located in small, regular nests at the dermo-epidermal junction (junctional Clark nevus). Occasionally one finds small nests of melanocytes in the papillary dermis as well (compound type of Clark nevus). In contrast to the "superficial" congenital nevus, these nests do not entirely fill the papillary dermis. A purely dermal Clark nevus does not exist.

This nevus is named after American pathologist Wallace H. Clark (5). He considered this nevus an intermediate step in the development of melanoma and therefore called them "dysplastic nevi". This concept is no longer tenable. Unfortunately Clark incorporated several different types of nevi in the term, with many of the nevi termed "dysplastic" by Clark actually being "superficial" or "superficial and deep" congenital nevi *(2.3)*. Many histopathologists continue to use the term "dysplastic" and continue to include various small congenital nevi under this name. Clark nevi may mimic melanoma and therefore occasionally require excision for diagnostic reasons. Prophylactic excision is not indicated because the risk of malignant transformation of a single Clark nevus is extremely low. The majority of melanomas arise de novo; they do not arise from a pre-existing nevus.

Congenital nevus

In the absence of further specification this is an ambiguous collective term used to mean different things by clinicians and pathologists. Clinicians refer to melanocytic nevi as congenital only when they are visible during or shortly after birth or when the size of the nevus does not permit any other differential diagnosis.

Depending on their size, these nevi are sub-divided into large (> 20 cm), medium-sized (1.5–19.9 cm) and small (< 1.5 cm) congenital nevi *(2.4)*. At the end of their period of growth, congenital nevi are usually raised above the skin and may be heavily or lightly pigmented. Sometimes, but not always, they have terminal hair. The majority of "small congenital nevi" appear after birth, i.e. usually during childhood and puberty. Their occurrence appears to be independent of exposure to ultraviolet rays.

The size of a congenital nevus is proportional to the likelihood of the nevus being visible at birth. When dermatopathologists refer to a congenital nevus they are usually talking about a nevus with a specific type of fine tissue architecture (arrangement and distribution of melanocytes), which obviously remains invisible to the clinician. Whether the nevus was present at birth or not, as well as its size, are of little importance to the dermatopathologist. The two types of congenital nevus are the "superficial" congenital nevus (Ackerman nevus) in which the accumulation of melanocytes is no deeper than the papillary dermis, and the "superficial and deep" congenital nevus (Zitelli nevus) in which melanocytes extend at least into the reticular dermis. Both types of congenital nevi are common – possibly as common as Clark nevi.

In dermatoscopy one is mainly interested in small congenital nevi. Many of the nevi termed "dysplastic" or "atypical" in patients with so-called "dysplastic nevus syndrome" are actually small congenital nevi *(2.5)*.

These patients are subject to a higher risk of melanoma because the number of congenital nevi is very likely an expression of a genetic predisposition. Many individuals have both small congenital nevi and Clark nevi *(2.6)*. As mentioned earlier, many dermatologists and dermatopathologists adhere to a different concept and refer to Clark nevi as well as "superficial" and "superficial and deep" congenital nevi as "dysplastic nevi". This creates the wrong impression that one is referring to the same type of nevus.

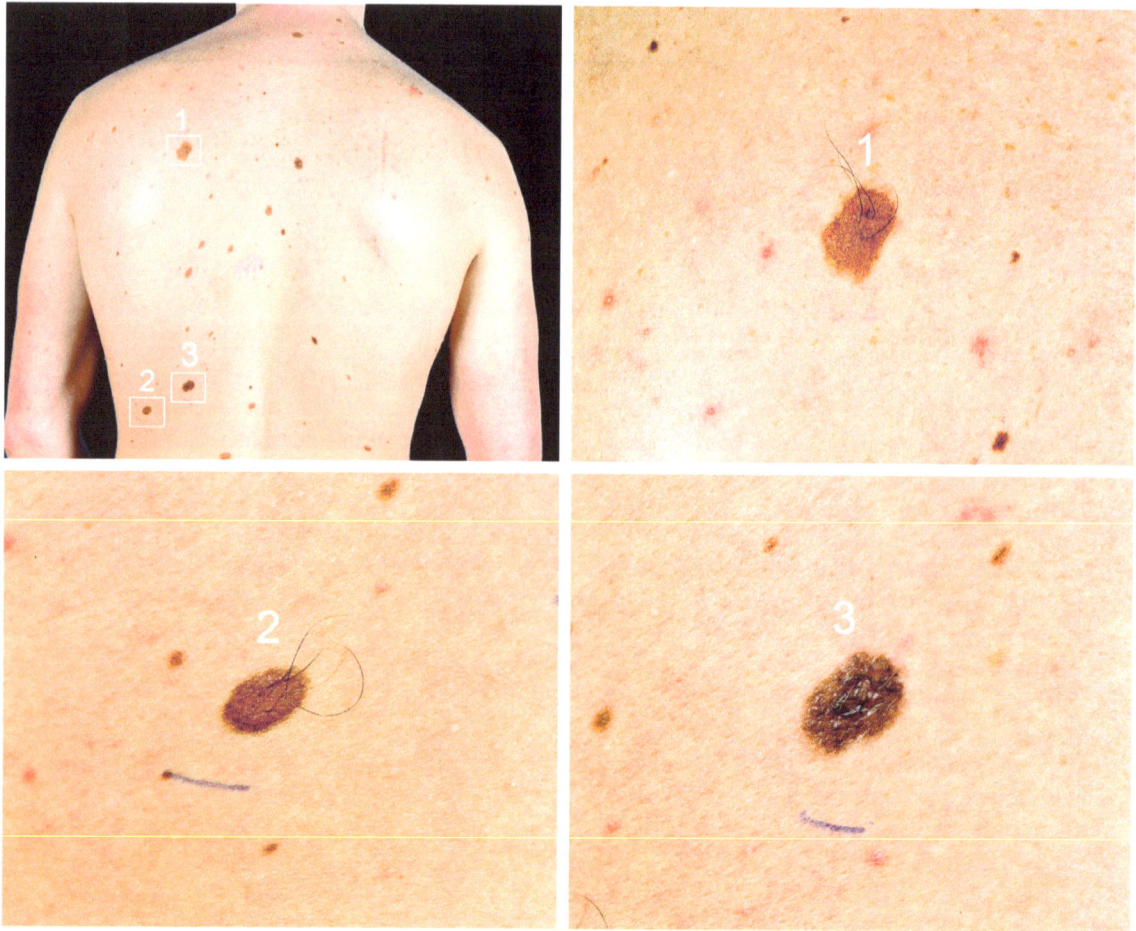

Figure 2.5: Three small congenital nevi in one patient.
The nevi numbered 1 and 2 have excess terminal hair, clearly indicating their congenital nature. Congenital nevus number 3 does not have an excess of terminal hair. These patients are diagnosed with a "dysplastic" or "atypical nevus syndrome", although some nevi such as those shown here are quite obviously congenital.

Figure 2.7 demonstrates the difficulties in distinguishing between Clark nevi and small congenital nevi when one relies on the clinical appearance alone. In the left column a Clark nevus is shown from a distance (A) and in detail (B). Adjacent to it (E, F) are corresponding photographs of a "superficial and deep" congenital nevus (Zitelli nevus). A distinction based on clinical criteria appears impossible. However, the difference is easily identified on dermatopathology. In Clark nevi (C, D) there are small nests of melanocytes at the dermo-epidermal junction (arrows in image D) while the papillary dermis is largely unaffected (the cells in the papillary dermis are inflammatory cells and melano-phages). The "superficial and deep" congenital nevus (G, H) has a different histopathological appearance. The melanocyte nests are large and are present in the papillary (therefore superficial) as well as the reticular

dermis (therefore deep). The arrow in Figure G points to a melanocyte nest in the reticular dermis. The arrows in Figure H point to nests in the papillary dermis. In a Clark nevus as we define it, nests of melanocytes are found no deeper than the papillary dermis.

Combined congenital nevus

When clinicians and dermatopathologists refer to a combined nevus they mean different things. For the clinician a combined nevus is a nevus that is pigmented in the junctional as well as the dermal portion. The junctional portion is brown and the dermal portion blue. (Melanocytes in the reticular dermis, filled with melanin, appear blue on the surface of the skin). In this case the term "combined" refers to the simultaneous occurrence of brown and blue. When a dermatopathologist (who, as a rule, is unaware of the clinical appearance) uses

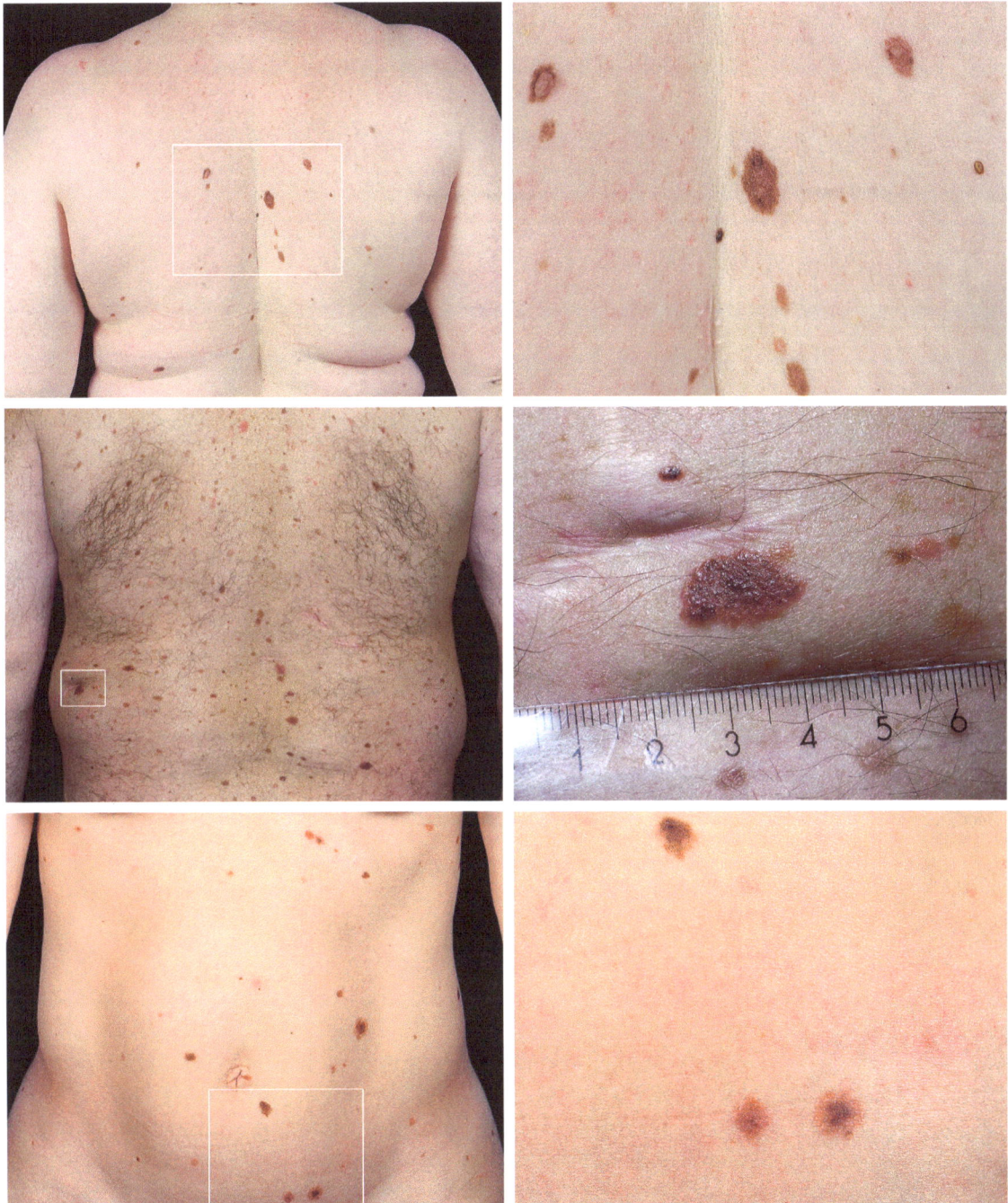

Figure 2.6: *Patients with multiple nevi, who in colloquial language are referred to as patients with "dysplastic nevus syndrome". These individuals not only have multiple nevi but also multiple types of nevi, namely Clark nevi, and "superficial" – as well as "superficial and deep" congenital nevi.*

the term "combined nevus" they are usually referring to a nevus composed of two or more cell populations. The term "combined" refers in this case to the cytology which, in turn, is not known to the clinician. In some cases the two viewpoints overlap, for instance when a nevus is composed of dermal spindle-shaped melano-cytes with melanin on the one hand; and small, round, junctional melanocytes on the other. Combined nevi, regardless of whether they are viewed from the clinical or the pathological perspective, are usually congenital. However, this does not always mean that they were visible at birth *(2.8)*.

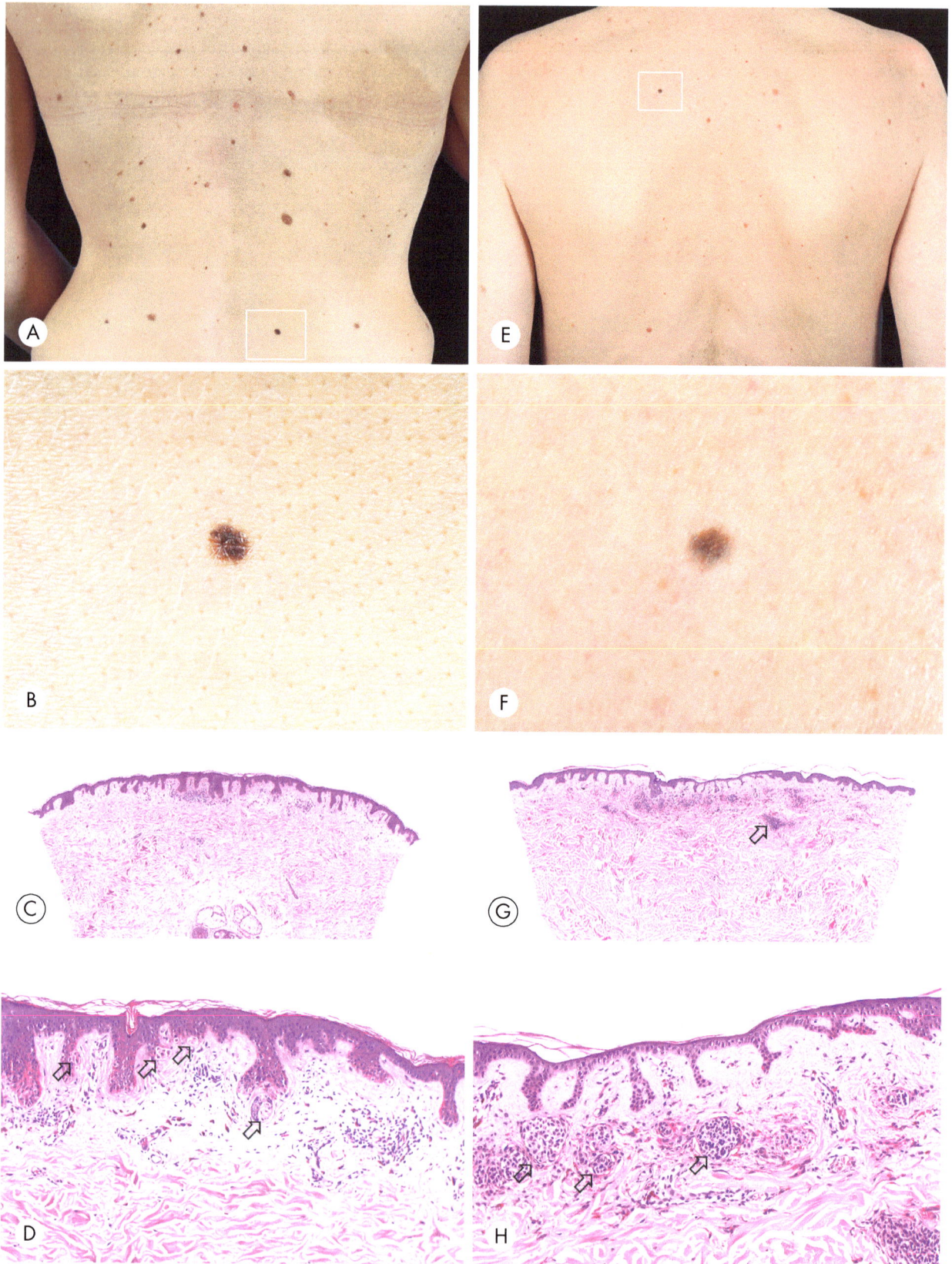

Figure 2.7: *Clark nevus (A, B, C, D) versus congenital nevus (E, F, G, H)*

Miescher nevus

Named after the dermatologist Guido Miescher (6), this nevus is a dome-shaped nodule on the face, usually skin-colored or light brown, rarely dark brown, and in some cases with terminal hair. On dermatopathology it has a characteristic silhouette with an accumulation of melanocytes in the dermis. The histopathological pattern is similar to that of a congenital nevus. However a Miescher nevus is not visible at birth, usually appearing around puberty. Clinicians frequently refer to it as a "dermal nevus" *(2.9)*.

Nevus spilus

Nevus spilus is a variant of a "superficial and deep" congenital nevus which appears variegate on clinical investigation *(2.10)*.

Reed nevus

This nevus was first reported by the American pathologist Richard Reed. Many authors describe it as a heavily pigmented variant of Spitz nevus (7). Others regard it as an independent entity that may be distinguished from Spitz nevus clinically, biologically (they differ with regard to their growth patterns), on dermatoscopy, and in terms of dermatopathology (8). We hold this view. Clinically a Reed nevus is a dark-brown to black pigmented papule or macule *(2.11)*. Like Spitz nevus, Reed nevus is most common in children and adolescents, but is also found in older adults. It appears quite often on the extremities. Because of their very heavy pigmentation, Reed nevi are examined much more frequently by dermatoscopy than Spitz nevi. Often they are excised for histopathological examination to exclude melanoma. The histopathological appearance of Reed nevus is quite specific. Reed nevi are rarely diagnosed in some regions such as Australia, but are diagnosed frequently in Europe and the USA. This may be due more to regional variation in patterns of histopathology reporting, rather than any true variation in incidence.

Recurrent nevus

Following incomplete excision, melanocytic nevi may recur in the scar *(2.12)*. This phenomenon is especially common after superficial removal (shave biopsy) or laser treatment of "superficial and deep" congenital nevi. Persistent melanocytes in deeper regions most likely migrate again into the epidermis via the follicular epithelium.

Spitz nevus

Named after the pathologist Sophie Spitz who described this nevus in the 1940s, Spitz nevus occurs most commonly in children and becomes vanishingly rare by old age. Because of its pleomorphic cytology, Spitz erroneously interpreted it as a melanoma (9). Today we know that it is a benign melanocytic lesion, with both pigmented and non-pigmented forms. The non-pigmented or lightly pigmented variant is seen as a rapidly growing reddish or skin-colored papule usually occurring on the face of children. These cases are rarely investigated by dermatoscopy because of the absence of pigmentation *(2.13)*. The pigmented type of Spitz nevus is a light-brown or dark-brown papule with no clear preference for a specific location *(2.14)*. The clinical appearance of pigmented Spitz nevi and Reed nevi can be very similar *(see figures 2.11 and 2.14)*, leading some authors to call them both Spitz nevi. On dermatoscopy and dermatopathology, however, one usually finds marked differences. In some cases it may be difficult or even impossible to distinguish Spitz nevus from melanoma not only clinically and dermatoscopically, but also on dermatopathology. This has given rise to ambiguous terms like "atypical Spitz nevus" or "MELTUMP" ("melanocytic tumor with uncertain malignant potential"). We do not use these terms in this book.

Sutton nevus (Halo nevus)

This nevus occurs mainly in children and adolescents, but is also seen in young adults. It is a small congenital nevus with a hypopigmented halo, also known as the halo phenomenon. Like vitiligo, it is most likely due to an immune reaction that may occasionally lead to complete disappearance of the nevus (10) *(2.15)*.

Unna nevus

This is a relatively common nevus that was named after the German dermatologist Paul Gerson Unna (6). While Miescher nevus nearly always occurs on the face, Unna nevus usually occurs on the trunk. Unna nevus is also referred to as a dermal nevus by clinicians. Characteristically this lesion is seen as a papillomatous, elevated, soft, occasionally pedunculated, skin-colored or brown papule. On dermatopathology it is marked by a characteristic silhouette and dermal arrangement of melanocytes. As in Miescher nevus, the pathological appearance is similar to that of a congenital nevus, but Unna nevus is also not seen at birth, appearing later in life *(2.16)*.

Common designations of melanocytic nevi which have not been used in this book are the following:

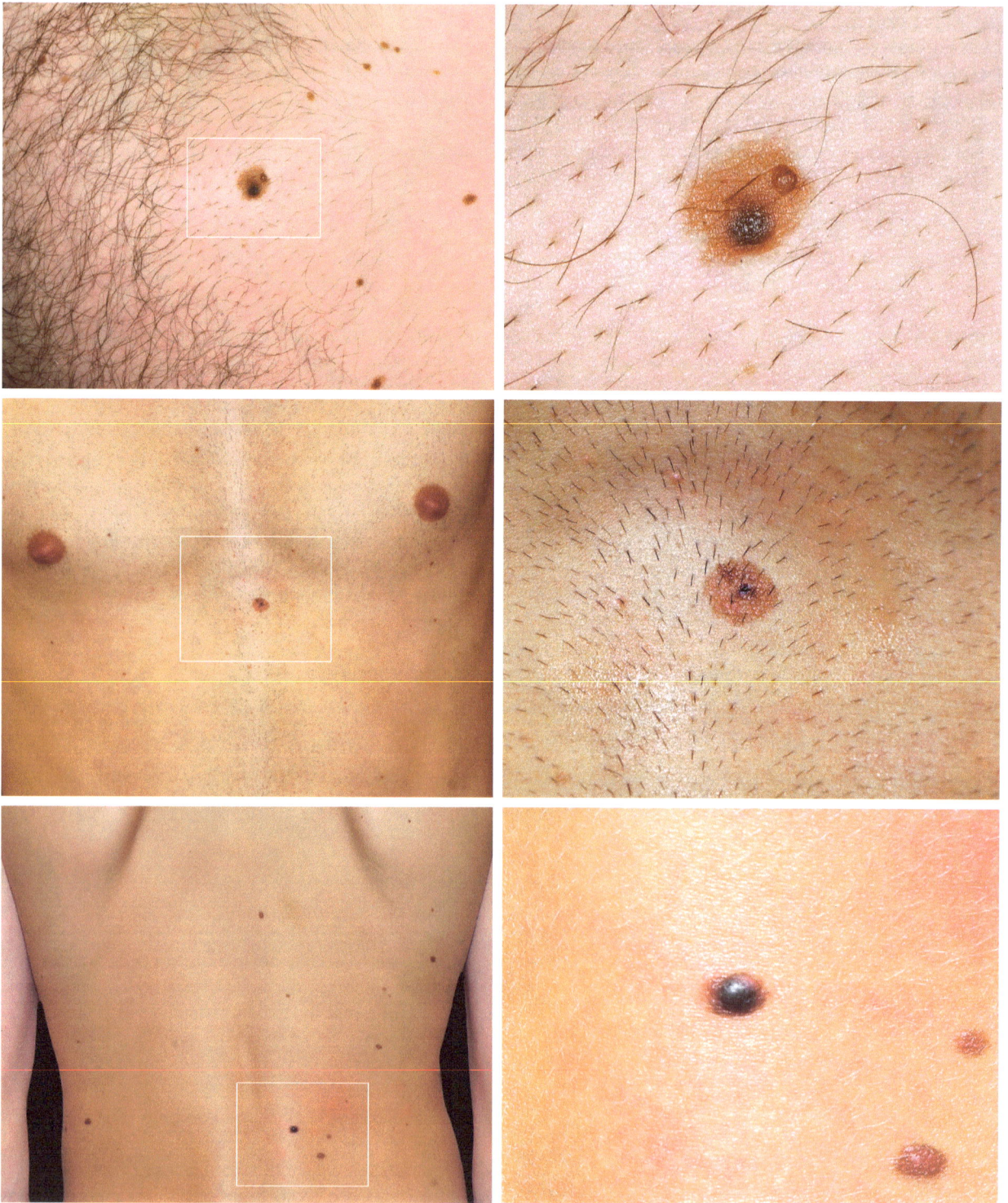

Figure 2.8: Combined congenital nevi.
The common feature of these combined congenital nevi is the joint occurrence of brown and blue portions. As the example in the first row shows, the blue portions may not be visible on clinical investigation. On histopathology, there are different populations of melanocytes. The blue portion corresponds to an accumulation of spindle-shaped melanocytes in the dermis, as in a "blue nevus", while the brown portion consists of melanocyte nests in the dermo-epidermal junction.

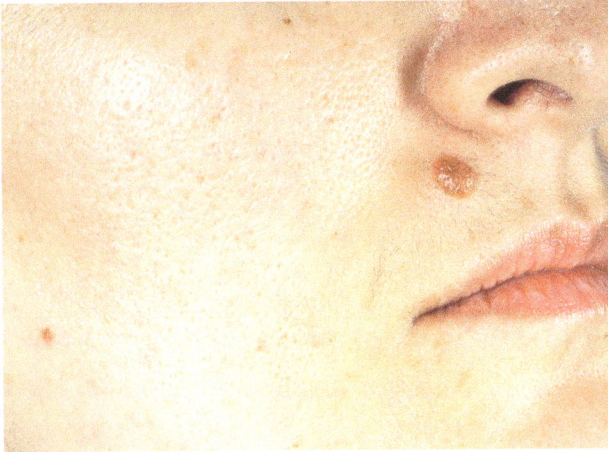

Figure 2.9: *Miescher nevus.*
Miescher nevus in a typical location.

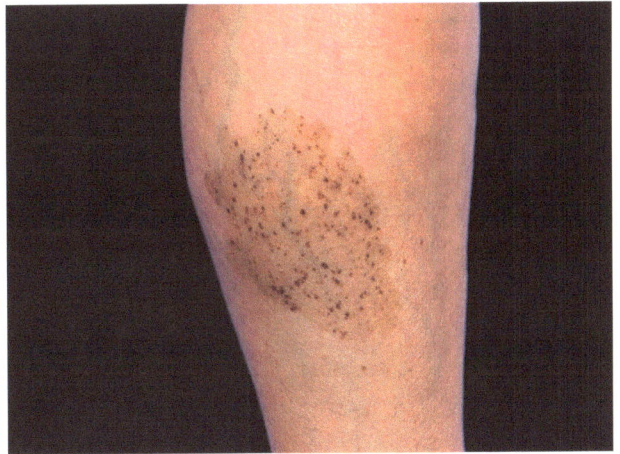

Figure 2.10: *Nevus spilus.*
A nevus spilus is a congenital nevus with variously pigmented portions. The hyperpigmented portions may be raised as shown here, or flat (nevus spilus maculosus).

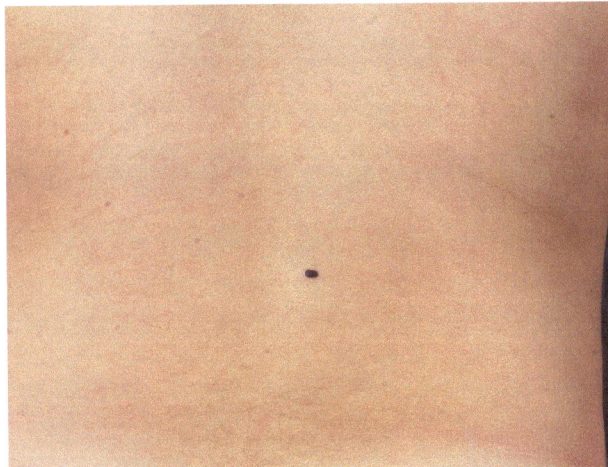

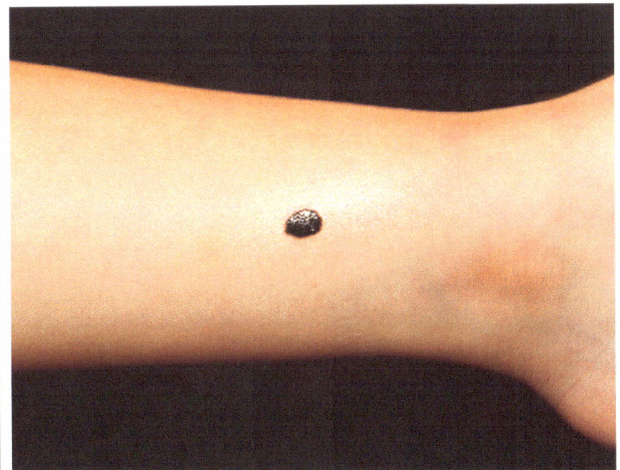

Figure 2.11: *Reed nevi.*
Two typical Reed nevi that appear as dark-brown or black papules or plaques on clinical investigation. The Reed nevus shown on the right is on the calf and is unusually large.

"Atypical nevus"

When clinicians refer to an "atypical nevus" they do not mean a specific type of nevus. Rather, it is an attempt to conceal diagnostic uncertainty. When clinicians refer to a "clinically atypical nevus" they mean that, morphologically, they are unable to confidently distinguish this entity from a melanoma. However, the term says nothing at all about the biological nature of the nevus. Although occasionally a melanoma may develop in association with a pre-existing nevus, the morphology of a nevus does not help predict which nevi are most likely to be affected. "Atypical nevi" are at no higher risk of developing into a melanoma; rather, the "atypical" nevus is more likely to actually be a melanoma.

"Dysplastic nevus"

When the dermatopathologist uses the term "dysplastic nevus" they also are not referring to a specific type of nevus. Rather, like its clinical companion "atypical", it conceals diagnostic uncertainty — the pathologist cannot entirely rule out melanoma. Some dermatopathologists use the term "dysplastic" in conjunction with gradations such as mild, moderate or high-grade (or severe). Again, this is merely an expression of the degree of the investigator's uncertainty, and these gradations are purely subjective.

The term "high-grade dysplastic nevus" means that, morphologically, the pathologist is unable to confidently distinguish between this entity and melanoma. The term says nothing about the biological nature of the nevus.

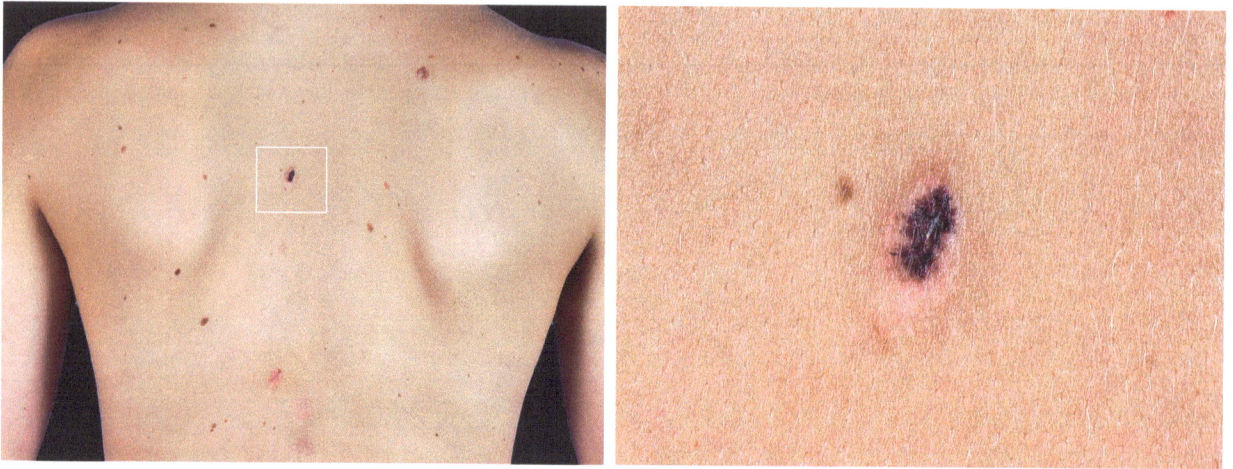

Figure 2.12: *Recurrent nevus.*
A recurrent nevus after incomplete excision may simulate a melanoma on clinical investigation. As this example shows, the visible pigmentation of a recurrent nevus typically does not extend beyond the region of the scar.

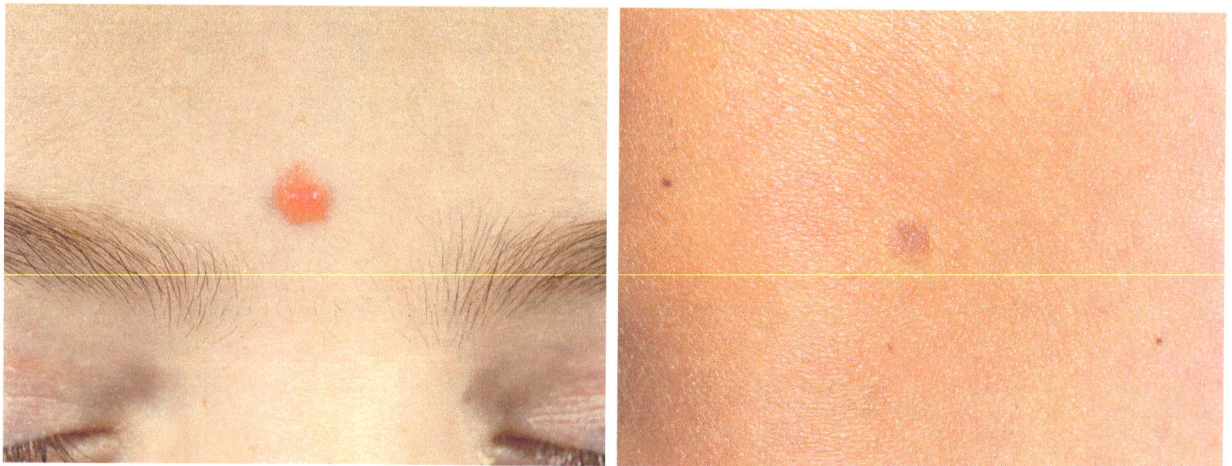

Figure 2.13: *"Classical" non-pigmented Spitz nevi*

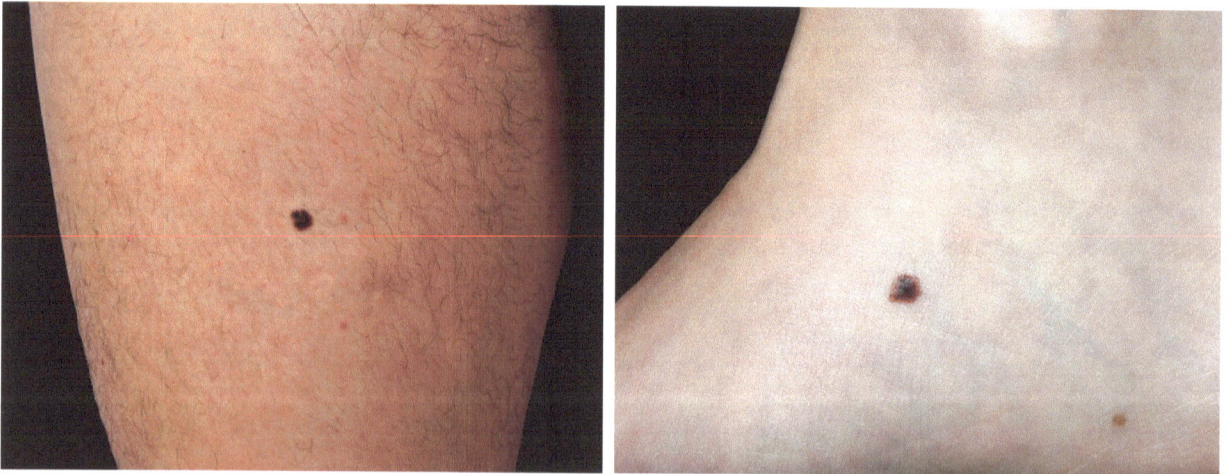

Figure 2.14: *Pigmented Spitz nevi*

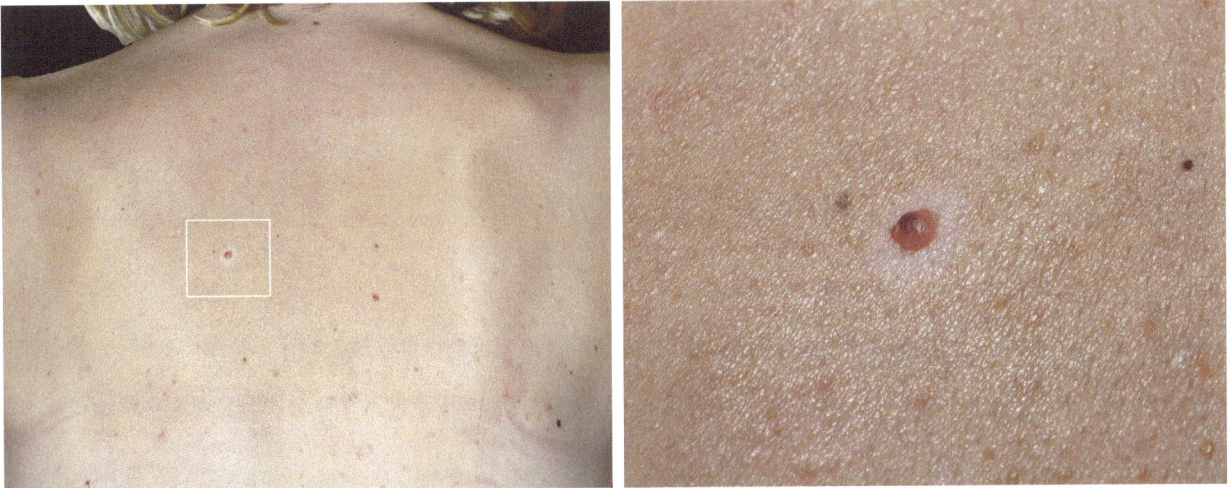

Figure 2.15: Halo nevus.
A hypopigmented zone around a small congenital nevus (halo nevus).

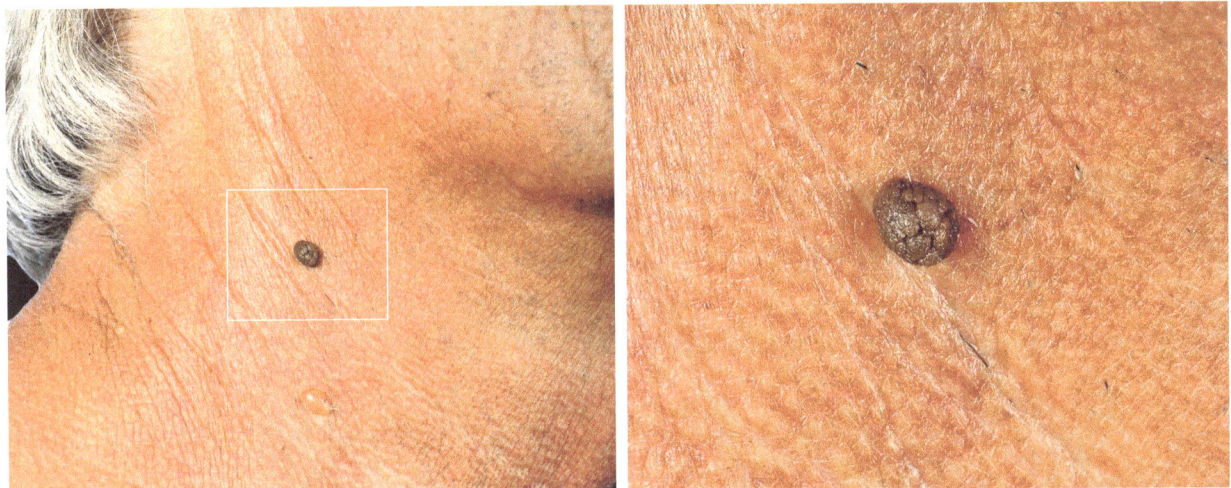

Figure 2.16: Unna nevus.
A typical characteristic of Unna nevus is its papillomatous surface. Unna nevi may be non-pigmented or, as in this illustration, light-brown to dark-brown in color.

"High-grade dysplastic nevi" are at no higher risk of developing into melanoma than any other nevi. Rather, a lesion diagnosed as a "high-grade dysplastic" nevus is more likely to actually be a melanoma. Occasionally the term "dysplastic" is used in the inflationary sense, i.e. all or nearly all excised flat nevi are termed "dysplastic". Used in this sense, the term loses any meaning it may have ever had.

Junctional, Compound and Dermal nevus
These terms only refer to the location of the melanocytes. They say nothing about the type of nevus. When melanocyte nests are exclusively located in the epidermis this is termed a junctional nevus. With melanocytes in the epidermis and the dermis, the nevus is referred to as a compound nevus. When melanocytes are exclusively located in the dermis, the nevus is known as a dermal nevus. One may refer to a junctional Clark nevus or a Clark nevus of the compound type, or make a distinction between a junctional Spitz nevus and a dermal Spitz nevus, but the terms junctional compound and dermal without specifying the type of nevus is as unspecific as the term "lentigo" and therefore they are not used in this book.

Other designations of melanocytic nevi not used in this book
Textbooks of dermatology and dermatopathology are full of different terms to describe nevi. An exhaustive list of all terms that have ever been used would make a

book of its own, but space is not the only reason why we do not list them all here. Some entities are controversial and ill-defined. Some are characterized pathologically but do not have a specific dermatoscopic appearance. For example, pathologists speak of "deep penetrating nevus" and "benign melanocytoma" but clinicians practically never do, because only pathologists are able to observe the specific features required to specifically diagnose these types of nevi. When examined with the unaided eye or with dermatoscopy both nevi usually look like blue nevi. On the other hand there are quite a number of nevi that have been defined by clinicians and dermatoscopists but do not show a specific pathology. Examples would be "eclipse nevus", a term that has been used for a type of congenital nevus, and "hypermelanotic nevus", a small Clark nevus with a hyperpigmented center (11). Other names are used to describe very specific circumstances, for example a Meyerson nevus (12) is a congenital nevus or, less

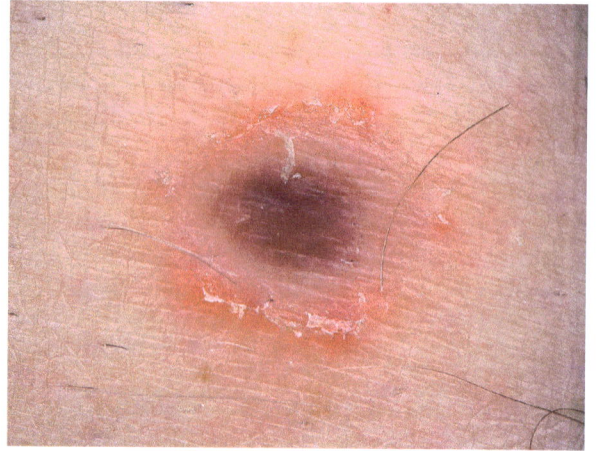

Figure 2.17: Meyerson nevus.
A Meyerson nevus is not a specific type of nevus. It is a nevus with a spongiotic ("eczematous") reaction. In this case, the inflamed nevus is most likely a "superficial and deep" congenital nevus. Ectatic blood vessels, redness and scales at the periphery are signs of inflammation.

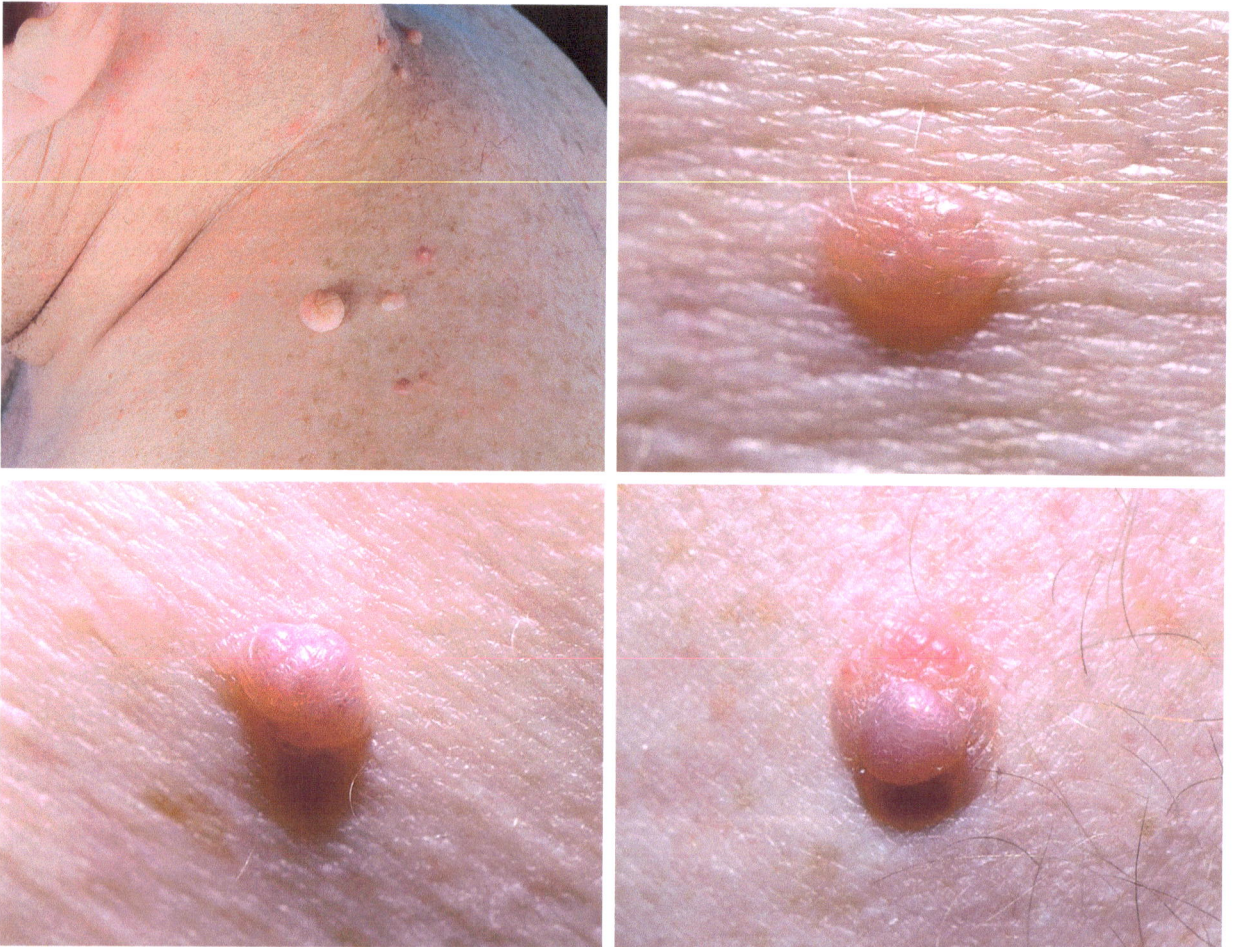

Figure 2.18: Nevi with BAP1 mutation ("BAPomas", "Wiesner nevi").
Nevi with BAP1 mutations in a patient with BAP1 germline mutation. The nevi look like "Unna nevi" clinically. Diagnosis requires histopathologic examination and immunohistochemistry to detect loss of BAP1 expression.

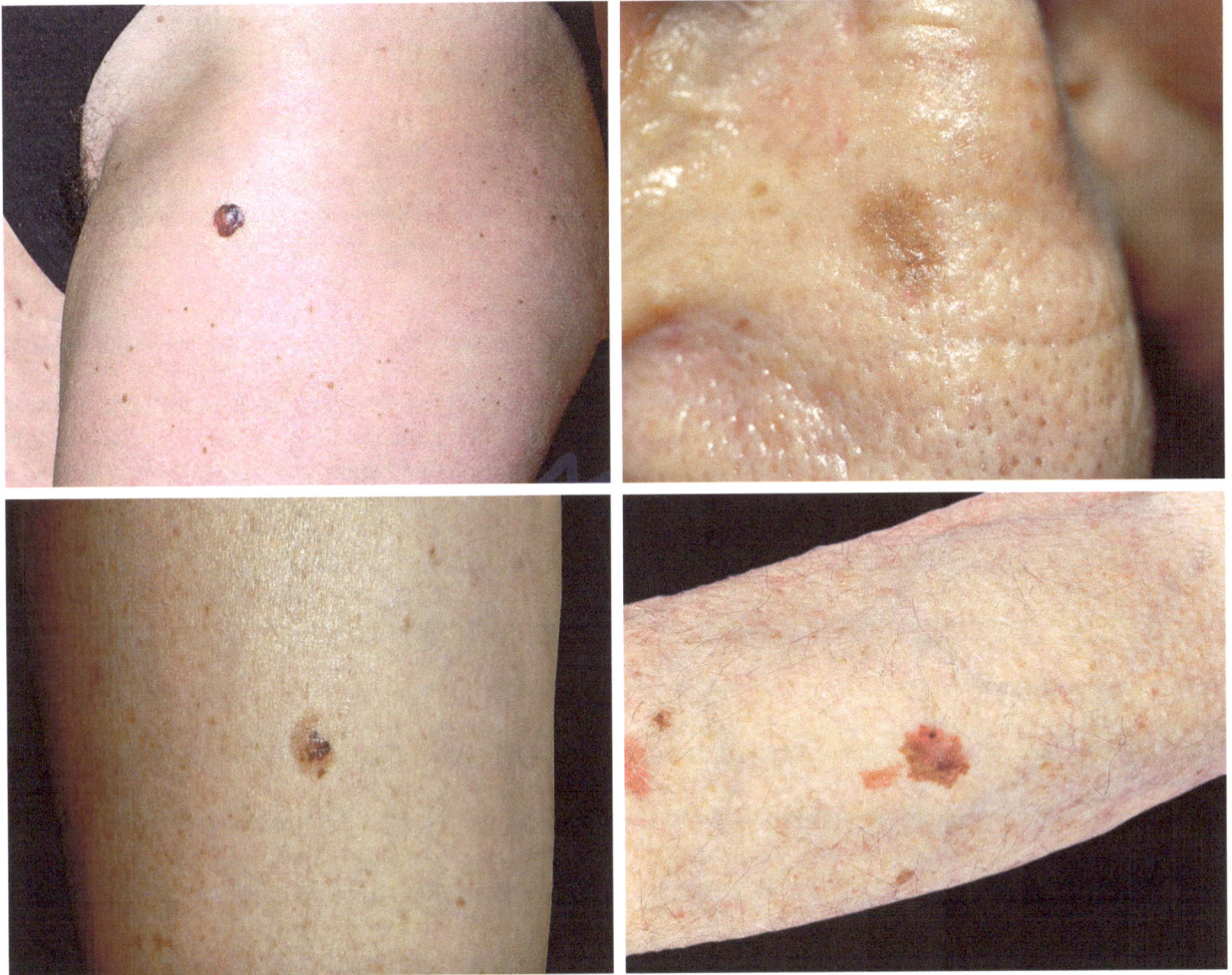

Figure 2.19: *Clinical photographs of four melanomas.*
Top left: *An asymmetrical, irregularly pigmented nodule (invasion thickness > 1 mm).* **Top right:** *An inconspicuous light-brown spot (in situ melanoma).* **Bottom left:** *A speckled, irregularly pigmented spot with a small brown papule (invasion thickness < 1 mm).* **Bottom right:** *An irregularly pigmented patch with irregular margins and signs of inflammation (in situ melanoma in regression).*

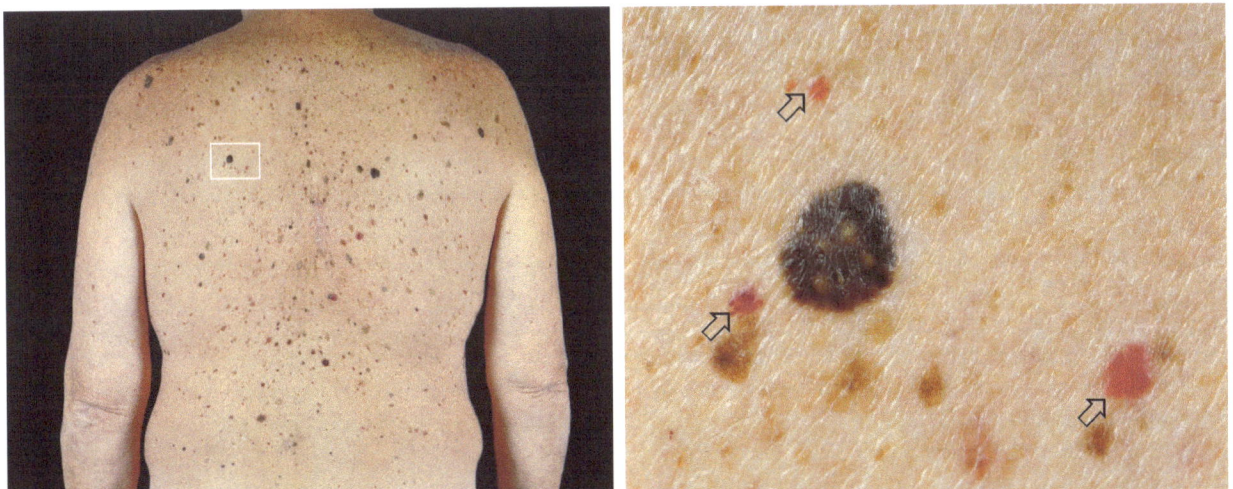

Figure 2.20: *Cherry angiomas.*
A patient with multiple solar lentigines, seborrheic keratoses and cherry angiomas. The detailed photograph (right) shows three cherry angiomas (arrows) surrounded by solar lentigines. A large dark-brown seborrheic keratosis is seen between the three angiomas.

frequently, a Clark nevus, with a spongiotic ("eczematous") reaction *(2.17)*.

The molecular revolution has seen an increasing availability of molecular data, allowing some nevi to be characterized genetically. For example, nevi that harbor mutations in the BAP1 gene ("BAPoma", "Wiesner nevus") have a peculiar cytomorphology with large melanocytes and abundant cytoplasm (13, 14). Clinically and dermatoscopically they resemble "Unna nevi" and are frequently referred to as "dermal nevi" by clinicians. When they appear in large number, they may indicate a germline mutation in the BAP1 gene, which predisposes to melanoma (especially ocular melanoma) and other malignant neoplasms *(2.18)*.

2.1.2 Melanoma

Melanoma is the only malignant neoplasia of melanocytes. In order to avoid ambiguities, in this book we use only this term. We do not use terms such as lentigo maligna, lentigo maligna melanoma, superficial spreading melanoma, nodular melanoma or acral lentiginous melanoma because these traditional classifications are inconsistent anatomically and histomorphologically, nor are they of any prognostic significance *(2.19)*. Nor do we use special designations based on pathological features, such as desmoplastic melanoma or nevoid melanoma. We acknowledge, however, that there are different manifestations of melanoma and that it is important to be familiar with these different manifestations. Melanomas can be non-pigmented. They may mimic nevi and viral warts. No two melanomas look alike.

While it may be useful to group melanomas into different categories, for example for therapeutic reasons, we do not think it is necessary to give a name to every manifestation of melanoma, like nevoid melanoma, verrucous melanoma, or animal-type melanoma, to name just a few of the terms that have been used. Every current classification of melanoma is arbitrary and currently all classifications have drawbacks. New classifications based on molecular data are emerging. It is not yet known whether this will lead to a rational basis for using one or more of the current classification systems, or to a new, purely molecular classification of melanoma. Most likely we will see a more meaningful and generally accepted classification that integrates morphologic, biologic and molecular data in the future. Until such a classification exists, we will call all melanomas just melanoma.

We do use the term "melanoma in situ", which refers to a non-invasive melanoma confined to the epidermis. A lentigo maligna is in fact one type of in situ melanoma. Throughout the book, legends to figures of invasive melanomas state whether the depth of the tumor (Breslow's invasion thickness) is < 1 mm or > 1 mm.

2.2 Non-melanocytic pigmented lesions

These lesions are included here because they may enter into the differential diagnosis of melanoma. Non-melanocytic does not mean non-pigmented or even not pigmented by melanin; non-melanocytic lesions may be pigmented by melanin or by hemoglobin or hemosiderin. Non-melanocytic lesions that are always non-pigmented are presented in chapter 6. As already mentioned the term "non-melanocytic" is problematic and artificial because it combines conditions that are entirely unrelated under one umbrella.

2.2.1 Vascular proliferations, vascular malformations and hemorrhage

The pigmentation of vascular proliferations or malformations and hemorrhage is not caused by melanin, but by the blood pigment hemoglobin or its degradation product hemosiderin. In the following, a distinction is made between hemangiomas, which represent a proliferation of blood vessels; and malformations of vessels such as nevus flammeus, which include dilatations of pre-existing vessels such as nevus araneus ("spider nevus") or angiokeratoma (15).

Hemangiomas

Hemangiomas are proliferations of blood vessels. Given the large number of different entities and the existing confusion of nomenclature, hemangiomas cannot be dealt with exhaustively in this book. So-called "senile" or tardive angiomas ("cherry angioma") are worthy of mention because they are common. These are cherry-red small papules which appear in large numbers. Like the much larger infantile hemangiomas ("strawberry hemangioma"), tardive angiomas have such a characteristic clinical appearance – merely because of their color – that they rarely pose difficulties in terms of differential diagnosis (e.g. traumatized or thrombosed angiomas) *(2.20)*.

Pyogenic granuloma is a benign, reactive (it often occurs after trauma or as a consequence of bacterial infection) vascular proliferation that presents clinically as a rapidly growing, usually eroded, reddish nodule. Melanoma mimics pyogenic granuloma far more frequently than any other proliferation of vessels. To avoid this grave error, tissue should always be submitted for histology when treating a "pyogenic granuloma" *(2.21)*.

Hemangiomas are more diverse from the pathologist's point of view than from the clinician's or dermatoscopist's

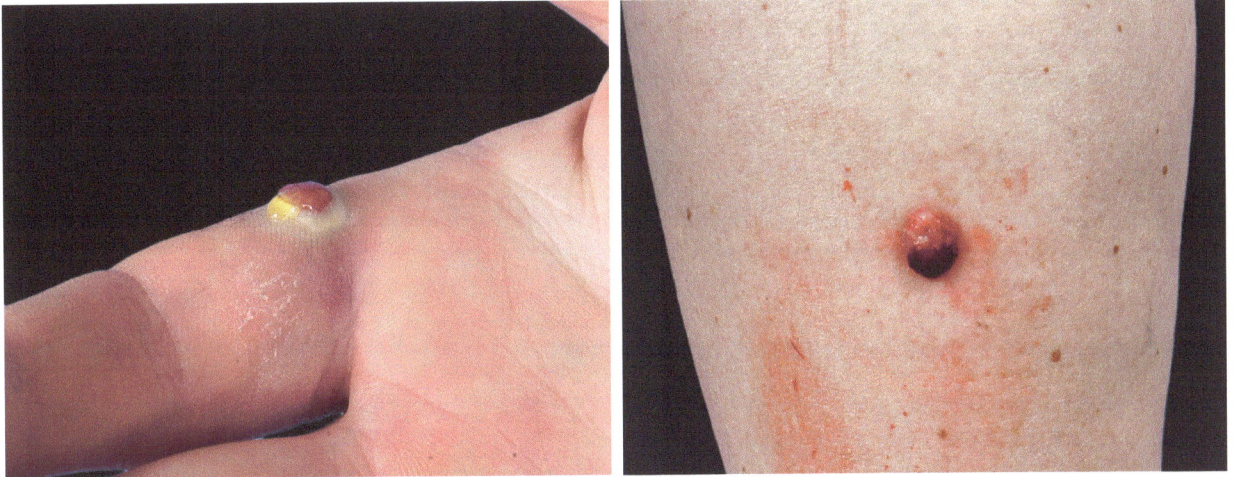

Figure 2.21: *Pyogenic granuloma.*
Two typical examples: Typical appearance is an erosive red or skin-colored hemorrhagic nodule. Malignancy, in particular amelanotic melanoma, may mimic pyogenic granuloma.

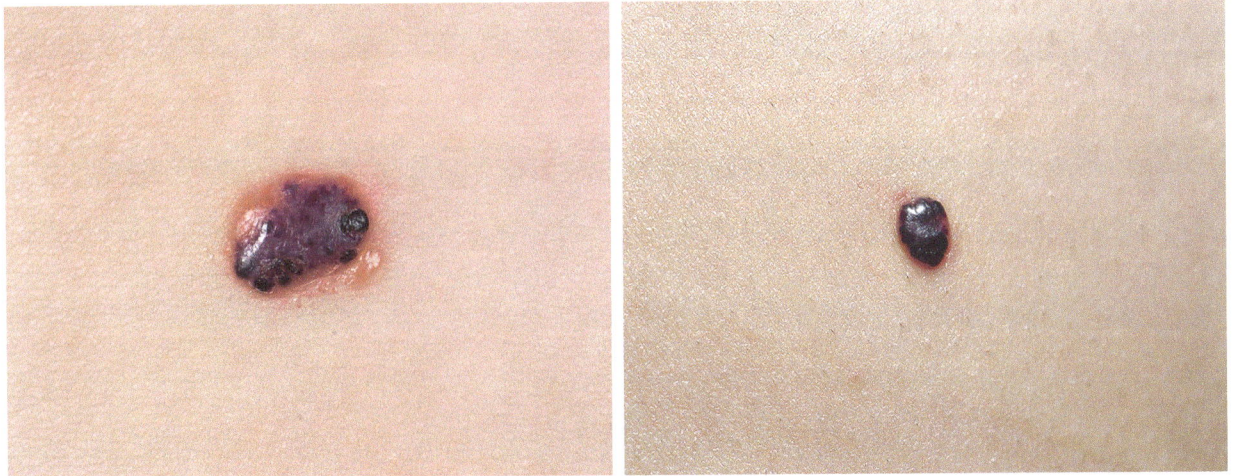

Figure 2.22: *Solitary angiokeratomas – two typical examples*

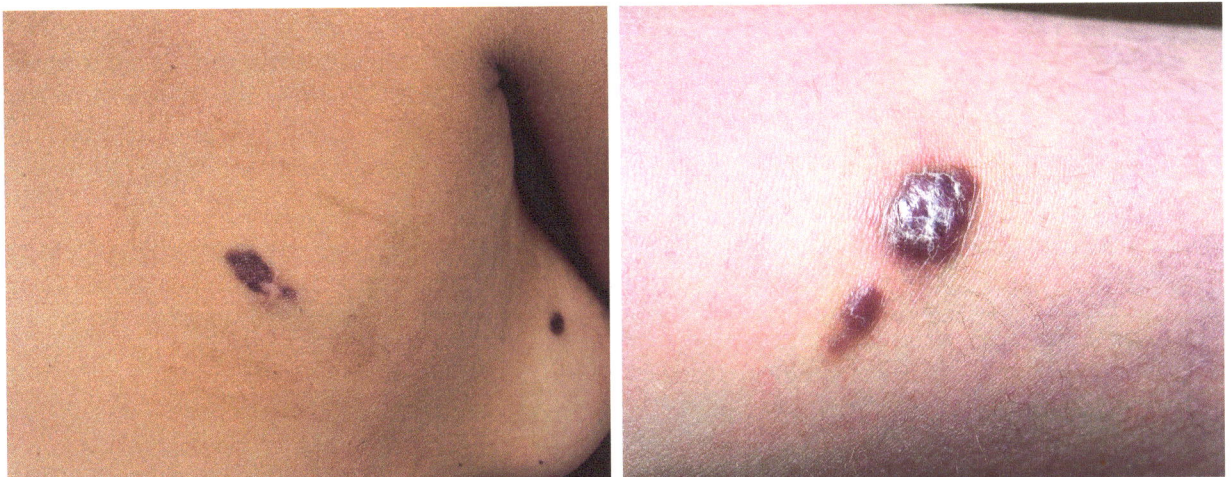

Figure 2.23: *Examples of skin lesions of Kaposi sarcoma.*
Left: *Purple-red plaques on a patient with dark skin.* **Right:** *Dark red plaques or nodules on a patient with lighter colored skin.*

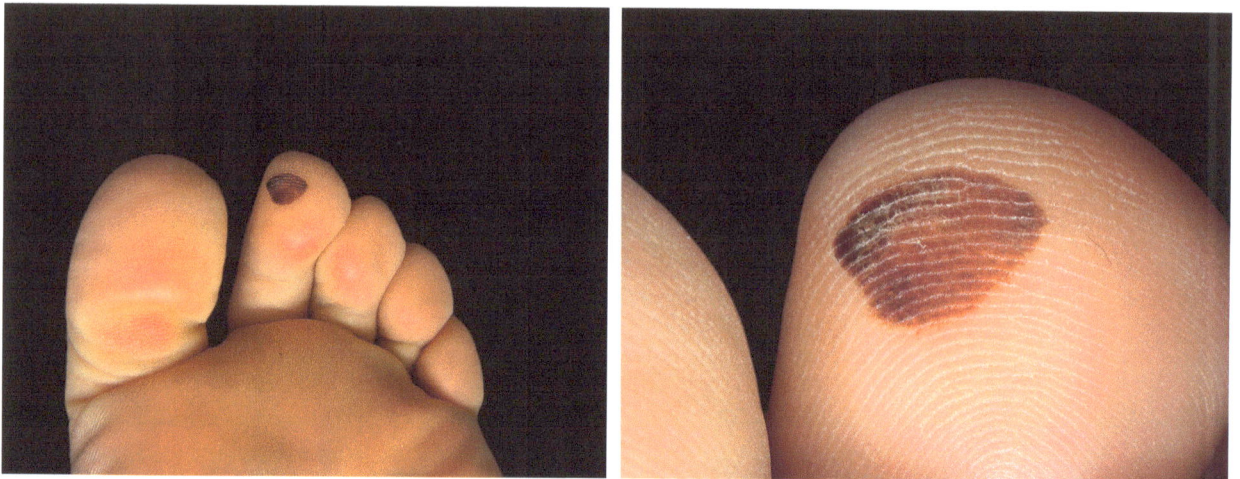

Figure 2.24: *Hemorrhage.*
Superficial hemorrhage in the stratum corneum of a toe.

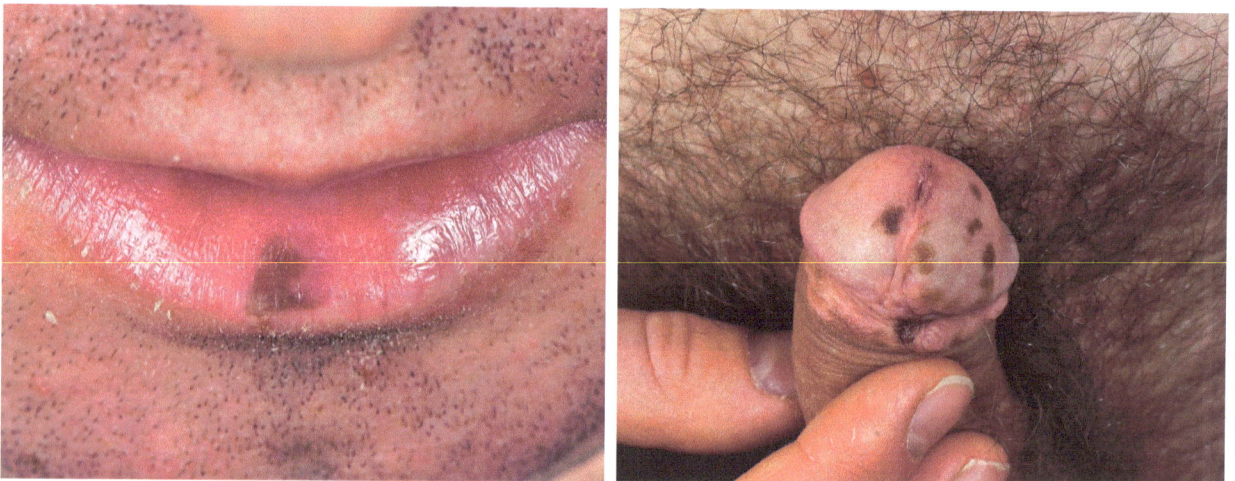

Figure 2.25: *Lentiginosis of the lip and genital lentiginosis*

point of view. Many benign vascular proliferations such as the targetoid hemosiderotic hemangioma, glomeruloid hemangioma and microvenular hemangioma can only be distinguished by the pathologist and will not be addressed here.

Vascular malformations

The nevus flammeus ("port-wine stain") is a common malformation of vessels with a characteristic clinical appearance. There is a pale, and subsequently darker, erythema caused by superficial telangiectasias. Predilection sites are the scalp, the neck, and the sacral region. As the clinical diagnosis is usually very clear, the nevus flammeus is rarely investigated by dermatoscopy.
The nevus araneus ("spider nevus") is composed of small superficial telangiectasias that arise from a central red papule. The latter is a small and extended arteriole. Nevus araneus may occur singly or multiply. In some cases this condition is believed to be associated with liver disease, pregnancy or hormone therapy.
Angiokeratomas are ectasias of the vessels of the upper vascular plexus with reactive hyperplasia of the epidermis. Various types of angiokeratomas exist. From the dermatoscopic point of view, the solitary type is most relevant. Clinically it is seen as a solitary, red, occasionally black nodule (or papule) with a hyperkeratotic surface *(2.22)*.

Kaposi's disease ("Kaposi sarcoma")

Kaposi sarcoma is actually not a sarcoma, i.e. a malignant neoplasm, but a reactive proliferation of vessels due to infection with the human herpes virus type 8

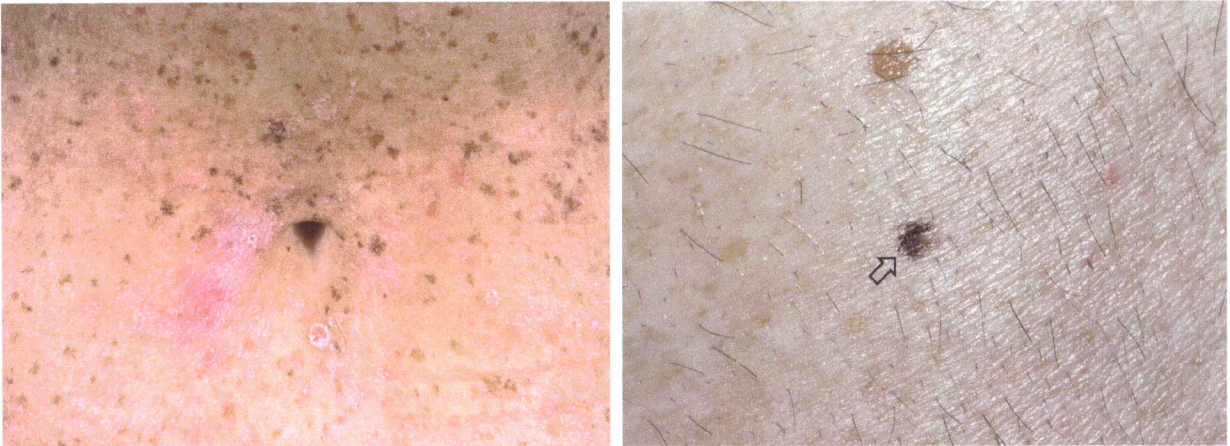

Figure 2.26: PUVA lentigines and ink-spot lentigo.
Left: Several PUVA lentigines in a patient with psoriasis after PUVA therapy. **Right:** Ink-spot lentigo seen as a solitary, sharply demarcated black macule.

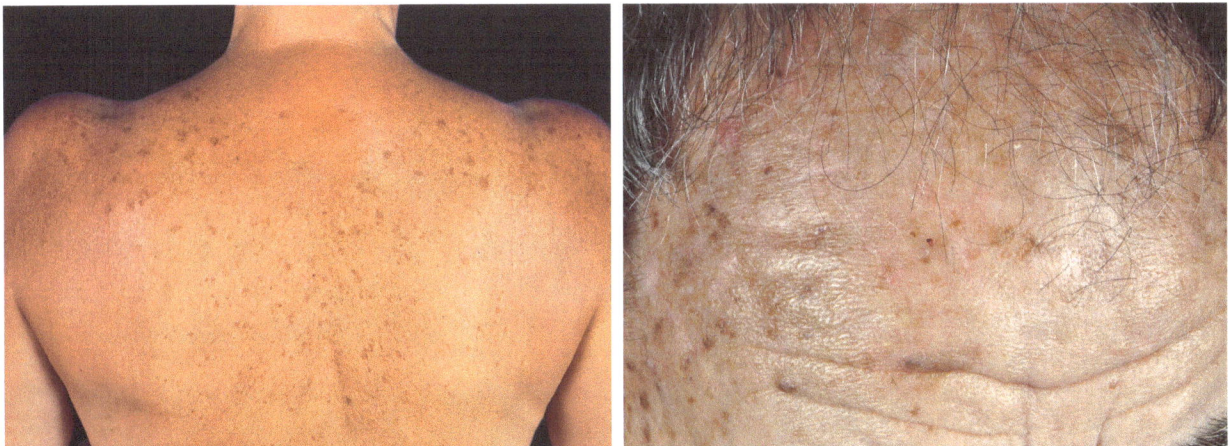

Figure 2.27: Solar lentigines.
Multiple solar lentigines on the back (**left**) and the scalp (**right**).

(HHV-8). The skin lesions in Kaposi sarcoma usually occur on the distal extremities, but when associated with HIV, Kaposi sarcoma may occur at any location. Clinically one finds multiple rust-brown or livid spots that may develop into plaques or nodules over time (2.23).

Hemorrhage
Hemoglobin and its degradation products produce the color of a hemorrhage. A fresh superficial hemorrhage usually appears red while older ones are brown or black. Hemorrhage becomes relevant to the dermatoscopist when it mimics melanoma. Hemorrhage in the nail-bed or bleeding in the stratum corneum of the epidermis (most frequent on acral skin) are the two conditions which commonly raise concern. The hemorrhage sometimes termed "black heel" is seen in figure (2.24).

2.2.2 Melanotic macules
Before we consider melanotic macules we must clarify the term "lentigo". Lentigo is an extremely vague term, derived from the word "lentil", which signifies no specific diagnosis on its own. Solar lentigo, mucosal lentigo, ink-spot lentigo, lentigo simplex and lentigo maligna have nothing in common except the word "lentigo". Lentigo simplex is the name given to a small junctional Clark nevus while lentigo maligna is an in situ melanoma. Both of these are melanocytic and are described in the section on melanocytic lesions. All other lesions termed lentigo are not melanocytic lesions.
The term "melanotic macule" includes all non-neoplastic lesions that are caused by hyperpigmentation of basal keratinocytes, but without significant increase in the number of melanocytes (16). This includes all types of

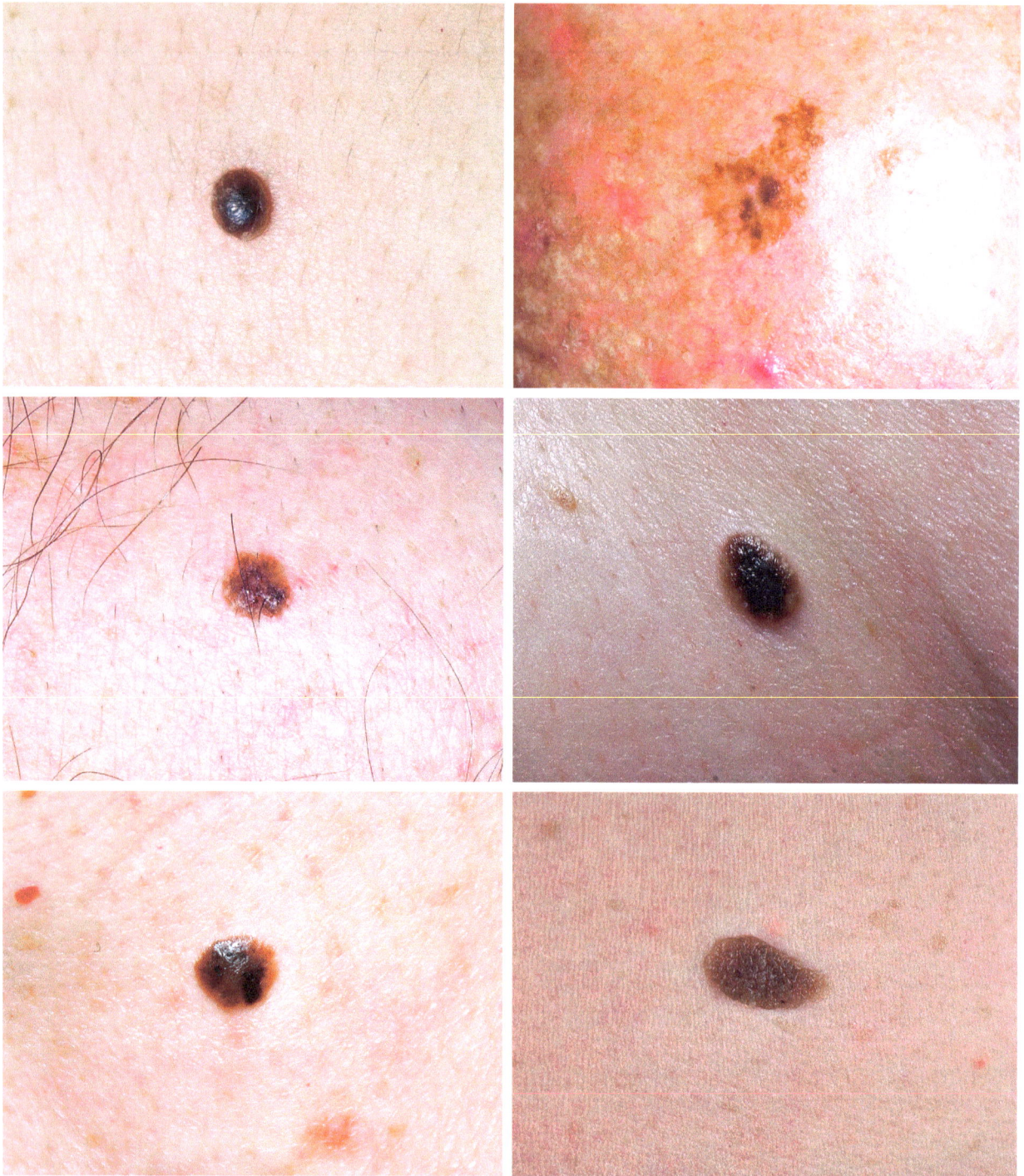

Figure 2.28: *Seborrheic keratoses.*
Various types of seborrheic keratoses: six examples.

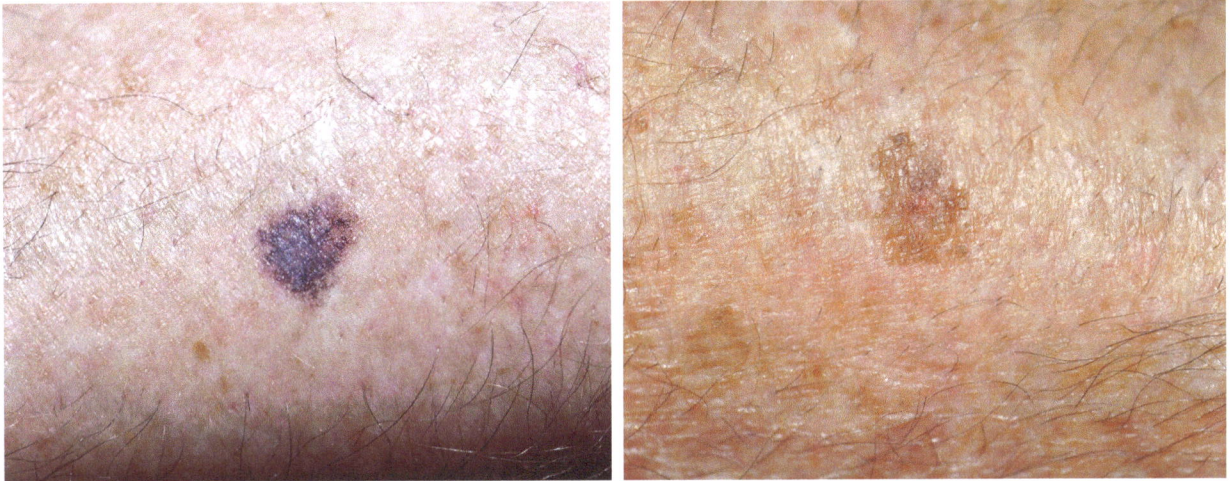

Figure 2.29: Lichen planus-like keratosis.
Two lichen planus-like keratoses on the forearm, surrounded by solar lentigines.

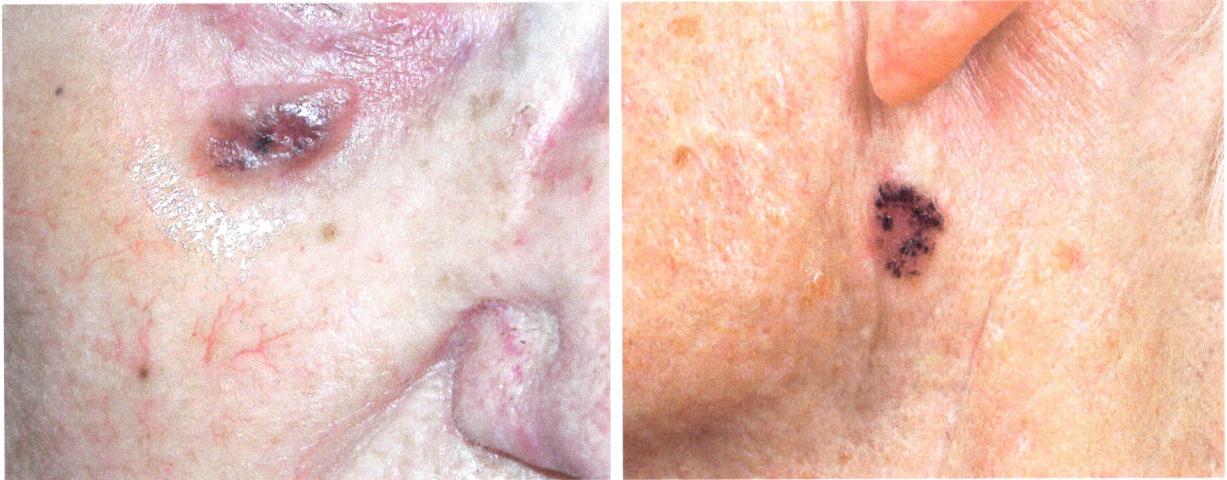

Figure 2.30: Pigmented basal cell carcinomas.
Left: A nodular pigmented basal cell carcinoma with central ulceration. **Right:** A rather flat, superficial pigmented basal cell carcinoma on the neck with no clinically visible ulceration.

genital lentiginosis and lentiginosis of the lip and the oral mucosa, PUVA lentigines, and ink-spot lentigo. Lentiginous lesions may also occur in the course of diseases such as Peutz-Jeghers syndrome, the LEOPARD syndrome, or the Laugier-Hunziker syndrome. Excluded from this list is solar lentigo, which is associated with epidermal hyperplasia and is therefore regarded, together with seborrheic keratosis, as a benign epithelial neoplasia.

Genital lentiginosis and lentiginosis of the lip and the oral mucosa

The relatively common genital lentiginosis and lentiginosis of the lip and the oral mucosa are also grouped under the term mucosal lentiginosis. Clinically one finds several light-brown or dark-brown spots. Genital lentiginosis is much more diverse in terms of morphology. As a reliable distinction between this entity and a mucosal melanoma cannot always be made on the basis of clinical features alone, these lesions are frequently biopsied (2.25).

PUVA lentigines and Ink-spot lentigo

The small dark pigmented macules that occur after PUVA radiation and ink-spot lentigo are similar lesions, probably induced by UV light. Because of their striking dark pigmentation, they are occasionally biopsied to histopathologically rule out melanoma (17). PUVA lentigines are usually multiple, whereas ink-spot lentigo is

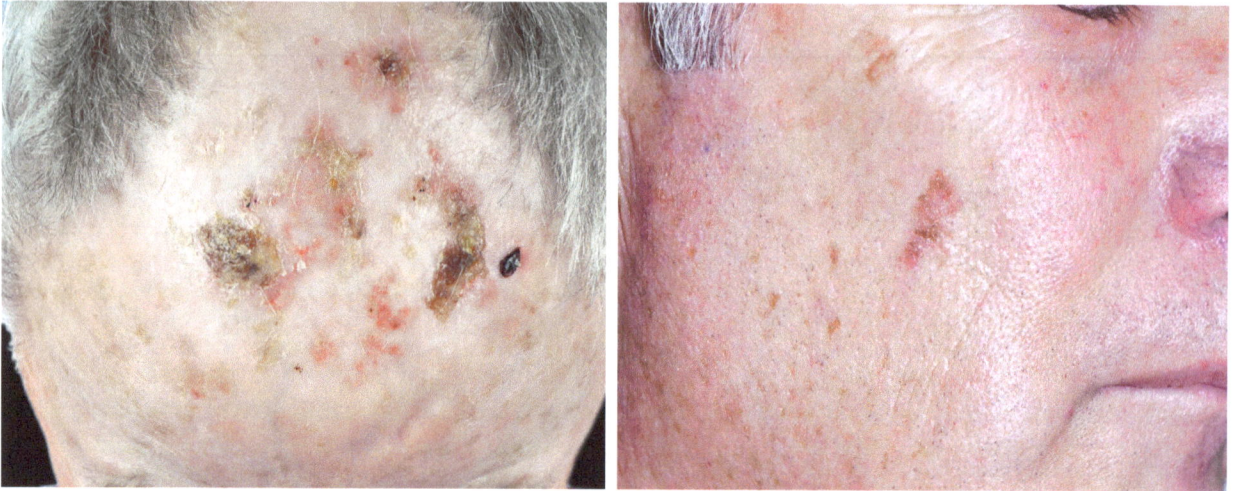

Figure 2.31: Actinic keratoses.
Left: *Numerous, partly erosive non-pigmented actinic keratoses on the scalp.* **Right:** *A solitary pigmented actinic keratosis on the cheek.*

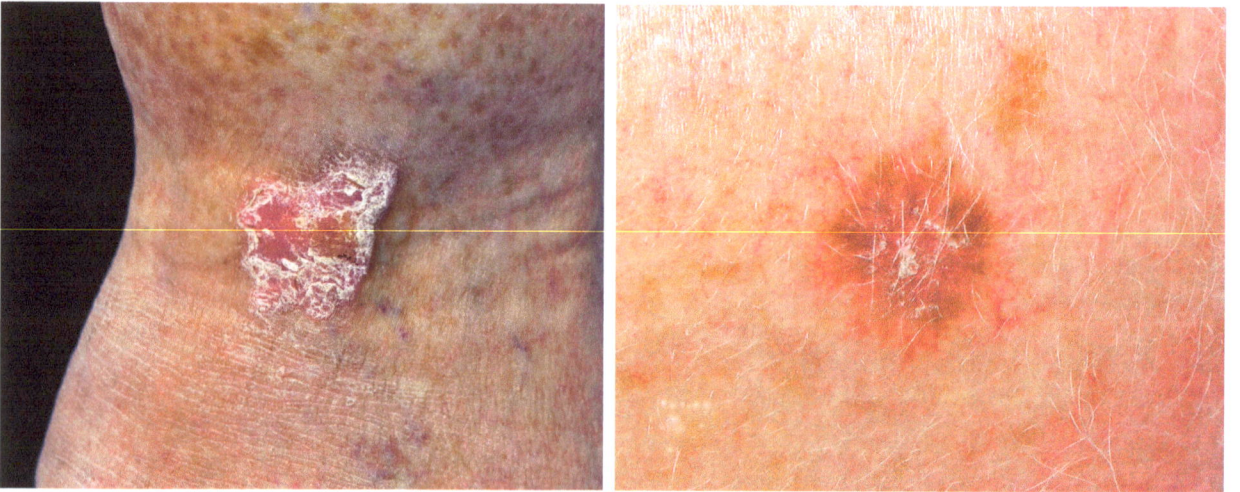

Figure 2.32: Bowen's disease ("intraepidermal carcinoma").
Left: *A solitary scaly plaque (non-pigmented Bowen's disease).* **Right:** *Mildly scaly light-brown plaque (pigmented Bowen's disease).*

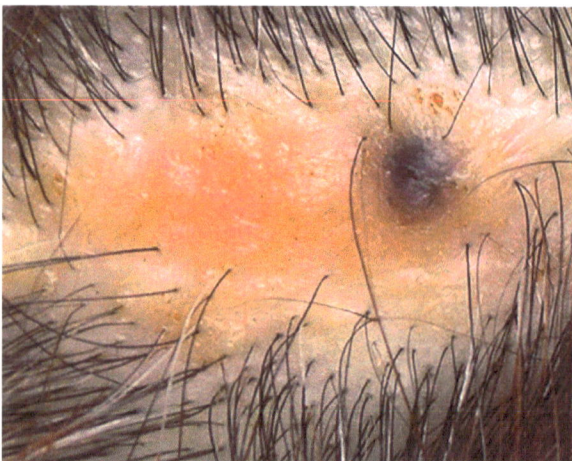

Figure 2.33: Pigmented trichoblastoma.
Pigmented trichoblastoma in a nevus sebaceous (image courtesy of Pedro Zaballos).

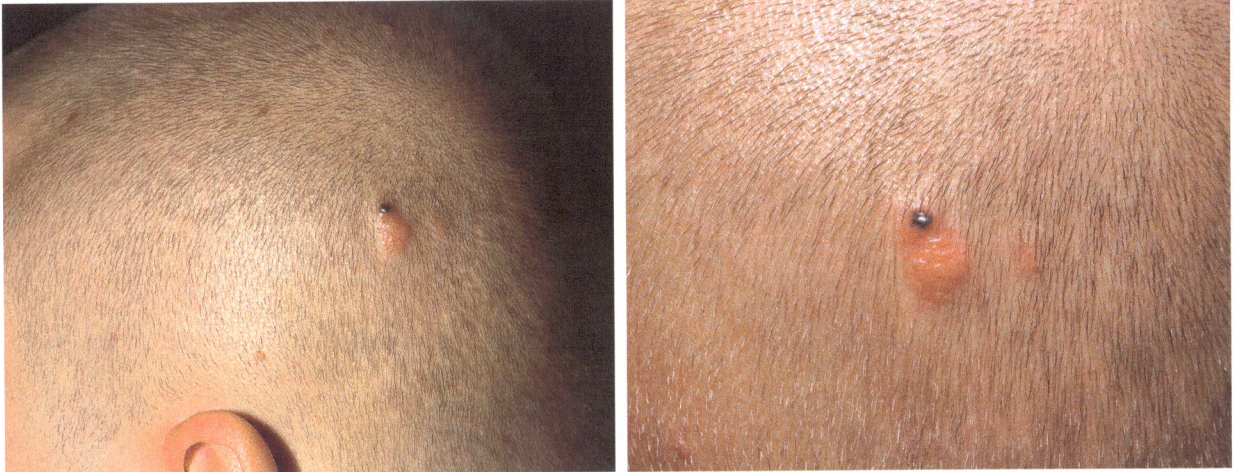

Figure 2.34: *Pigmented spiradenoma.*
Red to yellow pigmented plaque with eccentric blue pigmentation on the hair-bearing scalp.

commonly solitary. On histology the basal keratinocytes at the base of the rete ridges are strongly pigmented (18) *(2.26)*.

Lentigines in the course of diseases

Multiple lentigines may occur as part of syndromes such as Peutz-Jeghers syndrome, the LEOPARD syndrome, the Laugier-Hunziker syndrome, the Bannayan-Riley-Ruvalcaba syndrome, and the diseases grouped under the term "Carney complex" (19–23). Whether the lentigines of the various syndromes can be distinguished from each other on clinical examination, dermatoscopy or histopathology has not yet been investigated.

2.2.3 Benign epithelial neoplasms
Lentigo solaris

Solar lentigo is a circumscribed light-brown macule, usually multiple. They are also referred to as pigment spots, age spots, liver spots and "freckles" (although "freckle" is more correctly used for the ephilis). They usually occur on chronically UV-exposed skin and become more common with advancing age. Their brown color is due to concentration of melanin in basal keratinocytes (melanin produced by melanocytes is transferred to keratinocytes via melanocytic dendrites). These lesions are classified as non-melanocytic because number of melanocytes is only slightly increased, if at all. The epidermis is hyperplastic and has elongated rete ridges (except often on the face). Solar lentigines may develop into seborrheic keratoses and are regarded as a precursor of these by many authors (1) *(2.27)*.

Seborrheic keratosis

Seborrheic keratoses are extremely common epithelial neoplasms that often occur in large numbers. They mainly appear after age 40, becoming almost ubiquitous in later life (1). Colloquially they are rather inelegantly referred to as senile warts. The morphology of seborrheic keratoses is variable; it ranges from skin- to yellow-colored flat papules to dark brown plaques often with a verrucous surface. Several names exist for the different clinical and histological types, which possibly represent various stages of the lesion's development.

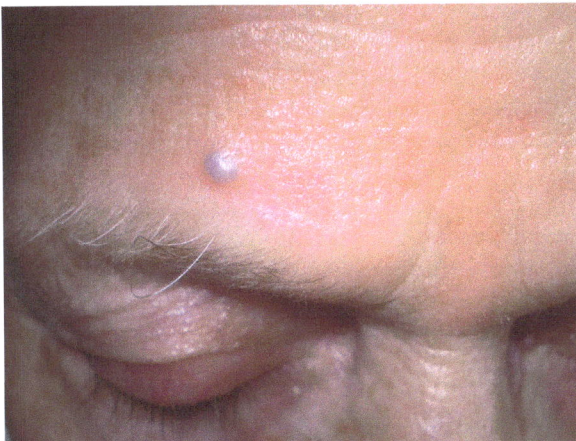

Figure 2.35: *Apocrine hidrocystoma.*
An apocrine hidrocystoma (apocrine cystadenoma) may appear as a blue nodule (image courtesy of Nisa Akay).

Another explanation for the morphological diversity may be various mutations and environmental factors. The main clinical significance of these harmless lesions is that occasionally they can mimic melanoma, and vice versa *(2.28)*.

Lichen planus-like keratosis
The term "lichen planus-like keratosis" was coined by Shapiro and Ackermann in 1966 (24). The term does not refer to a specific diagnosis but to a solar lentigo, or less often a seborrheic keratosis, in a stage of regression. Lichen planus-like keratosis usually occurs on chronic UV-exposed locations, such as the face or the dorsum of the hand. As a rule one finds a solitary lesion or more rarely an accumulation of several lesions. They are usually flat with sharply defined margins, colored brown and/or gray. Several solar lentigines are nearly always found in the vicinity of the lesion. Many lichen planus-like keratoses are biopsied because the clinical appearance raises the suspicion of a melanoma in regression, or of a basal cell carcinoma *(2.29)*.

2.2.4 Malignant epithelial neoplasms ("keratinocyte cancer")
Basal cell carcinoma and squamous cell carcinoma are commonly referred to together as "non-melanoma skin cancer", but for reasons already mentioned this is a problematic term. Alternative terms proposed to refer to basal cell carcinoma and squamous cell carcinoma collectively include "cutaneous malignant epithelial neoplasms" or "keratinocyte skin cancer", but these terms are also problematic. There are other cutaneous malignant epithelial neoplasms, not just basal cell carcinoma and squamous cell carcinoma, and traditionally neoplasms are classified according to their differentiation and not according to the cell of origin, which is often unknown. Strictly speaking, a basal cell carcinoma is an adnexal neoplasm with follicular differentiation and not "keratinocyte cancer".
It is best to avoid all these collective terms, whenever possible.

Basal cell carcinoma
The basal cell carcinoma is a malignant epithelial neo-plasm whose differentiation is similar to that of follicular epithelium. As already mentioned it is an adnexal neo-plasm with follicular differentiation. Another name for basal cell carcinoma is "trichoblastic carcinoma" but this is rarely used. Basal cell carcinoma is occasionally referred to as a semi-malignant lesion on the basis that while they grow in a locally destructive manner, they rarely metastasize. As basal cell carcinomas only occur

on hair-bearing skin, they are not found on the palms or the soles (except in a rare genodermatosis called the basal cell nevus or Gorlin-Goltz syndrome), the lips or the mucosa. A distinction is made between various types, but this classification differs according to the viewpoint. As is true for melanocytic nevi, clinicians and dermatopathologists speak different languages in this regard.
A basal cell carcinoma may be pigmented *(2.30)* but most are non-pigmented. The term "pigmented basal cell carcinoma" is used by clinicians, but not always by pathologists. A common pathological classification includes the following subtypes: nodular, superficial, morpheaform, fibroepithelial and infundibulocystic (1).

Squamous cell carcinoma
Superficial types of squamous cell carcinoma of the skin include actinic keratosis and Bowen's disease (1). Sometimes the term "intraepidermal carcinoma" is used instead of Bowen's disease. The causal role of UV exposure in all forms of squamous cell carcinoma is undisputed. The view that actinic keratoses are a variety of superficial squamous cell carcinoma is not universally accepted, with some preferring to call them "precancerous lesions". Actinic keratoses are usually numerous and mainly found in chronic UV-exposed areas. Clinically they appear as rough white hyperkeratoses on an erythematous base. Bowen's disease, another type of superficial squamous cell carcinoma, is usually a red scaly plaque which can easily be mistaken clinically for a psoriatic lesion or eczema. Both actinic keratosis and Bowen's disease are usually non-pigmented, but pigmented varieties also exist, and constitute an important differential diagnosis for melanoma. In contrast to superficial types, invasive cutaneous squamous cell carcinomas are only very rarely pigmented *(2.31 and 2.32)*.

2.2.5 Adnexal neoplasms
The general term adnexal neoplasm includes those with follicular, sebaceous, apocrine and eccrine differentiation. Although basal cell carcinoma is often lumped together with squamous cell carcinoma under umbrella terms like "non-melanoma skin cancer" or "keratinocyte cancer" it is an adnexal neoplasm with follicular differentiation. Most adnexal neoplasms are not pigmented and are therefore not mentioned in this glossary. Apart from basal cell carcinoma, trichoblastoma is the only adnexal neoplasm that is commonly pigmented *(2.33)*. Trichoblastoma is a benign neoplasm with follicular differentiation mostly occurring in conjunction with a nevus sebaceous. All other adnexal neoplasms are rarely or never pigmented. Images of pigmented spiradenoma

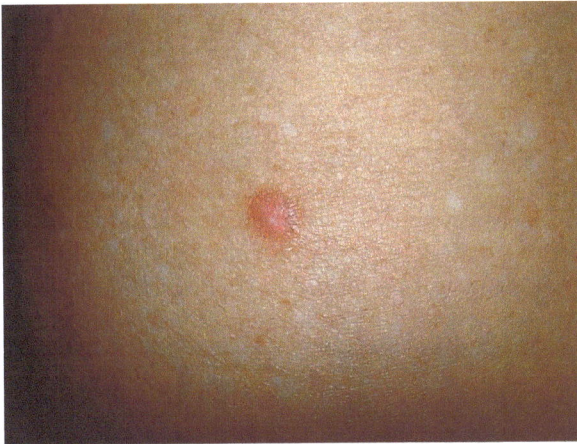

Figure 2.36: Dermatofibroma.
A brown papule in a typical location on the calf (dermatofibroma).

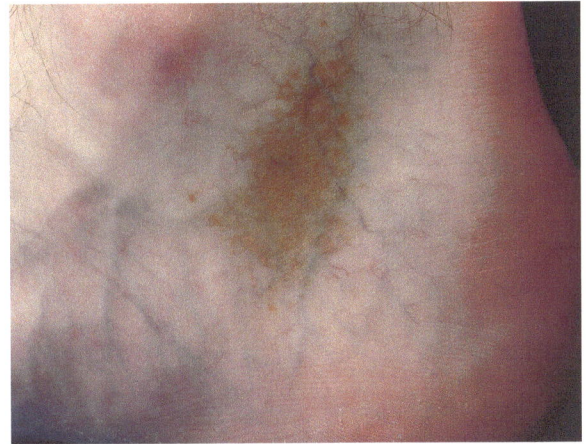

Figure 2.37: Pigmented purpura.
Reddish brown lesion on the ankle (pigmented purpura).

and pigmented eccrine poromas have been published (2.34). Rare cases of pigmented apocrine cysts have also been documented. They usually appear as blue nodules and may be confused with a blue nevus (2.35). Strictly speaking, apocrine cysts are cysts and not neoplasms.

2.2.6 Dermatofibroma

Dermatofibroma is not a neoplasm in the strict sense of the word, but a post-inflammatory tissue reaction associated with fibrosis of the dermis (1). For this reason, dermatofibromas are nodular and typically sink below skin level when squeezed between two fingers. Dermatofibromas occur most commonly on the calf, but they may occur at any location. With melanin hyperpigmentation of basal keratinocytes above the zone of dermal fibrosis, dermatofibromas are usually light-brown in color (2.36).

2.2.7 Other pigmented lesions relevant to dermato-scopy

Other pigmented skin lesions do not usually constitute a differential diagnosis for melanoma. They include urticaria pigmentosa, a special type of mastocytosis in which one finds several light-brown papules that are usually irregularly dispersed over the entire integument (1). Also worthy of mention are conditions arising from the group of purpura diseases associated with extravasation of erythrocytes. These include various types of pigmented purpura which are inflammatory skin diseases of unknown etiology, and stasis purpura (1) (2.37).

One should not forget exogenous pigmentation, such as silver nitrate (contained in cauterizing pens for the treatment of warts), and of course tattoos. Another condition is infection with the fungus *Hortaea werneckii*,

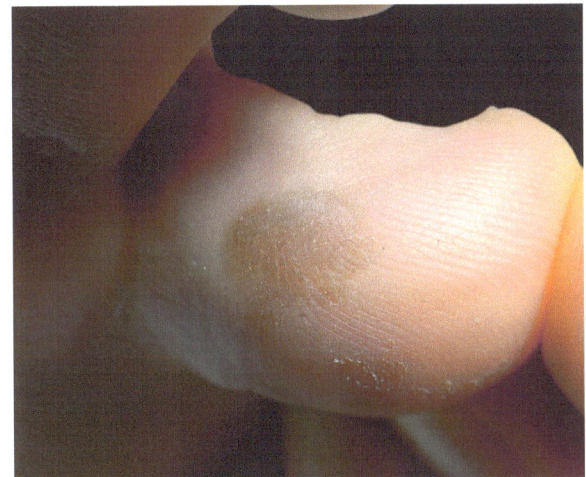

Figure 2.38: Tinea nigra.
Light-brown macule on the toe (Tinea nigra).

which causes a gray-black coloration of the skin and is therefore known as tinea nigra (25). Tinea nigra is important because it is a mimic of acral melanoma (2.38).

References

1   Ackerman AB, Kerl H, Sanchez J. A Clinical Atlas of 101 Common Skin Diseases: Ardor Scribendi; 2000.

2   Darlington S, Siskind V, Green L, Green A. Longitudinal study of melanocytic nevi in adolescents. J Am Acad Dermatol 2002; 46: 715–22.

3   Siskind V, Darlington S, Green L, Green A. Evolution of melanocytic nevi on the faces and necks of adolescents: a 4 y longitudinal study. J Invest Dermatol 2002; 118: 500–4.

4   Kachare SD, Agle SC, Englert ZP, Zervos EE, Vohra NA, Wong JH et al. Malignant blue nevus: clinicopathologically similar to melanoma. Am Surg 2013; 79: 651–6.

5   Clark WH, Jr., Reimer RR, Greene M, Ainsworth AM, Mastrangelo MJ. Origin of familial malignant melanomas from heritable melanocytic lesions. 'The B-K mole syndrome'. Arch Dermatol 1978; 114: 732–8.

6   Ackerman AB, Magana-Garcia M. Naming acquired melanocytic nevi. Unna's, Miescher's, Spitz's Clark's. Am J Dermatopathol 1990; 12: 193–209.

7   Reed RJ, Ichinose H, Clark WH, Jr., Mihm MC, Jr. Common and uncommon melanocytic nevi and borderline melanomas. Semin Oncol 1975; 2: 119–47.

8   Bar M, Tschandl P, Kittler H. Differentiation of pigmented Spitz nevi and Reed nevi by integration of dermatopathologic and dermatoscopic findings. Dermatol Pract Concept 2012; 2: 13–24.

9   Spitz S. Melanomas of childhood. Am J Pathol 1948; 24: 591–609.

10 Sutton RL. An unusual variety of vitiligo (leukoderma acquisitum centrifugum). J Cutan Dis 1916; 34: 797–801.

11 Schaffer JV, Glusac EJ, Bolognia JL. The eclipse naevus: tan centre with stellate brown rim. Br J Dermatol 2001; 145: 1023–6.

12 Meyerson LB. A peculiar papulosquamous eruption involving pigmented nevi. Arch Dermatol 1971; 103: 510–2.

13 Llamas-Velasco M, Perez-Gonzalez YC, Requena L, Kutzner H. Histopathologic clues for the diagnosis of Wiesner nevus. J Am Acad Dermatol 2014; 70: 549–54.

14 Wiesner T, Obenauf AC, Murali R, Fried I, Griewank KG, Ulz P et al. Germline mutations in BAP1 predispose to melanocytic tumors. Nat Genet 2011; 43: 1018–21.

15 Fritsch P. Dermatologie und Venerologie: Grundlagen. Klinik. Atlas. Berlin: Springer; 2003.

16 Sanchez J. Unifying Concept of Melanotic Macule: Synonymy for Melanotic Macule on Different Anatomic Sites. Dermatopathol: Pract & Conc 1998; 4: 2.

17 Bleehen SS. Freckles induced by PUVA treatment [proceedings]. Br J Dermatol 1978; 99: 20.

18 Bolognia JL. Reticulated black solar lentigo ('ink spot' lentigo). Arch Dermatol 1992; 128: 934–40.

19 Wilkes D, McDermott DA, Basson CT. Clinical phenotypes and molecular genetic mechanisms of Carney complex. Lancet Oncol 2005; 6: 501–8.

20 Fargnoli MC, Orlow SJ, Semel-Concepcion J, Bolognia JL. Clinicopathologic findings in the Bannayan-Riley-Ruvalcaba syndrome. Arch Dermatol 1996; 132: 1214–8.

21 Coppin BD, Temple IK. Multiple lentigines syndrome (LEOPARD syndrome or progressive cardiomyopathic lentiginosis). J Med Genet 1997; 34: 582–6.

22 McGarrity TJ, Amos C. Peutz-Jeghers syndrome: clinicopathology and molecular alterations. Cell Mol Life Sci 2006; 63: 2135–44.

23 Kanwar AJ, Kaur S, Kaur C, Thami GP. Laugier-Hunziker syndrome. J Dermatol 2001; 28: 54–7.

24 Shapiro L, Ackerman AB. Solitary lichen planus-like keratosis. Dermatologica 1966; 132: 386–92.

25 Schwartz RA. Superficial fungal infections. Lancet 2004; 364: 1173–82.

3 Pattern Analysis – Basic Principles

The method presented here for evaluating pigmented skin lesions is derived from pattern analysis. Nothing new is invented here; we have merely dispensed with the current proliferation of ill-defined metaphoric descriptions and given dermatoscopy a logical, well-defined and clearly structured system. If you are a newcomer to dermatoscopy, you will find it straightforward to learn the basic principles of this method. If you have experience but currently use another method, you will immediately notice the absence of fanciful descriptions and metaphoric terms. However, an unprejudiced and open-minded approach will rapidly demonstrate the advantages of revised pattern analysis. This system will serve as a basis to help you acquire a profound knowledge of dermatoscopy. One masters a technique by developing one's own style and the latter evolves from personal experience. However, in the absence of a system that helps to organize one's observations and catalog them appropriately, any experience on the subject is purely anecdotal.

What *is* novel here is the structured method of generating a description of lesions using simple geometrically defined terms. Importantly, generating this description guides the clinician along the diagnostic pathway.

3.1 Basic elements

Although skin lesions have an infinite variety of appearances, descriptions sufficient to derive the most accurate diagnosis possible can be formulated using arrangements of just five basic elements: *lines, pseudopods, circles, clods and dots* (3.1).

3.2 Basic patterns

A pattern consists of multiple repetitions of a single basic element. Every basic element may be part of a pattern, but only when they are repeated over a significant portion of a lesion. In other words, two or three dispersed lines, dots, clods, circles or pseudopods do not constitute a pattern. When assessing the pattern of a pigmented lesion one views it from a distance, as one does when assessing a histological specimen at scanning magnification. Details that are only apparent on close inspection are excluded from this initial assessment.

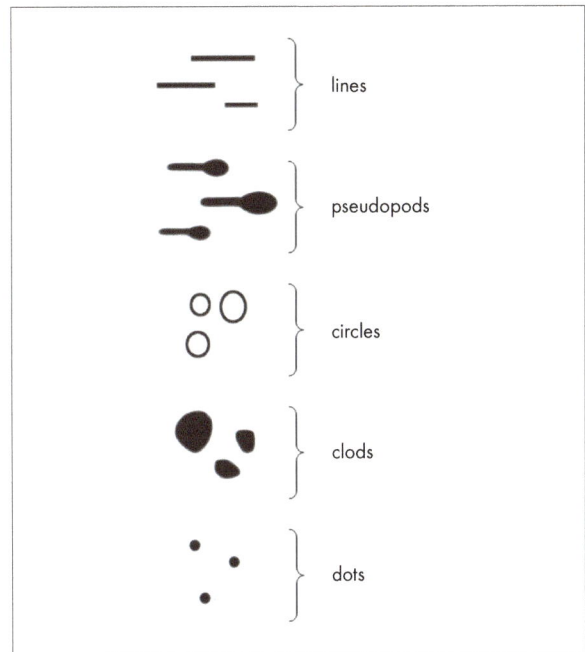

Figure 3.1: *Five basic elements.*
All patterns observed in dermatoscopy are composed of five simple geometric elements. These basic elements are lines, pseudopods, circles, clods, and dots. They are defined as follows: (1) Line – a two-dimensional continuous object with length greatly exceeding width, extending in one direction; (2) Pseudopod – a line with a bulbous end; (3) Circle – a curved line sensibly equidistant from a central point; (4) Clod – any well-circumscribed, solid object larger than a dot. Clods may take any shape; (5) Dot – an object too small to have a discernable shape (dots are not larger than the diameter of a terminal hair).

3.2.1 Pattern of lines

A pattern of lines consists of lines of one or more of the six types defined below, and is characterized by their arrangement and sometimes also by their shape (3.2).

Reticular lines

The lines are straight and arranged in such a manner that they intersect each other nearly at right angles in regular intervals to form a net-like structure. Reticular lines may be thin or thick. Thin reticular lines are narrower than the spaces they enclose, whereas thick lines are of the same width or wider than the enclosed spaces (3.3).

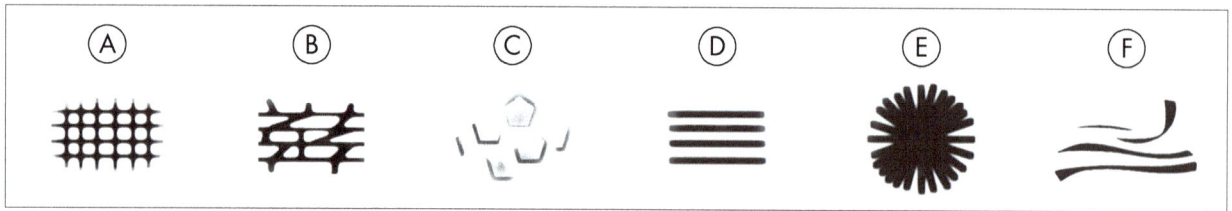

Figure 3.2: *Six possible patterns of lines.*
A, reticular; **B**, branched; **C**, angulated; **D**, parallel; **E**, radial; **F**, curved. *The pattern of radial lines always occurs in conjunction with another pattern. All other patterns of lines may occur alone.*

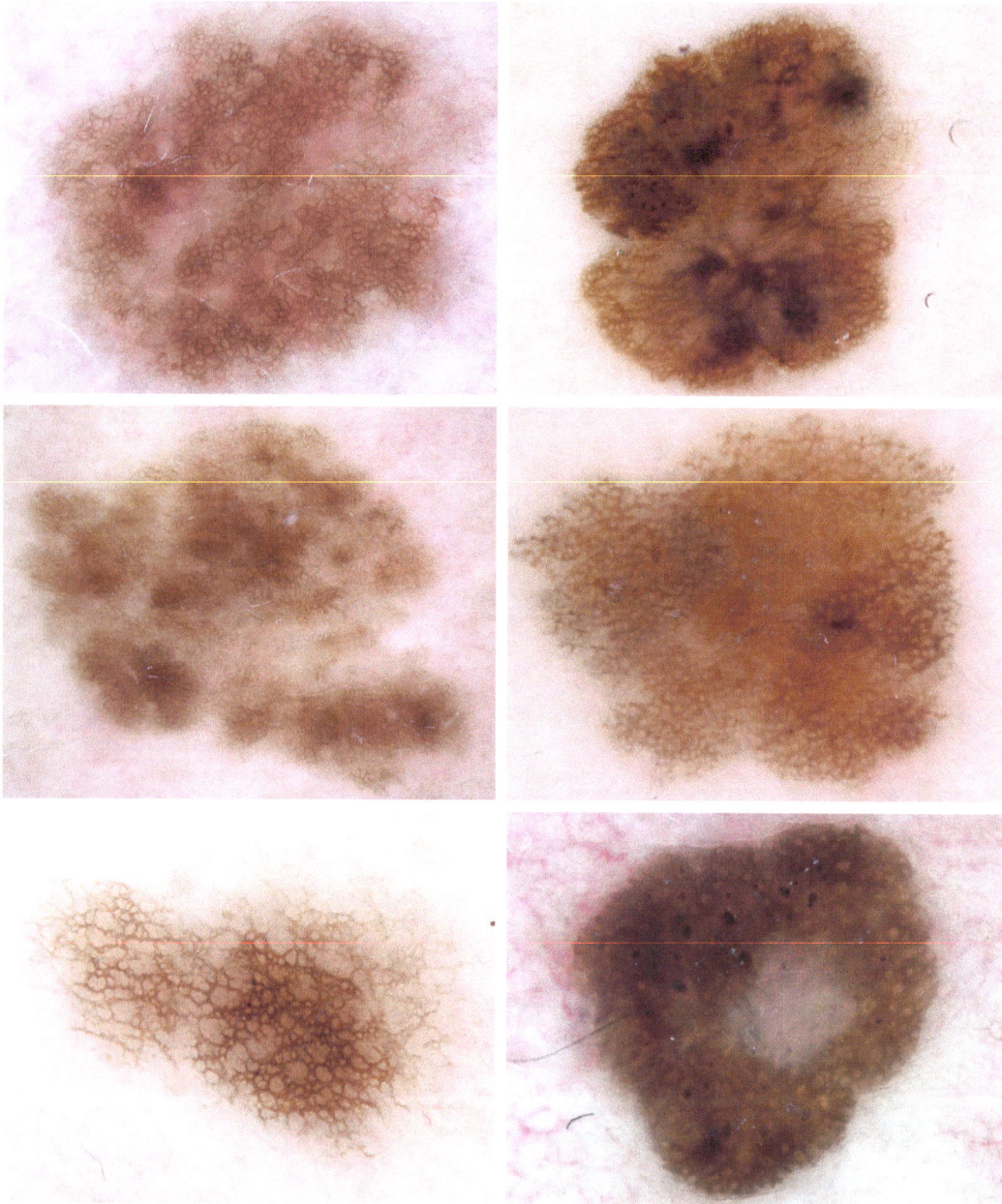

Figure 3.3: *Thin and thick reticular lines*
Left column: *thin reticular lines.* **Right column:** *thick reticular lines. Thin lines are narrower than the intervening hypopigmented spaces they enclose, whereas thick lines are at least equally wide. As is true for dermatoscopy in general, it is important to keep the overall picture (the pattern) in mind, rather than to assess the width of individual lines.*

Branched lines

The lines are straight and arranged such that they intersect each other, but not at regular intervals and not at right angles *(3.4).* One frequently finds thin and thick lines simultaneously. Several thin lines may originate from a thick line. The distinction between reticular and branched lines is not sharp; however distinguishing between these two patterns of lines is rarely of major importance for the diagnosis, as we will see later.

Angulated lines

The lines are straight, do not intersect, and meet at angles larger than 90° in such a way that they form complete or incomplete polygonal shapes *(3.5).*

Parallel lines

The lines are straight and arranged in parallel fashion, i.e. they do not intersect. Parallel lines are mainly found on acral skin, but also on the nails. On acral skin, parallel lines may be arranged on ridges, in furrows, or crossing the ridges and furrows *(3.6).* Parallel lines may, of course, be thick or thin.

Radial lines

Lines form the radial pattern when they converge at a single dot or clod, or if they would converge at a common point if extended (for example at the center of the lesion). Radial lines at a lesion's periphery may occupy the entire circumference, or be confined to one segment *(3.7).* The pattern of radial lines is always found in combination with another pattern.

Curved lines

The lines are not straight but curved, have few intersections, and may be parallel or distributed randomly. Parallel curved lines usually occur in pairs. Curved lines may be short or long, and thin or thick *(3.8).*
The patterns of the other basic elements and the structureless pattern are shown schematically in *figure 3.9.*

3.2.2 Pattern of pseudopods

This pattern consists of a collection of pseudopods at the periphery of the lesion or at the periphery of a well-defined structure within a lesion. Pseudopods may involve the entire periphery of the lesion, or be found in just a few segments. The pattern of pseudopods always occurs in combination with another pattern *(3.10).*

3.2.3 Pattern of circles

A collection of circles is termed a pattern of circles *(3.11).* Patterns of circles may, in principle, be found anywhere. However, they occur most commonly in pigmented lesions on the face. Circles may be densely arranged or sparse. When circles are so densely arranged or so wide that they coalesce with each other, the pattern of circles appears similar to the reticular pattern.

3.2.4 Pattern of clods

A pattern of clods is a collection of clods that, in contrast to dots, may have different sizes and may have different shapes i.e. an aggregation of clods of different size and shape still forms a pattern of clods. As in a pattern of dots, the individual clods in a pattern of clods may be densely arranged or sparse *(3.12).*

3.2.5 Pattern of dots

A pattern of dots is an accumulation of dots. It may be difficult to decide whether a single element is a dot or a clod. However, that is not the point; at this early stage of lesion analysis we only need distinguish between a pattern of dots and a pattern of clods. At the magnification of the handheld instrument dots are too small to have a discernable shape or to show sensible variation in size. In comparative terms, they are not larger than the diameter of a terminal hair. In contrast, on comparing individual clods within a collection of clods, one finds a range of different shapes and sizes. This distinction is usually quite obvious. A pattern of dots may be densely arranged or sparse *(3.13).*

3.2.6 Structureless pattern

The structureless pattern is a coherent area lacking basic elements, or where no basic element predominates *(3.14, 3.15, 3.16).* The requirement of a coherent area is critical.
For pigmented structures such as lines, pseudopods, circles, clods or dots to be clearly defined, they must be seen against some kind of background. Bearing in mind the general principle that structures are defined by pigment, this structureless background, by itself, should not be interpreted as constituting a structureless pattern. A structureless area need not be homogeneous or even completely without basic elements; one usually finds a certain degree of "noise". However – and this is the essential aspect – there are too few of any one basic element present to form a pattern of that element. Again following the general principle that structures are defined by pigment, the hypopigmented zones of the follicular openings are not part of a pattern; they disrupt the pattern. On the face for example, where the follicular openings are prominent, structureless pigmented zones are commonly interspersed with multiple hypopigmented "holes" (the follicular openings). This pattern should not be confused with thick reticular lines *(3.15).*

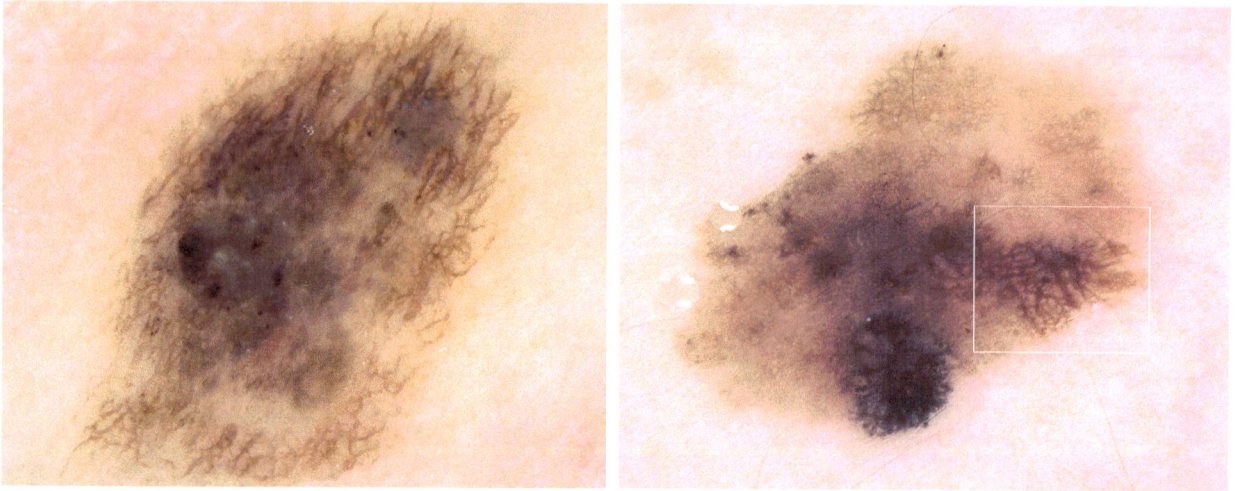

Figure 3.4: Branched lines.
Branched lines also intersect each other, but in contrast to reticular lines they do not always intersect at right angles. Typically one finds several thin lines originating from a thick one (right figure, white rectangle).

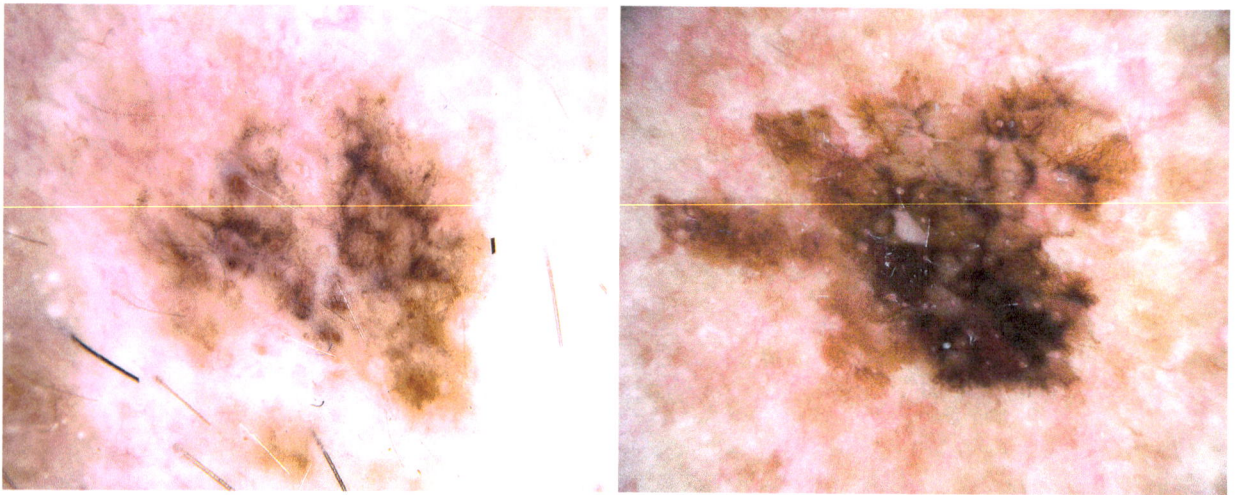

Figure 3.5: Angulated lines.
Left: Angulated lines (polygons) on facial skin. The angulated lines are surrounding the follicular openings. **Right:** The polygonal geometric shapes formed by angulated lines (polygons) of non-facial lesions are larger than the holes caused by individual follicular openings.

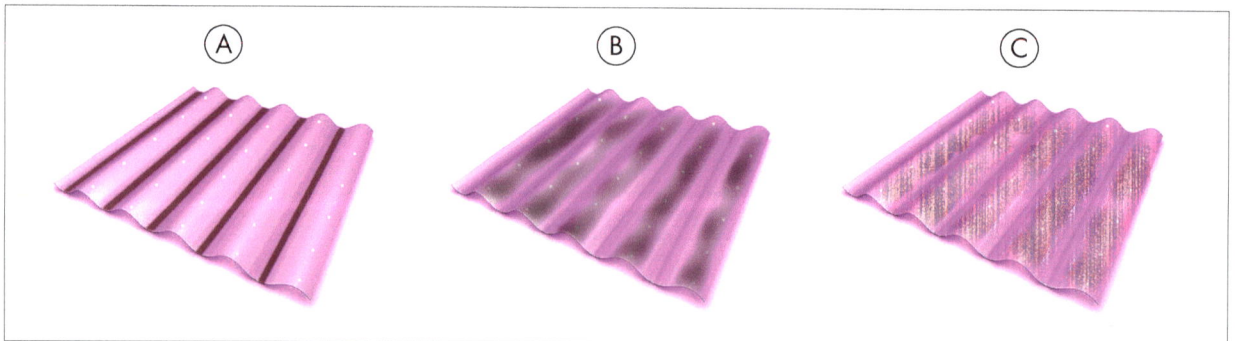

Figure 3.6: Schematic diagram of various types of parallel lines on acral skin. **A,** parallel lines in furrows; **B,** parallel lines on ridges, and **C,** parallel lines that cross ridges.

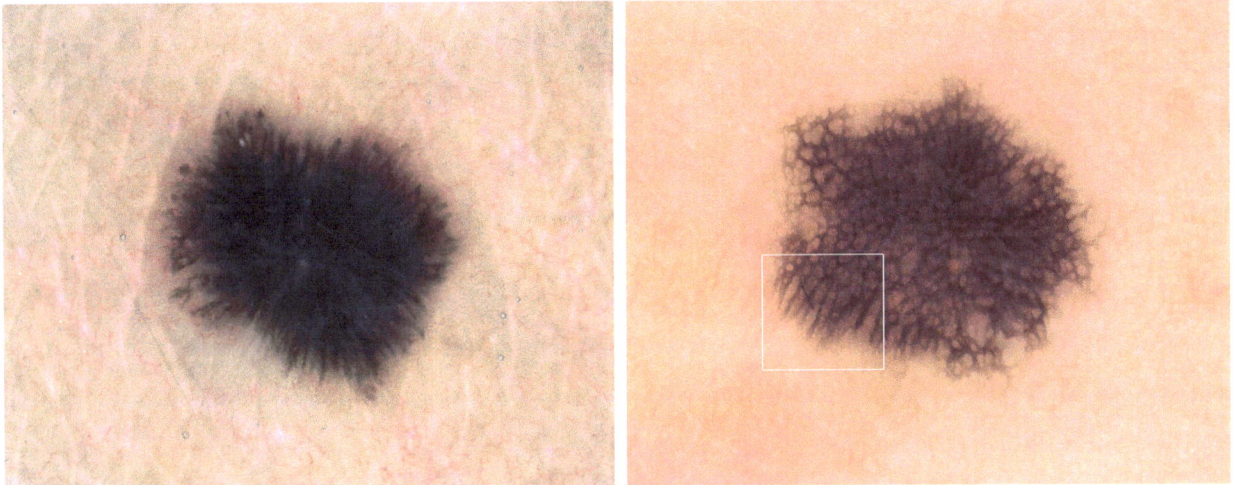

Figure 3.7: *Radial lines.*
Radial lines occur only in combination with other patterns. The left figure shows radial lines regularly distributed over the entire lesion. The center of the lesion is structureless. The lesion on the right has radial lines only in one segment (white rectangle). Radial lines are combined here with reticular ones.

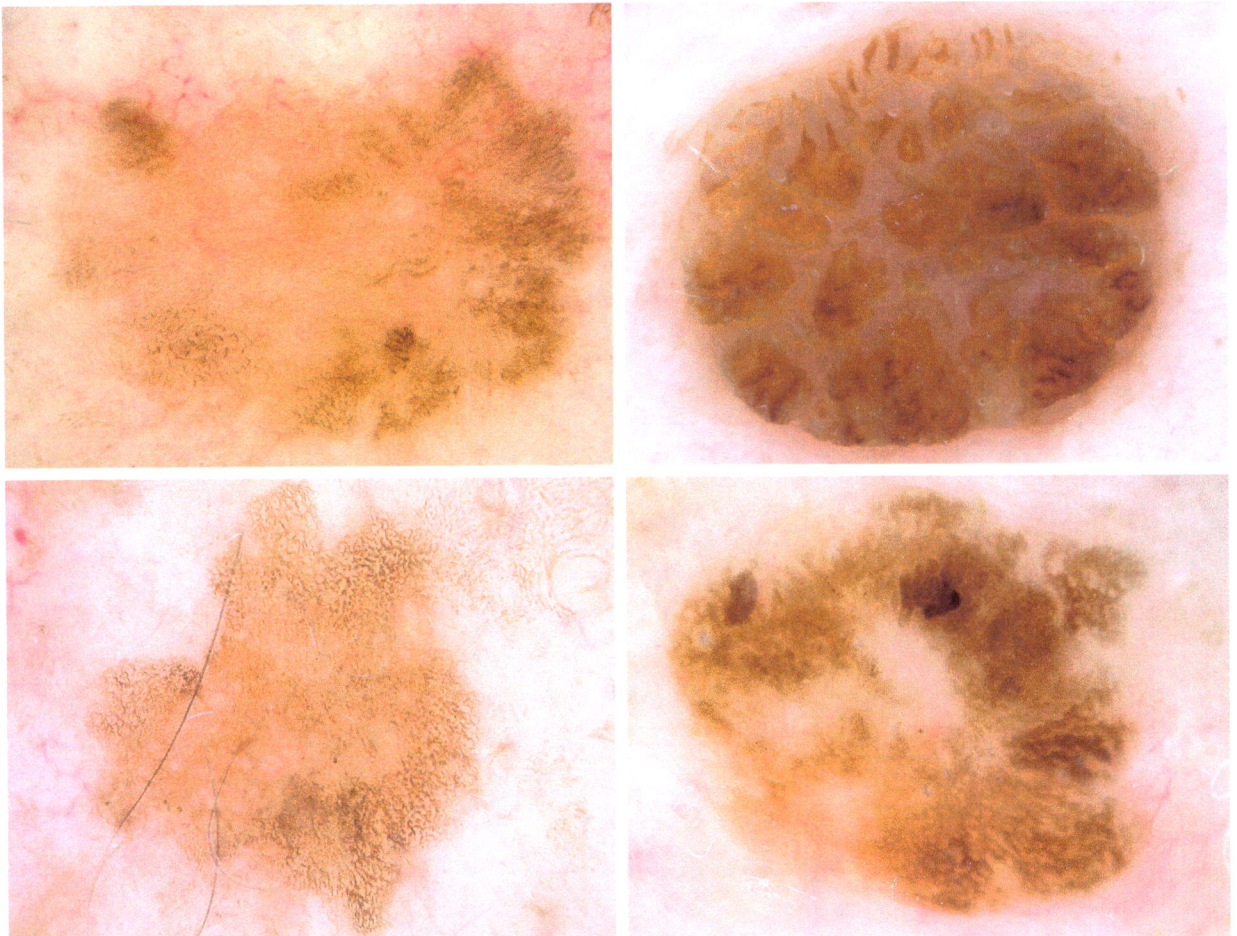

Figure 3.8: *Curved lines.*
Left column: *Thin curved lines.* **Right column:** *Thick curved lines.*

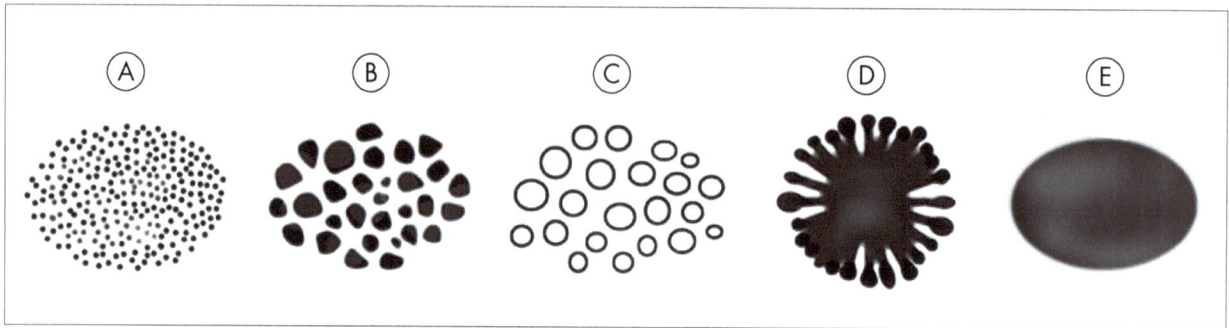

Figure 3.9: The remaining basic patterns.
*In addition to lines, aggregations of any of the other basic elements also constitute a pattern. **A,** Pattern of dots; **B,** Pattern of clods; **C,** Pattern of circles; **D,** Pattern of pseudopods. Like the radial pattern of lines, the pattern of pseudopods always occurs in combination with another pattern (e.g., structureless at the center). When an area has no basic elements, or has too few basic elements to constitute a pattern, the pattern in this area is termed structureless **(E).** Structureless does not mean featureless, only the absence of a predominant basic element.*

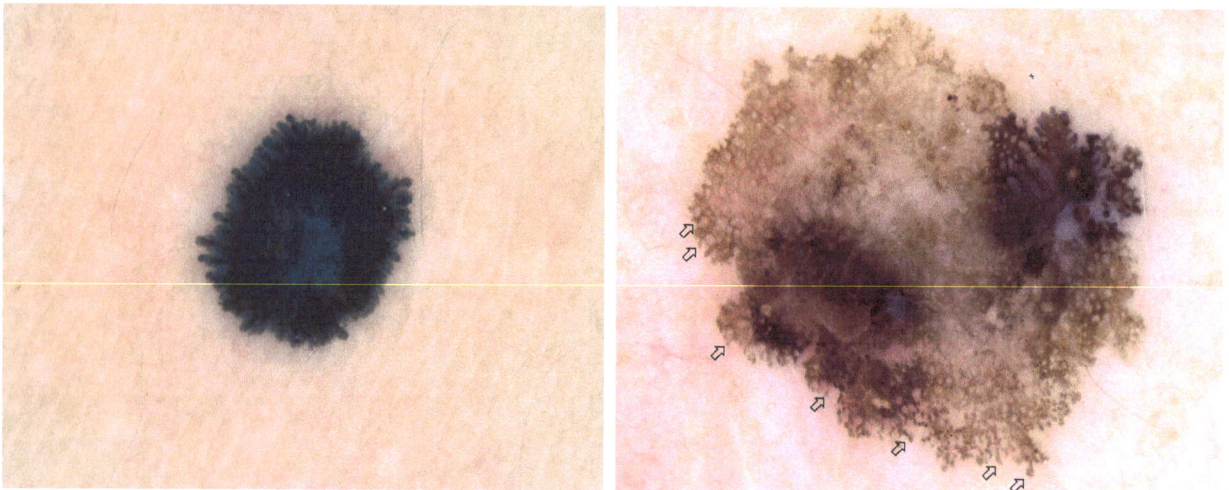

Figure 3.10: Pattern of pseudopods.
*Pseudopods are only seen at the periphery of a lesion and always occur in combination with another pattern. **Left:** Pseudopods are regularly distributed over the entire periphery of the lesion. In the center one finds a structureless pattern. **Right:** Pseudopods are located in some portions of the periphery. The rest of the lesion consists of thick reticular lines and white structureless zones.*

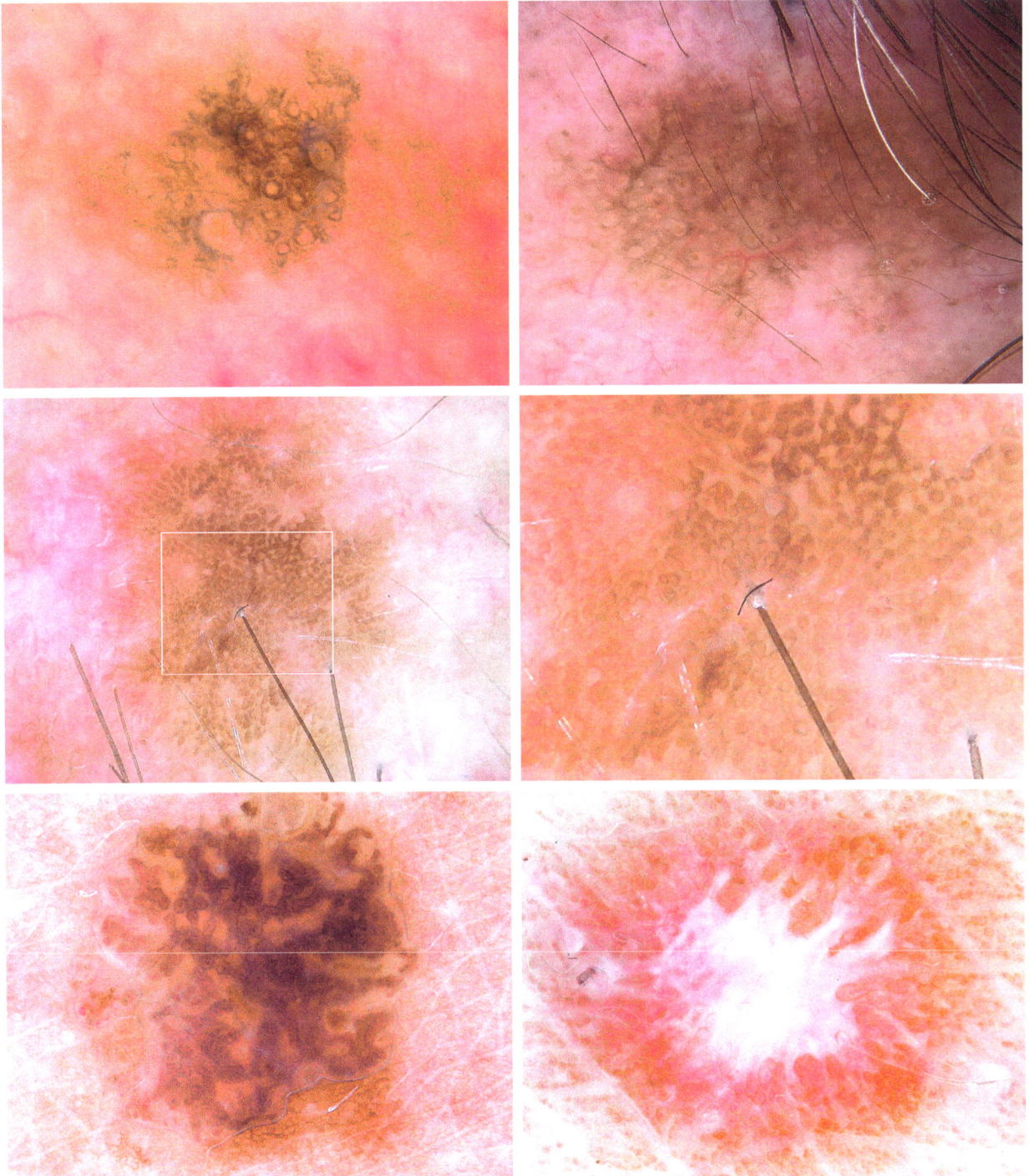

Figure 3.11: Pattern of circles.
Due to the large number of follicular openings and the absence of rete ridges, patterns of circles are usually seen on the face. However, pigmented circles may occur at any site of the body. **Top row:** *Two examples of patterns of circles on the face.* **Middle row:** *A pattern of circles in a non-facial lesion. In the overview on the left side the pattern of circles may be easily confused with a pattern of clods. The higher magnification of the center of the lesion on the right demonstrates that the pattern is composed of small circles.* **Bottom left:** *A pattern of small circles (with some curved lines) on non-facial skin.* **Bottom right:** *A pattern of large brown circles at the periphery of a lesion with a structureless white center.*

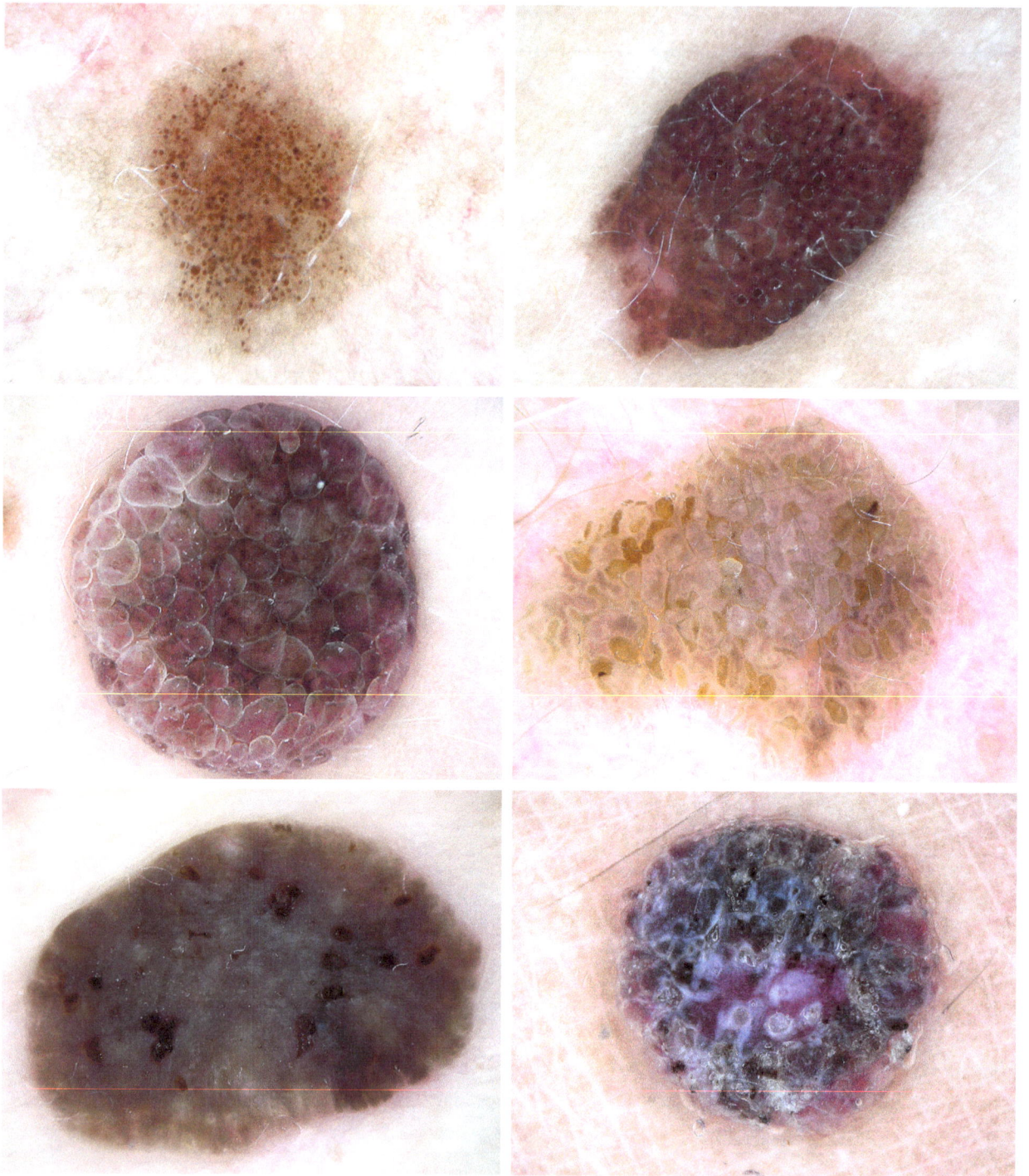

Figure 3.12: Pattern of clods.
Six examples of patterns of clods: Clods may be small or large; round, oval or polygonal; dense or sparse; brown, red, black, gray, blue, skin-colored or orange. **Top left:** small, brown clods, dense. **Top right:** large, brown clods, dense. **Middle left:** large, polygonal skin-colored and brown clods, dense. **Middle right:** orange and skin colored clods, dense. **Bottom left:** black clods, sparse. **Bottom right:** gray, red, blue, black clods; dense.

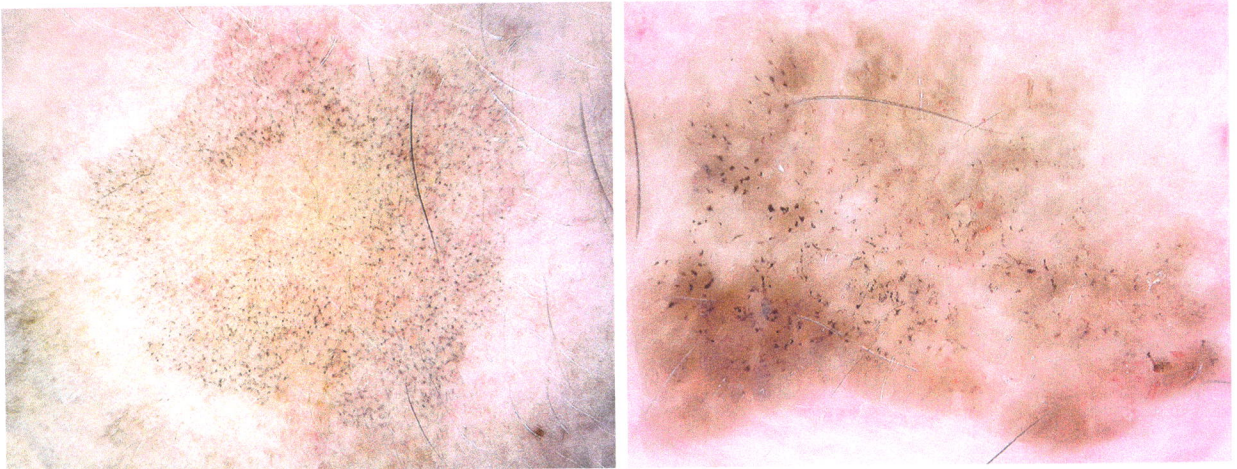

Figure 3.13: *Pattern of dots.*
Left: *Densely arranged gray dots.* **Right:** *Sparse accumulation of brown and gray dots distributed on a structureless tan background.*

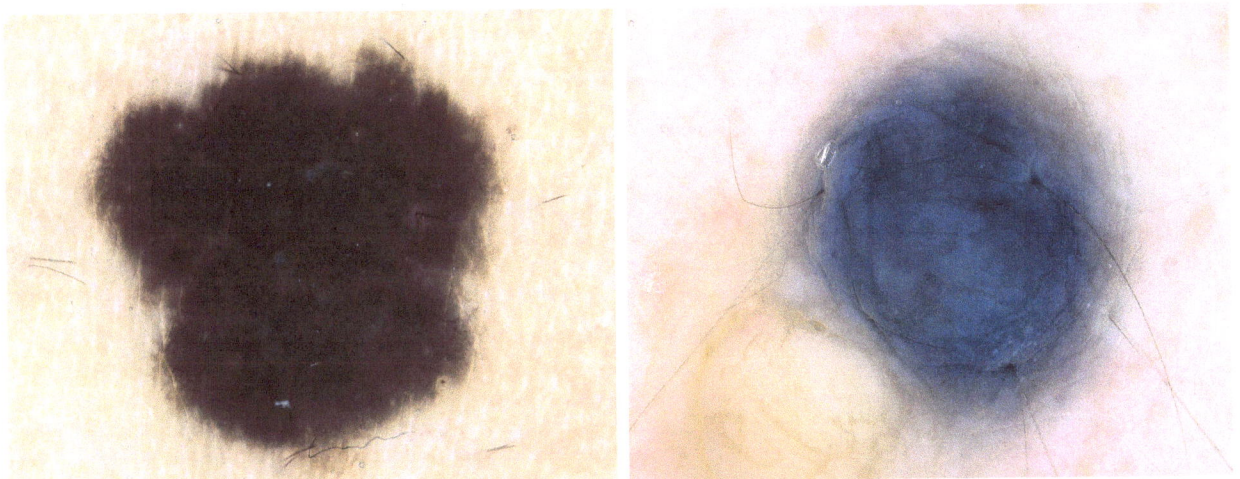

Figure 3.14: *Structureless pattern.*
Left: *Structureless dark brown (a few black dots in the center do not constitute a pattern).* **Right:** *Structureless blue.*

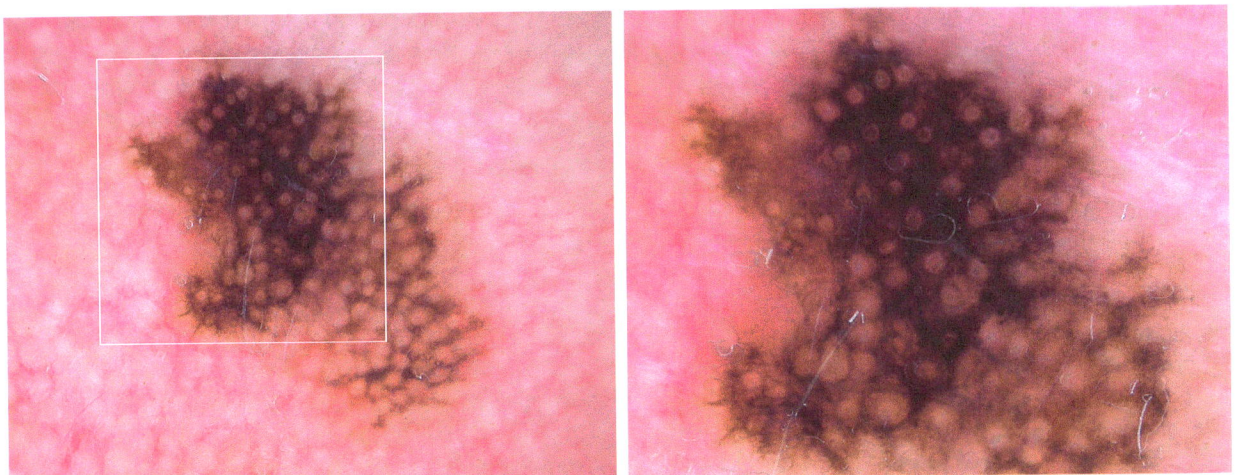

Figure 3.15: *Structureless pattern on the face.*
On the face, structureless pigmented zones are interspersed with multiple hypopigmented "holes" (follicular openings). This pattern should not be interpreted as thick reticular lines. The hypopigmented follicular openings are not part of the pattern; rather, they interrupt the pattern which is structureless.

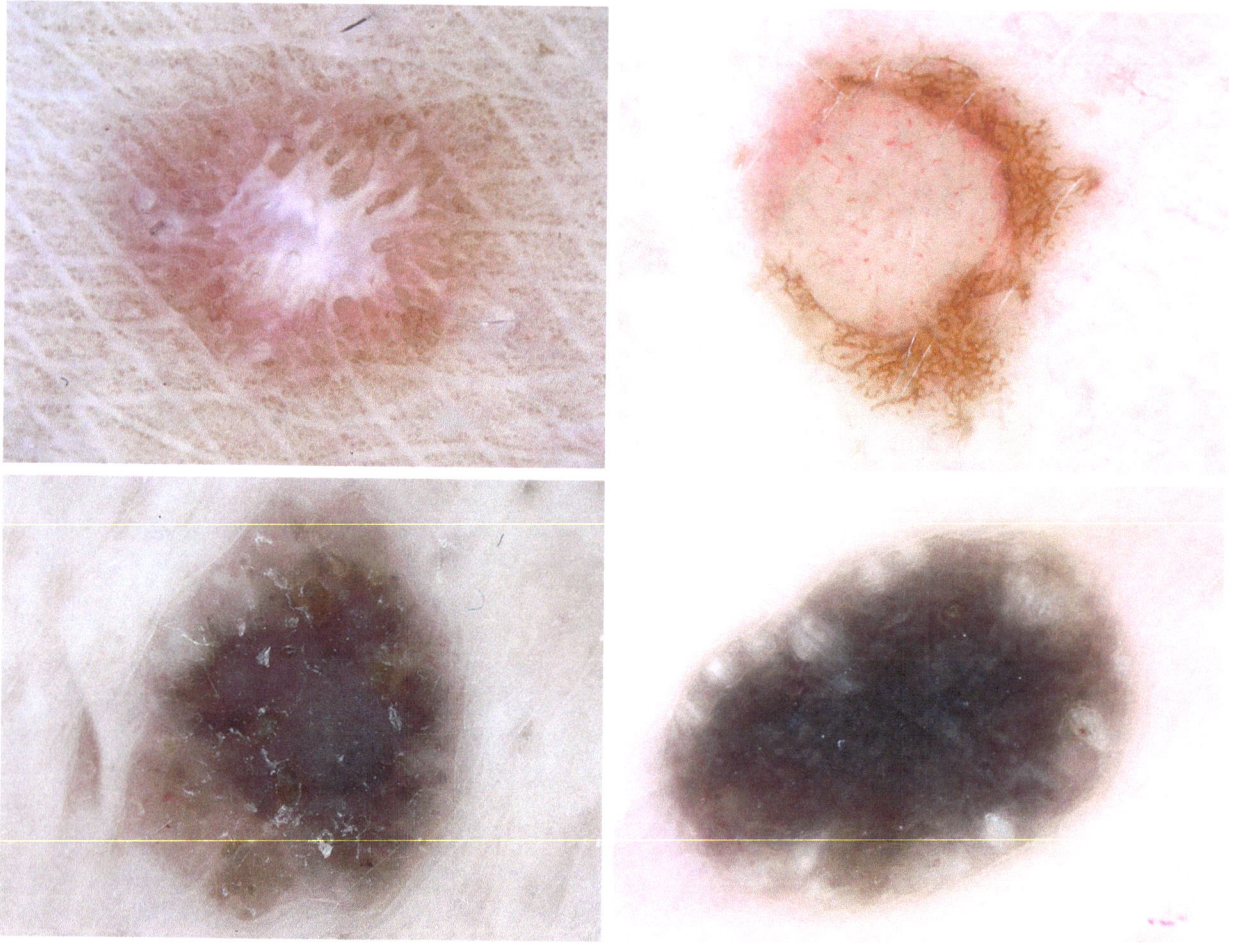

Figure 3.16: *Structureless in combination with other patterns.*
Top left: *Structureless white (defined as lighter than normal surrounding skin) centrally, circles at the periphery.* **Top right:** *Structureless skin-colored centrally, branched and reticular lines at the periphery (the vessels in the center should not be interpreted as structure).* **Bottom left:** *Structureless blue, brown and orange clods.* **Bottom right:** *Structureless blue and gray centrally, white clods peripherally.*

3.2.7 Combinations of patterns

A pigmented lesion may be composed of one or more patterns. In the latter case the combination of patterns may be symmetrical or asymmetrical. Symmetry exists when the lesion's pattern can be mirrored in any conceivable axis. Asymmetry exists when this is not the case. Symmetry is independent of the shape of the lesion; it is assessed on pattern. When assessing symmetry or asymmetry, one must remember that Nature does not make its designs on a drawing board; symmetry is only approximate and not exact.

When a lesion consists of two patterns there are three possible symmetrical combinations: a) one pattern at the center and the other at the periphery, or b) vice versa, or c) the elements of one pattern (usually dots or clods) are regularly distributed within the other pattern *(3.17).* All other combinations are, by definition, asymmetrical.

The number of possible asymmetrical combinations of patterns is, of course, infinite.

A pigmented lesion with three patterns is only symmetrical when the patterns are arranged concentrically. The more numerous the patterns, the greater is the likelihood of their being asymmetrical.

3.3 Colors
3.3.1 Melanin

A pigmented lesion is characterized not only by its pattern but also by its color *(3.18).* Melanin is the most important pigment. Depending on the layer of skin in which melanin is located, it may appear black (when located in the stratum corneum), brown (when located in the basal layers of the epidermis), gray (when located in the papillary dermis) or blue (when located in the reticular dermis).

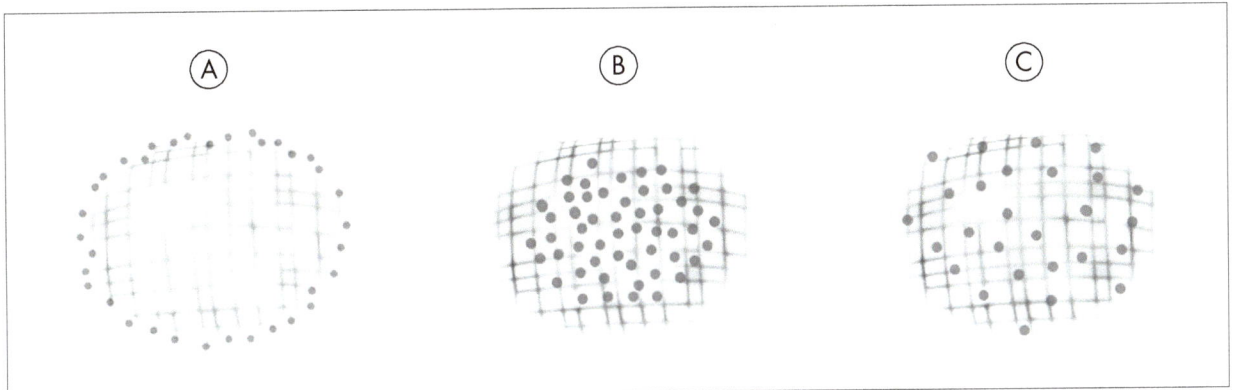

Figure 3.17: Combinations of patterns.
*While any pattern may be combined with another, in dermatoscopy there are only three ways in which two patterns may be arranged symmetrically. These illustrations use reticular lines and dots as an example. **A,** Dots peripherally, reticular lines centrally; **B,** Dots centrally and reticular lines peripherally; **C,** Regularly distributed dots on reticular lines. These three cases ensure symmetry in all axes. By definition, all other combinations in dermatoscopy are asymmetrical.*

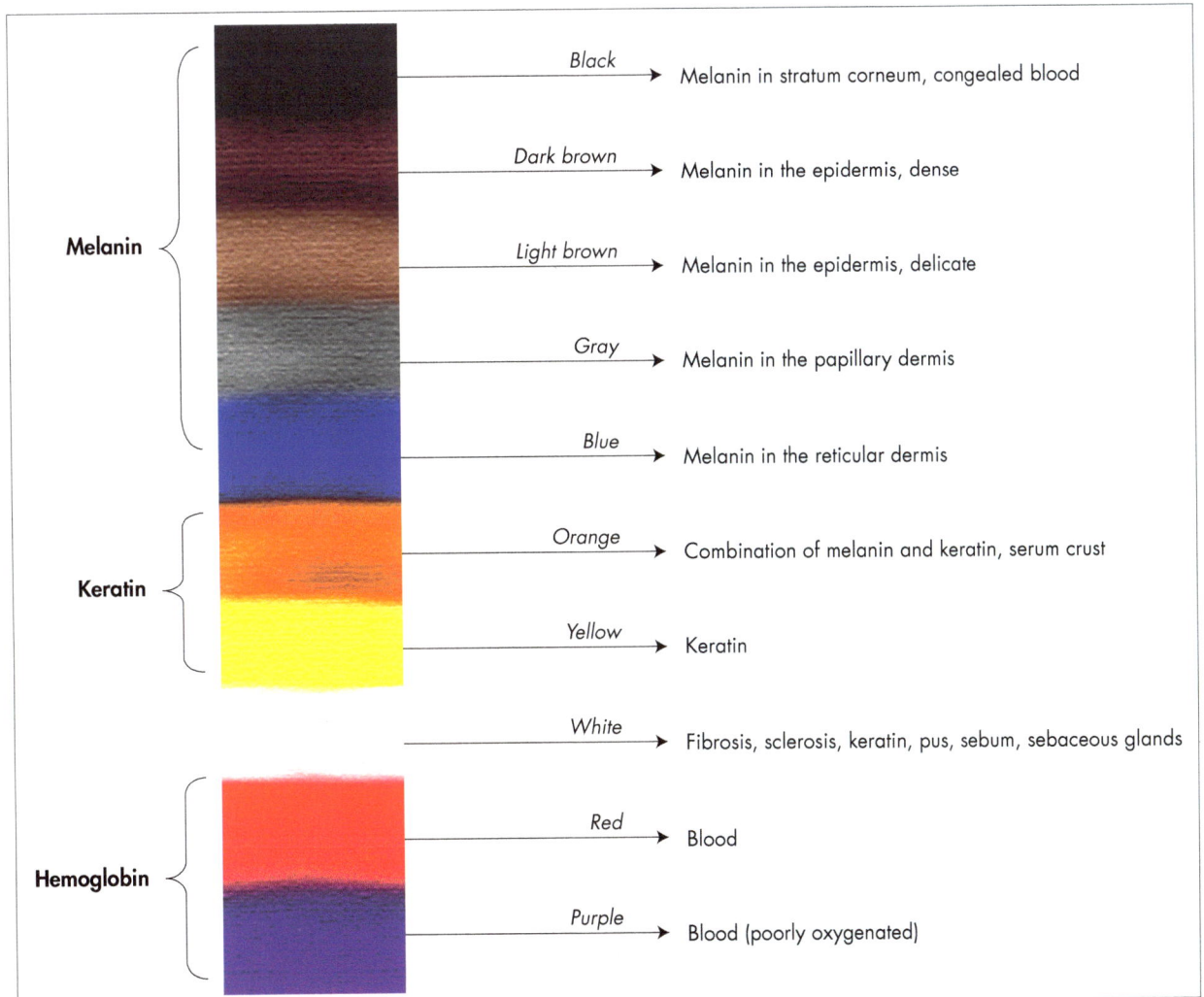

Melanin	*Black* →	Melanin in stratum corneum, congealed blood
	Dark brown →	Melanin in the epidermis, dense
	Light brown →	Melanin in the epidermis, delicate
	Gray →	Melanin in the papillary dermis
	Blue →	Melanin in the reticular dermis
Keratin	*Orange* →	Combination of melanin and keratin, serum crust
	Yellow →	Keratin
	White →	Fibrosis, sclerosis, keratin, pus, sebum, sebaceous glands
Hemoglobin	*Red* →	Blood
	Purple →	Blood (poorly oxygenated)

Figure 3.18: Colors in dermatoscopy

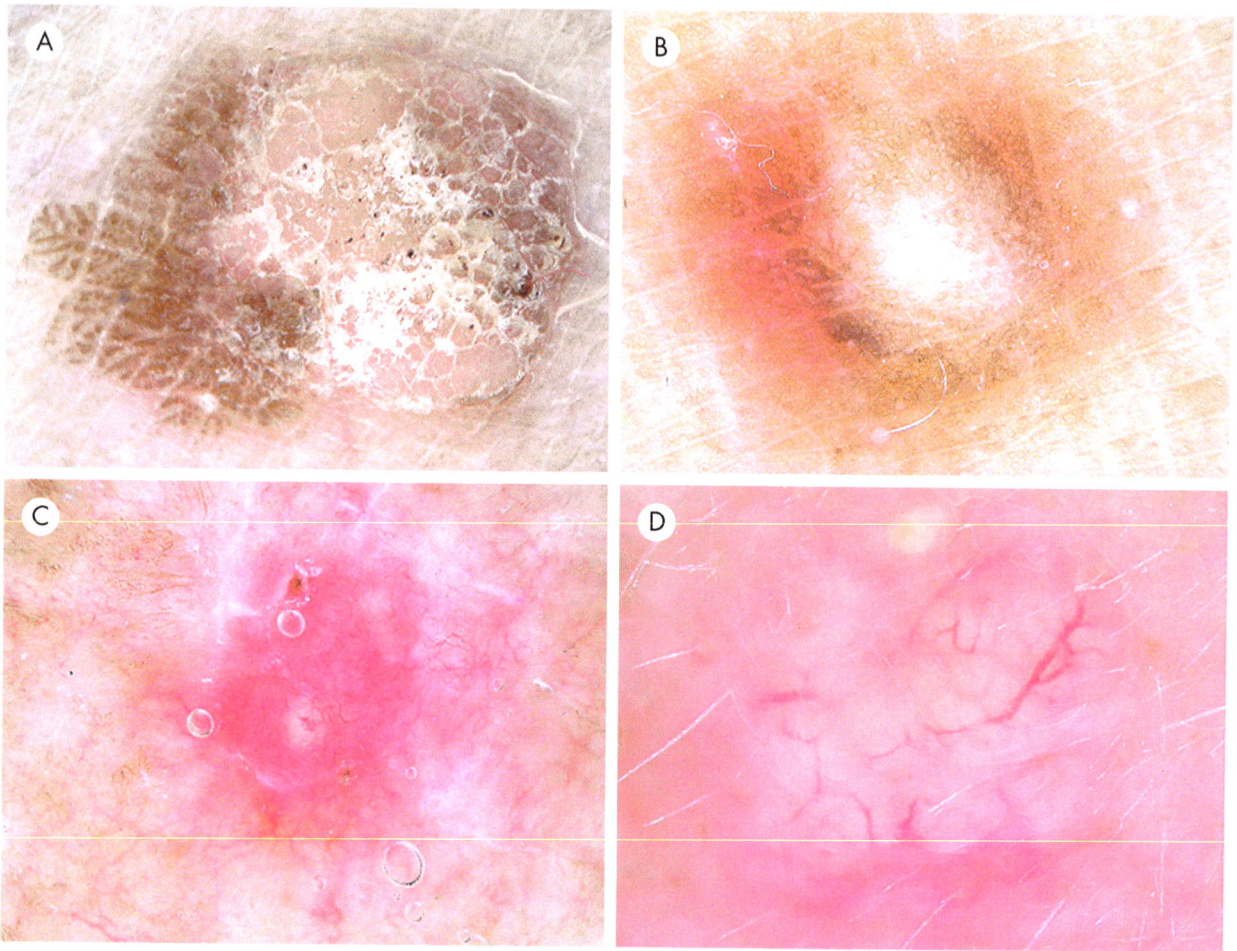

Figure 3.19: The "color" white in dermatoscopy.
*In dermatoscopy, white is defined as lighter than normal surrounding skin. **Top left:** In this seborrheic keratosis white corresponds to keratin (scale). **Top right:** White structureless center of a dermatofibroma corresponding to fibrosis and sclerosis of the dermis. **Bottom left:** White corresponding to pus in folliculitis. **Bottom right:** White corresponding to sebum and sebaceous glands in sebaceous gland hyperplasia. Note that the white of keratin and fibrosis is shiny whereas the white of pus and sebaceous glands is dull to pale yellow.*

Furthermore, the observed color depends on the density of melanin and the thickness of the epidermis. A dense accumulation of melanin in the basal layer of the epidermis may appear dark-brown or nearly black, a less dense accumulation would be light-brown. When the epidermis is thickened due to acanthosis (e.g. some seborrheic keratoses) melanin in the epidermis may appear blue.

It is often useful to divide pigmented lesions into those where melanin is the dominant pigment, and those where other pigments dominate.

3.3.2 Other pigments

Hemoglobin is the next most important pigment. Depending on the level of oxygen saturation, hemoglobin in vessels ranges from bright red to blue. When a massive extravasation of red blood cells occurs (i.e. hemorrhage), the entire coagulated blood is dark red, or may be black when it is in the stratum corneum (corneal bleeding). In the dermis, fresh blood may again be red to blue, but degradation of hemoglobin may give rise to various shades of color ranging from green to brown. In cases of ulcerated lesions, serum exudes from the surface, dries, and forms a crust. The serum is often mixed with red blood cells and is therefore orange. Keratin is white or yellow (when the stratum corneum is not pigmented it appears yellow). Mixture of the white or yellow of keratin with the brown of melanin gives rise to colors in the range orange to yellow which are characteristic of pigmented seborrheic keratoses. Fibrosis or sclerosis of the dermis also appears white. Pus, sebum and sebaceous glands also appear white

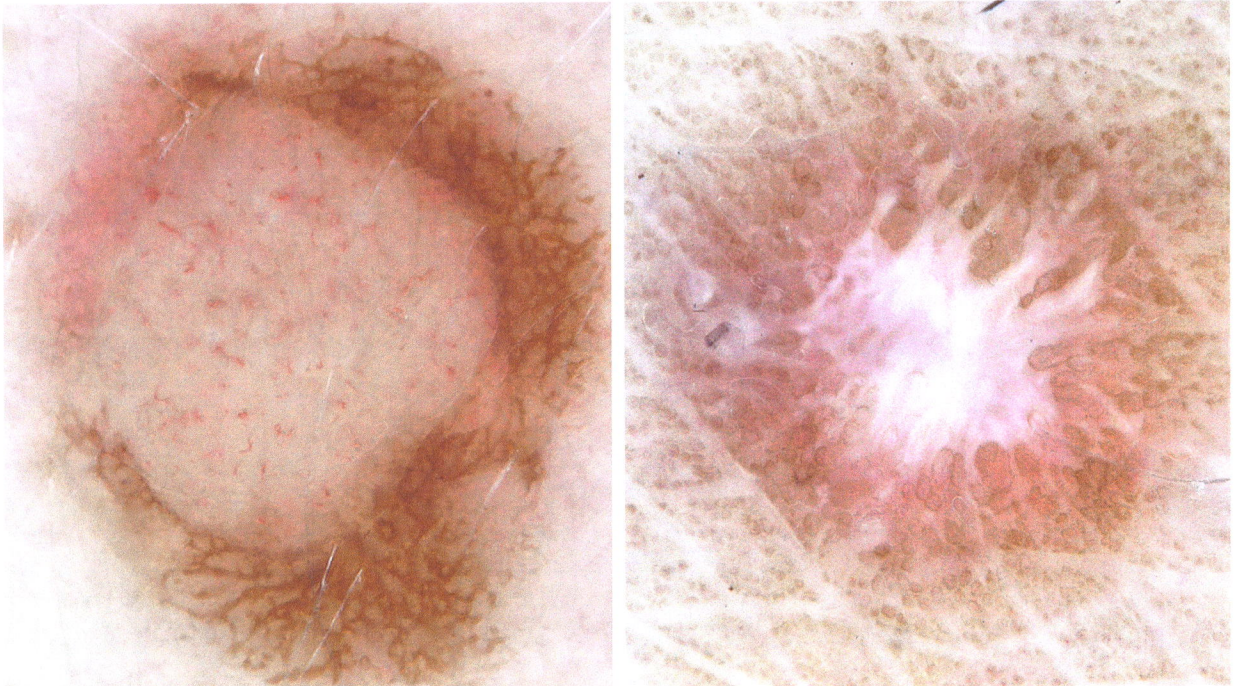

Figure 3.20: Skin color and the "color" white in dermatoscopy.
"White" is defined as lighter than the surrounding normal skin. The difference between skin color and white does affect diagnosis, despite similar patterns. **Left:** A "superficial and deep" congenital nevus with a skin-colored center. **Right:** A dermatofibroma with a white center.

in dermatoscopy. In contrast to keratin and fibrosis, which are shiny white, pus, sebum and sebaceous glands appear dull white *(3.19)*.

3.3.3 Color combinations

A pigmented lesion may be composed of one or several colors. As is true for patterns, colors may be arranged symmetrically or asymmetrically. With the exception of brown, variations in shade should not be interpreted as a separate color. It is diagnostically meaningful to distinguish between light-brown and dark-brown, but only in clear-cut cases and particularly when the transition between the two shades of brown is abrupt. It is very common to see lighter pigmentation at the periphery of a lesion, or around follicular openings; such lesions should still be classified as one color. The number of colors and the presence of specific colors are of immense importance in dermatoscopy. When evaluating colors (as patterns), the investigator should know when the observation should be very accurate and when it may be less exact. The color of normal skin varies from person to person, and even according to location on the body. While this normal skin color is not counted as a separate color, it is used as a reference to define "white"; white structures must be clearly lighter in color than surrounding normal skin *(3.20)*.

Distribution of color in lesions with a purely reticular pattern

It is usually sufficient to distinguish between symmetrical and asymmetrical arrangements of more than one color. Pigmented lesions that consist exclusively of a reticular pattern are, however, a special case, as three further specific arrangements are diagnostically significant. When a darker shade is seen in the center and a lighter one at the periphery, so that symmetry is retained, the lesion is considered to be centrally hyperpigmented. If the darker shade is seen at the periphery the lesion is called eccentrically hyperpigmented. If the colors within the lesions are distributed in such a way that areas of dark pigmentation alternate with areas of light pigmentation, the lesion is termed speckled or variegated *(3.21)*.

This can involve two shades of the single color brown (a single color because the transition is gradual), or two shades of brown plus black.

3.4 Descriptions of pigmented lesions on the basis of patterns and colors

Formulating a description of pattern(s) and color(s) is always the first step towards diagnosis. One first looks at the lesion from a distance. A pattern should

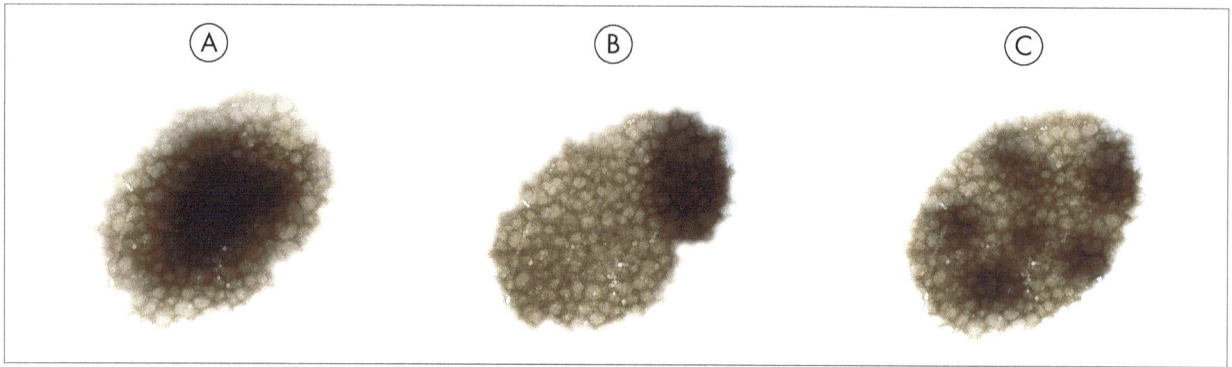

Figure 3.21: Possible distribution of color in lesions that consist exclusively of reticular lines. Centrally hyperpigmented (A), eccentrically hyperpigmented (B), speckled or variegated (C).

occupy a significant portion of the pigmented lesion; everything else may be initially ignored. Beginners tend to become immediately absorbed in details. However, at least at the initial step, single dots or single clods are of no importance. If necessary, these details can be incorporated later in the analysis.

Examples of pigmented lesions with a single pattern
Figures 3.22 and 3.23 show pigmented lesions with just one pattern.[1] Usually it is simple to decide which pattern is present. Occasionally it may be difficult to distinguish between reticular lines and branched lines, in which case one should prefer the more common reticular pattern.

In almost all cases, it is pigment that defines structure. A few examples will show how potential confusion can be avoided by keeping this principle in mind. The less pigmented areas between reticular lines are not a separate pattern, i.e. they are not clods. Hypopigmented areas between dots, clods, circles and all other lines should not be viewed as structureless areas. A circle of hypopigmentation around a hair follicle is not a structure, only an interruption to the pattern of the lesion. The few exceptions to pigment defining structure – mainly white structures – will be addressed in detail later.

For a zone to constitute the structureless pattern it must – as for patterns composed of basic elements – occupy a significant portion of the lesion. On the other hand, a sufficiently large zone does not have to be entirely devoid of pigmented structures to be considered structureless. Areas with visible structures which cannot be definitively classified as one of the basic elements are still correctly termed structureless, as are areas which

contain basic elements, but too few to constitute a pattern. In other words, not all pigment is structure, some is noise.

Examples of pigmented lesions with more than one pattern
Figure 3.24 shows pigmented lesions with more than one pattern. When assessing a lesion consisting of more than one pattern, the first question one should ask is whether the patterns are combined symmetrically or asymmetrically. When assessing symmetry one should exercise latitude, as symmetry in biology never reaches geometrical perfection. A beginner tends to over-interpret in favor of asymmetry. The examples in figure 3.24 will help the reader to develop a feeling for biological symmetry and asymmetry. The vast majority of lesions can be unequivocally classified as either symmetrical or asymmetrical. When (very rarely!) this cannot be done with certainty, one "investigates" in both directions, as we will see later.

3.5 Clues

Sometimes pigmented lesions can be unequivocally diagnosed on the basis of pattern(s) and color(s) alone. More often, assessment of pattern and color leads to a small differential diagnosis. In this case, one looks for clues. A clue is simply a feature which favors one possible diagnosis over another possible diagnosis. Sometimes a pattern may also constitute a clue, for example a structureless eccentric zone is both a pattern, and (in some contexts) a clue to the diagnosis of melanoma. Usually however, clues are features too localized to constitute a pattern, but nonetheless favoring one diagnosis over another. Clues include a special arrangement of basic elements, a typical color, a special combination of pattern and color, a characteristic pattern

---

1 As this chapter is mainly focused on a description of patterns and colors rather than diagnosis, only the dermatoscopic images are shown here. Clinical and dermatoscopic appearances are shown simultaneously in most of the remaining chapters.

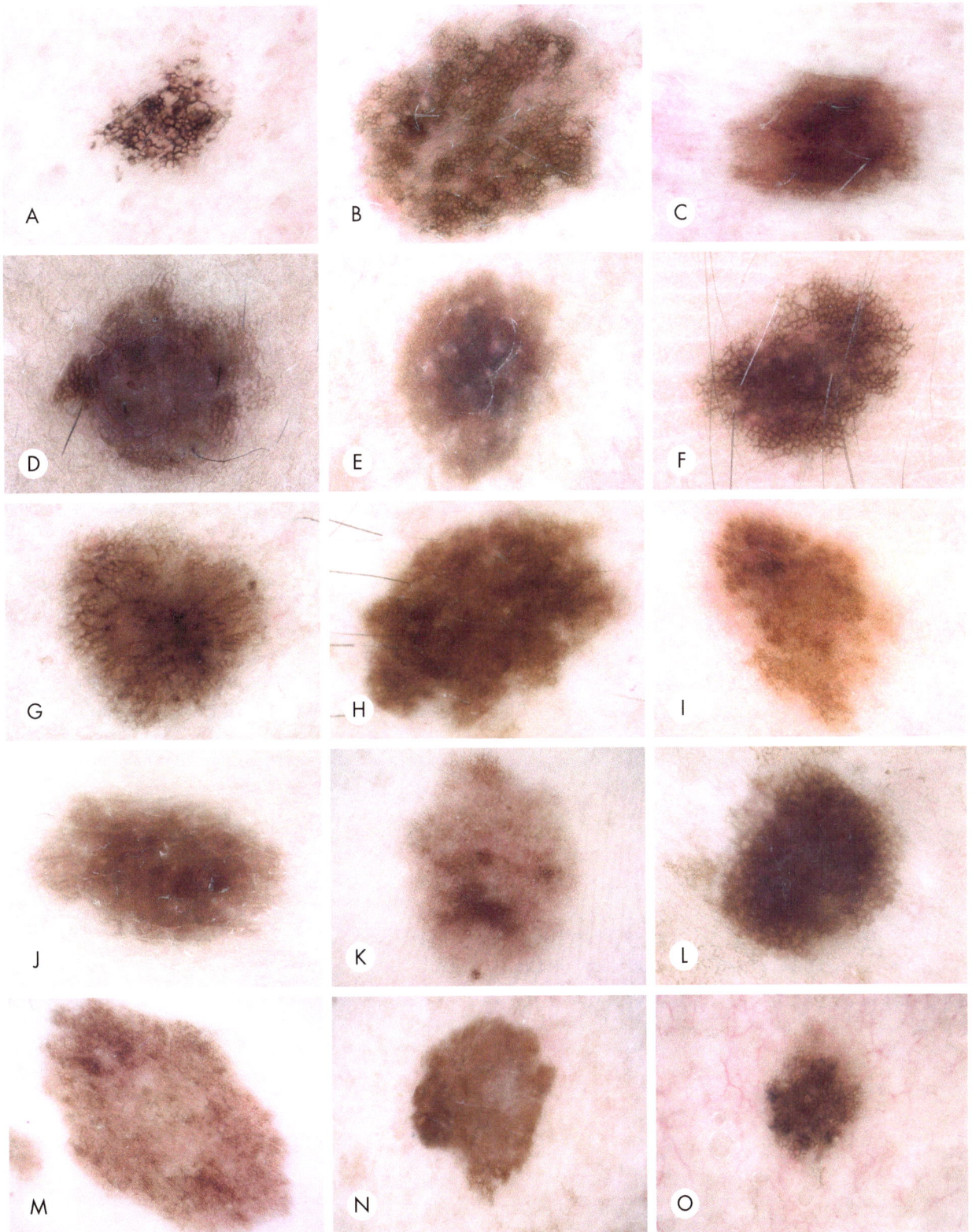

Figure 3.22: Pattern analysis (one pattern).
A: *reticular, dark-brown or black,* **B:** *reticular, light-brown,* **C:** *reticular, centrally hyperpigmented,* **D:** *reticular, variegate (a few dots do not constitute a separate pattern),* **E:** *reticular, centrally hyperpigmented,* **F:** *reticular, centrally hyperpigmented,* **G:** *reticular (or branched) lines, centrally hyperpigmented,* **H:** *reticular, variegate (best interpretation of color distribution),* **I:** *reticular, eccentrically hyperpigmented,* **J:** *reticular, centrally hyperpigmented,* **K:** *reticular, variegate,* **L:** *reticular (thick reticular lines!), centrally hyperpigmented,* **M:** *reticular, variegate (best interpretation of color distribution),* **N:** *reticular, hypopigmented,* **O:** *reticular, dark-brown.*

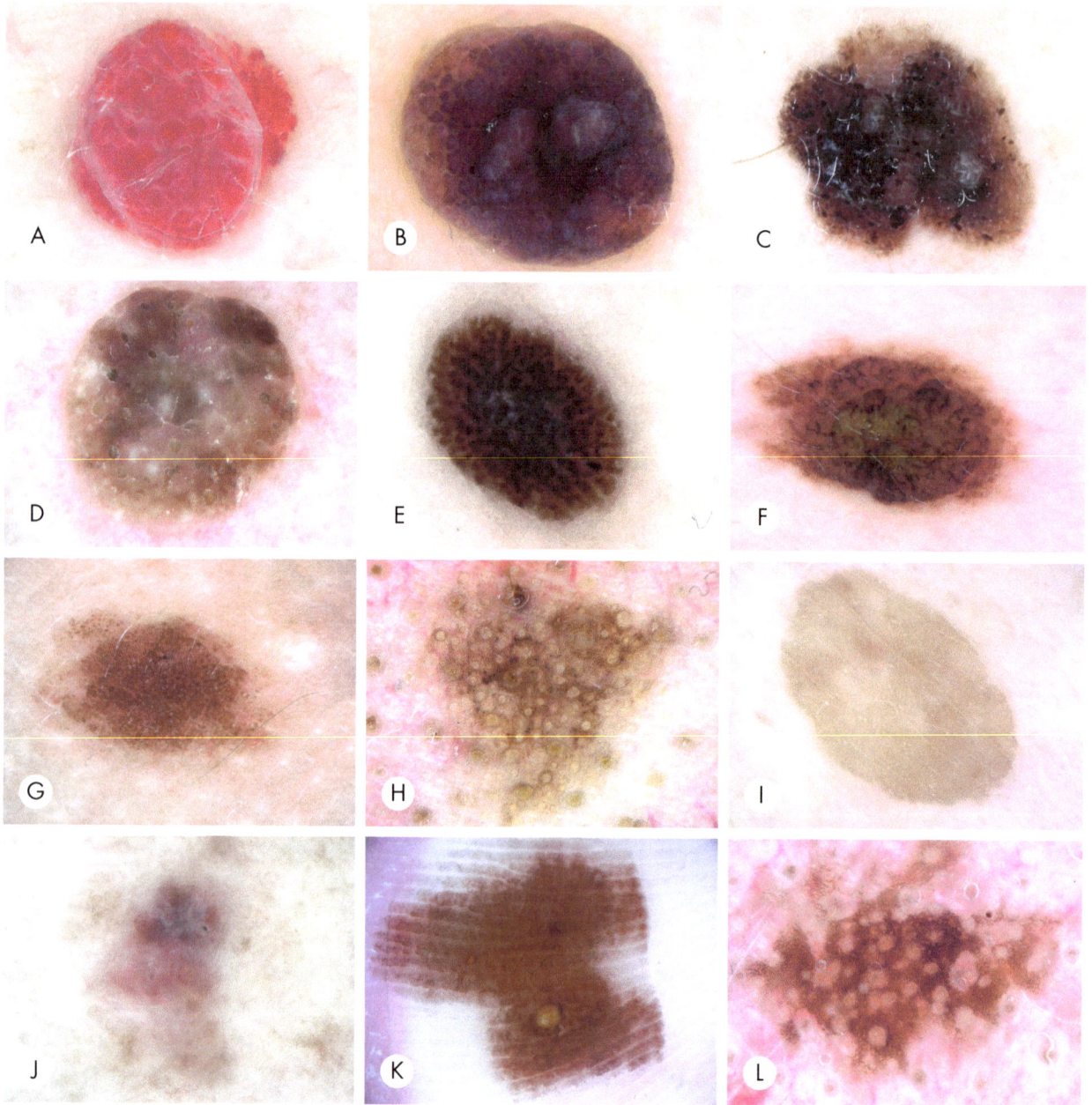

Figure 3.23: Pattern analysis (one pattern).
A: *Clods (large), red,* **B:** *Clods (large and polygonal), light-brown and dark-brown,* **C:** *Clods (small), various shades of melanin (brown, gray, black),* **D:** *Clods (large), orange, yellow, white, brown,* **E:** *Clods (small), brown,* **F:** *Clods (large), brown and yellow,* **G:** *Clods (very small), brown,* **H:** *Circles, brown (the orange clods do not belong to the lesion because they are also present in the surrounding healthy skin),* **I:** *Structureless, light-brown,* **J:** *Structureless, brown and pink,* **K:** *Lines, parallel, on the ridges,* **L:** *Lines, reticular. In contrast to the pattern of circles in H, one finds reticular lines here between the non-pigmented follicular openings. Hypopigmented follicular openings are not circles; rather, they are interruptions to the pattern. Only circular pigmentation around the follicular openings, as shown in figure 3.12 (top row), should be called circles in facial lesions.*

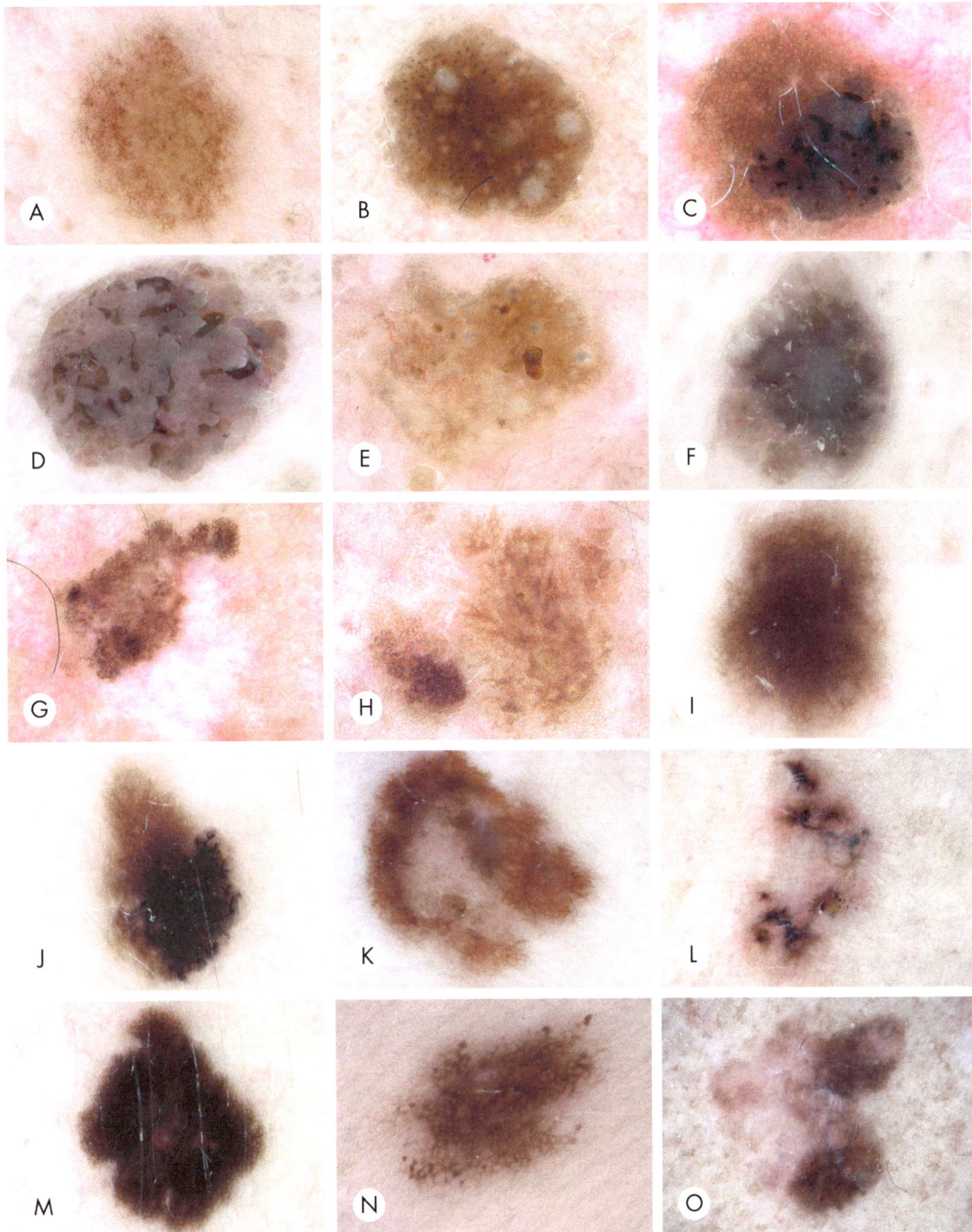

Figure 3.24: Pattern analysis (more than one pattern).
A: *Reticular peripherally, structureless centrally, symmetrical (one color, light-brown),* ***B:*** *White clods (the white clods are not whiter than the surrounding skin because the image has been taken with polarized dermatoscopy) and brown dots, asymmetrical,* ***C:*** *Reticular and black clods, asymmetrical,* ***D:*** *Brown clods and thick curved lines, asymmetrical,* ***E:*** *Reticular lines, orange clods and structureless, asymmetrical,* ***F:*** *Orange clods, structureless blue, asymmetrical,* ***G:*** *Reticular lines, structureless white, asymmetrical,* ***H:*** *Curved lines, circles, orange clods, asymmetrical,* ***I:*** *Reticular lines peripherally, brown dots centrally, symmetrical,* ***J:*** *Reticular lines, black structureless area, pseudopods, asymmetrical,* ***K:*** *Reticular lines, skin-colored structureless area, brown dots, asymmetrical,* ***L:*** *Blue and brown clods, skin-colored structureless area, asymmetrical,* ***M:*** *Reticular lines peripherally, dark-brown structureless area centrally,* ***N:*** *Reticular lines centrally, brown clods peripherally, symmetrical,* ***O:*** *Reticular lines, skin-colored structureless area, asymmetrical.*

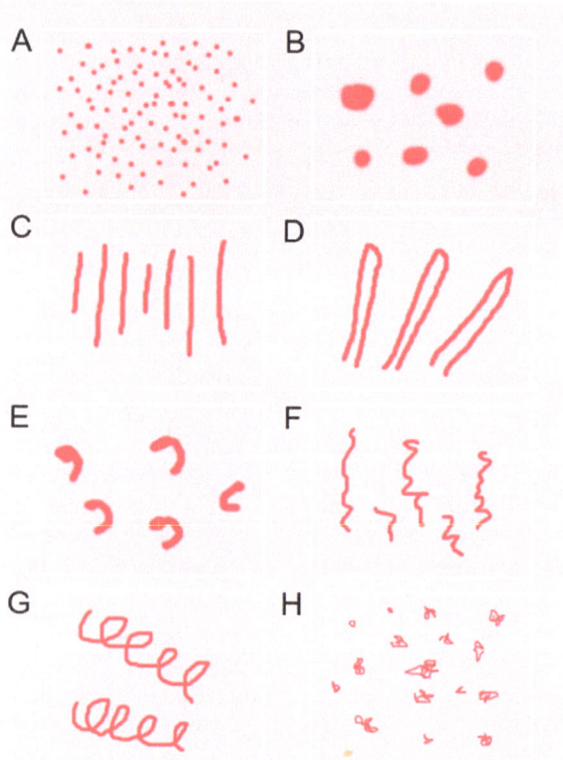

Figure 3.25: Types of vessels.
*Vessels may be seen as dots (**A**), clods (**B**), or lines (**C–H**). Lines may be straight (**C**), looped (**D**), curved (**E**), serpentine (**F**), helical (**G**), or coiled (**H**).*

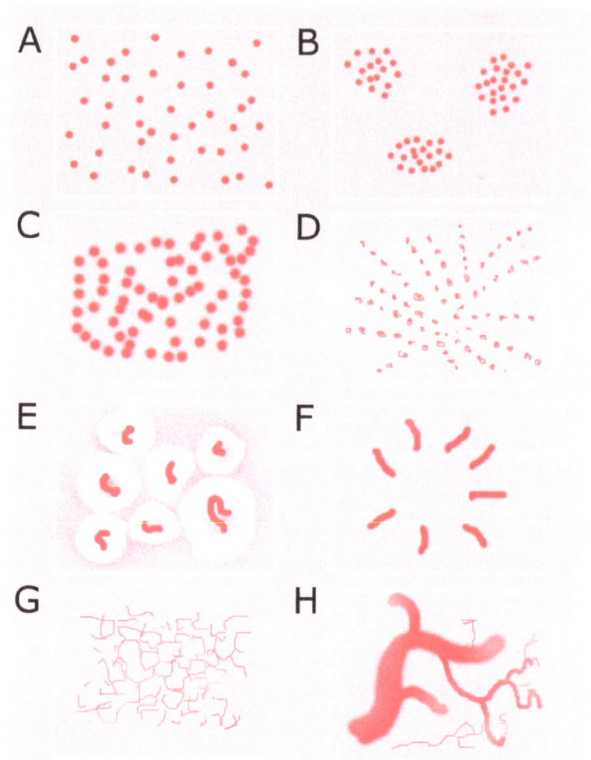

Figure 3.26: Arrangements of vessels.
*Vessels may be randomly distributed (**A**), clustered (**B**), serpiginous (**C**) linear (**D**), centered (**E**), radial (**F**), reticular (**G**), or branched (**H**).*

of vessels, or even absence of a feature. Clues may, but need not necessarily, be present. The more numerous the clues that support a diagnosis (and the fewer that support an alternative diagnosis), the more likely that specific diagnosis is correct. Pattern and color limit the differential diagnoses, but clues confirm a diagnosis or rule it out. Often however, clues are weak, or even contradictory. For these cases, judgement is required in deciding how much weight to assign to each clue, and hence which final diagnosis should be favored. This is discussed in greater detail in chapter 7. As a general principle, more weight should be given to the pattern overall than to any single clue. The most difficult part of dermatoscopy is to correctly assign weight to clues, and particularly to avoid overvaluing an unreliable or misleading clue. This is the role of experience in dermatoscopy.

Pattern of vessels

Blood vessels are visible dermatoscopically due to the hemoglobin they contain. Analysis of vessel pattern(s) often serves as an additional clue to diagnosis. Pat-

terns of vessels are most conspicuous in the absence of pigmentation. In cases of dense melanin pigmentation, vessels are difficult or impossible to visualize.

Patterns formed by vessels are usually much less specific than patterns formed by melanin. As a general principle, whenever pigment is present one should attempt to reach a diagnosis on the basis of these pigmented structures, and relegate blood vessel analysis to the status of a clue to diagnosis. However, when diagnosing non-pigmented lesions, one has to rely on analysis of vessels and keratin structures to reach a diagnosis. Blood vessels are described using the same geometrically defined basic elements used to describe pigmented structures. Like pigmented structures, vessels may appear as dots, clods or lines. Additional line types (looped, curved, serpentine, helical and coiled) are defined for vessels, as these are not seen in pigmented structures. Analogous to patterns formed by pigment, a collection of vessels of the same type gives rise to a pattern of vessels.

Linear vessels are classified based on the number and type of curves *(3.25)*. Those with no curves are termed

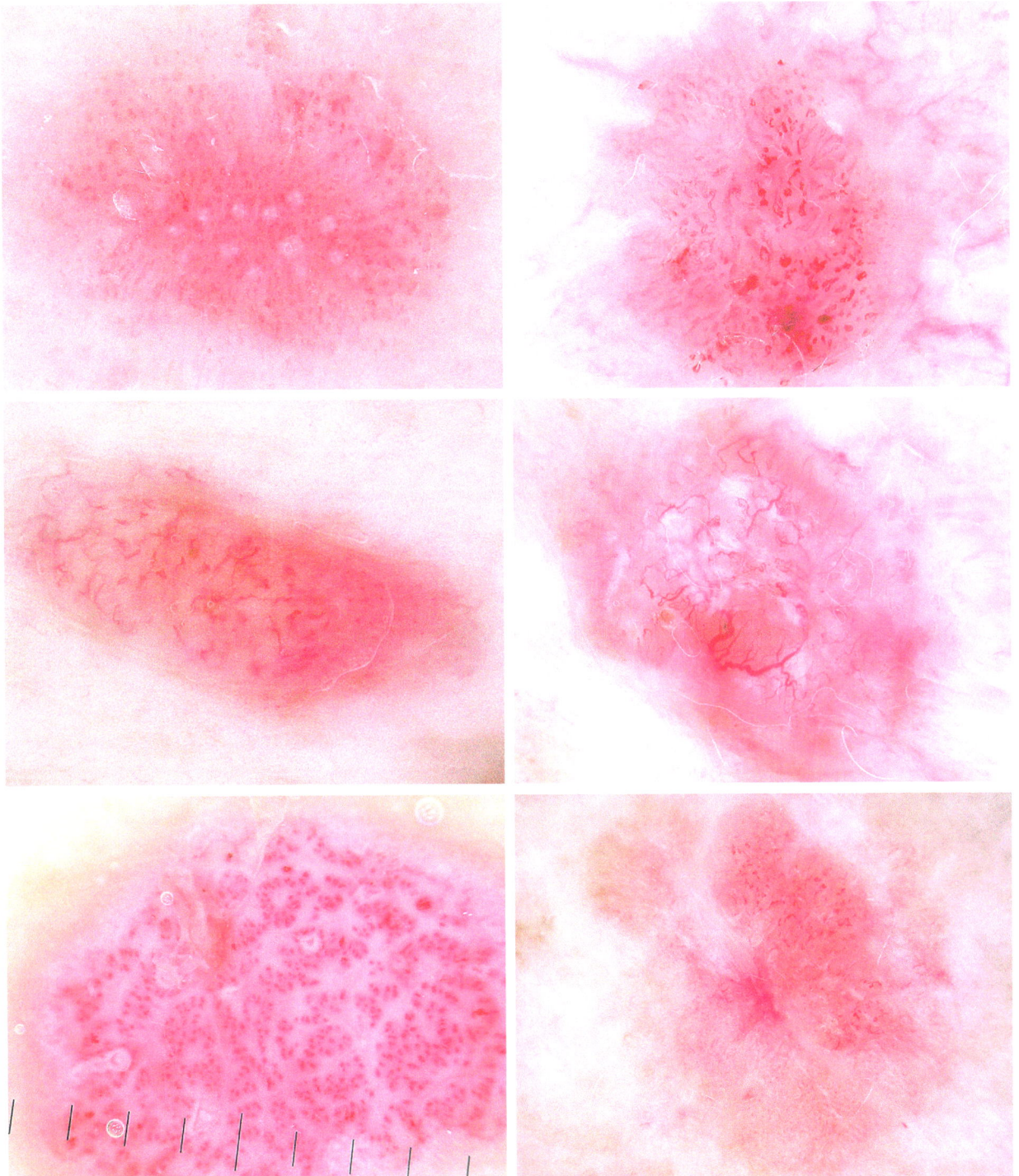

Figure 3.27: Patterns of vessels.
Top left: *Monomorphous, small coiled vessels, random arrangement.* **Top right:** *Polymorphous, coiled and serpentine vessels, random arrangement.* **Middle left:** *Polymorphous; serpentine and curved vessels and vessels as dots, arranged randomly.* **Middle right:** *Monomorphous; serpentine vessels, branched.* **Bottom left:** *Monomorphous; small coiled vessels, arranged in a serpiginous manner.* **Bottom right:** *Polymorphous, vessels as dots and various types of linear vessels, random arrangement.*

"straight". Those with one curve are termed *"looped"* when the bend is so sharp that two sections are formed which are sensibly parallel. A vessel with a single obtuse bend is termed *"curved"*. Vessels with more than one bend are termed *"serpentine"*. A serpentine vessel is termed *"helical"* when the curves are focused on a central axis. Vessels are called *"coiled"* when convoluted compactly.

"Thick" or "thin" and "short" or "long" are additional attributes one may use to describe linear vessels. Logically, the use of these terms is limited to linear vessels. Usually these additional terms contribute nothing to the diagnostic process. However, in exceptional cases these distinctions might provide useful information. Generally, vessels are "thick" only when they are much thicker than normal nail fold capillaries. Vessels are "long" only when they cross a significant part of the lesion and so applies only to straight, serpentine, or helical vessels. Conversely, vessels are "short" only when their length does not greatly exceed their breadth. This applies – if at all – only to straight, curved and serpentine linear vessels.

In addition to the morphology of individual vessels, their arrangement relative to one another and to the lesion as a whole is also important *(3.26)*. In the majority of cases, vessels appear to be distributed randomly, i.e. not arranged in any specific manner throughout the lesion. However, a few important exceptions exist. Vessels as dots or coils may be arranged as lines. When vessels as dots or coils are arranged in straight lines, this arrangement is termed *"linear"* (it is important not to confuse linear vessels with linear arrangement of vessels). When these vessels are arranged in serpentine lines the pattern is known as *"serpiginous"*. When vessels are not uniformly distributed but are much more dense at some sites than others, this arrangement is termed *"clustered"*. Linear vessels of any type at the periphery that are oriented towards but do not cross the center are termed *"radial"*. The arrangement of linear vessels (most commonly curved, sometimes serpentine or looped) in the center of skin colored or light brown clods is termed "centered". As for pigmented lesions, we term straight linear vessels that intersect each other nearly at right angles *"reticular"*. Finally, serpentine vessels may be arranged such that multiple vessels originate from one common vessel; the derivative vessels typically originate from a thicker vessel. This arrangement is termed *"branched"*. Equipped with these definitions, one may describe the morphology of, and classify, all vascular patterns. Patterns of vessels are described using the same general principles as those used to describe the patterns formed by pigment *(3.25, 3.26)*.

A pattern of vessels is composed of multiple vessels of the same type. When one vessel type predominates over the others, we term the pattern of vessels *"monomorphous"*. When more than one pattern of vessels is present we use the term *"polymorphous"*.

Evaluation of the vascular pattern is not always simple. Sometimes one is unable to conclusively assign individual vessels to a specific type. Rather than becoming absorbed in details one should observe the general pattern; the assessment of individual vessels is rarely useful *(3.27, 3.28)*. For instance, in some melanomas one finds – to the extent that pigment allows the vascular pattern to be inspected at all – a mixture of short and straight, short and curved, short and serpentine, and coiled serpentine vessels. The exact classification of individual vessels is not important in this instance; the overall impression is important and that is of polymorphous vessels.

It may be difficult or even impossible to distinguish vessels as dots from vessels as small coils *(3.27 top left)*. At higher magnifications nearly all vessels will have discernable shape; vessels that are dots at magnifications equivalent to the handheld dermatoscope are classified as dots, regardless of their appearance at higher magnifications. Vessels on large, skin colored clods are usually of the linear type; either curved, serpentine or looped *(3.29)*. If each clod contains multiple linear vessels the arrangement is clustered *(3.29 top row)*. If each clod contains a single linear vessel (usually of the curved type) the arrangement is centered *(3.29 bottom row)*.

As regards the occasionally difficult distinction between curved vessels and short serpentine ones, one should remember that curved vessels are usually much thicker than short serpentine ones. Sometimes it is also difficult to decide if there is a specific arrangement of vessels or not. In these doubtful cases it is better to assume that the vessels are arranged randomly. One should also make a distinction between vascular patterns and erythema. Erythema is not a pattern of vessels but a reddening caused by vasodilatation (usually due to inflammation) which, in contrast to a red structureless area, does not cover pigmented structures but gives the background skin a red hue.

Correct technique is critical for dermatoscopic imaging of vessels. Strictly speaking, we do not see the vessels themselves, we see hemoglobin in blood. Too much pressure on the glass plate compresses the vessels and, with blood thus excluded, renders the vessels invisible. For optimum evaluation of vessels one should use a contact medium of higher viscosity, such as ultrasound gel, which is retained between the lesion and the glass plate of the dermatoscope without the use of

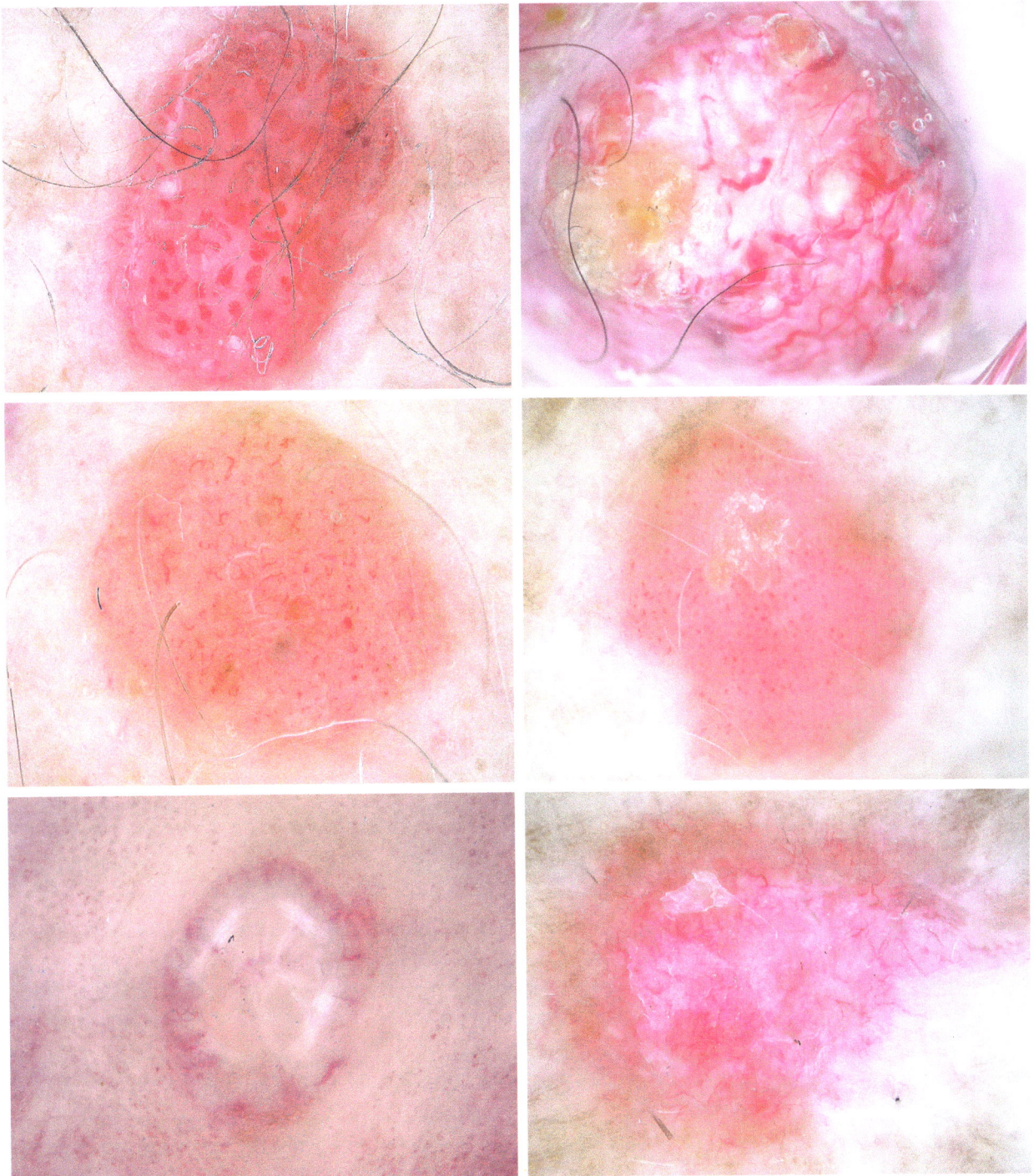

Figure 3.28: *Patterns of vessels.*
Top left: *Monomorphous, large coiled vessels, random arrangement.* **Top right:** *Monomorphous, serpentine vessels, branched arrangement.*
Middle left: *Polymorphous; serpentine, curved and coiled vessels; arranged randomly.* **Middle right:** *Monomorphous; vessels as dots, random arrangement.* **Bottom left:** *Polymorphous; straight and serpentine vessels, radial arrangement.* **Bottom right:** *Monomorphous, serpentine vessels, random arrangement.*

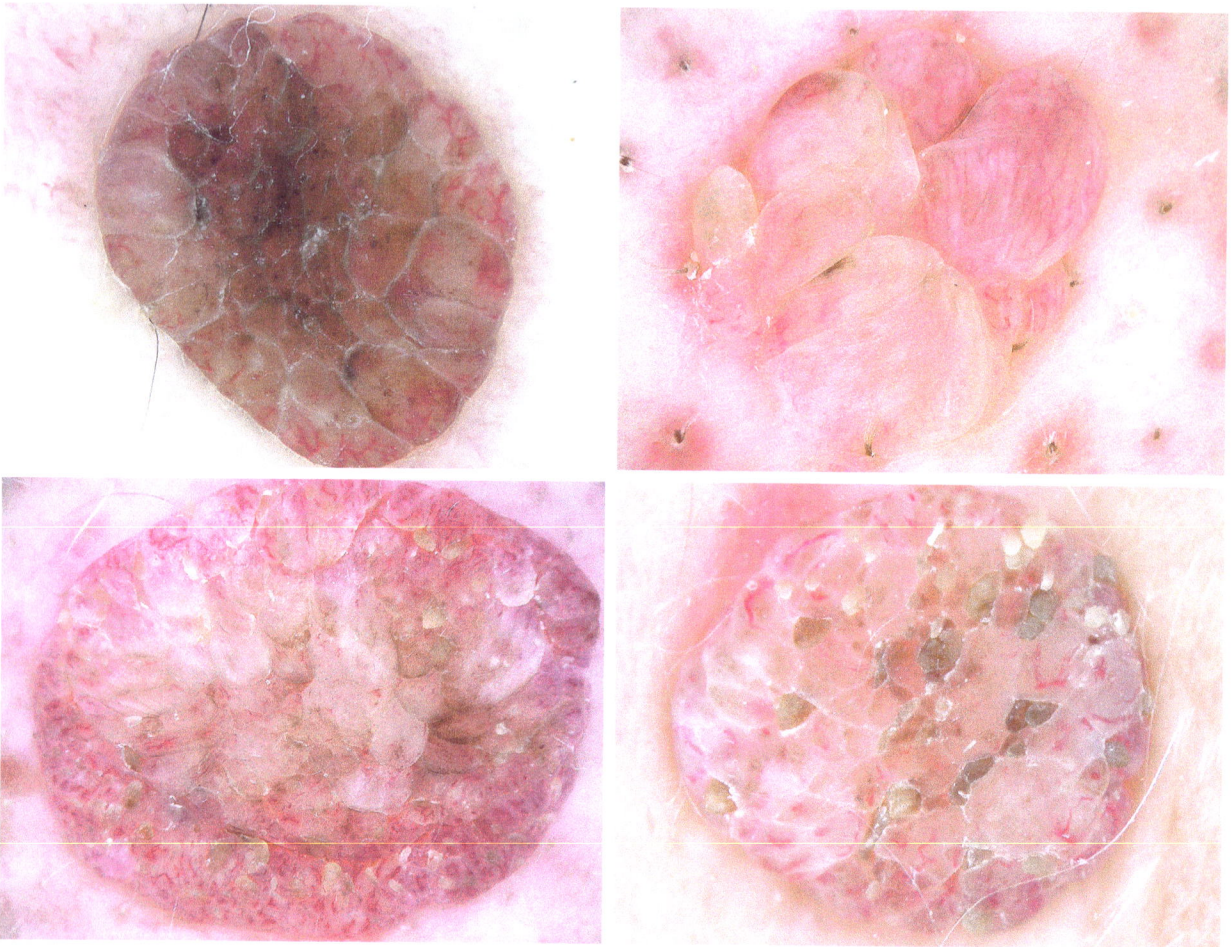

Figure 3.29: Vessels on large skin colored clods.
Top: *Multiple serpentine vessels on each skin-colored clod is a clustered arrangement.* **Bottom:** *Individual curved vessels in the center of each skin-colored clod is a centered arrangement.*

pressure. Alternatively, contact with the skin surface (and thus vessel compression) can be avoided entirely by using a polarizing dermatoscope with the contact plate removed. In some cases vessels may be obscured by polarizing-specific white lines and clods, and in these cases they may be visualized more clearly with non-polarizing (contact) dermatoscopy.

Other clues

Vascular patterns are only one of many clues that we use to establish the diagnosis when assessment of pattern and color alone are insufficient. These clues will be addressed in the following chapters describing the principal pigmented lesions. It should be mentioned here that a stepwise description – first of pattern, then color, and finally clues, is the best way of arriving at the diagnosis.

Pattern + Color + Clue = Diagnosis

3.6 Characteristic features of pigmented non-melanocytic lesions

3.6.1 Proliferation of vessels
Hemangiomas and vascular malformations
Hemangiomas and vascular malformations arguably have the most distinctive dermatoscopic appearance of all lesions. There is one pattern, clods, with color ranging between red and purple, depending on the degree of oxygenation of the blood in the vessels *(3.30, 3.31)*. Black clods are caused by thrombosis of vessels or are indicative of older blood crusts due to exogenous trauma. Other basic elements are completely absent, i.e. there are no lines, pseudopods, circles or dots. In some instances one may find a structureless area adjacent to the clods. Hemangioma should not be diagnosed when any vessels as lines or dots are found within red or purple clods, as this pattern may be seen in amelanotic melanoma.

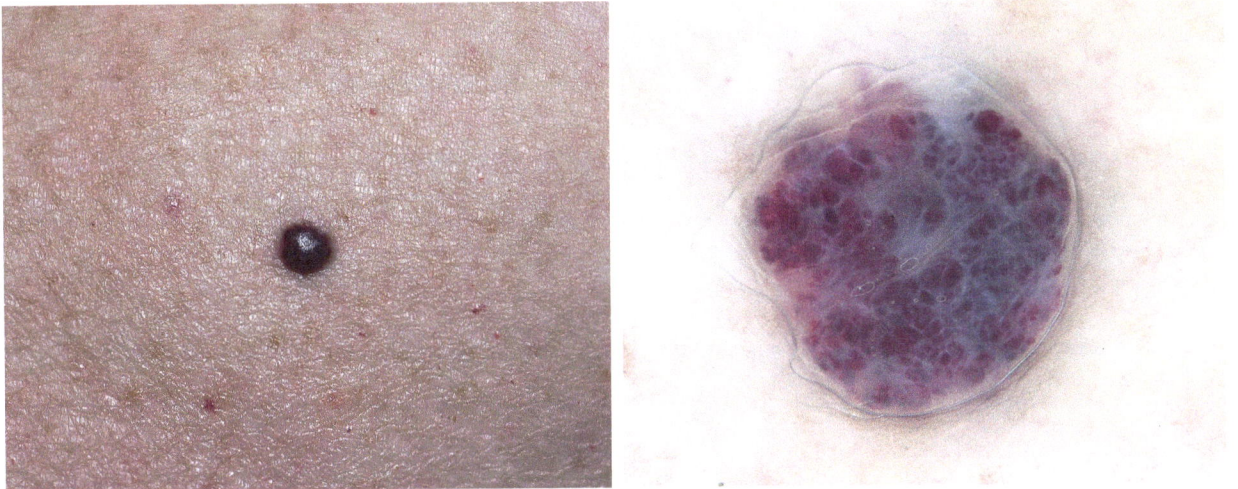

Figure 3.30: Hemangioma.
*Clinical **(left)** and dermatoscopic **(right)** view of a hemangioma. The right figure shows the characteristic dermatoscopic appearance of a hemangioma: one pattern, red or purple clods.*

Hemangioma

Pattern	Colors	Clues
Typical: Only clods Occasional: Clods and structureless	Typical: Red and/or purple Occasional: Black	None

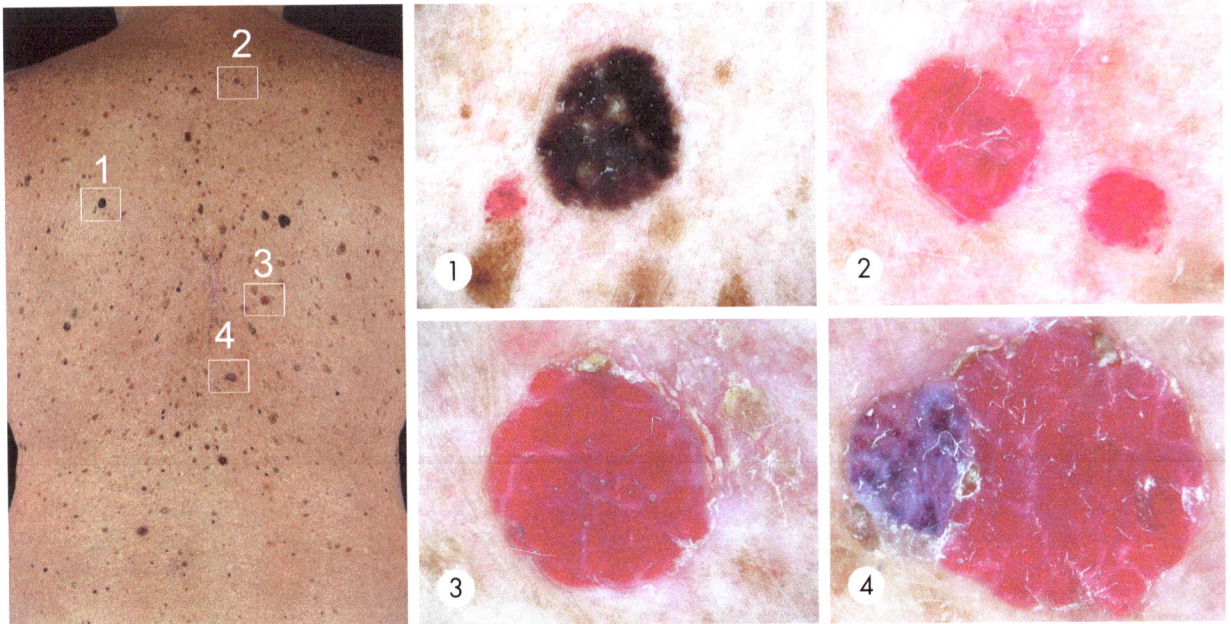

Figure 3.31: "Senile" angiomas (cherry angiomas).
*The overview shows a patient's back dotted with "senile angiomas" (cherry angiomas) and seborrheic keratoses. The first dermatoscopy image **(1)** shows a large and relatively heavily pigmented seborrheic keratosis. To its left is a tiny cherry angioma that already demonstrates the characteristic pattern of red clods. Images **2**, **3** and **4**: on dermatoscopy, angiomas present with only one pattern, namely red clods or, as in example 4, red and purple clods.*

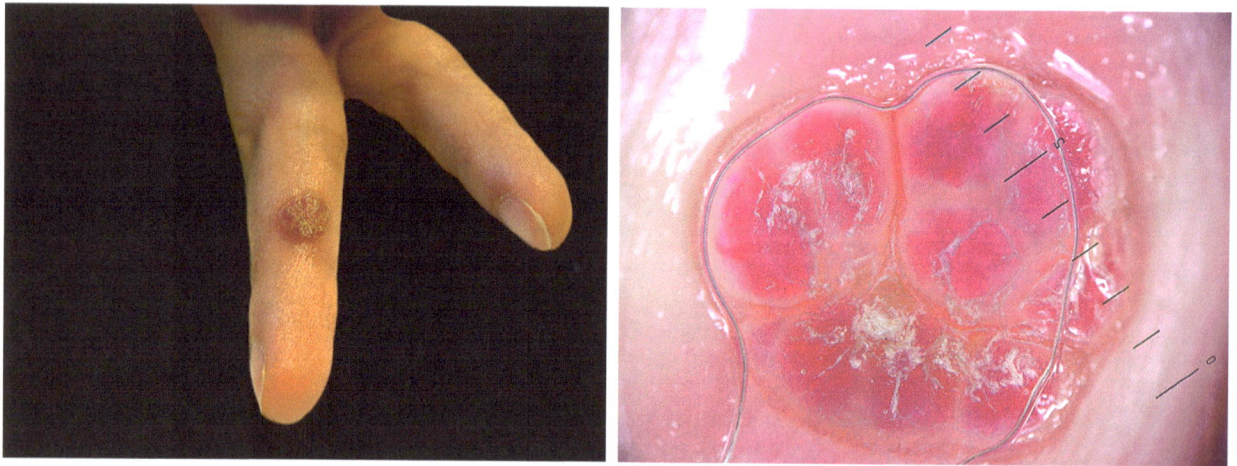

Figure 3.32: Pyogenic granuloma.
Clinical (left) and dermatoscopic (right) view of a pyogenic granuloma. Large pink clods separated by thick skin-colored or white lines and a peripheral white rim are typical of this lesion.

Pyogenic granuloma		
Pattern	Colors	Clues
Typical: Clods and structureless	Typical: Pink, red, white	Typical: The clods are separated by thick white or skin-colored lines, and the tumor is surrounded by a white or light-brown margin. Occasional: Erosions and ulcerations, which are seen as orange, dark-red or black clods or structureless areas.

Correlation between dermatoscopy and dermatopathology
Red or purple clods correspond to dilated and blood-filled vessels in the dermis. The color depends on the oxygenation of blood and the location of the proliferation of vessels. Vessels located higher in the dermis are red whereas deeper ones tend to be purple.

Pyogenic granuloma
The pyogenic granuloma is a reactive proliferation of vessels. Its pattern is similar to that of hemangiomas, but the clods are usually pink or bright-red and typically separated from each other by thick, white or skin-colored lines *(3.32)*. Occasionally pyogenic granuloma has a white or light-brown periphery. As pyogenic granuloma is frequently eroded, one may find orange, dark-red or black clods or structureless areas.

Correlation between dermatoscopy and dermatopathology
The pink clods represent dense proliferations of vessels in the dermis, which are separated by septa of connec-tive tissue (thick, white or skin-colored lines). Pyogenic granuloma is frequently eroded and therefore coated with a crust of blood or serum. These erosions may be seen as orange, red or black clods or structureless areas.

Solitary angiokeratomas
Solitary angiokeratomas reveal a similar pattern of vessels as hemangiomas or senile angiomas. However, in contrast to hemangiomas which are usually marked by bright red clods, solitary angiokeratomas have dark-red, purple or black clods *(3.33)*. Structureless areas are also more common in angiokeratomas than in hemangiomas. Sometimes there is marked hyper-keratosis *(3.34)*. Occasionally it may be difficult to differentiate the purple clods of angiokeratoma from the blue clods pigmented by melanin (like for exam-ple in basal cell carcinoma). As a rule of thumb, one should assume that the pigment is hemoglobin if most of the other clods are red, and assume the pigment is melanin when found associated with brown. Of course it is prudent to assume the pigment is melanin in equivocal cases.

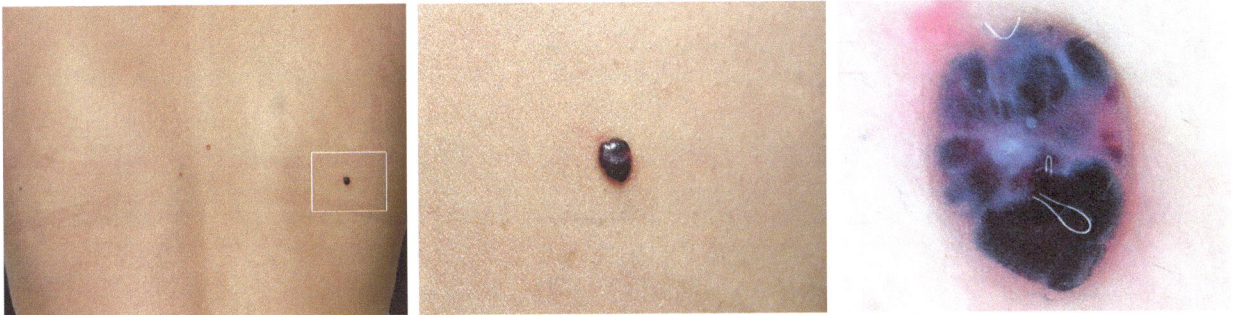

Figure 3.33: Angiokeratoma.
*Clinical view of an angiokeratoma: overview (**left**) and detailed view (**middle**). On dermatoscopy (**right**): there is only one pattern, clods, red or black.*

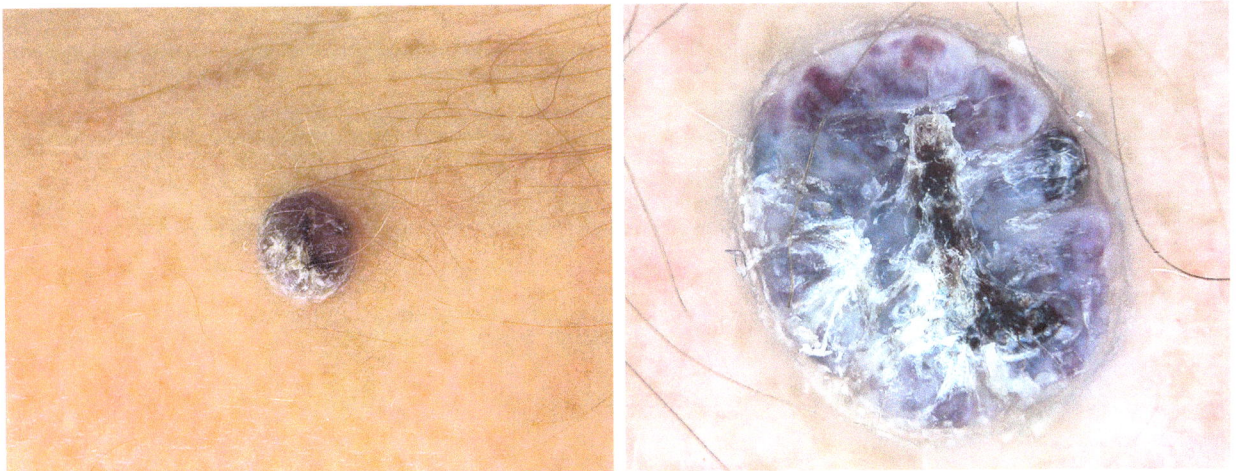

Figure 3.34: Angiokeratoma.
***Left:** Clinical view of an angiokeratoma. **Right:** Dermatoscopy. There are clods, and their colors are red, purple, and black. Sometimes it may be difficult to differentiate purple clods (pigmented by hemoglobin) from blue clods (pigmented by melanin). If most of the other clods are red, one should assume that the pigment is hemoglobin and not melanin. Note the white structureless zone that corresponds to hyperkeratosis.*

3.6.2 Intracorneal hemorrhage

Hemorrhage in the stratum corneum usually occurs on acral skin because the stratum corneum is sufficiently thick at this site. In cases of recent hemorrhage one finds a red or reddish-brown structureless area, or red or reddish-brown clods. However, in case of older hemorrhage the color is black. Typical features of intracorneal hemorrhage are a larger structureless area with a sharply demarcated border *(3.35),* sometimes surrounded by small satellite clods. At acral sites the pattern may also be of parallel lines following the ridges. In such instances, subcorneal hemorrhage must be differentiated from acral melanoma. At non-acral sites, subcorneal hemorrhage may show the pattern of curved lines.

Correlation between dermatoscopy and dermatopathology
The structureless area, clods and parallel lines represent accumulations of red blood cells in the stratum corneum.

3.6.3 Solar lentigo, seborrheic keratosis and lichen planus-like keratosis
Solar lentigo
The appearance of solar lentigo depends on its location. The most common pattern on the trunk is reticular or curved lines *(3.36, 3.37),* alone or in combination. Occasionally small brown circles may be superimposed. In facial solar lentigines we can find the structureless pattern, curved lines, a reticular pattern or, albeit rarely, regularly spaced brown circles. Solar lentigines on the forearm and the dorsum of the hand are often structureless and light-brown, sometimes with superimposed brown dots *(3.38).*

At all sites, the border of solar lentigines is well-demarcated and scalloped (with multiple concavities). This quality of the border is an important clue to solar lentigo.

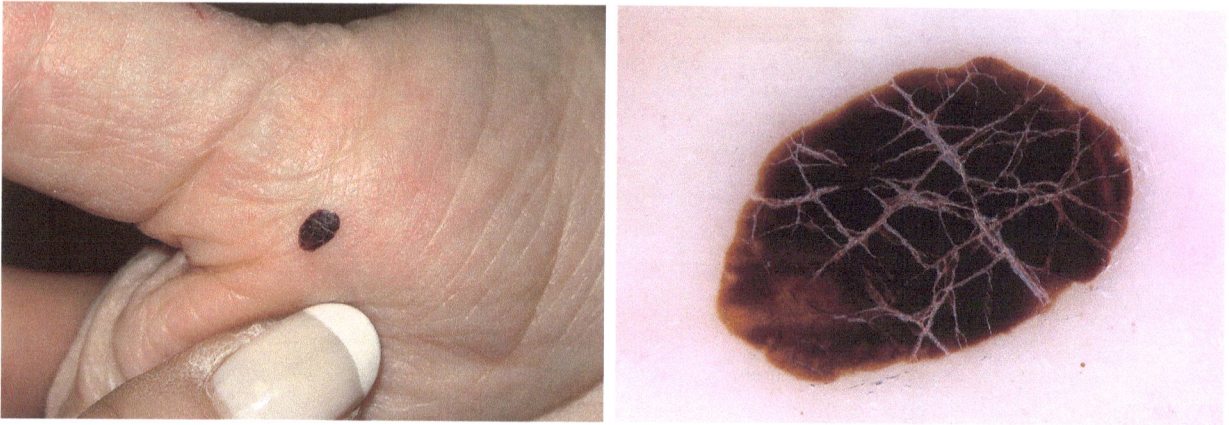

Figure 3.35: Hemorrhage in the stratum corneum.
This hemorrhage on the palm of the hand is seen on dermatoscopy (right) as a reddish-brown or black structureless area. It is sharply delineated from its surroundings.

Intracorneal hemorrhage

Pattern	Colors	Clues
Typical: Structureless, clods or parallel lines on the ridges	*Typical:* Red, reddish-brown (recent), black (old)	*Typical:* Sharp contours Small satellite clods detached from the main lesion

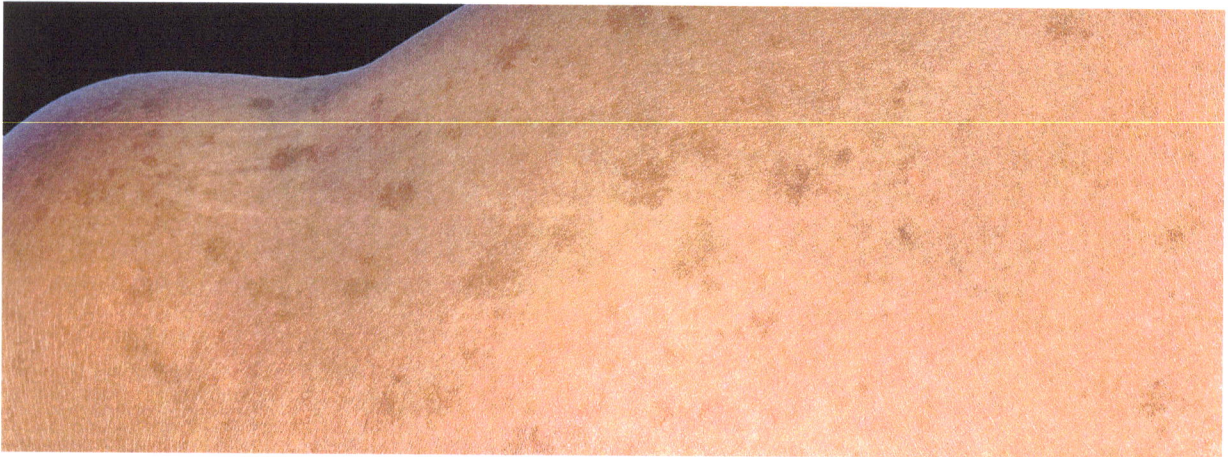

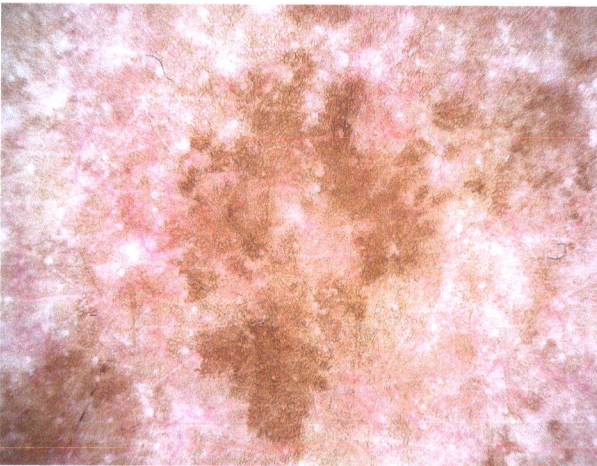

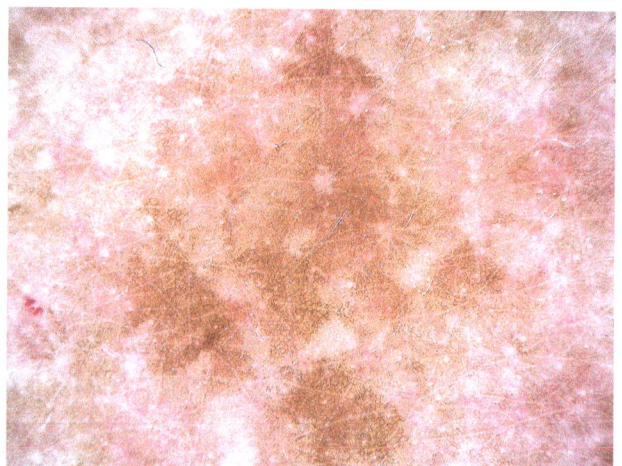

Figure 3.36: Solar lentigines.
Multiple solar lentigines on the back. On dermatoscopy (**bottom row**) the reticular pattern is predominant. Reticular lines are thin and light-brown.

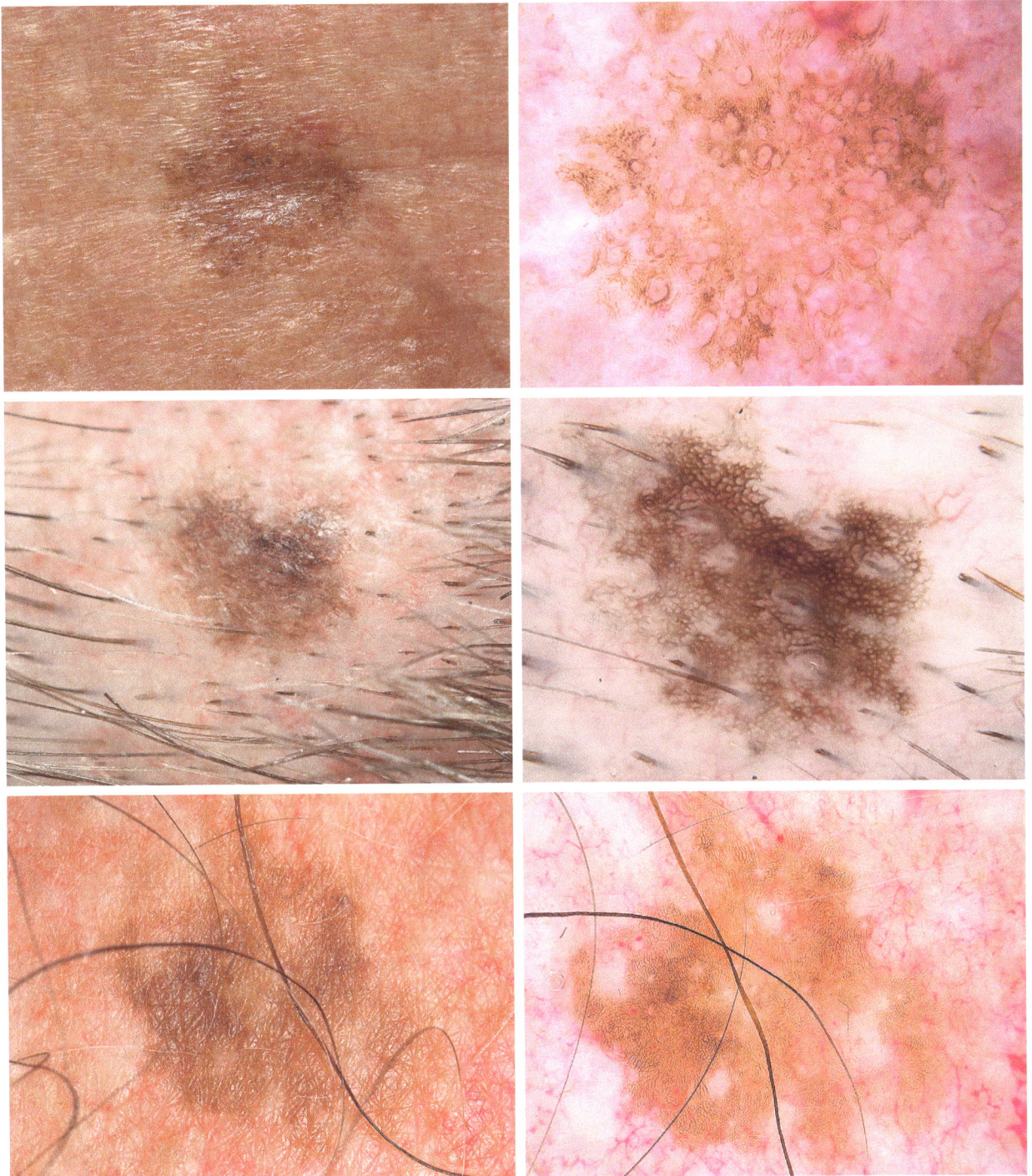

Figure 3.37: *Solar lentigines.*
Clinical **(left)** *and dermatoscopic* **(right)** *view of solar lentigines.* **Top right:** *Solar lentigo with curved lines and circles.* **Middle right:** *solar lentigo with reticular lines.* **Bottom left:** *Solar lentigo with curved lines.*

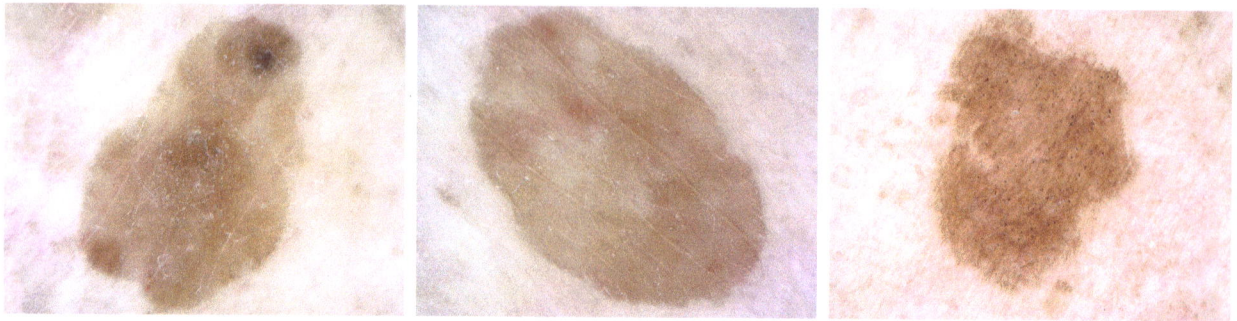

Figure 3.38: Dermatoscopic view of solar lentigines on the forearm.
On the forearm, common patterns are structureless, **(left and middle)** or structureless with superimposed dots **(right)**.

Solar lentigo		
Pattern	Colors	Clues
Typical: Trunk: Reticular and/or curved lines Face: Structureless, reticular or curved lines Forearm and dorsum of the hand: Structureless and/or dots	*Typical:* Light-brown	*Typical:* Sharply demarcated, scalloped (with multiple concavities) border

Correlation between dermatoscopy and dermatopathology

The brown reticular and curved lines are due to hyperpigmentation of basal keratinocytes when rete ridges are present. The structureless brown pattern corresponds to hyperpigmentation of basal keratinocytes when the epidermis is flat (rete ridges are absent). This is usually the case on chronic sun-damaged skin.

Seborrheic keratosis

No other benign lesion shows the diversity of dermatoscopic appearances seen in seborrheic keratosis *(3.39–3.43).* Except for the pseudopod pattern, any pattern or color may be found.

Flat seborrheic keratoses (and the flat portions of raised types) on the trunk show similar patterns to solar lentigo, i.e. light-brown reticular or curved lines. With early acanthosis (thickening of the epidermis) and hence thickening of the lesion, thin curved lines (frequently arranged as parallel pairs) and circles become more prominent. With advanced acanthosis, the predominant structures become thick curved lines and clods.

In early acanthosis, brown and orange (or yellow) are the predominant colors seen. Verrucous types when heavily pigmented are marked by thick curved lines in combination with brown and/or orange clods and/or a structureless area in shades of brown, blue or gray. In less heavily pigmented verrucous types the predominant feature is often orange, yellow or skin-colored clods.

White dots or clods are seen in all types of seborrheic keratosis, but become more common in more raised lesions, i.e. with more advanced acanthosis. As with all aggregations of basic elements, white clods or dots must be multiple to form a pattern (though lesser numbers may still constitute a clue).

In addition to white dots or clods, a sharply demarcated border, a scalloped border and looped and/or coiled vessels are important clues to seborrheic keratosis.

Correlation between dermatoscopy and dermatopathology

As in solar lentigo, the brown lines and circles of flat seborrheic keratoses result from hyperpigmentation of basal keratinocytes. Reticular lines may become thick with acanthosis of the epidermis. The hypopigmented areas between lines are dermal papillae and infundibula of the hair follicles. Thick curved lines, clods and circles of raised or verrucous seborrheic keratoses represent invaginations of the epidermis filled with keratin (thick lines and clods) or infundibula (clods and circles) filled with keratin. As white or yellow keratin may be mixed with melanin, the spectrum of colors of lines and clods ranges from yellow (no melanin) to orange (moderate quantity of melanin), brown (large quantity of melanin), and in exceptional cases even black.

White dots or clods correspond histopathologically to cysts filled with keratin. The blue or gray structureless area of some verrucous seborrheic keratoses is due to acanthosis of the epidermis, which causes epidermal melanin to appear blue.

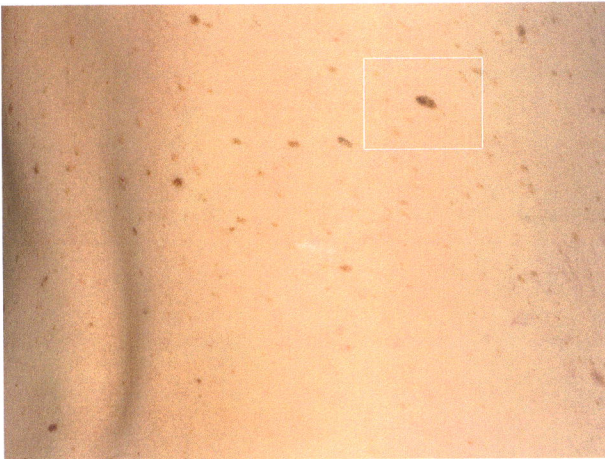

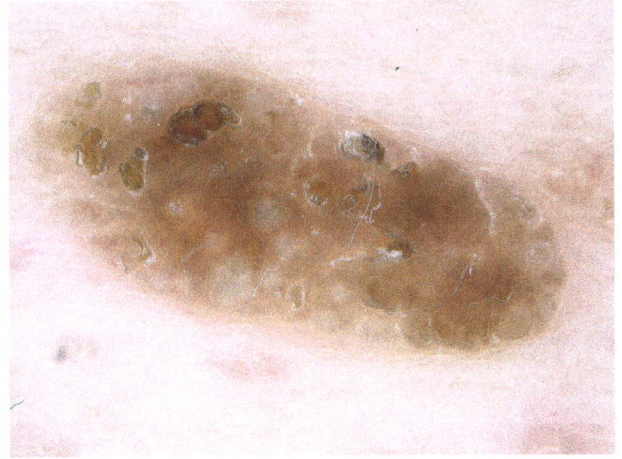

Figure 3.39: Seborrheic keratosis with only one pattern, namely yellow, orange and white clods

Lichen planus-like keratosis

Lichen planus-like keratosis is actually a solar lentigo (or sometimes a seborrheic keratosis) in regression and may therefore show the same dermatoscopic features as these lesions. Two additional features are clues to lichen planus-like keratosis; erythema (a sign of inflammation) and gray dots and/or clods *(3.44)*.

Once the solar lentigo has disappeared and the inflammation has subsided, complete regression is marked by gray dots and/or clods with no sign of the pre-existing lesion. In this case, of course, other differential diagnoses must be considered, including a fully regressed melanoma. In most cases the distinction is obvious because several lichen planus-like keratoses occur together at typical sites (forearm, dorsum of the hand, face and back). However, a diagnostic biopsy may be necessary in some cases.

Correlation between dermatoscopy and dermatopathology
On histopathology the gray clods or dots represent accumulations of melanophages in the papillary dermis.

3.6.4 Dermatofibroma

The most common patterns of dermatofibroma on dermatoscopy are reticular lines peripherally and structureless white centrally *(3.45)*. Peripheral reticular lines are usually brown and always thin – never thick. Instead of reticular lines there may be dense light-brown circles or, more rarely, regularly arranged radial lines distributed over the entire circumference. Thick white lines in place of the central structureless zone is also a common variant. If the center of the dermatofibroma is brown or red structureless one can also find (polarizing-specific) perpendicular white lines in the center.

There are also other less common patterns of dermatofibroma. For instance, the central white structureless zone may be entirely absent. Instead, one may find a few smaller eccentrically located structureless zones that may be white or skin-colored. Another uncommon dermatofibroma variant has no peripheral lines or circles, consisting entirely of brown, white and skin-colored structureless zones. Usually dermatofibroma have a symmetric combination of patterns and colors but exceptions like the one shown in *figure 3.46* exist. The firm consistency on palpation is an additional clinical clue to the diagnosis of dermatofibroma.

Correlation between dermatoscopy and dermatopathology
Thin reticular lines or circles are caused by elongation of rete ridges and melanin hyperpigmentation of basal keratinocytes. White structureless zones, thick white reticular lines and perpendicular white lines are caused by dermal fibrosis. Red or pink pigmentation is caused by inflammation and dilated blood vessels.

3.6.5 Melanotic macules
Ink-spot lentigo

The characteristic pattern of ink-spot lentigo is reticular lines (more rarely branched lines) that may be quite thick, but always have a uniform dark-brown or black pigmentation *(3.47)*. A clue is that the reticular lines within the lesion may be interrupted at various sites, and tend to end abruptly at the margin.

Correlation between dermatoscopy and dermatopathology
The reticular pattern of ink-spot lentigo is caused by marked hyperpigmentation (therefore dark-brown or black) of basal keratinocytes at the rete ridges.

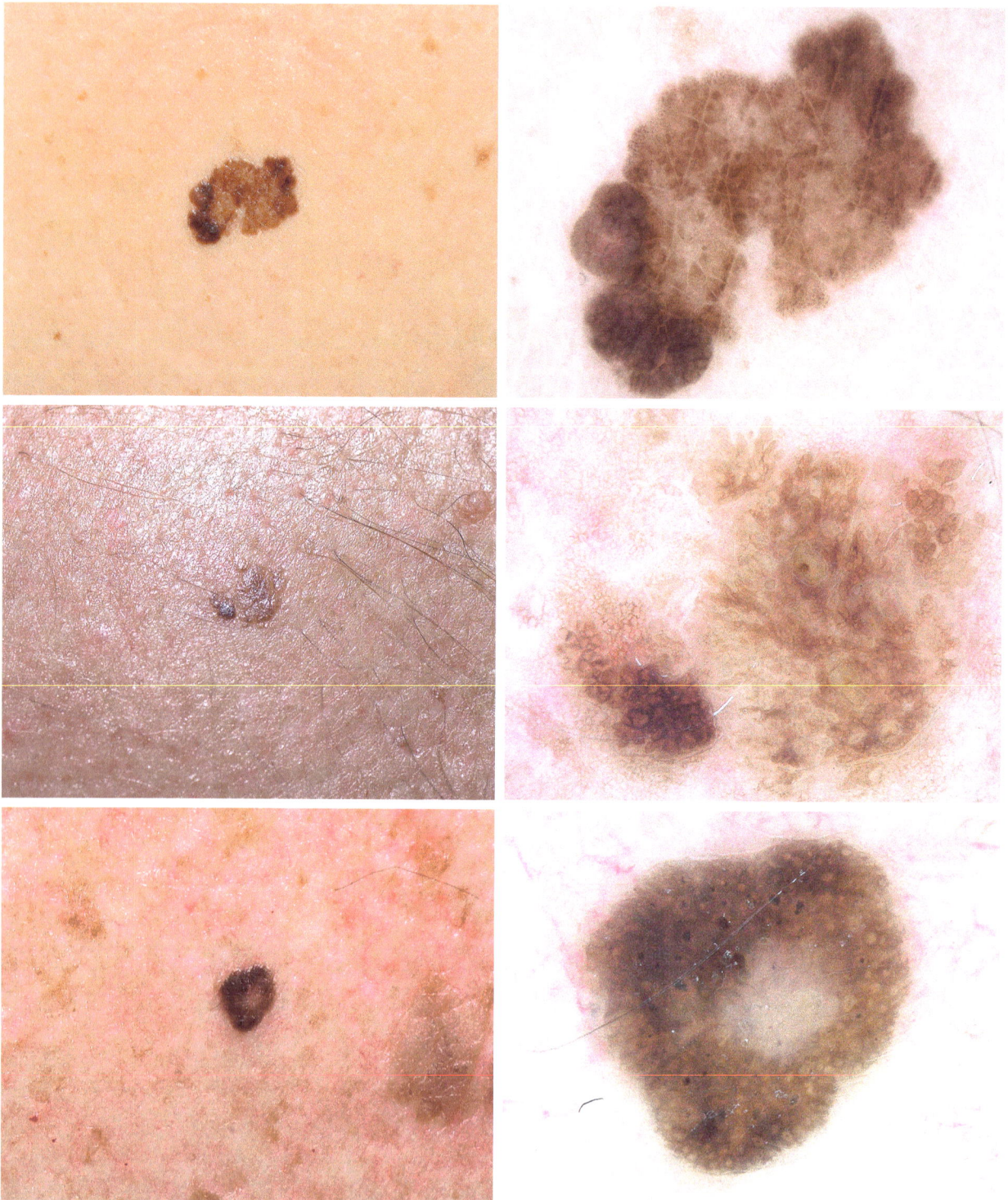

Figure 3.40: *Seborrheic keratoses.*
Top row: *Based on the clinical appearance* **(left)** *alone, it is difficult to make a distinction between seborrheic keratosis and a melanocytic lesion. On dermatoscopy* **(right)** *one finds a pattern of reticular lines (between 6 o'clock and 9 o'clock) and a structureless area. A clue is the well demarcated and scalloped border.* **Middle row:** *Seborrheic keratosis with circles and curved lines in a typical paired parallel arrangement. Additionally there are yellow clods.* **Bottom row:** *Seborrheic keratosis with reticular lines. The dark-brown, yellow and orange clods constitute a clue.*

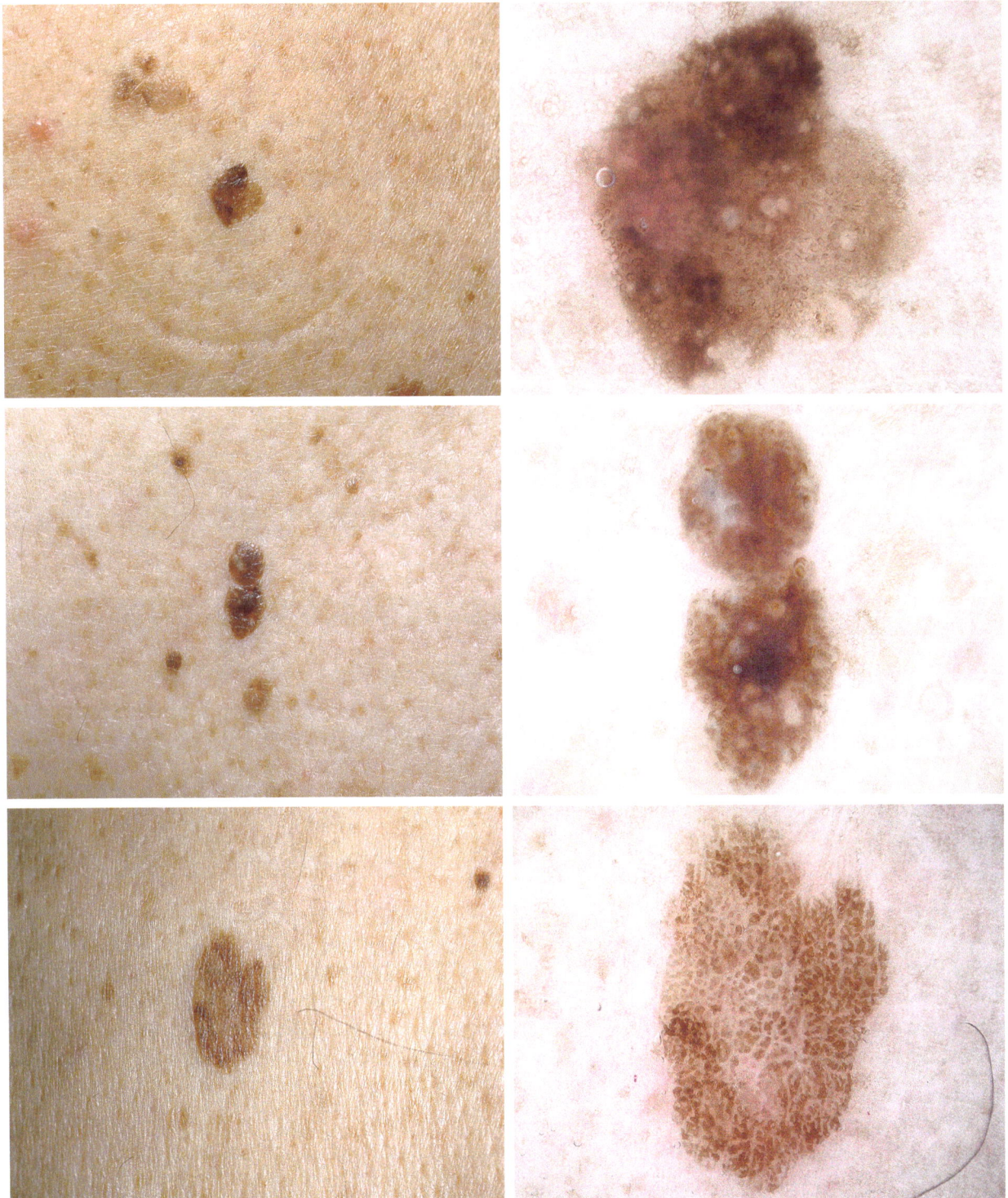

Figure 3.41: *Seborrheic keratoses.*
Top row: *On dermatoscopy* (**right**) *one finds two patterns, circles and structureless. The "circles" may be distorted into ellipses.* **Middle row:** *The pattern of circles is predominant in this seborrheic keratosis. Occasional curved lines constitute a clue.* **Bottom row:** *A seborrheic keratosis with one pattern, brown clods. The only clue here is the presence of very sparse curved lines.*

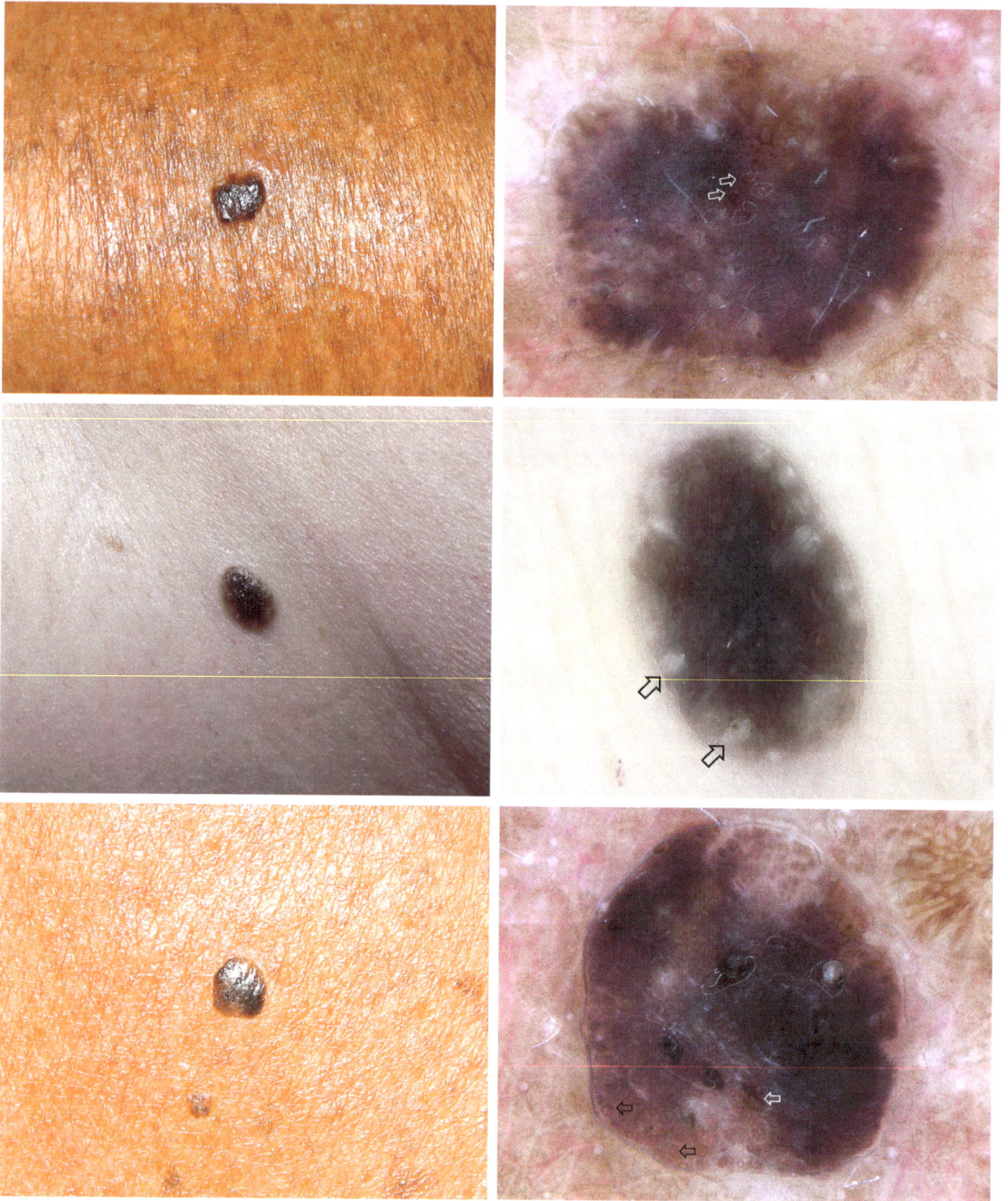

Figure 3.42: *Predominantly structureless seborrheic keratoses.*
Top row: *The structureless pattern is predominant. It is very unspecific. The clue to the diagnosis is the sparse circles (arrows).* **Middle row:** *Two patterns, structureless brown or dark-gray in the center, and large white clods at the periphery (arrows).* **Bottom row:** *Two patterns, structureless and circles (black arrows), and a few dark-brown and even orange clods (white arrow).*

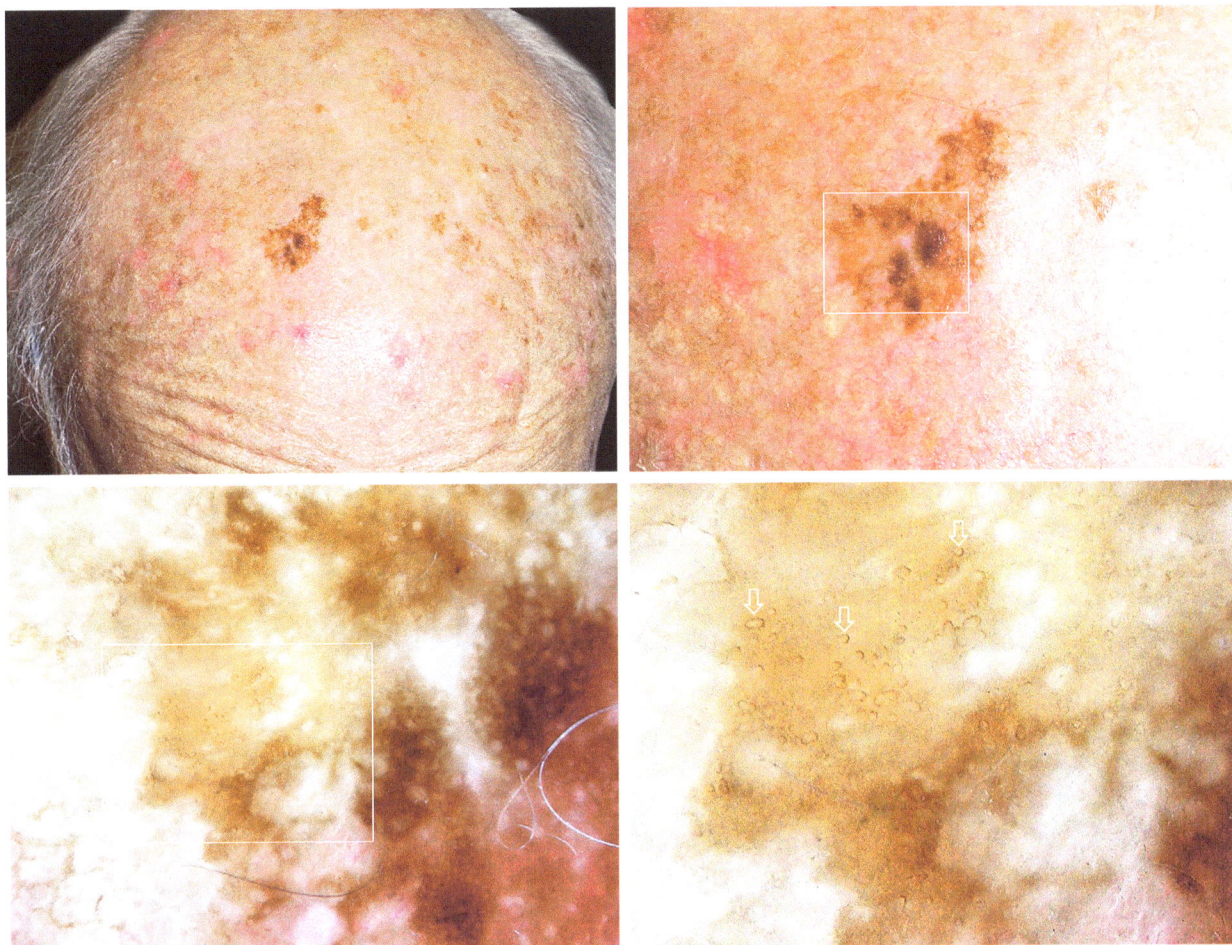

Figure 3.43: Seborrheic keratosis on the scalp.
This seborrheic keratosis can be confidently diagnosed on dermatoscopy; the clues being a few circles (arrows) and a well-demarcated, scalloped border.

Seborrheic keratosis

Pattern	Colors	Clues
Typical: Flat: Reticular or curved lines, circles Moderately raised: Curved lines, clods, circles Verrucous: Clods, thick curved lines, structureless	*Typical:* Lines: Brown Circles: Brown Clods: White, skin-colored, orange, brown, occasionally the pigmentation may be so dense that black clods are found. Structureless area in heavily pigmented types: Brown, blue and gray.	*Typical:* White dots or clods Sharp border – in cases of flat types, a scalloped border (with multiple concavities). Looped or coiled vessels

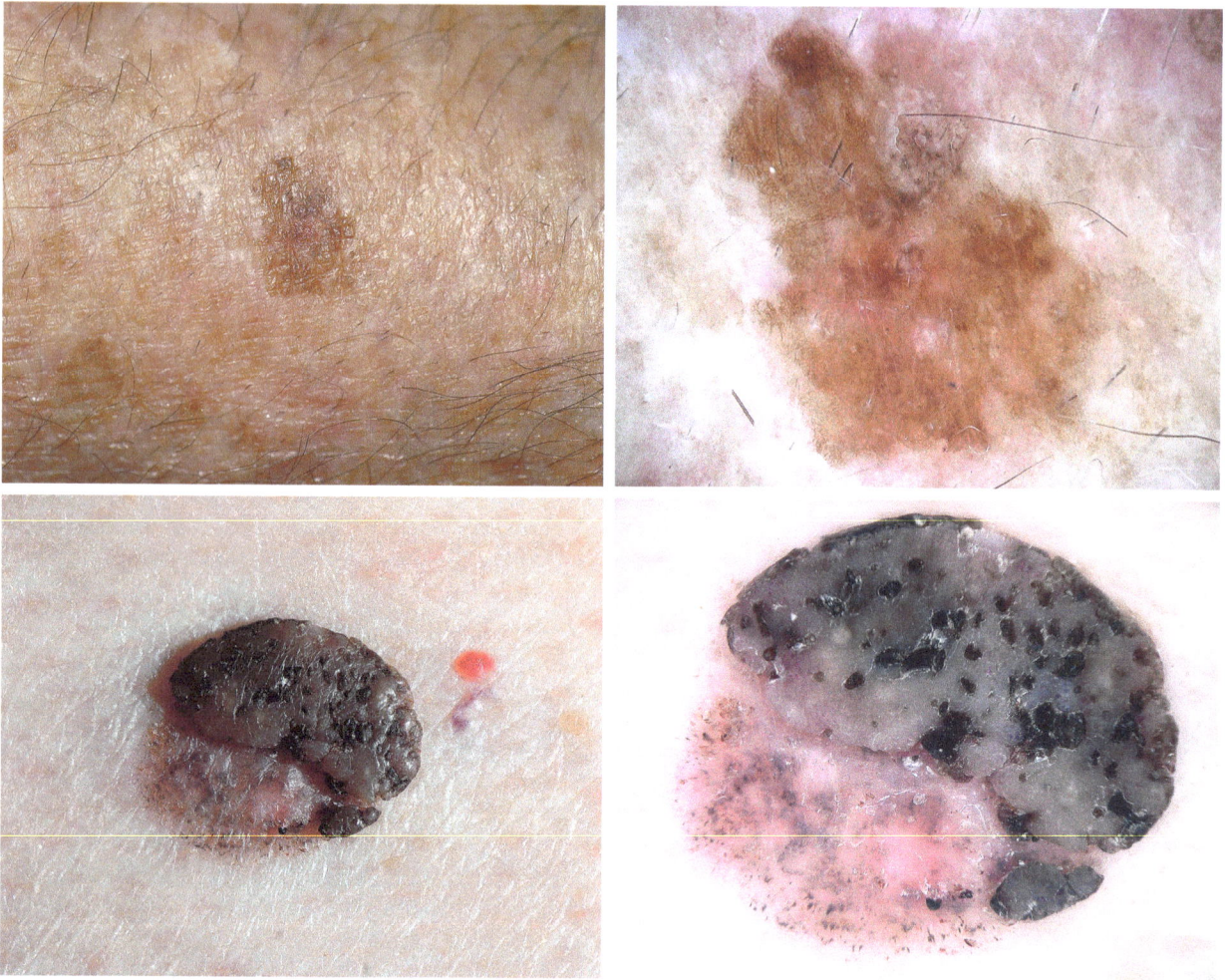

Figure 3.44: Lichen planus-like keratoses.
Top row: On dermatoscopy **(right)** one finds criteria of solar lentigo (reticular lines) as well as gray dots (solar lentigo in a stage of regression). **Bottom row:** Seborrheic keratosis with regression (Lichen planus-like keratosis), clinical view **(left)** and dermatoscopy **(right)**. The raised part of the lesion shows the typical features of seborrheic keratosis, in the flat part one finds grey dots.

Lichen planus-like keratosis

Pattern	Colors	Clues
Typical: Pattern of a pre-existing solar lentigo or a seborrheic keratosis	*Typical:* Gray, light-brown	*Typical:* As in solar lentigo/seborrheic keratosis plus gray dots and/or clods

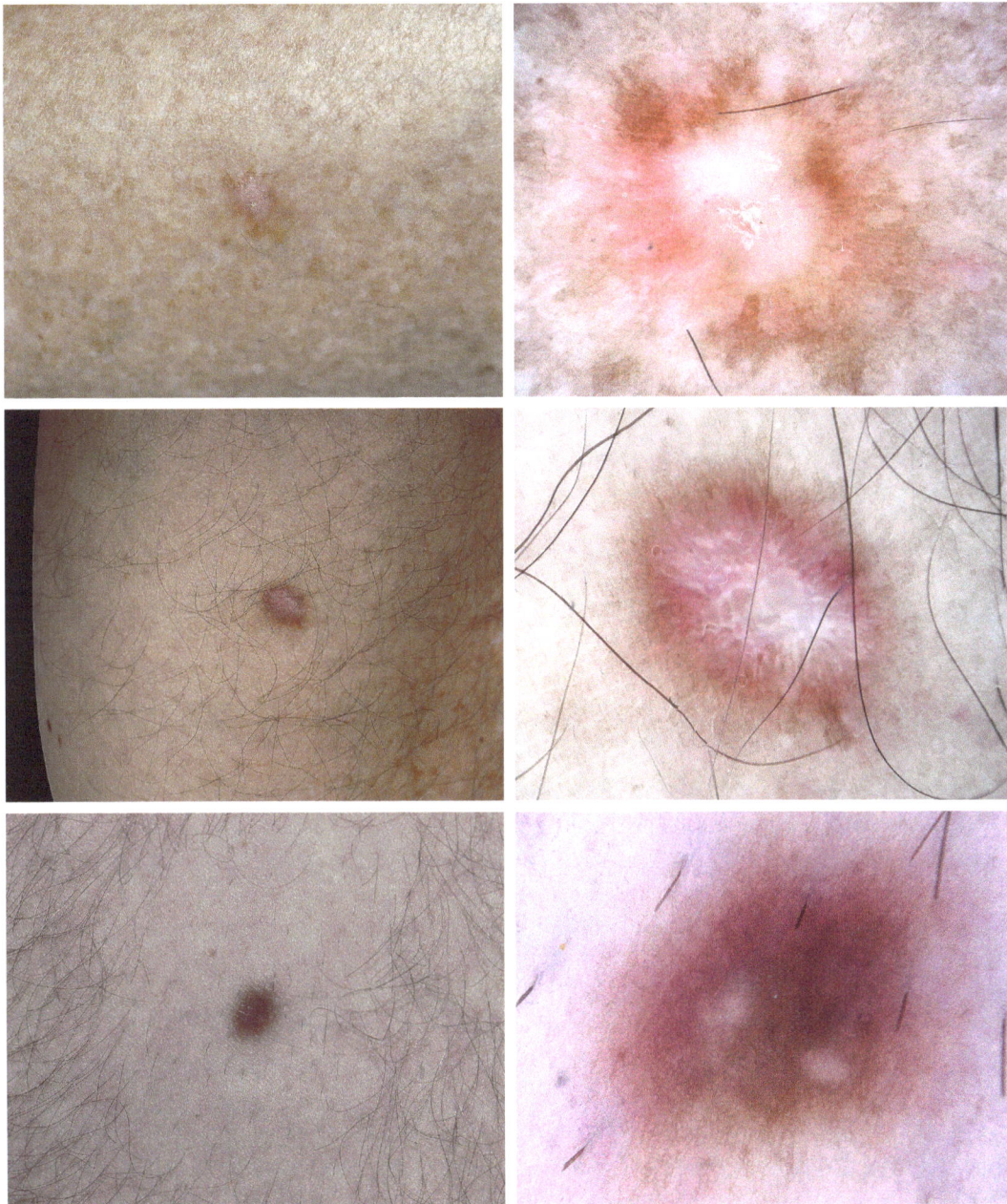

Figure 3.45: Dermatofibromas.
Top row: *Thin reticular lines at the periphery and a white structureless zone in the center constitute the typical dermatoscopic appearance of a dermatofibroma.* **Middle row:** *Instead of the structureless white center there may be thick reticular and perpendicular white lines.* **Bottom row:** *Rarely, several small hypopigmented structureless zones replace the usual single structureless zone.*

Dermatofibroma

Pattern	Colors	Clues
Typical: Reticular and structureless *Variants:* Instead of thin brown reticular lines there may be densely arranged light-brown circles; instead of the structureless white center there may be thick, white reticular lines. *Rare:* Completely structureless or radial lines at the periphery (on the entire circumference).	*Typical:* Reticular lines and circles are light-brown, structureless zones are either white or skin-colored.	*Typical pattern:* Reticular (or circles) at the periphery, structureless (or white reticular lines) or white perpendicular lines (only visible with polarized dermatoscopy) in the center.

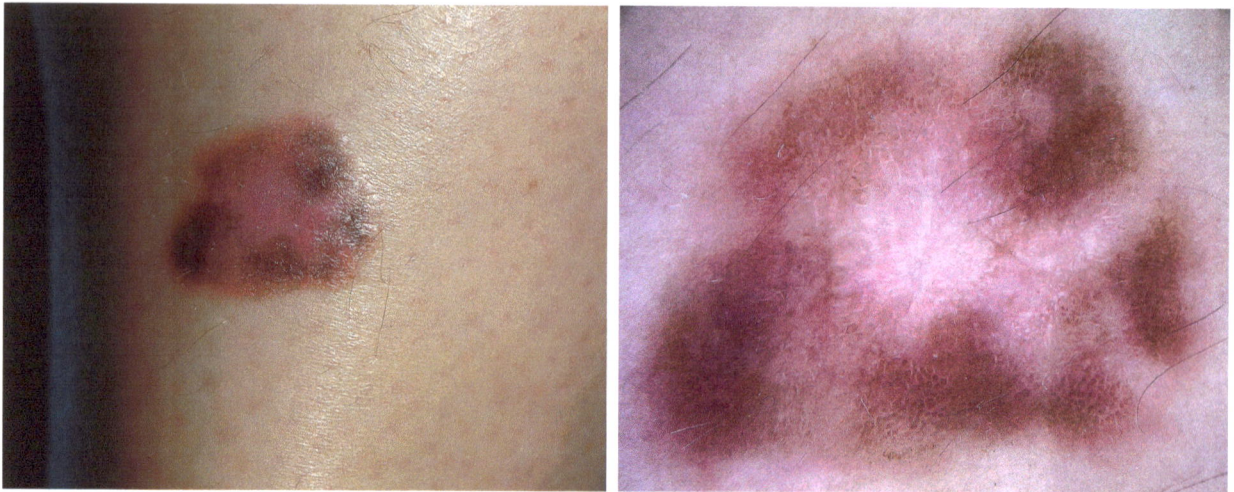

Figure 3.46: Unusually large dermatofibroma.
On dermatoscopy this large dermatofibroma is chaotic (asymmetry of pattern and color). It is typified by white structureless center, white perpendicular lines, and reticular white lines. In addition the typical brown reticular lines can be found at the periphery.

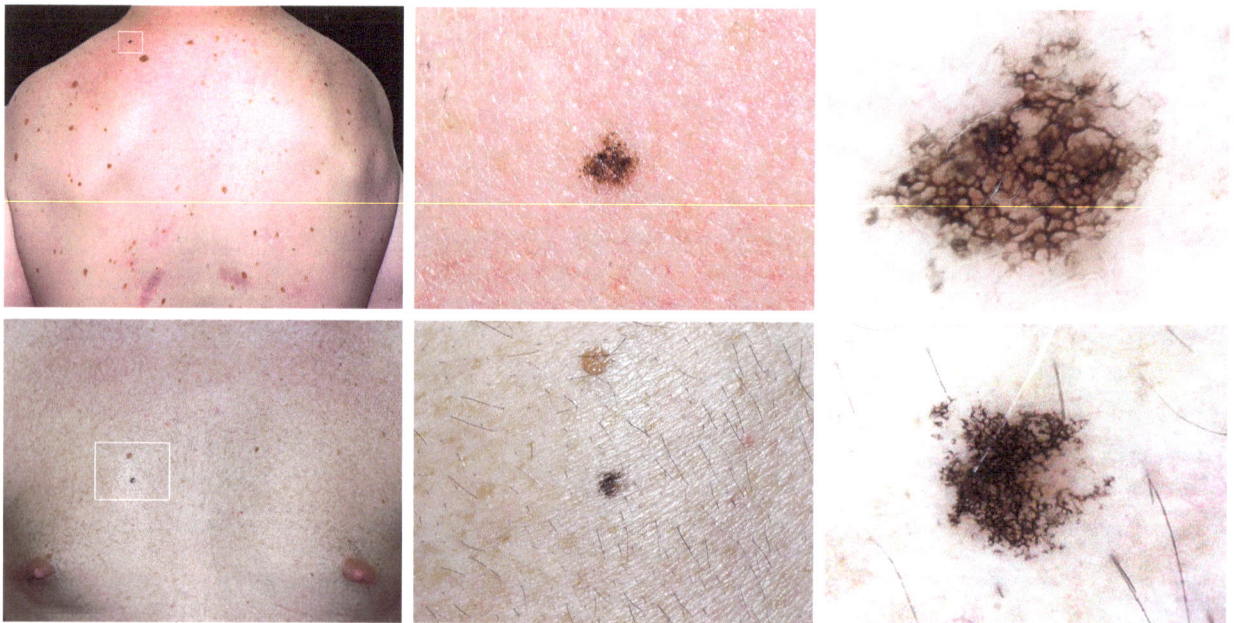

Figure 3.47: Ink-spot lentigo.
Two typical examples of "ink-spot lentigo". In both cases one finds only one pattern, reticular lines, that are typically dark-brown or black. The lines end abruptly at the margin and also within the lesion some lines end abruptly.

Ink-spot lentigo		
Pattern	Colors	Clues
Typical: Reticular lines	Typical: Black or dark-brown	Typical: Reticular lines within the lesion, some interrupted, and abrupt break-off of pigmentation at the margin

Genital lentigo, labial lentigo
Regardless of whether labial or genital lentigines occur in isolation or as part of a syndrome, they are characterized by three different patterns: 1. structureless 2. curved parallel lines, and 3. circles. The pigmentation ranges from light-brown to dark-brown *(3.48)*.

Correlation between dermatoscopy and dermatopathology
The structureless pattern correlates with hyperpigmentation of basal keratinocytes in areas where rete ridges are absent or flattened (e.g. on the lip). Patterns of parallel lines and circles are probably due to the special anatomy of the epidermis on the vulva and the penis and of the transition zone between keratinizing epidermis and mucosa.

3.6.6 Pigmented basal cell carcinoma
Pigmented basal cell carcinomas have a diverse, but usually characteristic, dermatoscopic appearance, showing patterns composed only of radial lines, dots, clods and structureless zones *(3.49, 3.50)*. A common pattern and color combination is blue clods that are usually, but not always, of different sizes and shapes. This may occur in isolation or in combination with brown clods, gray, blue and/or brown dots, white structureless zones, and radial lines. All other arrangements of lines (reticular, branched, curved and parallel), as well as pseudopods and circles do not occur in basal cell carcinoma. These structures are all very strong clues against the diagnosis of basal cell carcinoma. The pigmentation of basal cell carcinoma is caused by melanin. The pigmented tumor cell aggregates of basal cell carcinoma appear brown or gray when they are superficial, and blue when they lie deeper. An orange-colored structureless area correlates with an erosion or ulcer coated with serum crusts. Structureless zones are usually central and are skin-colored or white. Clues include peripheral radial lines, seen segmentally (as opposed to occupying the entire circumference). These radial lines may be thin or thick and nearly always have a common base. Radial lines may also converge at a central hyperpigmented dot or clod. These latter structures may be seen centrally as well as peripherally. Both these patterns of radial lines constitute very strong clues to the diagnosis of basal cell carcinoma.
Blue clods constitute a relatively specific feature, not only as a pattern, but also as a clue (when only one or two blue clods are present).
The pattern of vessels in basal cell carcinoma (both pigmented and non-pigmented) is an important clue. The typical vessel pattern of basal cell carcinoma is branched serpentine vessels that originate from a thick

stem (branched pattern of vessels). However, while this pattern is common in nodular basal cell carcinomas it is usually absent in superficial basal cell carcinomas, which are characterized by a polymorphous pattern of vessels consisting of thin, serpentine vessels that are not branched, and occasionally coiled vessels. Reticular lines and vessels as dots are not seen in basal cell carcinoma and when seen constitute a clue against the diagnosis. Ulceration, which is relatively common in basal cell carcinoma can induce the full variety of polymorphous vessel types including dot vessels, but a pattern of dot vessels is not expected.

Correlation between dermatoscopy and dermatopathology
Blue, gray and brown clods correspond to pigmented tumor cell aggregates. When they are located deep they appear gray or blue. In superficial location they are brown. Radial lines with a common base and radial lines that converge in a central clod arise when several epithelial tumor strands originate from one follicular structure. The histopathological correlate of skin-colored or white structureless zones is the fibrous stroma. In sclerosing basal cell carcinoma, this stroma may constitute most of the lesion. Orange clods or orange structureless areas are usually a sign of erosion coated with serum.

3.6.7 Squamous cell carcinoma
Invasive cutaneous squamous cell carcinoma is rarely pigmented, but pigmentation is not uncommon in both Bowen's disease and actinic keratosis.

Pigmented actinic keratosis
Pigmented actinic keratoses usually occur on the face. On dermatoscopy they may show a variety of patterns *(3.51)*. Most commonly there are gray and brown dots arranged between the follicular openings. Other common patterns of facial pigmented actinic keratosis are angulated lines, structureless and circles (grey dots arranged around follicular openings). Frequently one can find dermatoscopic criteria of a solar lentigo in addition, for example curved lines or a well demarcated, scalloped border *(3.51 bottom row)*.
The dermatoscopic pattern of gray dots between or around follicular openings can equally be seen in melanoma in situ and solar lentigo in regression (lichen planus-like keratosis). Sometimes these three entities cannot be clearly distinguished from each other on dermatoscopy alone. Clues to pigmented actinic keratosis are scale, white circles and 4 white dots in a square (4-dot clod, *3.51*). The latter clue can only be seen with polarized dermatoscopy.

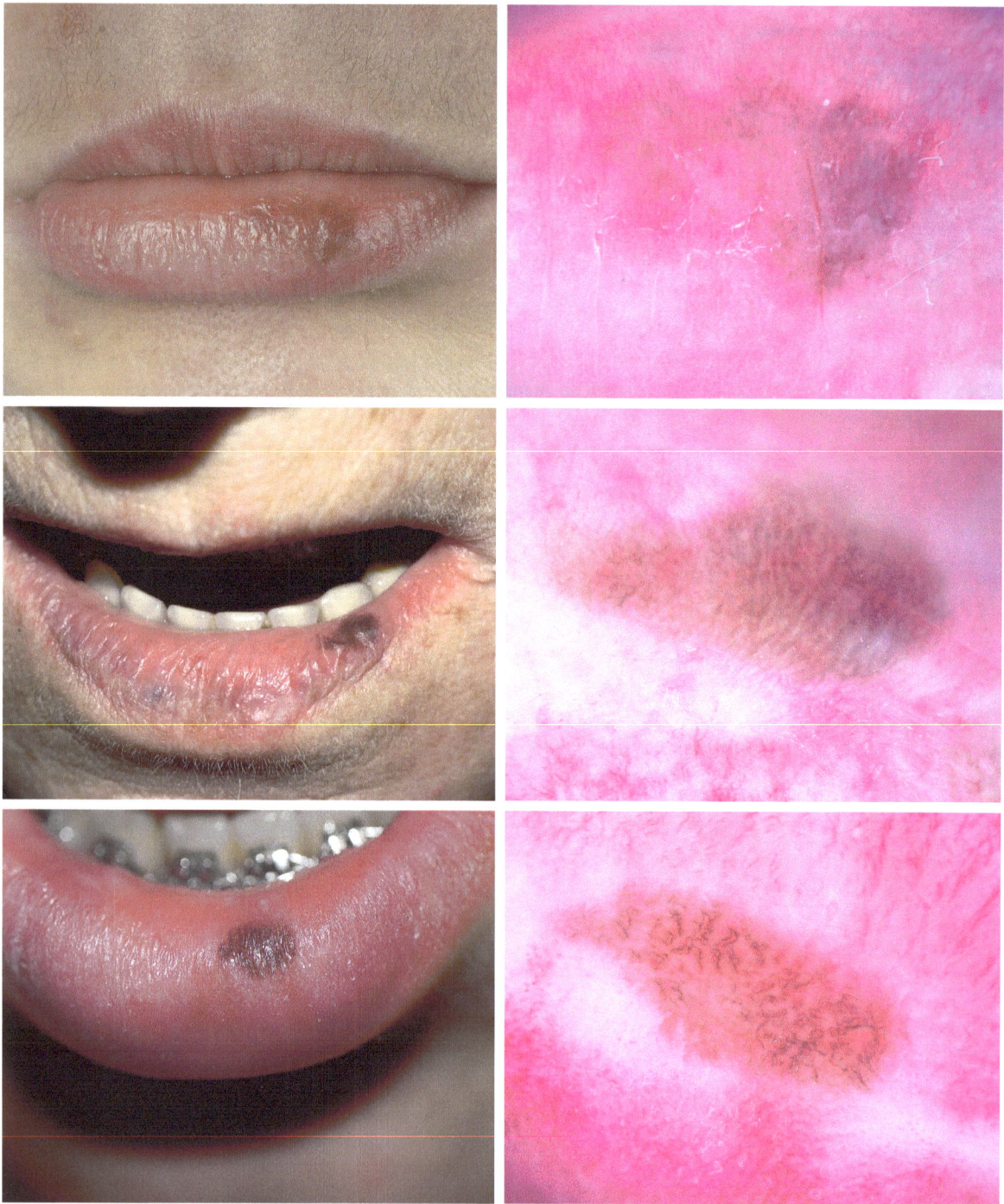

Figure 3.48: Labial lentigines.
Top row: labial lentigo with the structureless pattern. **Middle and bottom rows:** labial lentigines with two dermatoscopic patterns, brown curved lines and circles.

Genital lentigo, Labial lentigo		
Pattern	Colors	Clues
1. Structureless 2. Parallel lines, curved 3. Circles	*Typical:* Light-brown to dark-brown, rarely with gray or black	None

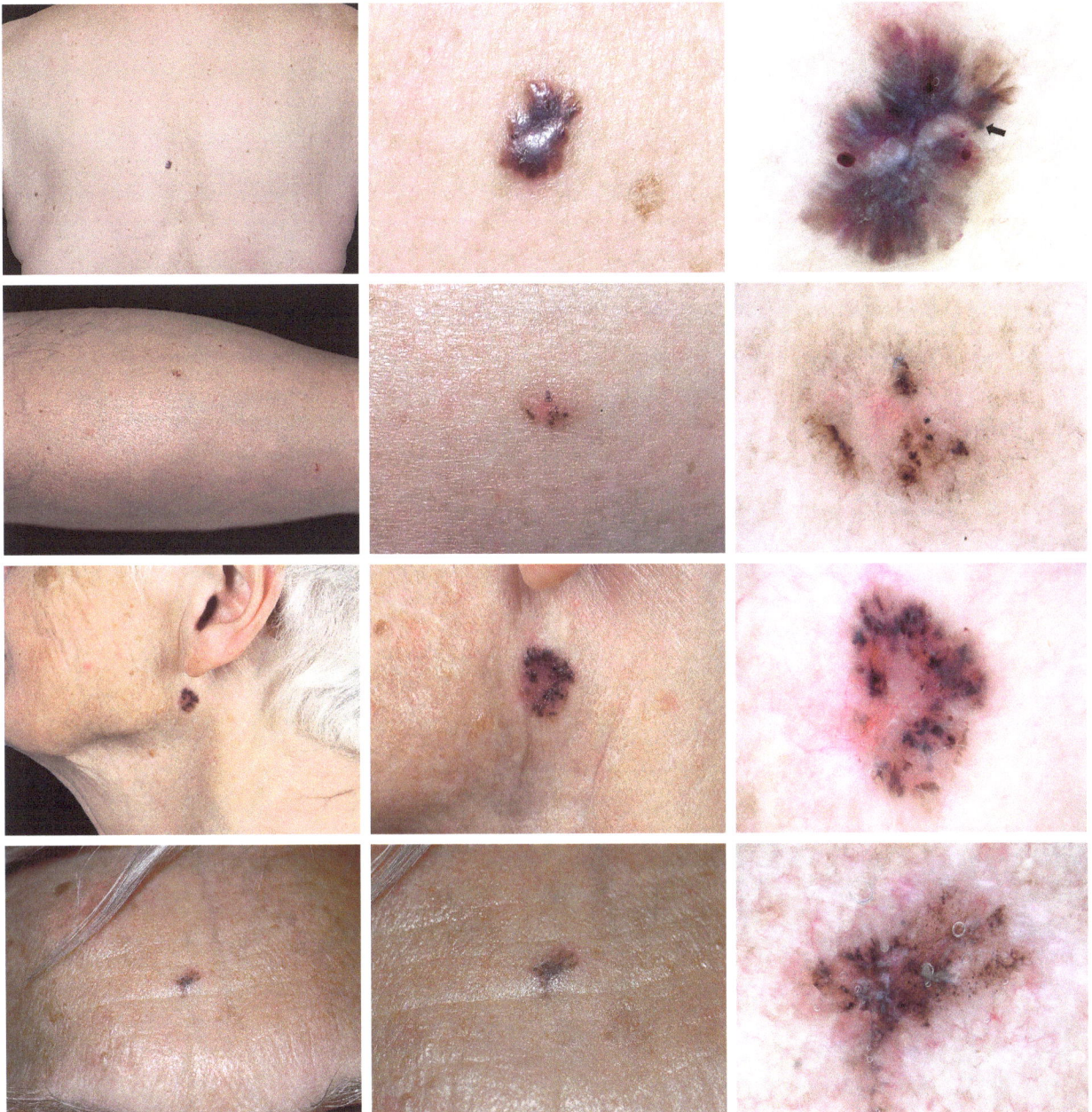

Figure 3.49: Pigmented basal cell carcinomas.
Dermatoscopy in **right column.**
Top row: *The pattern is a combination of radial lines at the periphery (white arrow) and a large structureless zone. Clues include a few blue clods (black arrow) and red clods as a sign of ulceration with hemorrhage.* **Second row:** *Two patterns, structureless (skin-colored) and clods, some of which are blue and gray. The vessels are serpentine but not branched (the definition of branched requires that the vessel of origin be thicker than the branches).* **Third row:** *In this basal cell carcinoma the clod pattern is predominant. These clods vary in size and shape, and are predominantly blue, with only a few being brown. The vessels are serpentine, with some branched.* **Bottom row:** *A typical pattern of pigmented basal cell carcinoma; clods which are blue, grey and brown.*

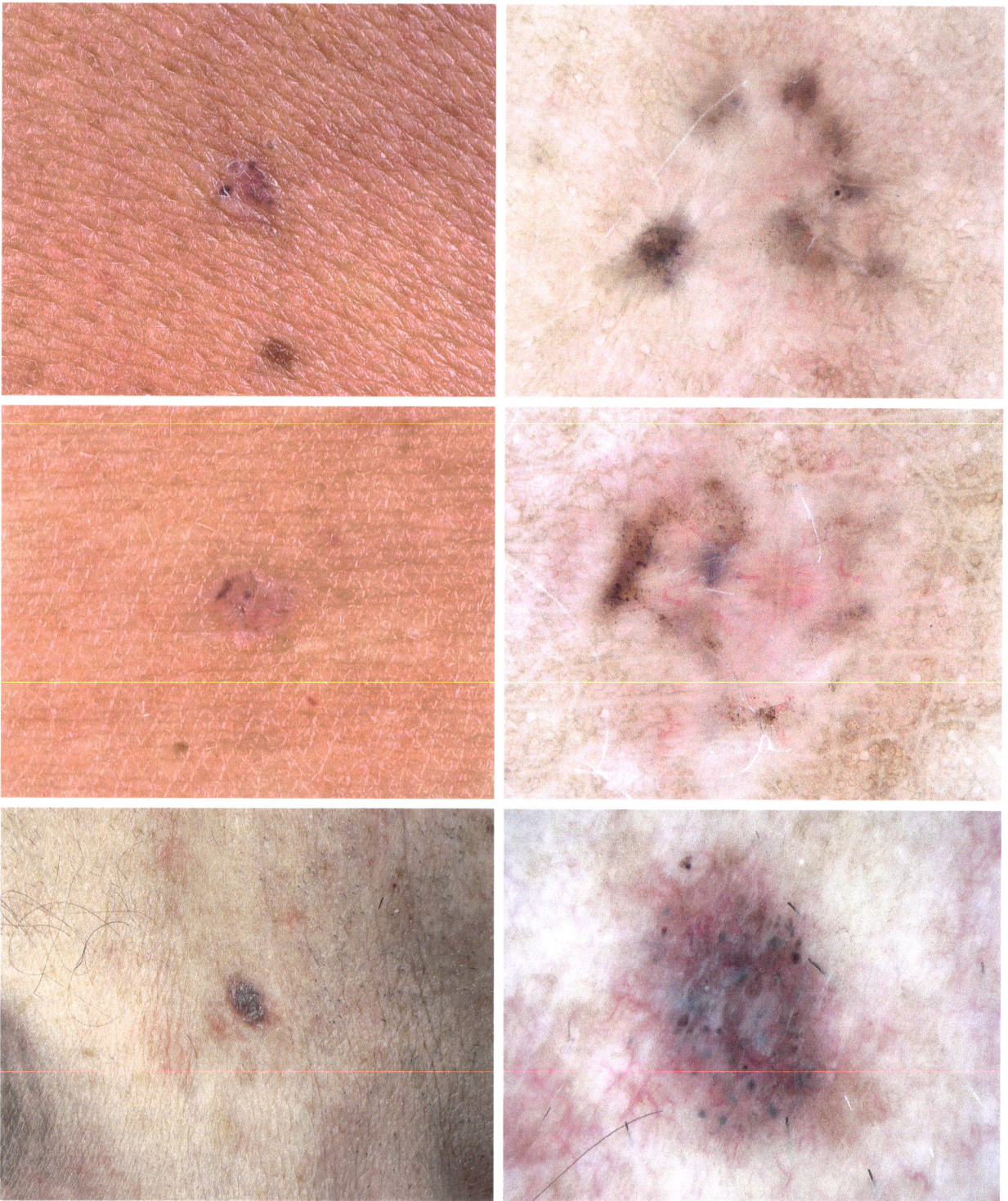

Figure 3.50: *Pigmented basal cell carcinoma.*
Top row: *This typical basal cell carcinoma on the trunk has two patterns on dermatoscopy, structureless and radial lines, combined asymmetrically. Clues to the diagnosis of basal cell carcinoma are: gray dots, the radial lines converge to a common base, a few blue clods (at 9 o'clock position) and central serpentine vessels.* **Middle row:** *Two patterns, structureless and dots, arranged asymmetrically, and serpentine vessels, yield the diagnosis of a basal cell carcinoma.* **Bottom row:** *One pattern: blue clods, and serpentine branched vessels, are typical characteristics of a pigmented basal cell carcinoma.*

Pigmented basal cell carcinoma		
Pattern	*Colors*	*Clues*
Typical:	*Typical:*	*Typical:*
1. Clods of different sizes and shapes	Clods = blue, gray, or brown	1. Peripheral radial lines with a common base
2. Peripheral radial lines (occasionally)	Dots = gray or blue, occasionally brown	2. Radial lines that converge at a central dot
3. Dots	Structureless area = skin-colored, white or	or clod
4. Structureless	orange	3. Blue or gray clods
The pattern of clods and structureless may	Radial lines = brown	4. Orange structureless area
occur alone or in combination with other		5. Blue or gray dots
patterns. Radial lines, on the other hand,		6. Central structureless area, white or
occur in basal cell carcinoma only in com-		skin-colored
bination with other patterns.		7. Branched vessels or thin serpentine vessels

Pigmented Bowen's disease

Pigmented Bowen's disease shows two common patterns. The most common is structureless and brown *(3.52)*. Less common, but more specific is an asymmetric combination of brown and/or gray dots (or more rarely small brown clods), and a hypopigmented (pink, white, or skin colored) structureless area. Vessels are coiled and usually seen in hypopigmented zones *(3.53)*. At 10x magnification these vessels may resolve as dots rather than coils. Arrangement of vessels may be linear, random or clustered. A few white clods may be seen, being a dermatoscopic sign of surface scale. The arrangement of brown and/or gray dots as radial lines is an important clue *(3.53)*. Coiled vessels may also be incorporated into these radial lines.

Reticular lines should be absent, their presence being a strong clue to consider an alternative diagnosis. If they are present they usually indicate a collision with solar lentigo. For lesions on lighter skin phototypes, the presence of black pigmentation is also a clue against the diagnosis of pigmented Bowen's disease. The dermatoscopic presentation of pigmented Bowen's disease is the same irrespective of whether it has been induced by UV radiation, chemicals such as arsenic, or, by human papilloma virus (HPV) infection as shown in *figure 3.54*.

Correlation between dermatoscopy and dermatopathology

The gray dots of pigmented actinic keratoses and Bowen's disease correspond to melanophages in the papillary dermis. The predominance of the structureless pattern in both lesions indicates the absence of rete ridges (a frequent consequence of heavy UV exposure). The circular arrangement of dots in facial pigmented actinic keratosis is due to the fact that the round openings (infundibula) of hair follicles are non-pigmented and melanophages tend to be arranged around the follicle. The brown dots in pigmented Bowen's disease correspond to accumulations of melanin in an angiocentric location in the dermal papillae this being the reason red dots in linear array may merge into pigmented dots in the same linear arrangement.

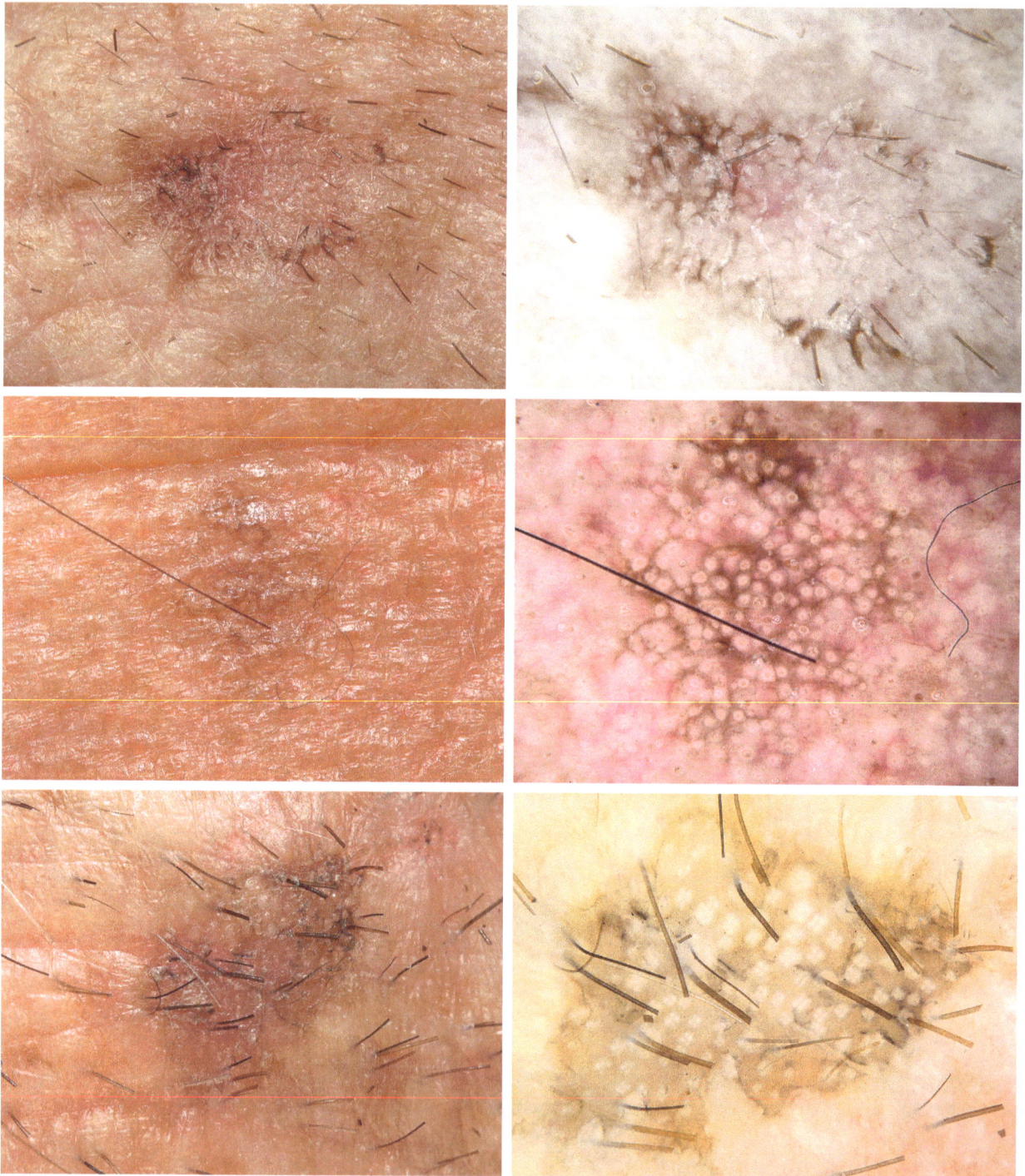

Figure 3.51: *Facial pigmented actinic keratosis.*
Dermatoscopy, **right column.** Pigmented actinic keratosis is typically located on the face. **Top row:** *Angulated lines and structureless dom-inate this actinic keratosis. The structureless pattern is interrupted by the hypopigmented follicular openings. There are some sparse gray dots and prominent scale, which is a good clue to actinic keratosis.* **Middle row:** *Angulated lines and gray dots between hypopigmented follicular openings are the patterns of this pigmented actinic keratosis. This pattern can also be seen in melanoma in situ or in lichen pla-nus-like keratosis but the clue of prominent white circles points to the diagnosis of actinic keratosis.* **Bottom row:** *Actinic keratosis with a structureless brown pattern and gray dots on dermatoscopy. The clue here is the presence of multiple 4-dot clods (4 white dots arranged in a square). These structures are only seen with polarized dermatoscopy. The sharply demarcated border indicates a collision with solar lentigo.*

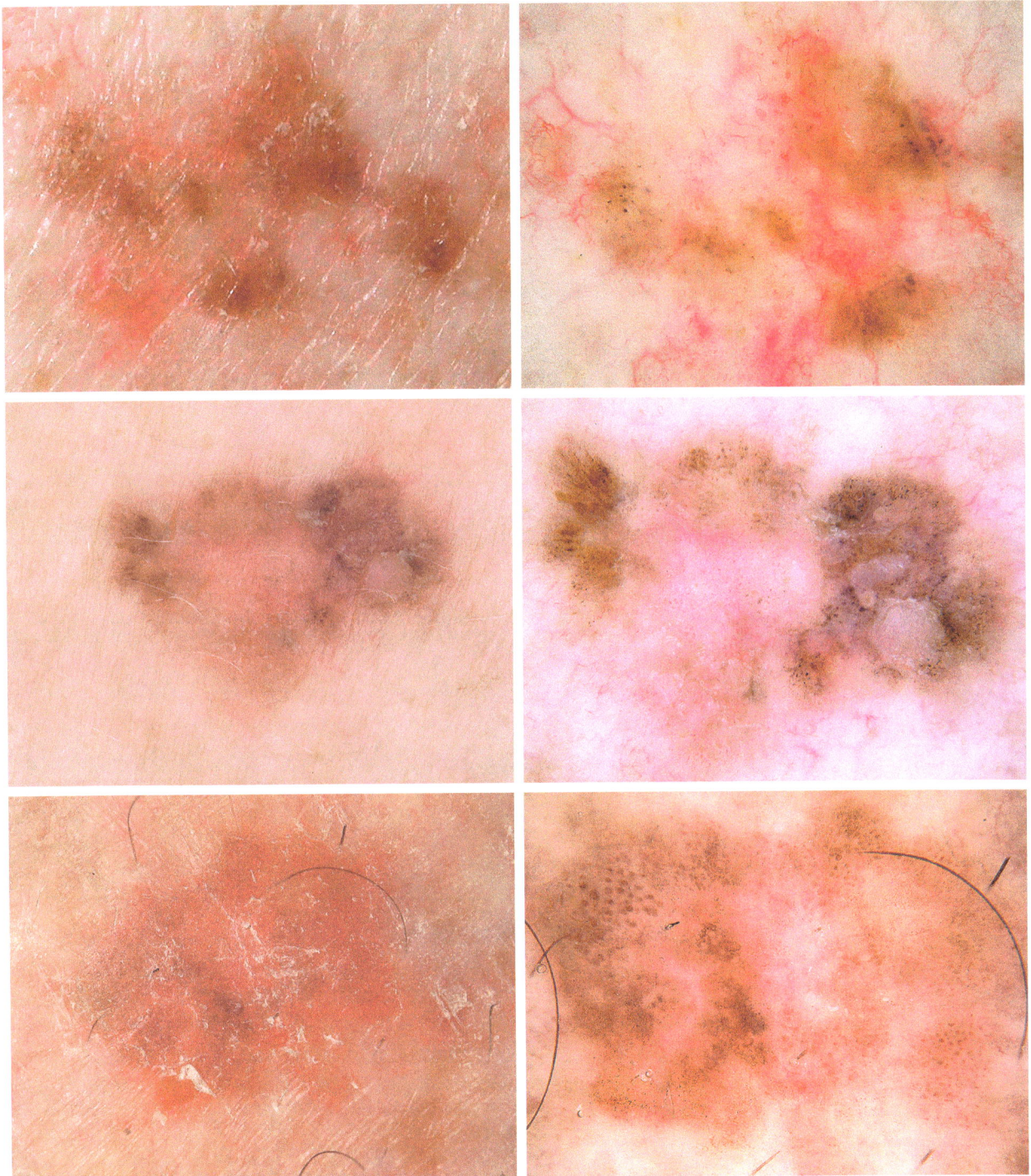

Figure 3.52: Pigmented Bowen's disease.
Dermatoscopy, **right column. Top row:** The most common pattern of pigmented Bowen's disease is structureless brown. The clue of coiled vessels allows a diagnosis of pigmented Bowen's disease. **Middle row:** On dermatoscopy there is more than one pattern (dots and structureless). The dots are gray and brown and peripherally they are, in part, arranged as radial lines (between 9 o'clock and 11 o'clock). **Bottom row:** On dermatoscopy there is more than one pattern (structureless, dots and small clods). The clue of coiled vessels is suggestive of Bowen's disease.

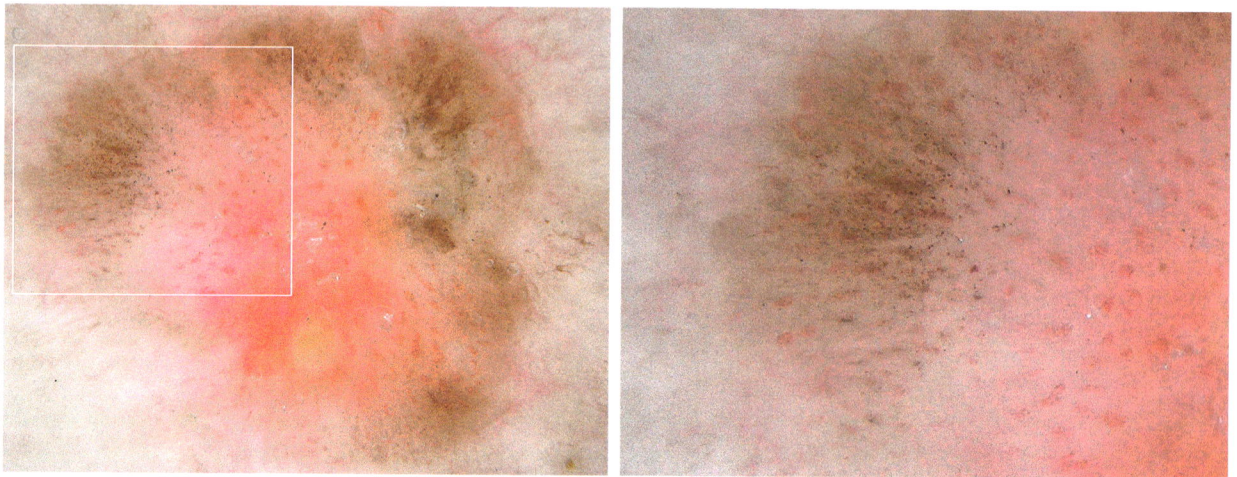

Figure 3.53: Dots and coiled vessels arranged in lines in Bowen's disease.
The dermatoscopic overview on the left shows two patterns (dots and structureless). Brown dots and coiled vessels are arranged in lines in the periphery. The close-up on the right shows a higher magnification of brown dots arranged in lines.

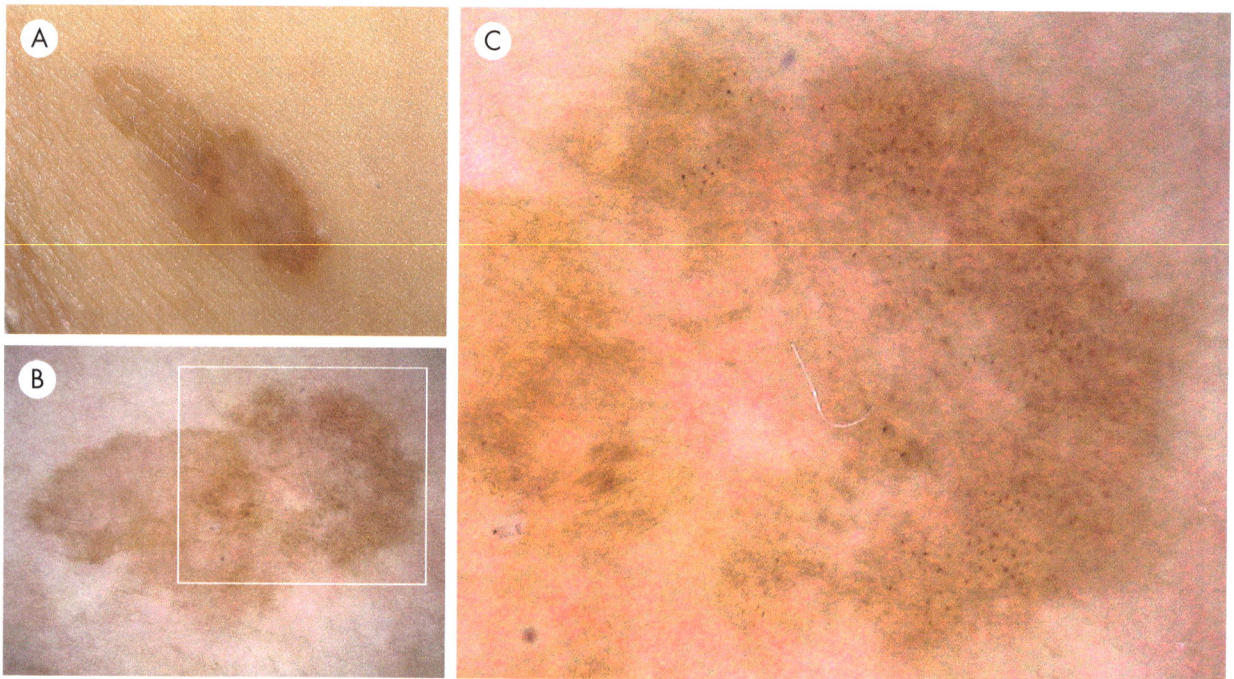

Figure 3.54: Pigmented Bowen's disease induced by human papilloma virus (HPV).
Clinical examination (**A**) reveals a brown plaque with a scalloped border. Dermatoscopically (**B**) there are two patterns (structureless and dots). The higher magnification (**C**) shows brown dots arranged in lines. This clue permits a specific diagnosis.

Pigmented actinic keratosis and pigmented Bowen's disease

	Pattern	Colors	Clues
Actinic keratosis, pigmented (face)	*Typical:* Structureless, angulated lines, dots, and occasionally circles	*Typical:* Brown (structureless part), Gray (dots)	Scale, white circles, 4-dot clod (4 white dots arranged in a square), which is visible only with polarized dermatoscopy
Bowen's disease, pigmented	*Typical:* Dots (dots arranged in lines may appear as radial lines in lower magnification), structureless	*Typical:* Brown, occasionally gray. Structureless areas = skin-colored or light-brown	*Typical:* Dots are arranged in lines radially at the periphery. Coiled vessels, clustered or arranged in lines, scale.

3.7 Characteristic features of melanocytic lesions

3.7.1 Melanocytic nevi

Clark nevus

The most common acquired nevus is the Clark nevus. While on dermatoscopy it shows remarkably diverse morphology, there are specific features which distinguish the Clark nevus both from other benign nevi on the one hand and melanoma on the other *(3.55–3.59)*. However the range of appearances of Clark nevi does overlap with both superficial congenital nevi and melanoma (especially in situ melanoma) to an extent that differential diagnosis may be quite difficult even with dermatoscopy. This does not mean that a biological zone of overlap actually exists; rather this should be viewed as a limitation of the method.

The reticular pattern usually predominates in the Clark nevus; indeed most often thin reticular lines is the only pattern *(3.55)*. In the growth phase, the reticular pattern may be combined with peripheral dots or clods *(3.56)*. These peripheral structures usually regress as the nevus matures. Clark nevi consisting solely of brown dots or small brown clods are exceptions. Less common again is the combination of the reticular pattern with a structureless zone, nearly always hyperpigmented and located centrally.

In general – as one expects in benign lesions – combinations of patterns are arranged symmetrically in the Clark nevus. The same is not true for arrangements of colors, which may be symmetrical or asymmetrical. As the proliferation of melanocytes in the epidermis is the essential architectural feature of the Clark nevus, the colors are those of melanin in the epidermis: light-brown, dark-brown and black. The commonest arrangements of colors in the Clark nevus are uniform brown pigmentation, and brown peripherally with central hyperpigmentation. This pattern of central hyperpigmention of a reticular lesion is a clue to the diagnosis of Clark nevus. Pigmentation may also be variegate, or eccentrically hyperpigmented. This pattern of Clark nevi overlaps morphologically with in situ melanoma.

Other features, especially those of melanoma, are usually absent. Occasionally one finds a few gray dots (melanophages in the dermis), erythema (a sign of inflammation) or peripheral radial lines occupying the whole circumference.

Very rarely there may be skin-colored or white reticular lines. It should be noted that grey dots and white lines are also clues to melanoma. In these rare cases it may not be possible to confidently reach a diagnosis of Clark nevus. In general, pattern and color, and the symmetry of their combinations, should be given greater importance than any single clue to melanoma. The pattern of vessels in Clark nevi is unremarkable: it usually consists of a pattern of dots occasionally interspersed with short vessels, either straight or curved. Distinguishing between a Clark nevus and a "superficial" or a "superficial and deep" congenital nevus is usually simple. Clark nevi are flat clinically while "superficial" or "superficial and deep" congenital nevi are raised. The reticular pattern is predominant in Clark nevus, the clod pattern is usually (but not always) predominant in congenital nevi. Clark nevi are either uniformly pigmented or marked by central or eccentric hyperpigmentation, while small congenital nevi are usually centrally hypopigmented or variegate (see the section on this entity). Confusion arises because most dermatopathologists do not make this distinction, describing both Clark nevi and small congenital nevi as "dysplastic" junctional or compound nevi or simply as a junctional or compound nevus.

Correlation between dermatoscopy and dermatopathology

The 2-dimensional horizontal projection of the 3-dimensional rete ridges causes the characteristic reticular pattern on the surface of the skin. The pigmented lines correspond to vertically arranged rete ridges while the hypopigmented center represents the dermal papillae. The brown pigmentation of lines is primarily due to deposits of melanin in basal keratinocytes. Often the melanocytes themselves are not sufficiently pigmented to be visible on dermatoscopy. If they are, they appear as brown dots or clods that correspond to smaller or larger nests of melanocytes at the dermoepidermal junction.

"Superficial" and "superficial and deep" congenital nevi

Like Clark nevi, "superficial" and "superficial and deep" congenital nevi are extremely diverse morphologically, but have specific clues that usually make diagnosis straightforward. Again, it should be remembered that in this context the term "congenital" does not necessarily mean that the nevus was visible at birth. As mentioned in chapter 2, "superficial" and "superficial and deep" congenital nevi have a different architecture to Clark nevi and are usually easy to distinguish from the latter by histopathology.[2] As we have described above, this is also true – with certain limitations – of dermatoscopy. While the reticular pattern is predominant in Clark nevus, the clod pattern is predominant in congenital nevi *(3.60, 3.61)*. The clod pattern occurs either alone

---

2 Regrettably, this distinction is not made by many dermatopathologists. Both types of nevi are termed "dysplastic compound nevi" or "compound nevi".

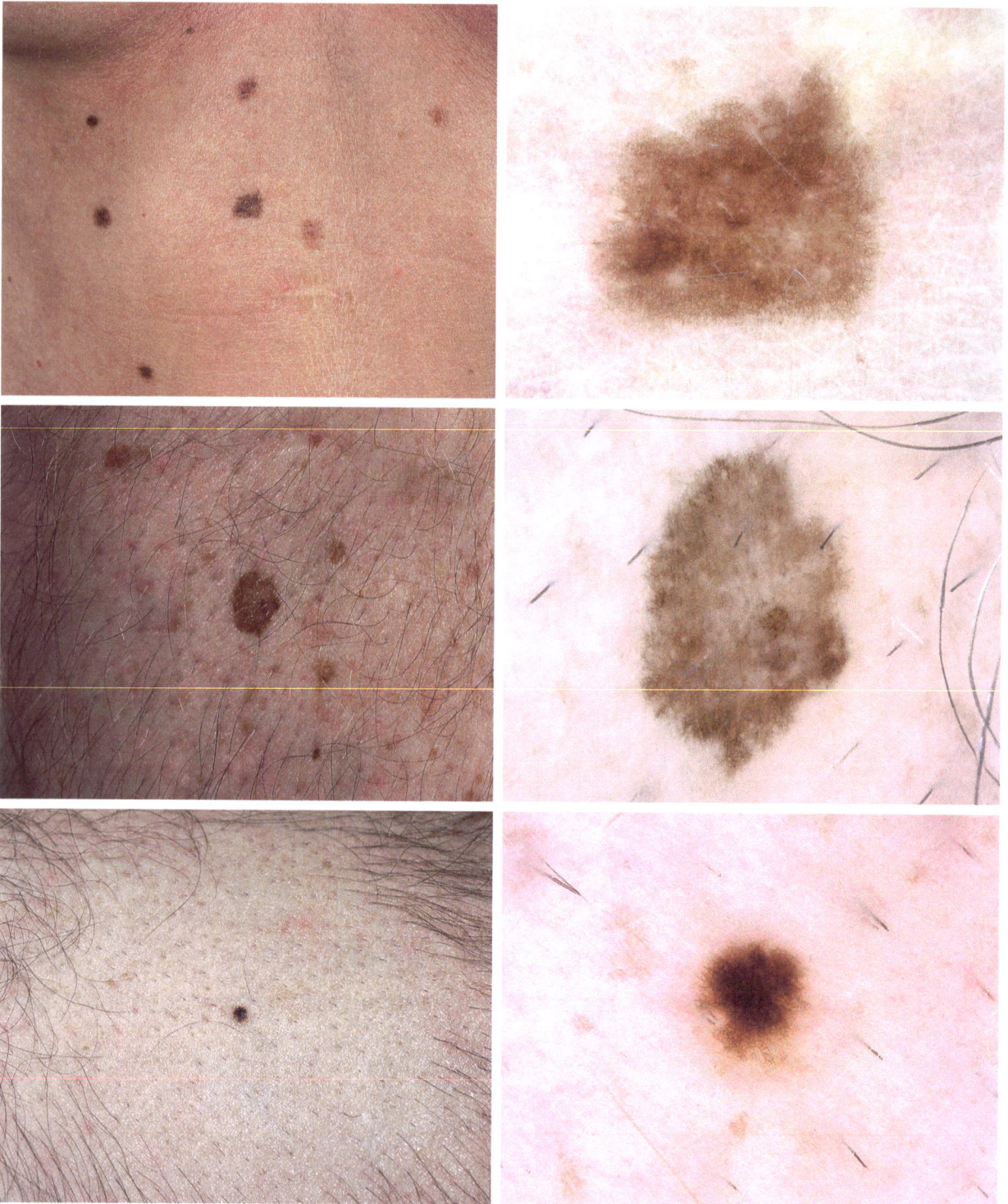

Figure 3.55: Typical Clark nevi.
Dermatoscopy **right column. Top row, right:** *One pattern, reticular, uniformly light-brown.* **Middle row, right:** *One pattern, reticular, uniformly light-brown.* **Bottom row, right:** *One pattern, reticular, centrally hyperpigmented.*

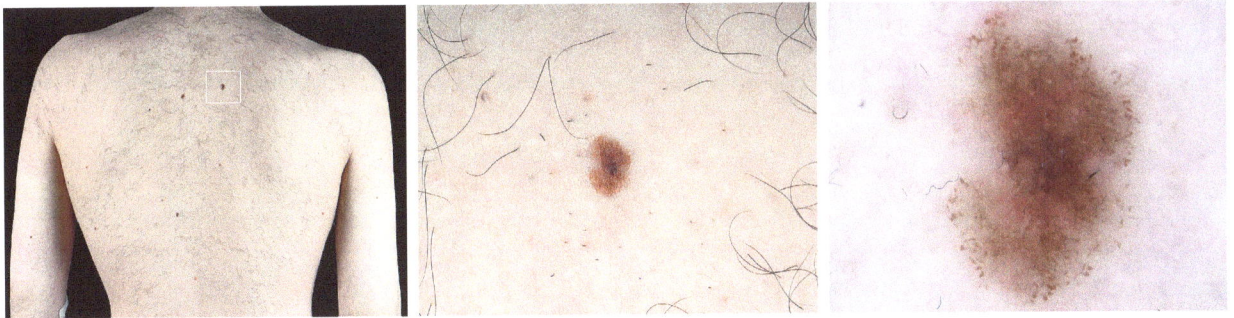

Figure 3.56: Growing Clark nevus.
On dermatoscopy a Clark nevus in the growing phase is typically seen as a symmetrical combination of the reticular pattern in the center and clods peripherally.

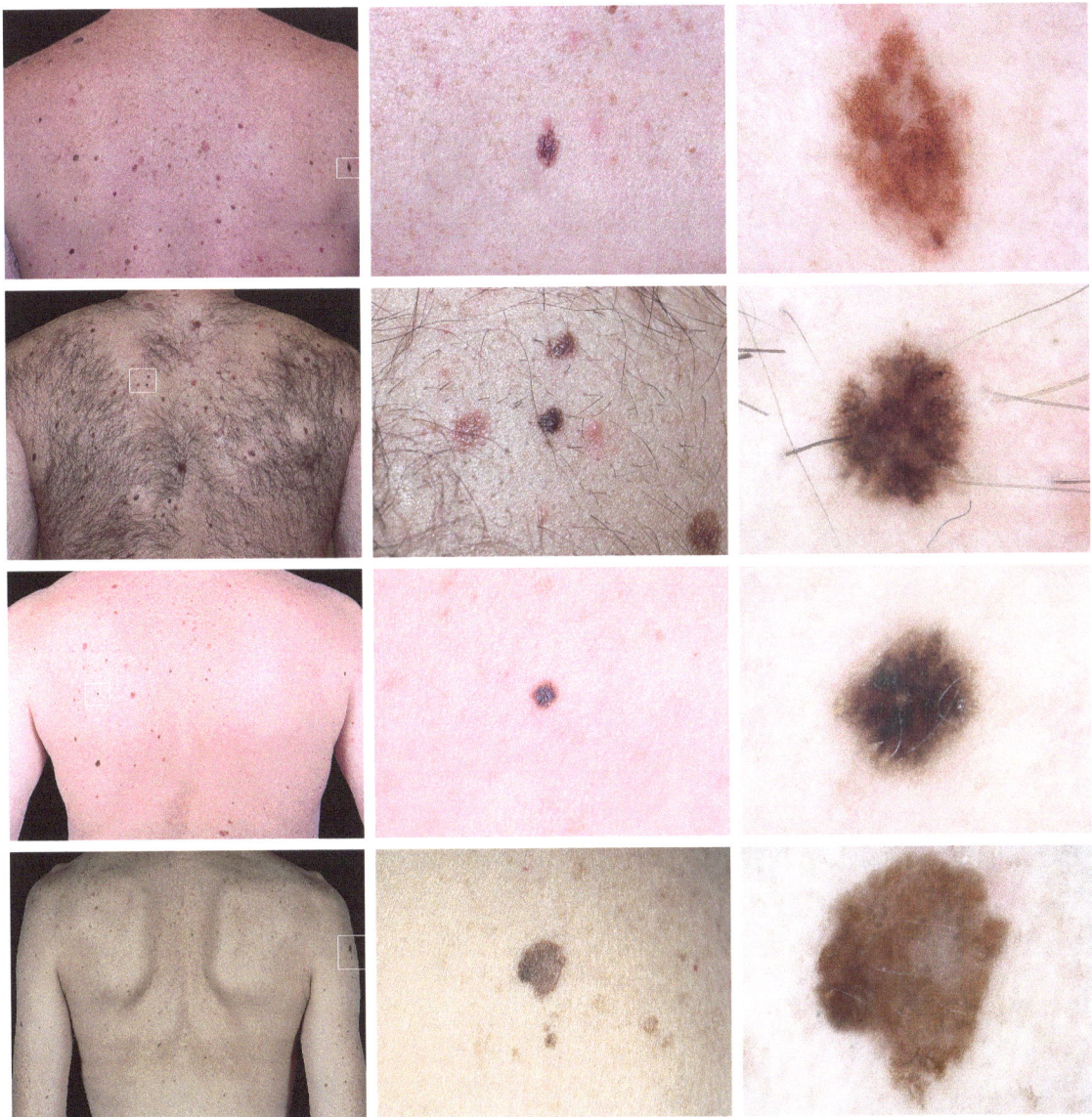

Figure 3.57: Clark nevi on the trunk.
Dermatoscopy, **right column. Top row:** One pattern, reticular lines, light-brown (the hypopigmented structureless area is too small to be interpreted as a pattern). **Second row:** One pattern, reticular, variegate. **Third row:** More than one pattern, reticular peripherally, structureless centrally, symmetrically combined, and central hyperpigmentation. **Bottom row:** One pattern, reticular, eccentric hyperpigmentation.

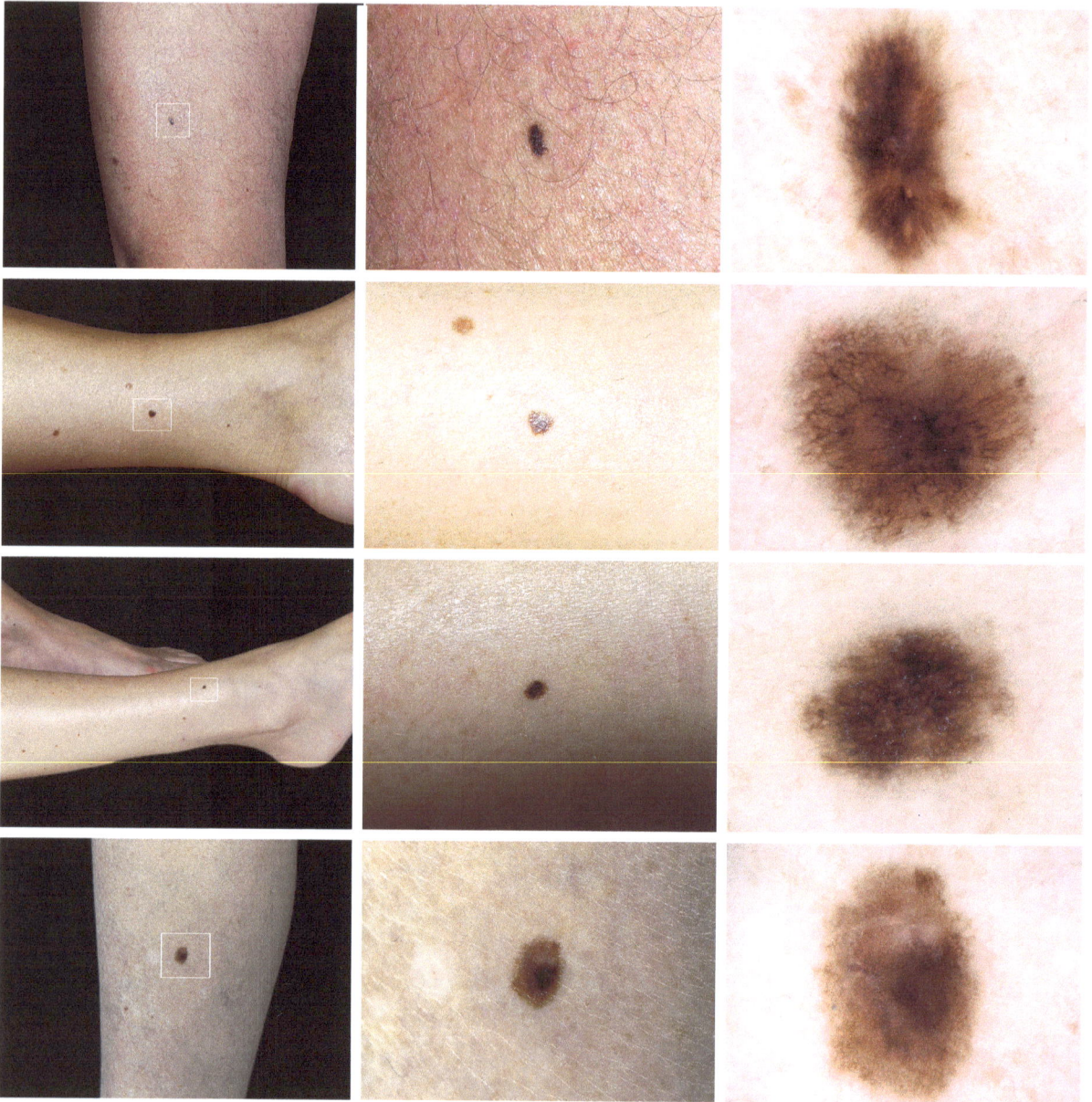

Figure 3.58: Clark nevi on the extremities.
Dermatoscopy, **right column. Top row:** More than one pattern, reticular and radial lines peripherally, structureless in the center. The patterns are symmetrically arranged and there is central hyperpigmentation. **Second row:** One pattern, reticular, centrally hyperpigmented. **Third row:** One pattern, reticular, centrally hyperpigmented. **Bottom row:** More than one pattern, reticular and dots, asymmetrically combined, eccentric hyperpigmentation.

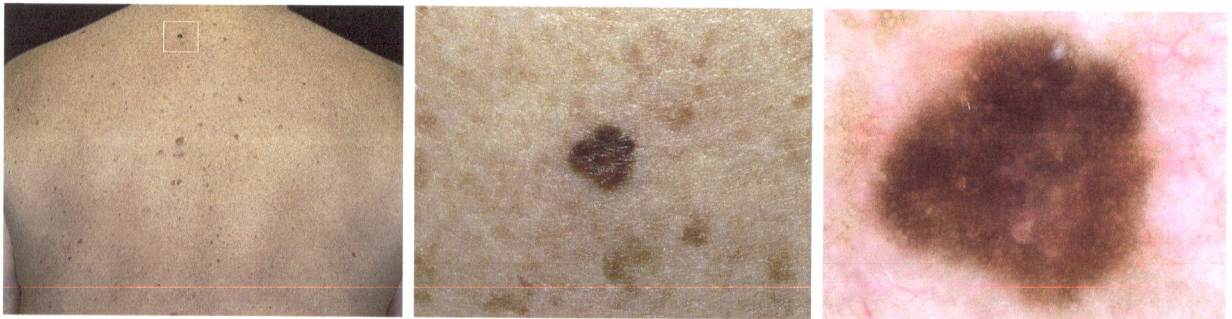

Figure 3.59: Clark nevus.
Clinically one finds an irregularly pigmented, dark-brown lesion. The differential diagnosis is melanoma versus Clark nevus. On dermatoscopy there is one pattern, namely reticular lines, and eccentric hyperpigmentation, but no unequivocal clue to melanoma. Therefore the diagnosis is Clark nevus.

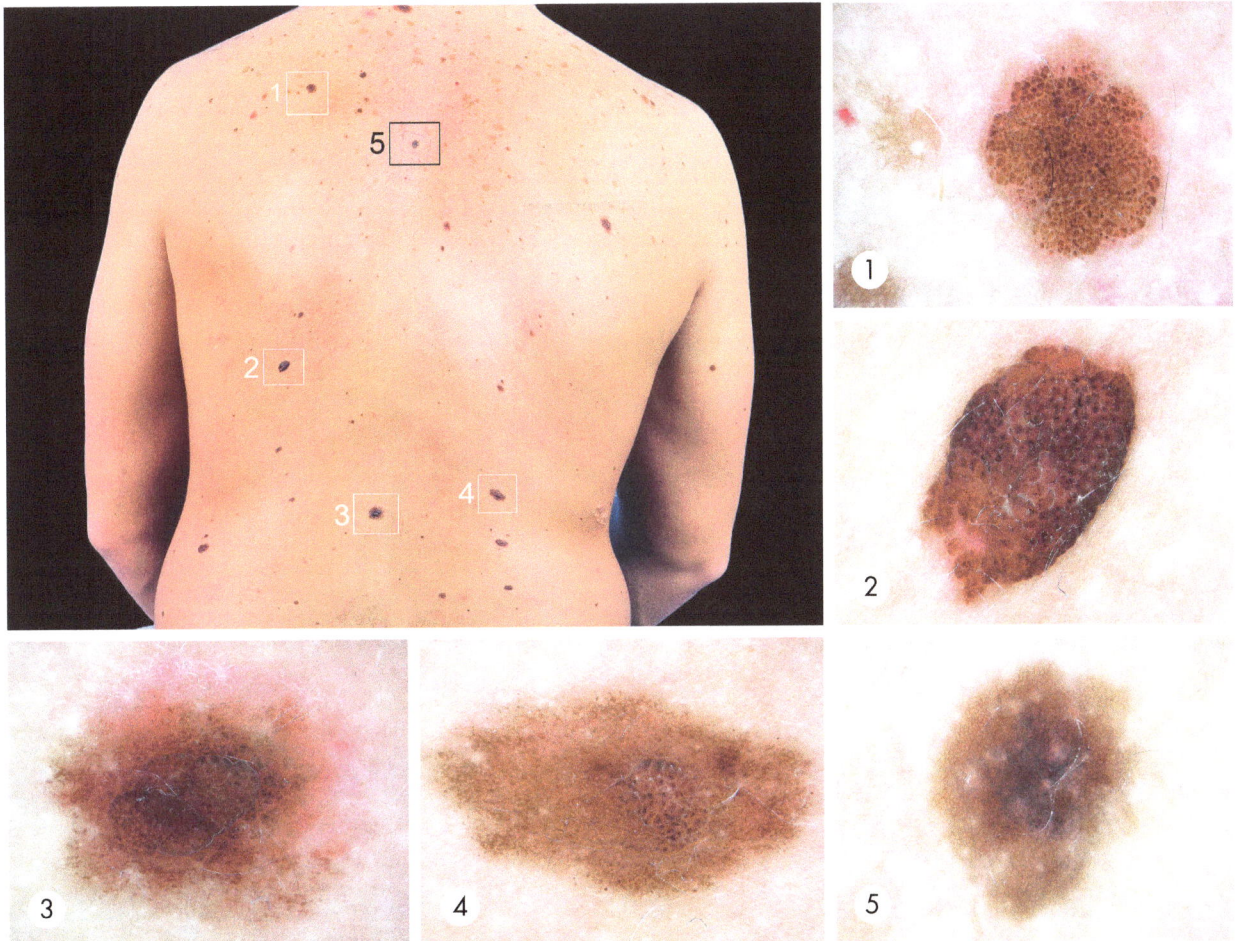

Figure 3.60: Congenital nevi and Clark nevi.
"Superficial and deep" congenital nevi and Clark nevi frequently occur together, as in this patient. While "superficial and deep" congenital nevi are marked by a clod pattern on dermatoscopy (lesions **1 to 3**), the Clark nevus shows a reticular pattern with central hyperpigmentation (lesion **5**). Lesion **4** has two patterns, namely reticular peripherally and clods centrally. Thus, it is also a "superficial and deep" congenital nevus.

Clark nevus: Characteristic features

Pattern	Colors	Clues
Typical: 1. Reticular 2. Reticular with dots or clods (in cases of growing Clark nevi these are typically peripheral). *Occasional:* 1. Reticular peripherally and structureless centrally, central hyperpigmentation 2. Combination of reticular lines and/or clods with a skin-colored structureless area *Rare:* 1. Only brown dots or small brown clods 2. Brown circles (instead of reticular lines) 3. Brown structureless Patterns are usually combined symmetrically.	*Typical:* Uniform light-brown or various shades of brown with central hyperpigmentation *Occasional:* Variegate, various shades of brown, or eccentric hyperpigmentation	*Typical:* Reticular lines, usually thin, small dots or clods of the same size and nearly the same shape; peripheral dots or clods are larger in the early phase of growth *Occasional:* When visible, usually a monomorphous vascular pattern with vessels as dots, occasional erythema *Rare:* Peripheral radial lines over the entire circumference, black dots on reticular lines

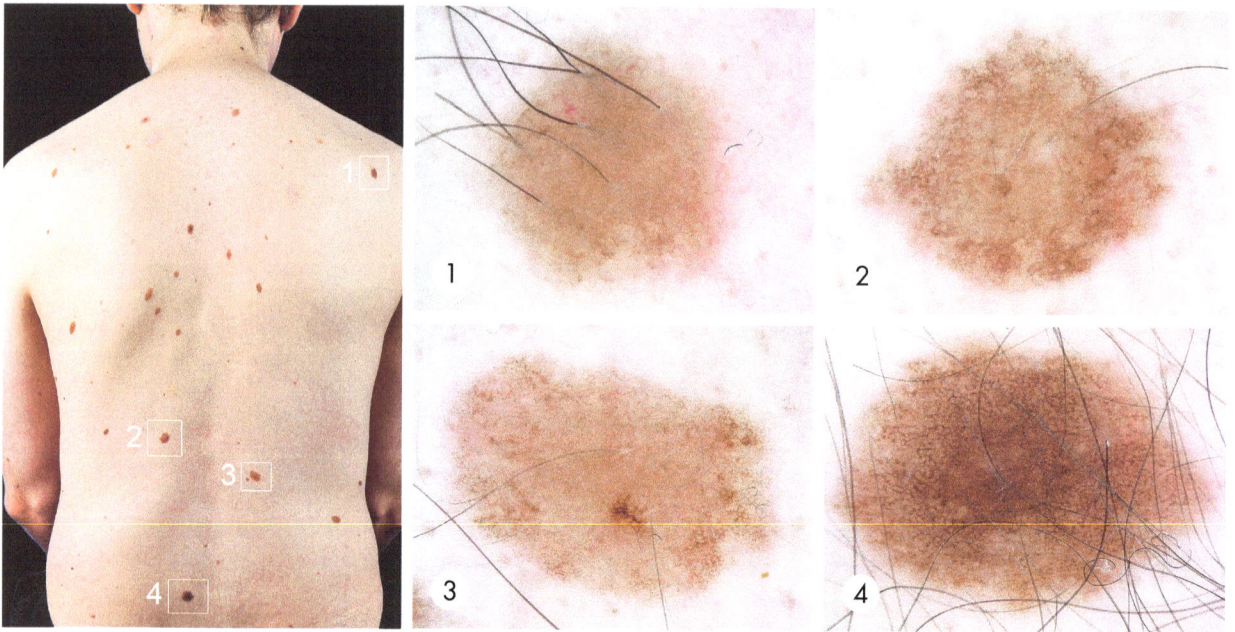

Figure 3.61: *A patient with several "superficial and deep" congenital nevi.*
On dermatoscopy one finds various patterns: (1) Structureless and brown (2) Reticular at the periphery, structureless in the center (3) Reticular at the periphery, structureless in the center (4) Reticular (differential diagnosis: Clark nevus).

"Superficial" and "superficial and deep" congenital nevi: Characteristic features

Pattern	Colors	Clues
Typical: 1. Only clods 2. Reticular lines (or branched lines) and clods; the clods are larger than those in Clark nevus, typically light-brown or skin-colored, and usually in the center of the lesion. *Occasional:* 1. Reticular (or branched) lines peripherally and structureless centrally, central hypopigmentation 2. Combination of three patterns: reticular lines, clods and a (usually skin-colored) structureless area *Rare:* Only reticular or branched, or only structureless. All combinations of patterns are usually symmetrical.	*Typical:* Uniformly brown, skin-colored and brown (centrally hypopigmented) or, when reticular, variegate	All of these are only occasionally present: 1. Terminal hair 2. Large polygonal, skin-colored to light-brown clods in the center 3. White dots (milia) 4. Orange clods 5. Small brown clods, dots or vessels as dots in a hypopigmented center of reticular lines 6. Curved lines 7. Small and closely adjacent circles

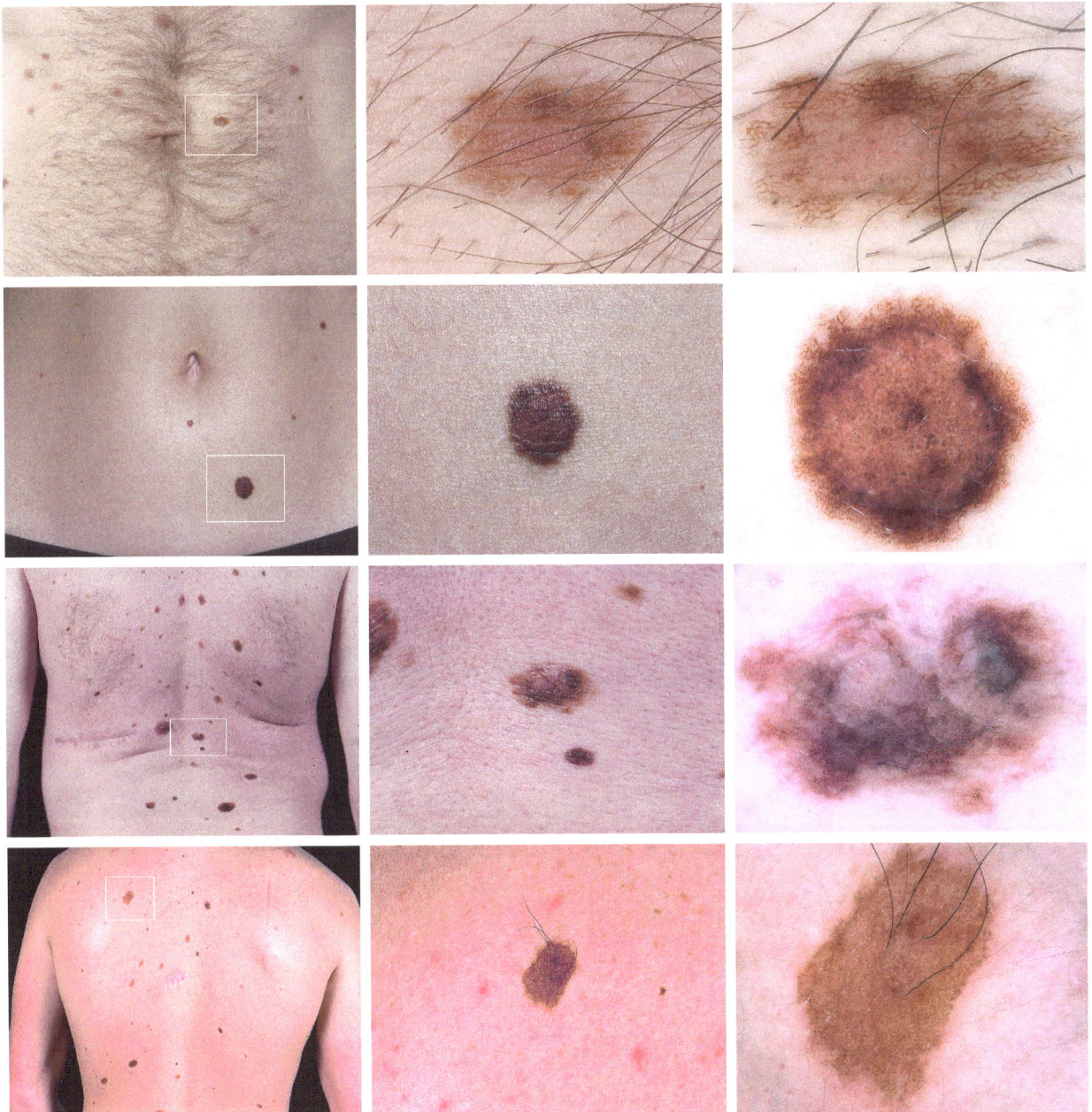

Figure 3.62: "Superficial and deep" congenital nevi.
Dermatoscopy, **right column. Top row:** More than one pattern, symmetrical, structureless in the center, reticular at the periphery. In contrast to most Clark nevi, which show central hyperpigmentation, this "superficial and deep" congenital nevus shows central hypopigmentation. **Second row:** More than one pattern, symmetrical, clods centrally, reticular peripherally. **Third row:** More than one pattern, large skin-colored clods in the center, reticular and dots at the periphery, relatively symmetrical. **Bottom row:** One pattern, clods, a specific clue is the excess number of terminal hairs.

or in combination with other patterns, usually reticular or less often structureless. When clods are combined with the reticular pattern, the clods are usually found centrally and not, as in the (growing) Clark nevus, peripherally. Occasionally, congenital nevi with exclusively reticular or curved lines may be found, usually on the extremities. As in Clark nevus, combinations of patterns are usually symmetrical in both "superficial" and "superficial and deep" congenital nevi.

A further clue to "superficial" and "superficial and deep" congenital nevi, especially the more common clod or clod-reticular types is that they are either uniformly brown or hypopigmented in the center. The less common purely reticular types, on the other hand, often have variegate pigmentation. The dermatoscopic presentation of "superficial" and "superficial and deep" congenital nevi is more protean than that of Clark nevi *(3.62)*.
The most specific clue to the diagnosis of congenital nevus is terminal hairs, in greater numbers, or longer and darker, than on surrounding skin. This clue is, however, seen only in a minority of cases. Some "superficial" or "superficial and deep" congenital nevi show dermatoscopic features of seborrheic keratosis, most often white dots or clods, and occasionally orange clods between skin-colored clods. Occasionally there is also peri-infundibular hyperpigmentation (brown circles around the infundibula). Other less specific dermatoscopic clues are clods or vessels as dots located in the center of reticular lines, curved lines (primarily in combination with reticular or branched lines), and densely arranged aggregations of small circles.
Occasionally it may be difficult to distinguish between a Clark nevus and a congenital nevus on dermatoscopy, as the reticular pattern may occur alone or in combination

with other patterns in both types of nevus. There also is a morphological zone of overlap with melanoma. Clues to melanoma, especially gray dots and white reticular lines, may be found in some congenital nevi. Occasionally, histopathology is required to make this distinction.

Correlation of dermatoscopy and dermatopathology
The histological correlate of reticular lines was explained in the section on Clark nevi. Brown clods correspond to nests of melanocytes at the dermo-epidermal junction, which are usually larger in congenital nevi than in the Clark nevus. Skin-colored clods arise due to lightly pigmented or non-pigmented nests of melanocytes in the papillary dermis.
The widened dermal papillae filled with melanocytes cause the epidermis to protrude outward, which gives rise in metaphorical terminology of a cobblestone pattern. When the nests of melanocytes are somewhat deeper, i.e. below the dermal papillae, the surface of the is seen as a skin-colored or light-brown structureless area.

Combined congenital nevi
Combined congenital nevi are those showing features of both a "blue nevus" and either a "superficial" or "superficial and deep" congenital nevus *(3.63)*. The dermatoscopy is exactly what one would expect from such a combination. In most cases there is a central blue structureless area (blue nevus), surrounded by brown reticular lines or brown clods (or both). If the blue structureless area is located eccentrically rather than centrally, it is difficult to distinguish a combined nevus from a melanoma. Occasionally, instead of a blue structureless area one sees blue clods, which rarely may be distributed over the entire lesion.

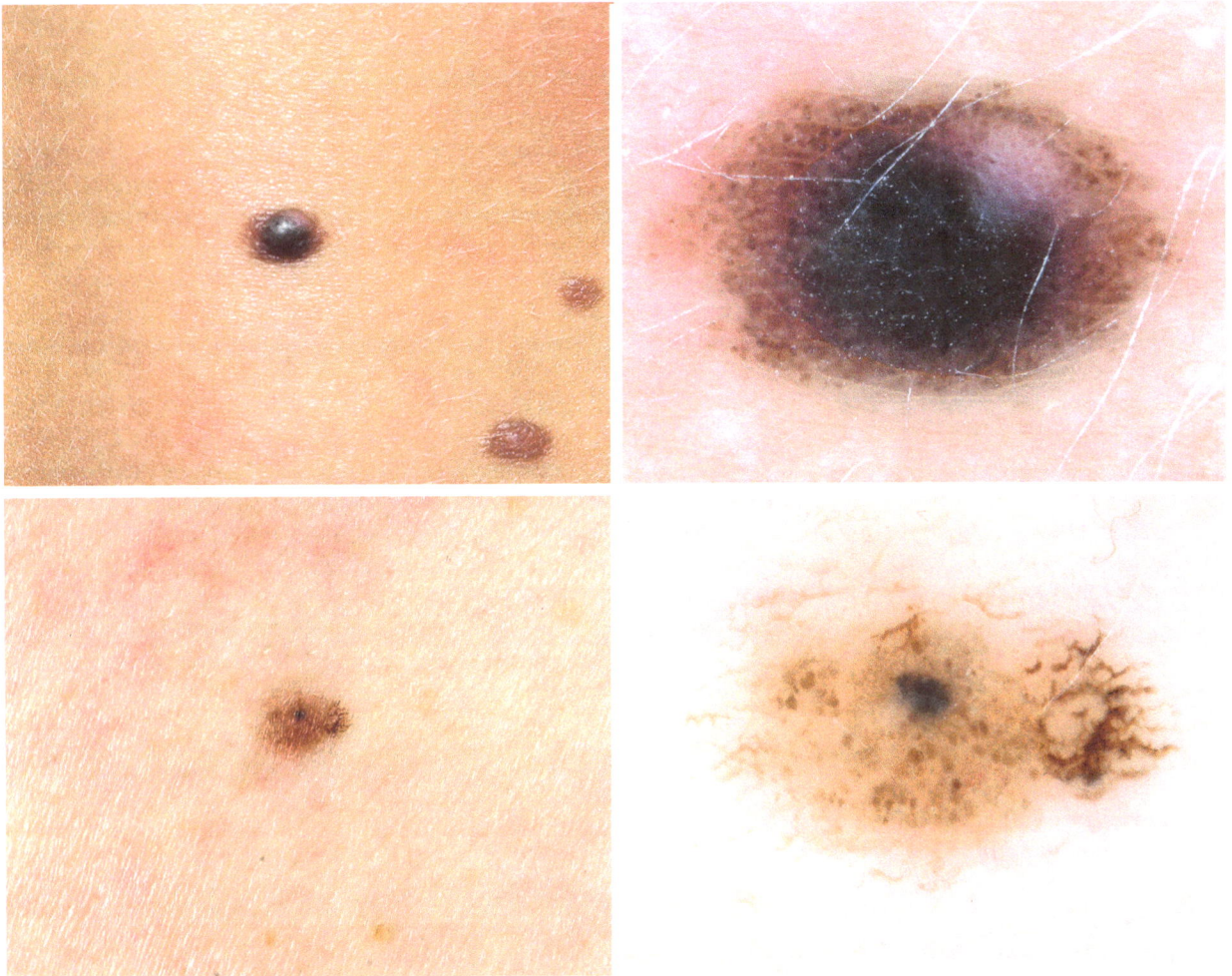

Figure 3.63: Combined congenital nevi.
Dermatoscopy, **right column. Top:** *More than one pattern, symmetrical, clods peripherally, structureless blue in the center.* **Bottom:** *More than one pattern, branched lines and clods peripherally, structureless blue in the center, relatively symmetrical.*

Combined congenital nevi		
Pattern	Colors	Clues
Typical: Structureless, reticular lines, clods Combinations of patterns are usually symmetrical	*Typical:* Structureless area: blue Reticular lines and clods: brown *Occasional:* Blue clods	The structureless blue area is in the center.

Correlation between dermatoscopy and dermatopathology
Refer to the above sections regarding blue nevi and "superficial" or "superficial and deep" congenital nevi.

Recurrent nevus

On dermatoscopy one typically sees a hypopigmented (lighter than surrounding skin) structureless zone, corresponding to the scar after excision *(3.64)*. The recurrent nevus is within this area. Common patterns seen are peripheral radial lines, pseudopods, and brown clods of different sizes. Radial lines and pseudopods are of course clues to melanoma. In contrast to local recurrence of a melanoma, the recurrent nevus usually does not extend beyond the scar.

Correlation between dermatoscopy and dermatopathology
The radial lines and pseudopods correspond to fascicles of pigmented melanocytes at the dermo-epidermal junction.

Spitz nevus

The "classical" Spitz nevus as described by Sophie Spitz is non-pigmented or only lightly pigmented. On dermatoscopy one most often finds skin-colored or light-brown clods and perpendicular white lines *(3.65)*. Alternatively when the lines seen between the clods are lighter than the normal skin, they are termed white reticular lines. This pattern is also seen in some melanomas and dermatofibromas. In non-pigmented or lightly pigmented Spitz nevi one may find vessels as dots.
The patterns seen in pigmented Spitz nevi are brown clods peripherally; centrally gray or blue-gray clods or structureless *(3.66 A, B)*. This central area is occasionally interspersed with thick, light-gray reticular lines and/or polarizing-specific white lines.
Spitz nevi are nearly always easily distinguished from Reed nevi. Clinically Spitz nevi are nodular or papular and Reed nevi are flat or only slightly raised. Dermatoscopically, the patterns of established Reed nevi are pseudopods or radial lines. Only in the early stages of growth may one see clods in Reed nevi. *(3.66 C, D)*.

Correlation between dermatoscopy and dermatopathology
Like the previously described nevi, brown clods correspond to pigmented melanocyte nests in the epidermis. White lines are most likely due to zones of fibrosis in the papillary dermis. The gray reticular lines in the center of pigmented Spitz nevi are probably due to the combination of relatively heavily pigmented nests of melanocytes and acanthosis of the epidermis.

Reed nevus

Serial dermatoscopic photography shows that an early Reed nevus consists solely of dark-brown clods. The characteristic pattern of radial lines or pseudopods at the periphery only develops during subsequent growth *(3.67)*. The radial lines or pseudopods are symmetrically distributed over the entire periphery while there is a black, black-gray or dark-brown structureless area in the center, or occasionally thick, gray reticular lines. Occasionally there are black dots or clods peripherally. Once growth ceases, the radial lines and pseudopods disappear. A Reed nevus is then identical to a darkly pigmented Clark nevus with reticular lines peripherally and a structureless hyperpigmented center, or reticular lines only. One plausible theory suggests this is followed by transepidermal elimination of melanocytes and the disappearance of the nevus. Combinations of patterns in Reed nevus are usually symmetrical. If the pseudopods in a Reed nevus are only seen in some segments of the circumference, it cannot be distinguished from a melanoma dermatoscopically.

Correlation between dermatoscopy and dermatopathology
The pseudopods and radial lines at the periphery are fascicles of pigmented melanocytes at the dermo-epidermal junction that have spread centrifugally.

Blue Nevi

Most blue nevi can be diagnosed easily. As we noted in chapter 2, the term "blue nevus" includes various entities which can be distinguished by dermatopathology, but not by dermatoscopy or clinical examination. As this book is primarily focused on dermatoscopy, specific sub-classification will not be performed and the general term "blue nevus" will be used.
The dermatoscopic pattern of all blue nevi is structureless *(3.68)*. Blue nevi usually have only one color, most commonly blue or gray. (When assessing color one exercises latitude: slight variations in shade should not be interpreted as a separate color.) Occasionally one sees variegate blue and gray. Less common again are blue nevi with shades of gray and blue flanked by brown regions. It may then be difficult or even impossible to distinguish between this entity and a combined congenital nevus on dermatoscopy.
Occasionally grey lines or dots may be seen against a blue background. Applying the basic principle that

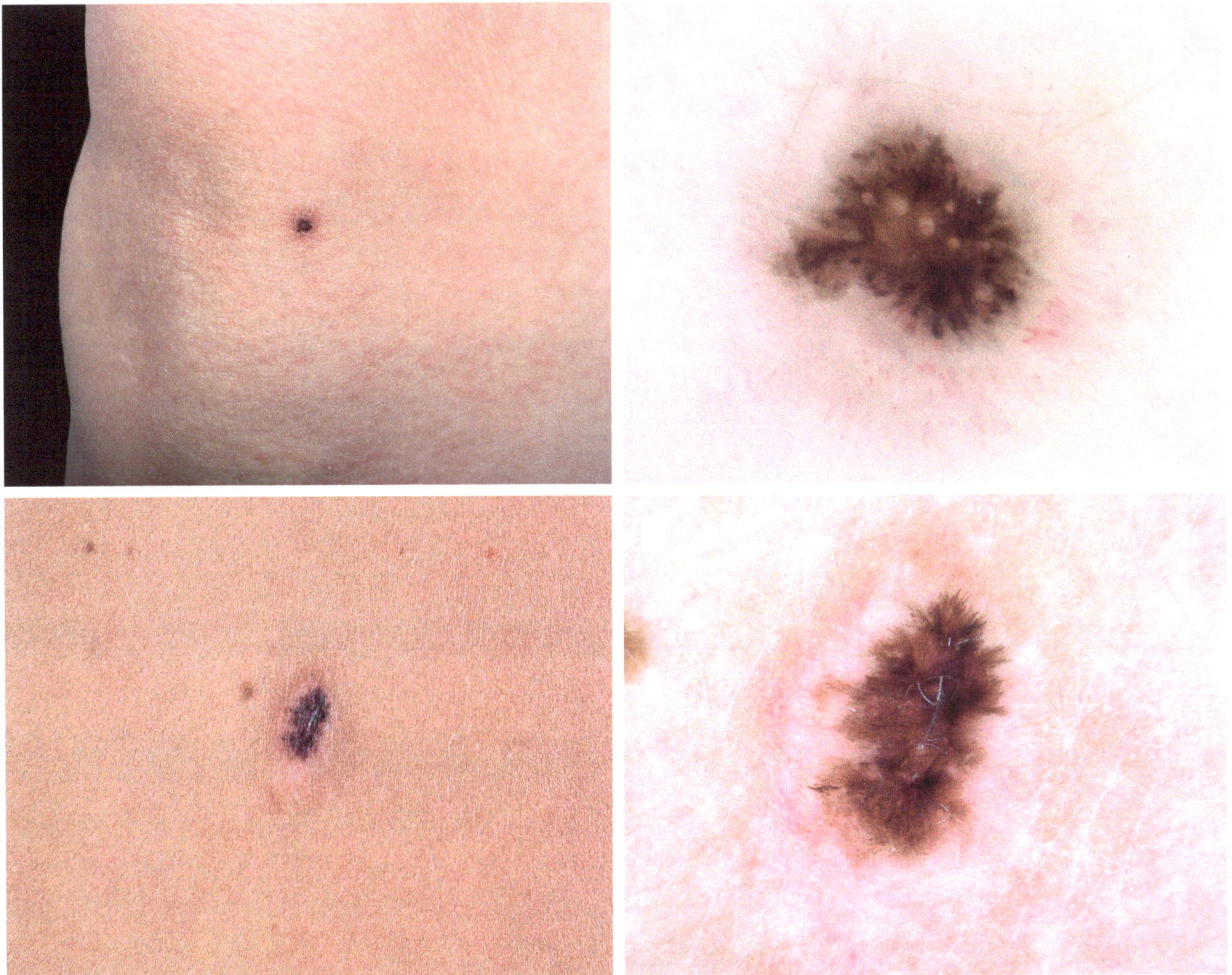

Figure 3.64: *Recurrent nevi.*
*Dermatoscopy, **right column. Top:** More than one pattern, clods and pseudopods, asymmetrical (differential diagnosis: melanoma). The pigmentation does not extend beyond the scar (skin-colored structureless area with vessels as coils and loops. **Bottom:** More than one pattern, radial lines peripherally, structureless in the center, quite symmetrical. The pigmentation does not extend beyond the scar.*

Recurrent nevi: Characteristic features		
Pattern	Colors	Clues
Typical: Radial or pseudopods but other patterns may occur	Typical: Brown	The pigmentation does not reach beyond the scar

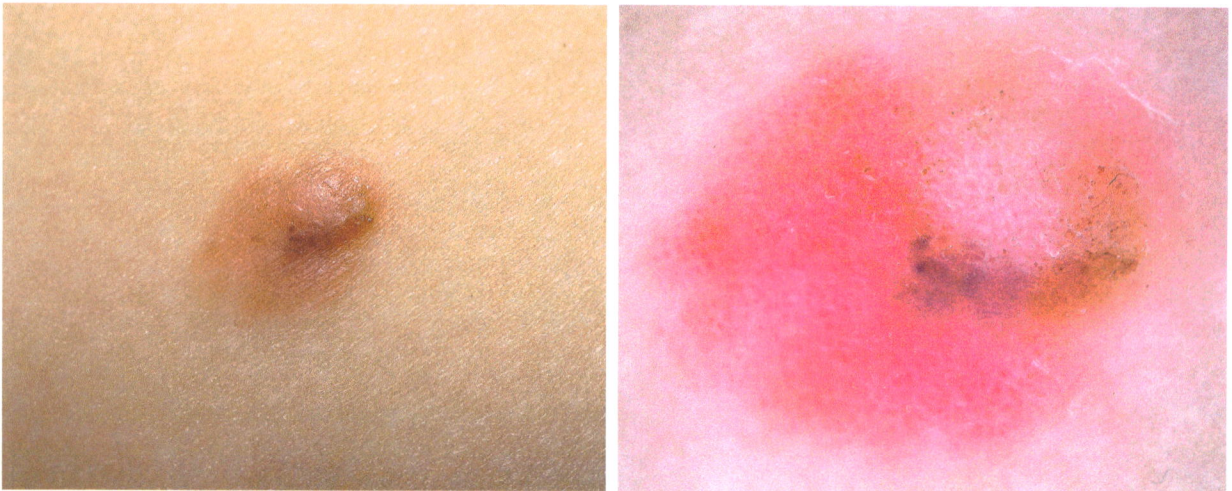

Figure 3.65: *"Classical", lightly pigmented Spitz nevus.*
*Clinical view on the left reveals a pink papule. Dermatoscopic view (**right**) shows a structureless pattern, pink color, perpendicular white lines in the raised part and vessels as dots.*

Spitz nevus: Characteristic features

	Pattern	Colors	Clues
Classical, lightly pigmented or non-pigmented type	*Typical:* Clods or structureless	*Typical:* Skin-colored or light-brown	*Typical:* Short, white, polarizing-specific perpendicular lines; reticular white lines, vessels as dots
Pigmented Spitz nevus	*Typical:* Clods *Occasional:* Structureless in the center	*Typical:* Clods = brown Center (both clods and structureless variants) = gray or gray-blue	*Occasional:* Thick, gray reticular lines in a hyperpigmented center. Short, white, polarizing-specific perpendicular lines in the center.

Reed nevus: Characteristic features

Pattern	Colors	Clues
Early phase: Brown clods Subsequent growth phase: peripheral radial lines or pseudopods are regularly distributed over the entire surface and there is a central structureless area. Late phase (the growth phase has been concluded): 1. Reticular lines at the periphery and structureless hyperpigmented center 2. Only reticular lines Combinations of patterns are usually symmetrical, but asymmetrical combinations of patterns do occur.	*Typical:* Black or dark-brown	*Occasional:* Within the structureless area in the center there are thick, gray reticular lines.

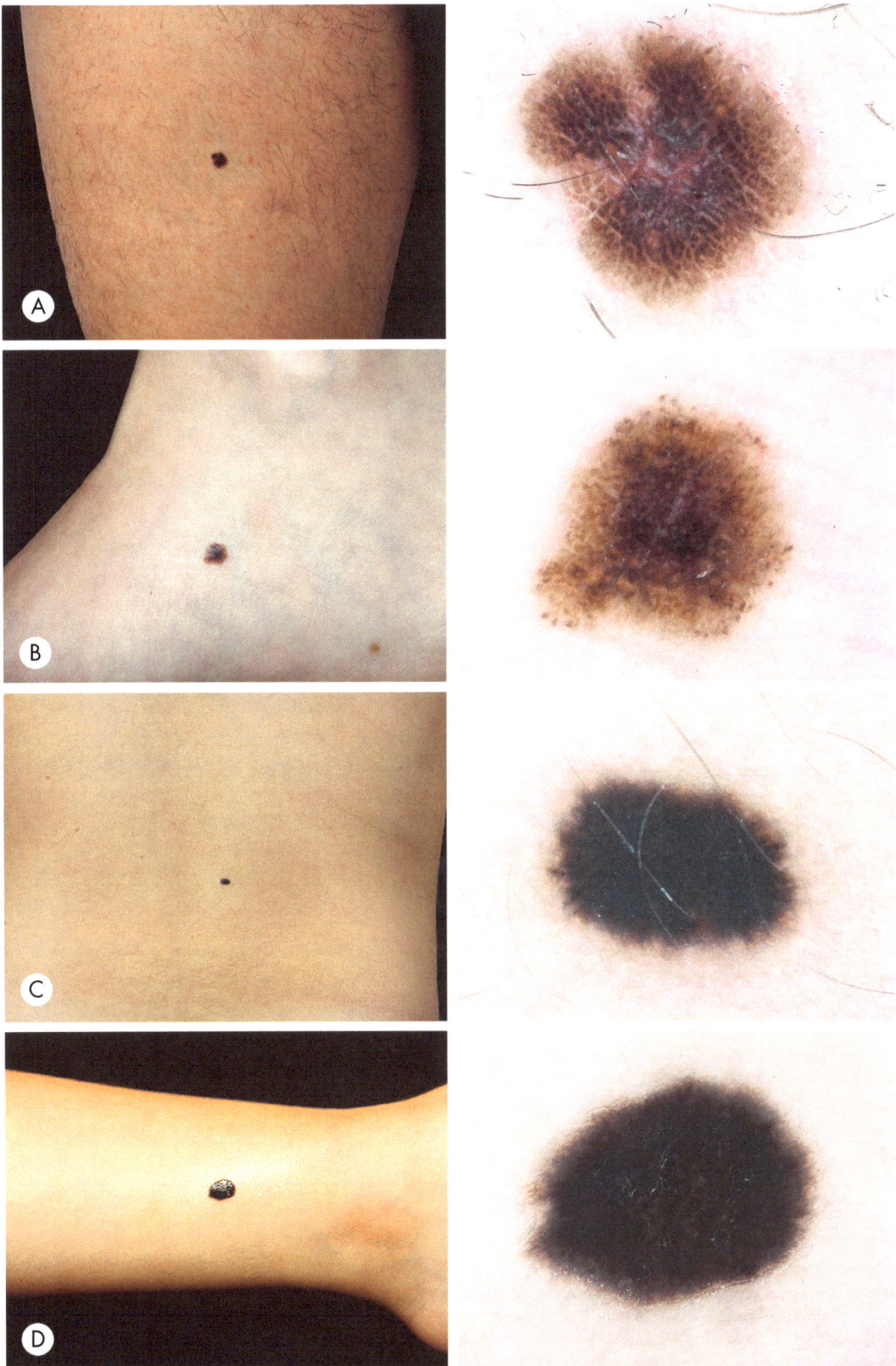

Figure 3.66: Pigmented Spitz nevi and Reed nevi.
Pigmented Spitz nevi and Reed nevi differ on dermatoscopy. Pigmented Spitz nevi usually demonstrate a clod pattern where the clods in the center may be gray (**A**) or brown (**B**). Typical Reed nevi (**C, D**) are structureless in the center, dark-brown or black, and show either radial lines or pseudopods, or more rarely reticular lines peripherally.

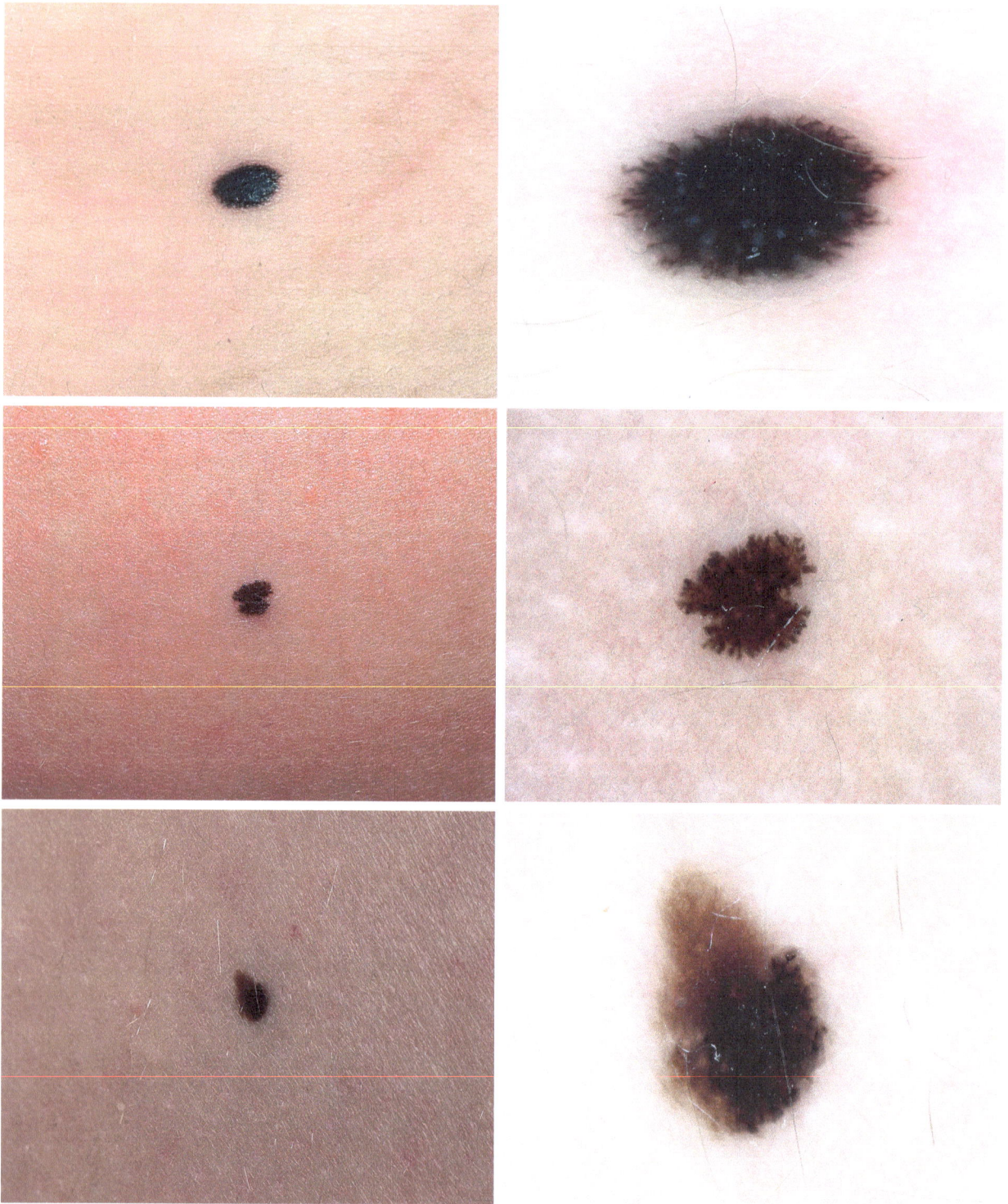

Figure 3.67: *Reed nevi.*
These Reed nevi are marked by radial lines or pseudopods peripherally. **Top:** *More than one pattern, symmetrical, structureless in the center, radial lines peripherally.* **Middle:** *More than one pattern, symmetrical, structureless in the center, pseudopods at the periphery.* **Third row:** *More than one pattern, asymmetrical, reticular lines and pseudopods at the periphery, but these do not occupy the entire circumference (differential diagnosis: melanoma).*

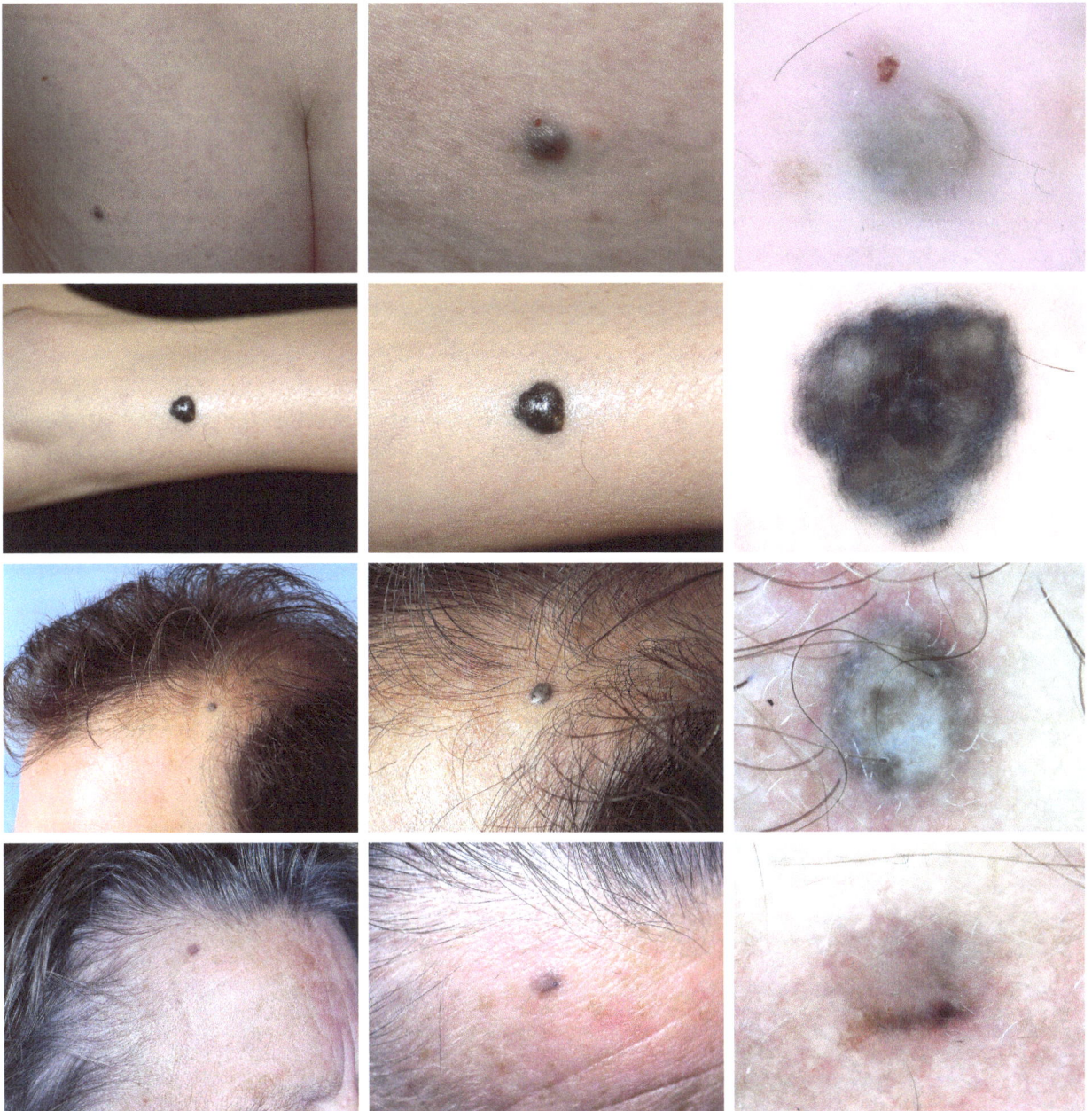

Figure 3.68: *Blue nevi.*
Blue nevi have only one pattern, structureless; and usually only one color, blue. Occasionally there may be gray or white structureless zones instead of or in addition to blue ones.

Blue nevi: Characteristic features

Pattern	Colors	Clues
Typical: Structureless Occasionally one finds white or gray lines or dots within the blue structureless area; these should not be interpreted as a pattern	Typical: Blue Occasional: Additionally brown, gray or white	None

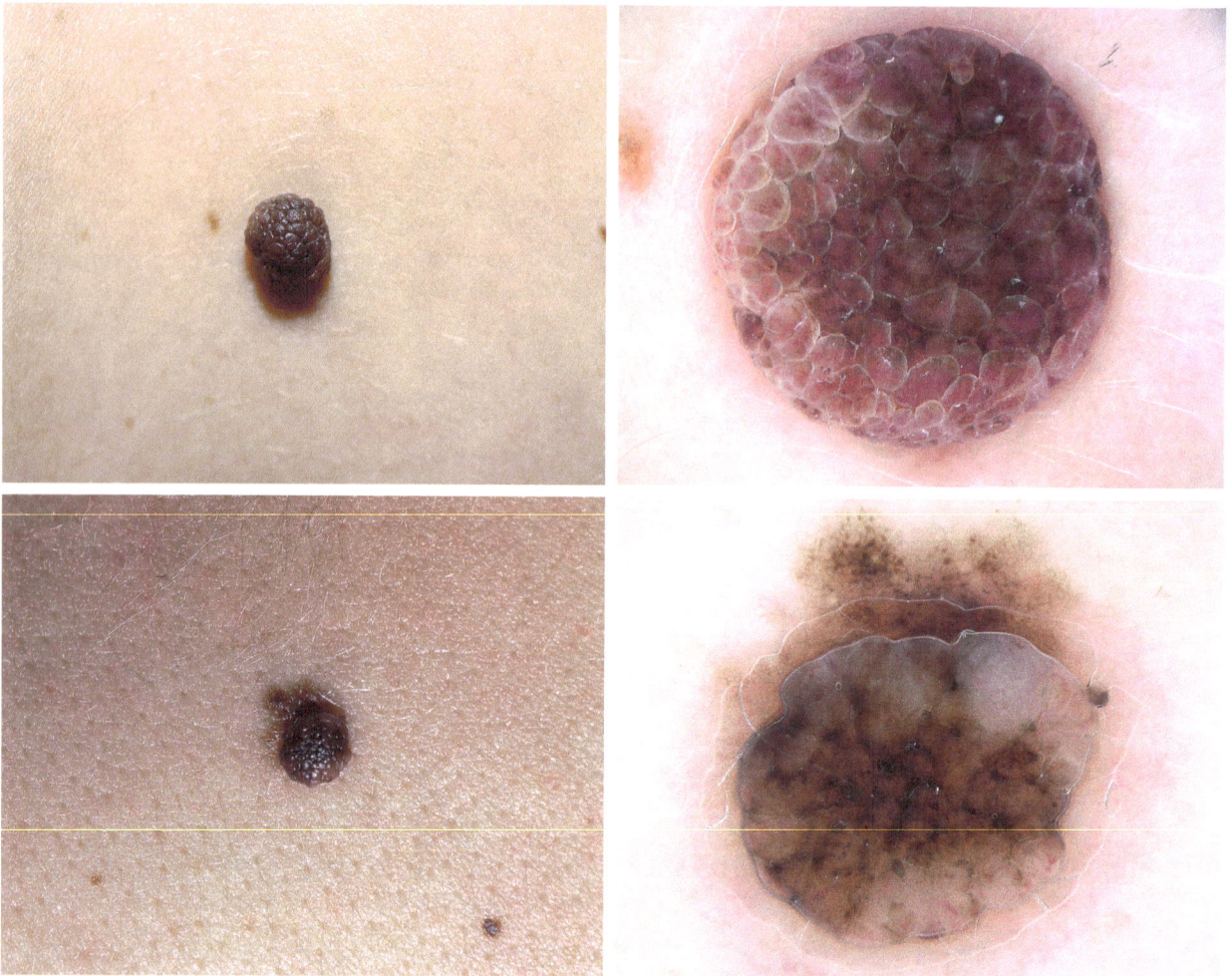

Figure 3.69: Unna nevi.
Top: Unna nevus with typical large polygonal skin-colored or light-brown clods. **Bottom:** Unna nevus (skin-colored large clods interspersed with small orange and dark-brown clods) in combination with a superficial congenital nevus with a reticular pattern and small clods.

Unna and Miescher nevi: Characteristic features

Pattern	Colors	Clues
Typical: Clods *Occasional:* Structureless; in Miescher nevus also circles	*Typical:* Skin-colored or brown	The clods are large and polygonal. White dots or orange clods Thick curved vessels in the clods (centered vessels) Terminal hair

pigment defines structure and acknowledging that gray structures are less densely pigmented than blue structures, one should not interpret such gray regions as a separate pattern.

Correlation between dermatoscopy and dermatopathology
Dermal melanocytes filled with melanin appear as a blue or gray structureless zone. When the melanocytes contain little or no melanin the structureless area appears light gray or even skin colored.

Unna and Miescher nevi
Both these nevi are primarily dermal proliferations of melanocytes. Although they appear after birth, histopathologically they are marked by a congenital growth pattern. For both Unna and Miescher nevus, the diagnosis is usually based on clinical appearance, with dermatoscopy providing little extra information. The typical dermatoscopic appearance of Unna nevus is of large polygonal skin-colored or light-brown clods (3.69). Between these clods there may be orange clods, and white dots and/or clods may be seen through the lesion. In such cases, the dermatoscopic appearance may resemble seborrheic keratosis. If skin-colored clods are poorly demarcated, the impression of a structureless pattern may be created.

The best clue to Unna nevus is short, thick and curved vessels in the center of skin-colored or light brown clods. Occasionally one may find brown dots or small brown clods. Very rarely there may be reticular brown lines at the periphery of the Unna nevus, which represent a junctional component.

Miescher nevus only occurs on the face. Features at dermatoscopy are similar to Unna nevus. Due to the anatomy of the facial skin and its prominent hair follicles, heavily pigmented types may have circles instead of clods. A strong clue to the diagnosis of Miescher nevus is excess numbers of terminal hairs, which also underlines the congenital nature of this nevus.

Correlation between dermatoscopy and dermatopathology
Polygonal clods correspond to widened dermal papillae filled with melanocytes, which cause the epidermis to protrude outward. In the invaginations between these epidermal protrusions there may be accumulations of keratinous material (orange clods) while exophytic growth may lead to the formation of epidermal inclusion cysts (milia), which appear as white dots. The curved vessels are located in the widened dermal papillae.

3.7.2 Melanoma
The dermatoscopy of melanoma is unique in that any pattern and any color may be seen (3.70–3.76). The more patterns and the more colors a lesion has, the more likely it is to be a melanoma. The question of the minimal features ever seen in melanoma is more about the limitations of dermatoscopy rather than the biology of the lesion. Melanomas can be diagnosed dermatoscopically at a stage when they have only one pattern, but by the time they have a specific clue to melanoma they will normally have more than one color. Melanomas can only be diagnosed earlier than this by monitoring for change (or by luck!). More advanced melanomas generally have two or more patterns which are nearly always arranged asymmetrically. In revised pattern analysis, the diagnosis of melanoma requires either more than one pattern or more than one color (chaos) and at least one clue to melanoma. This is a similar schema to the algorithm for the diagnosis of melanoma proposed by Menzies.

However, the clues used are somewhat different, and pattern analysis can be used regardless of lesion location; i.e. it may also be used to diagnose facial and acral melanomas.

Revised pattern analysis defines nine primary clues to melanoma:
1. Eccentric structureless zones of any color (except skin color)
2. Gray circles, lines, dots or clods
3. Black dots or clods at the periphery
4. Pseudopods or radial lines at the periphery, which do not occupy the entire circumference
5. White lines
6. Thick reticular lines
7. Polymorphous vessels
8. Parallel lines on the ridges
9. Angulated lines (polygons)

Clues to melanoma are shown in figures 3.70 to 3.76 and described in the figure legends. As mentioned in chapter 2, in this book we make no distinction between the types of melanoma, namely nodular, superficial spreading, acral lentiginous and lentigo maligna melanoma, because this classification is illogical and inconsistent. The nine clues to melanoma apply regardless of the histopathological growth type, size, and intensity of pigmentation.

Due to the specific anatomy of rete ridges on acral skin, the clue "parallel lines on ridges" refers only to acral melanomas. However, all other clues to melanoma are also clues to acral melanomas. While parallel lines on the ridges is the commonest clue to acral melanoma, it is not necessary to make the diagnosis.

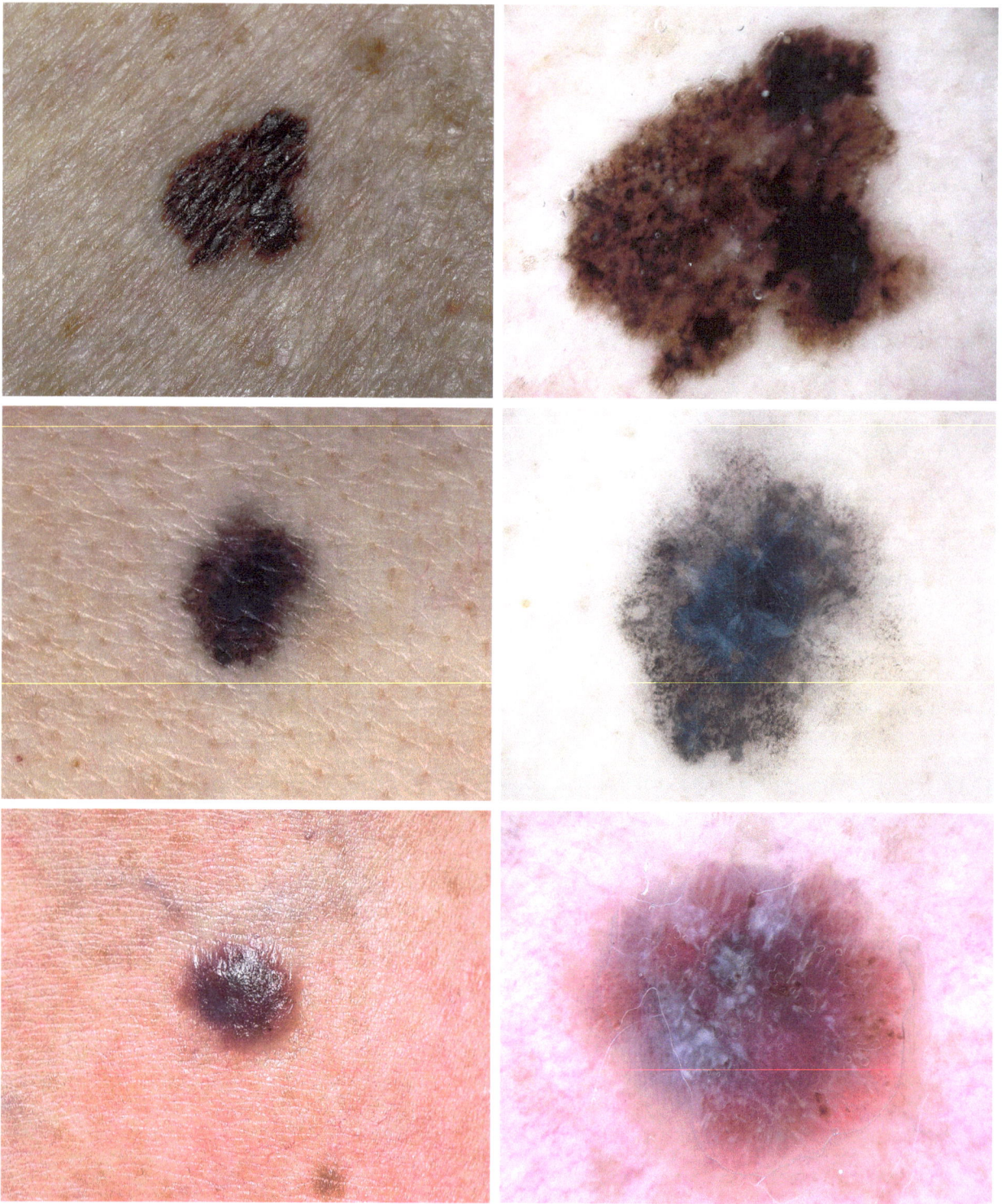

Figure 3.70: Melanomas and their clues.
Dermatoscopy, **right column. Top:** More than one pattern (reticular and structureless), more than one color; clue to melanoma: eccentric black structureless zone. **Middle:** More than one pattern (dots, clods and structureless), more than one color; clues to melanoma: 1. eccentric blue structureless zone, 2. gray dots and clods. **Bottom:** One pattern, clods, more than one color; clues to melanoma: 1. gray clods and gray lines, 2. white lines.

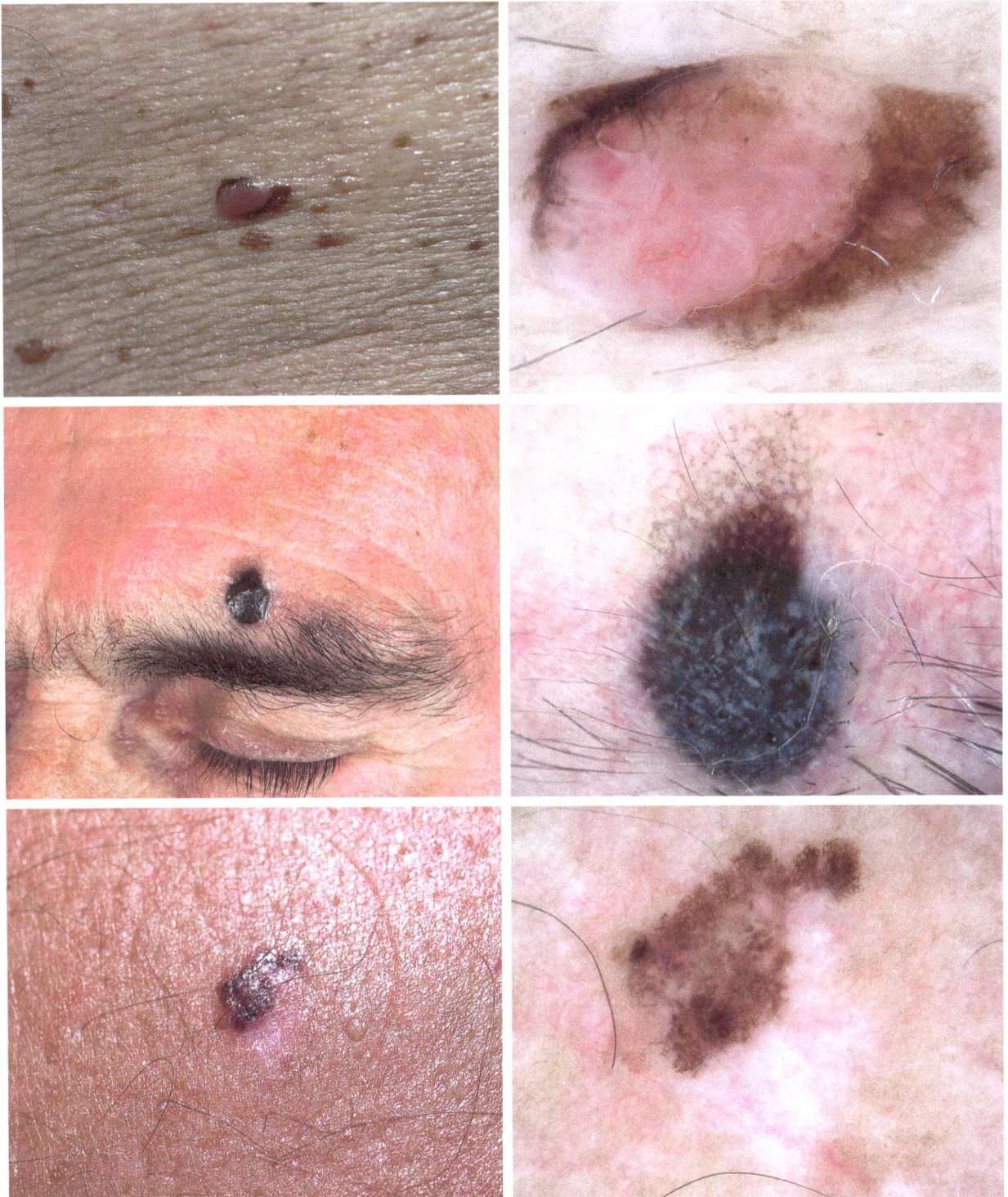

Figure 3.71: *Melanomas and their clues.*
Dermatoscopy, **right column.** **Top row:** *More than one pattern (reticular and structureless), more than one color; clue to melanoma: poly-morphous vascular pattern.* **Middle row:** *More than one pattern (dots, circles and structureless), more than one color; clues to melanoma: 1. eccentric blue structureless zone, 2. gray dots and clods.* **Bottom row:** *More than one pattern (reticular and structureless), more than one color; clue to melanoma: eccentric white structureless zone.*

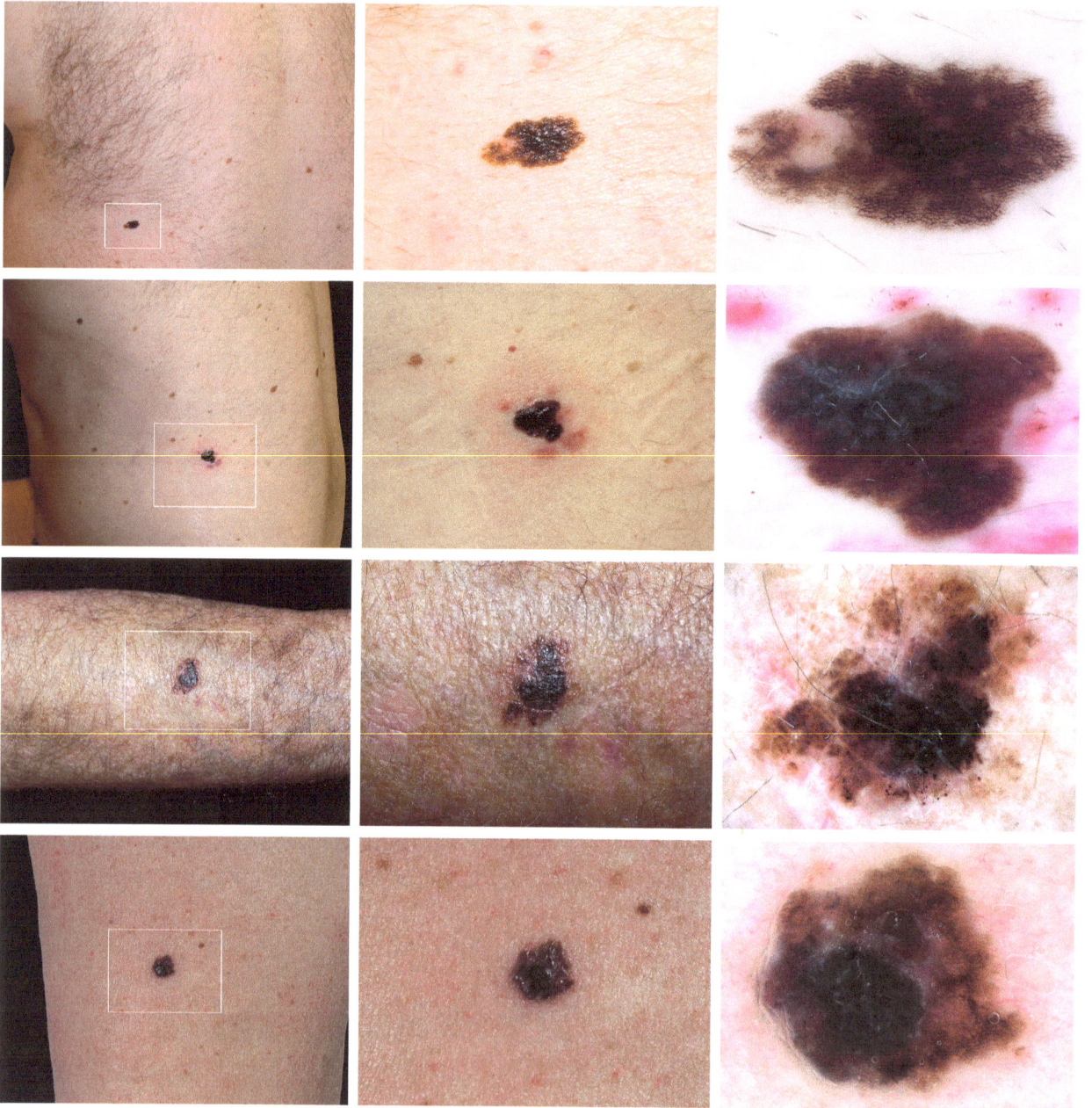

Figure 3.72: *Relatively large and heavily pigmented melanomas.*
Dermatoscopy, **right column. Top row:** *More than one pattern (reticular and structureless), arranged asymmetrically, more than one color; clue to melanoma: thick reticular lines.* **Second row:** *More than one pattern (reticular, structureless and clods), arranged asymmetrically, more than one color; clue to melanoma: eccentric gray structureless zone.* **Third row:** *More than one pattern (clods and structureless), arranged asymmetrically, more than one color; clue to melanoma: eccentric black structureless zone.* **Bottom row:** *More than one pattern (reticular and structureless), arranged asymmetrically, more than one color; clue to melanoma: eccentric black structureless zone.*

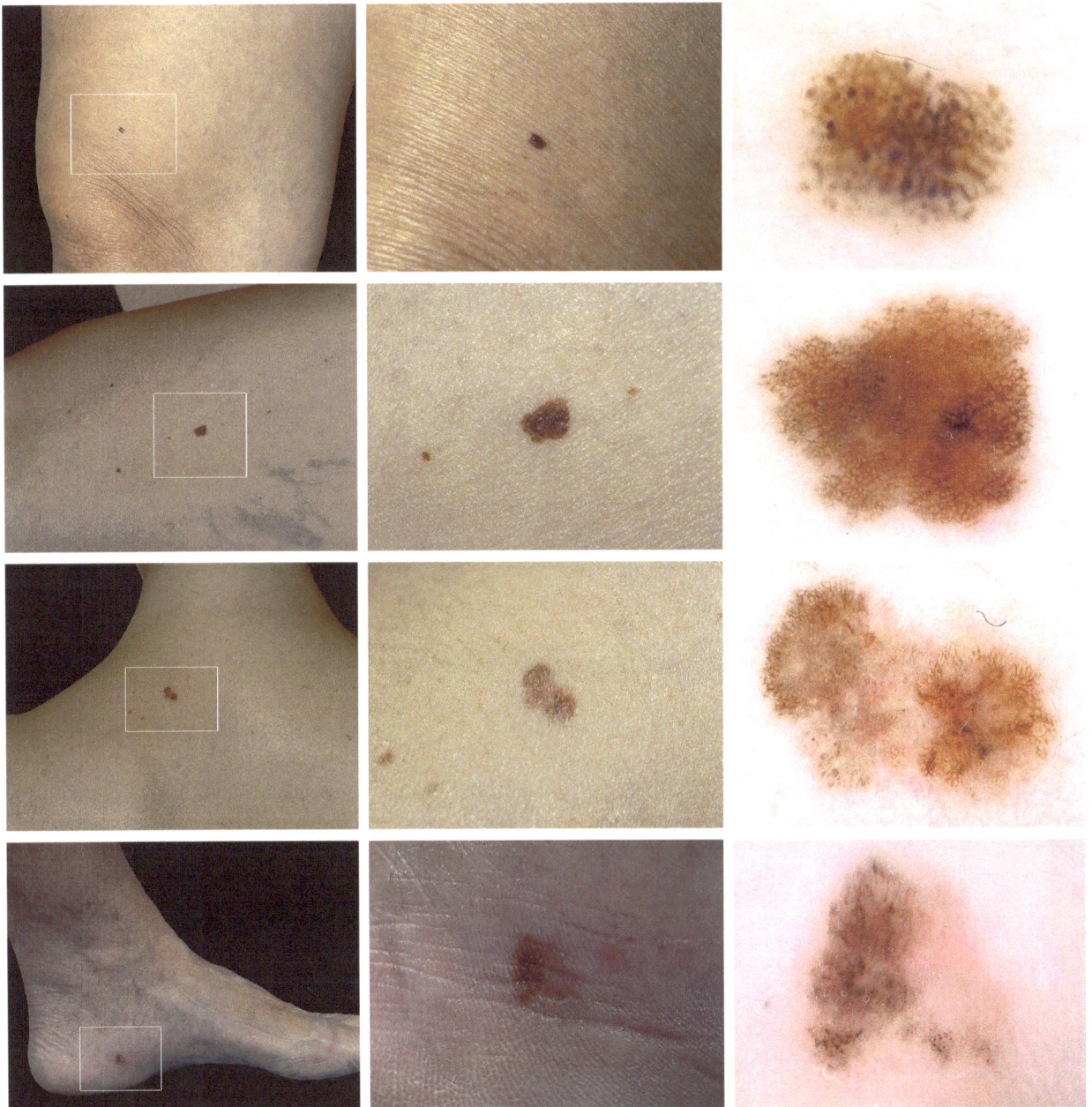

Figure 3.73: *Relatively small melanomas.*
Dermatoscopy, **right column. Top row:** *More than one pattern (reticular and clods), arranged asymmetrically, more than one color; clue to melanoma: thick reticular lines.* **Second row:** *One pattern (reticular), eccentric hyperpigmentation; clue to melanoma: thick reticular lines.* **Third row:** *One pattern (reticular), eccentric hyperpigmentation; clue to melanoma: thick reticular lines.* **Bottom row:** *More than one pattern (dots and structureless), arranged asymmetrically, more than one color; clues to melanoma 1. peripheral black dots, 2. gray dots.*

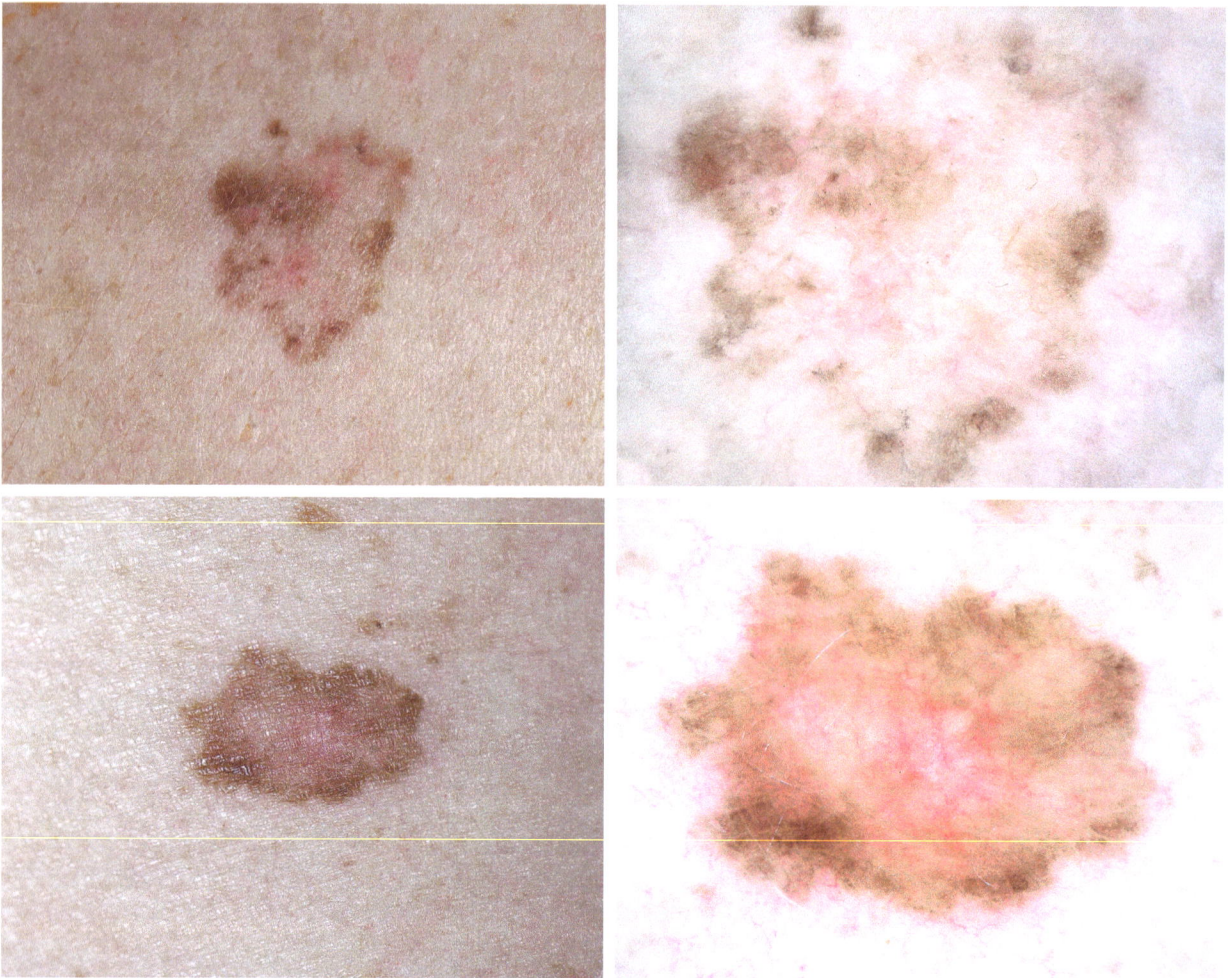

Figure 3.74: Less heavily pigmented melanomas.
Top: More than one pattern (reticular and structureless), arranged asymmetrically, more than one color; clue to melanoma: white lines.
Bottom: One pattern (structureless), eccentric hyperpigmentation; clues to melanoma: 1. white lines, 2. polymorphous vessels.

Melanoma: Characteristic features	
Pattern	Clues
More than one pattern or more than one color arranged asymmetrically (chaos)	1. Eccentric structureless zone of any color (except skin color) 2. Gray or blue structures (lines, circles, dots or clods) 3. Black dots or clods, peripheral 4. Radial lines or pseudopods, segmental 5. White lines 6. Reticular or branched lines, thick 7. Polymorphous vessels 8. Parallel lines on the ridges, or chaotic on the nails 9. Angulated lines (polygons)

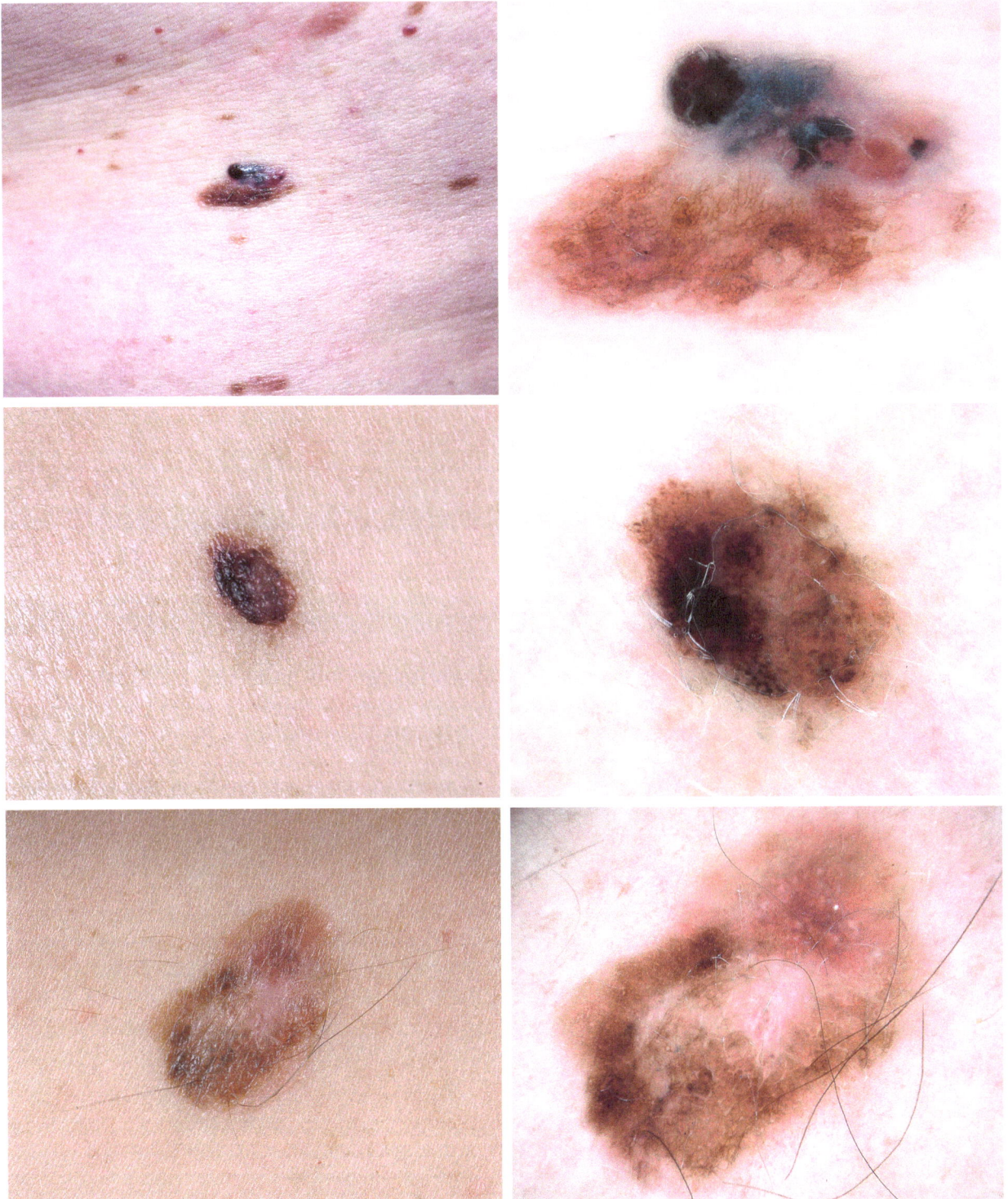

Figure 3.75: *Melanomas in a pre-existing nevus.*
Most melanomas arise de novo and not in a nevus. When a melanoma does arise in a pre-existing nevus it usually is a superficial and deep congenital nevus. **Top:** *More than one pattern (reticular and structureless), arranged asymmetrically, more than one color; clue to melanoma: eccentric blue and black structureless zone. The reticular region corresponds to a pre-existing "superficial and deep" congenital nevus.* **Middle:** *More than one pattern (reticular, clods, structureless), arranged asymmetrically, more than one color; clue to melanoma: eccentric black structureless zone. The region with large brown clods (right) corresponds to a pre-existing "superficial and deep" congenital nevus.* **Bottom:** *More than one pattern (reticular, structureless), arranged asymmetrically, more than one color; clue to melanoma: white reticular lines. The region with the thin brown reticular lines corresponds to a pre-existing "superficial and deep" congenital nevus.*

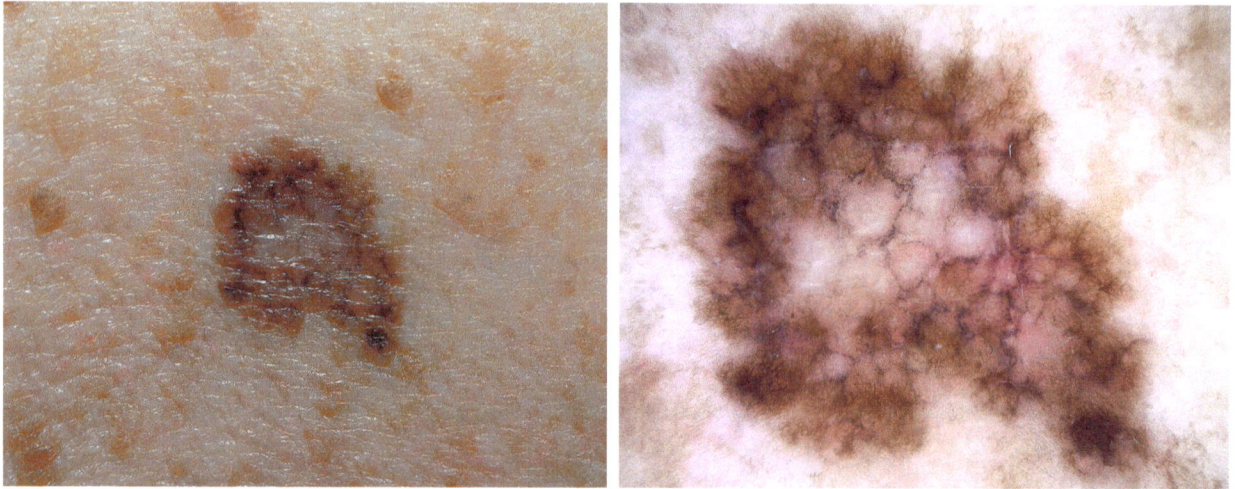

Figure 3.76: Melanomas and their clues.
A flat melanoma on chronic sun-damaged skin (non-facial) with angulated lines (polygons) as a clue to melanoma.

The same is true for melanomas on the face (lentigo maligna in common nomenclature when they are in situ, and lentigo maligna melanoma when they have become invasive). Flat melanomas on the face often show the pattern of gray circles, or gray dots arranged as circles, or angulated lines. Angulated lines (polygons) are also a specific clue for non-facial flat melanomas on chronic sun damaged skin *(3.76)*. The polygonal geometric shapes formed by angulated lines of non-facial lesions are larger than the holes caused by individual follicular openings, whereas in facial lesions the angulated lines are framing the hypopigmented follicular openings.

Correlation between dermatoscopy and dermatopathology

Histological correlates of the basic elements and the colors of melanin have already been addressed. Here we will only address some of the clues to melanoma. The histological correlate of an eccentric structureless zone varies according to its color. A black structureless zone is caused by a dense accumulation of melanin in the epidermis, usually in the stratum corneum. Brown structureless zones are usually due to lentiginous arrangements of pigmented melanocytes at the dermo-epidermal junction.

However, this is only seen when the rete ridges are flattened; if the rete ridges were intact there would be reticular lines instead of the brown structureless zone.

Blue and gray structureless zones are caused by melanin in the dermis and/or orthohyperkeratosis (and in most cases hypergranulosis as well) of the overlying epidermis. White structureless areas are caused by a zone of fibrosis in the dermis, which usually indicates regression. Gray structures are produced by an accumulation of melanophages in the dermis. These melanophages may be aggregated to form dots or clods, or be arranged in lines along the rete ridges, or in circles around hair follicles. Black dots or clods correspond to either nests of melanocytes or accumulations of melanin in the stratum corneum.

As in Reed nevus, peripheral pseudopods or radial lines are caused by fascicles of melanocytes at the dermo-epidermal junction that have spread centrifugally. White lines are a sign of fibrosis in the dermis. Thick brown reticular lines correspond to widened rete ridges filled with pigmented atypical melanocytes.

Parallel lines on the ridges are caused by a tendency in acral melanoma for melanocytes to proliferate along the crista profunda intermedia. Angulated lines of facial lesions correspond to deposition of melanin in the papillary dermis around follicular openings and proliferation of pigmented melanocytes in follicular epithelium. The histopathological correlate of angulated lines of non-facial lesions is not currently known. One plausible explanation is that they correspond to angiocentric deposition of melanin in proximity to the vessels of the superficial dermal plexus.

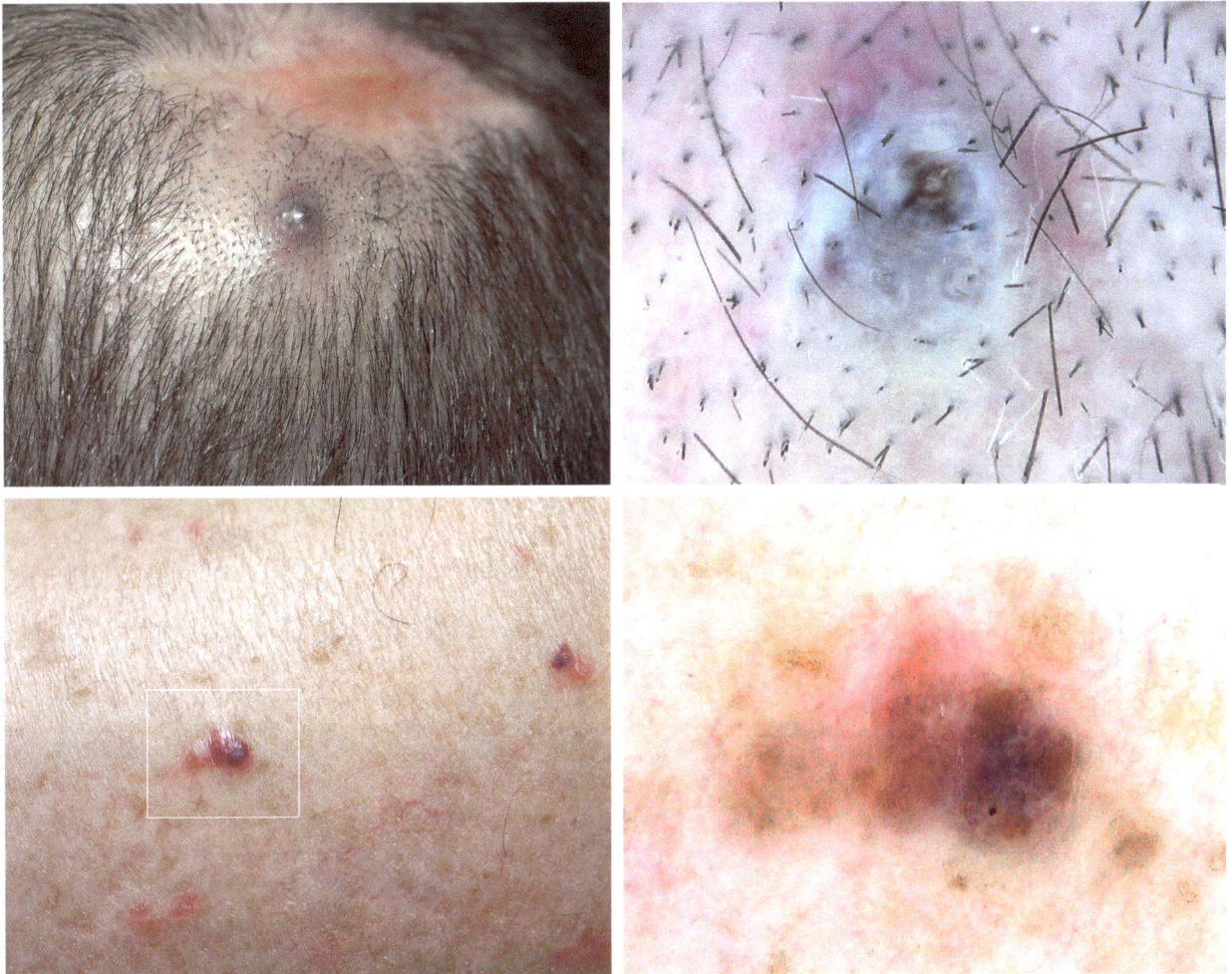

Figure 3.77: Metastases of melanoma, pigmented.
Top: *Metastasis of melanoma that simulates a blue nevus. Pattern: structureless and blue. The only subtle clue to the true diagnosis is the orange structureless zone that, on histopathology, corresponds to an erosion with a serum crust.* **Bottom:** *Metastasis of melanoma. One pattern, structureless, brown and gray pigmented; clue to melanoma: a polymorphous pattern of vessels.*

3.7.3 Metastases of melanoma

Cutaneous metastases of melanoma, when pigmented, usually demonstrate a structureless pattern *(3.77)*. Occasionally there may be clods. They are usually blue but also may be brown or gray. Usually the past history of melanoma and the presence of multiple lesions makes diagnosis straightforward. Differential diagnoses for solitary melanoma metastases include blue nevi and combined nevi. Pigment tends to conceal blood vessels. Non-pigmented metastases of melanoma (see Chapter 6) may have a polymorphous pattern of vessels and tend to simulate vascular proliferations.

Suggested readings sorted by topics

Pyogenic Granuloma
Zaballos P, Llambrich A, Cuéllar F, Puig S, Malvehy J. Dermoscopic findings in pyogenic granuloma. Br J Dermatol.
2006 Jun; 154(6): 1108–11.

Angiokeratoma
Zaballos P, Daufí C, Puig S, Argenziano G, Moreno-Ramírez
D, Cabo H, Marghoob AA, Llambrich A, Zalaudek I,
Malvehy J. Dermoscopy of solitary angiokeratomas: a
morphological study. Arch Dermatol. 2007 Mar; 143(3):
318–25.

Intracorneal Hemorrhage
Zalaudek I, Argenziano G, Soyer HP, Saurat JH, Braun RP.
Dermoscopy of subcorneal hematoma. Dermatol Surg.
2004 Sep; 30(9): 1229–32.

Solar lentigo, seborrheic keratosis and lichen planus like keratosis
Braun RP, Rabinovitz HS, Krischer J, Kreusch J, Oliviero M,
Naldi L, Kopf AW, Saurat JH. Dermoscopy of pigmented
seborrheic keratosis: a morphological study. Arch Dermatol. 2002 Dec; 138(12): 1556–60.
Zaballos P, Blazquez S, Puig S, Salsench E, Rodero J, Vives
JM, Malvehy J. Dermoscopic pattern of intermediate
stage in seborrhoeic keratosis regressing to lichenoid
keratosis: report of 24 cases. Br J Dermatol. 2007 Aug;
157(2): 266–72.

Dermatofibroma
Zaballos P, Puig S, Llambrich A, Malvehy J. Dermoscopy of
dermatofibromas: a prospective morphological study of
412 cases. Arch Dermatol. 2008 Jan; 144(1): 75–83.
Kilinc Karaarslan I, Gencoglan G, Akalin T, Ozdemir F.
Different dermoscopic faces of dermatofibromas. J Am
Acad Dermatol. 2007 Sep; 57(3): 401–6.

Ink-spot lentigo
Argenziano G. Dermoscopy of melanocytic hyperplasias:
subpatterns of lentigines (ink spot). Arch Dermatol. 2004
Jun; 140(6): 776.

Genital lentigo, Labial lentigo
Blum A, Simionescu O, Argenziano G, Braun R, Cabo H,
et al. Dermoscopy of pigmented lesions of the mucosa
and the mucocutaneous junction: results of a multicenter
study by the International Dermoscopy Society (IDS).
Arch Dermatol. 2011 Oct; 147(10): 1181–7.

Pigmented Basal Cell Carcinoma
Menzies SW, Westerhoff K, Rabinovitz H, Kopf AW, McCarthy
WH, Katz B. Surface microscopy of pigmented basal cell
carcinoma. Arch Dermatol. 2000 Aug; 136(8): 1012–6.
Lallas A, Apalla Z, Argenziano G, Longo C, Moscarella E et
al. The dermatoscopic universe of basal cell carcinoma.
Dermatol Pract Concept. 2014 Jul 31; 4(3): 11–24.

Pigmented Actinic Keratosis
Akay BN, Kocyigit P, Heper AO, Erdem C. Dermatoscopy
of flat pigmented facial lesions: diagnostic challenge
between pigmented actinic keratosis and lentigo maligna.
Br J Dermatol. 2010 Dec; 163(6): 1212–7.

Pigmented Bowen's Disease
Cameron A, Rosendahl C, Tschandl P, Riedl E, Kittler H. Der-
matoscopy of pigmented Bowen's disease. J Am Acad
Dermatol. 2010 Apr; 62(4): 597–604.

Squamous Cell Carcinoma
Rosendahl C, Cameron A, Argenziano G, Zalaudek I, Tschandl
P, Kittler H. Dermoscopy of squamous cell carcinoma and
keratoacanthoma. Arch Dermatol. 2012 Dec; 148(12):
1386–92.
Zalaudek I, Giacomel J, Schmid K, Bondino S, Rosendahl C et
al. Dermatoscopy of facial actinic keratosis, intraepidermal carcinoma, and invasive squamous cell carcinoma:
a progression model. J Am Acad Dermatol. 2012 Apr;
66(4): 589–97.

Clark Nevus, "superficial" and "superficial and deep" congenital nevi
Clark WH Jr, Reimer RR, Greene M, Ainsworth AM, Mastran-
gelo MJ. Origin of familial malignant melanomas from
heritable melanocytic lesions. 'The B-K mole syndrome'.
Arch Dermatol. 1978 May; 114(5): 732–8.
Kittler H, Tschandl P. Dysplastic nevus: why this term should
be abandoned in dermatoscopy. Dermatol Clin. 2013
Oct; 31(4): 579–88
Rosendahl CO, Grant-Kels JM, Que SK. Dysplastic nevus:
Fact and fiction. J Am Acad Dermatol. 2015 Sep; 73(3):
507–12.
Hofmann-Wellenhof R, Blum A, Wolf IH, Zalaudek I, Piccolo
D, Kerl H, Garbe C, Soyer HP. Dermoscopic classification
of Clark's nevi (atypical melanocytic nevi). Clin Dermatol.
2002 May-Jun; 20(3): 255–8.
Argenziano G, Zalaudek I, Ferrara G, Hofmann-Wellenhof R,
Soyer HP. Proposal of a new classification system for mela-
nocytic naevi. Br J Dermatol. 2007 Aug; 157(2): 217–27.

Combined congenital nevi

De Giorgi V, Massi D, Salvini C, Trez E, Mannone F, Carli P. Dermoscopic features of combined melanocytic nevi. J Cutan Pathol. 2004 Oct; 31(9): 600–4.

Recurrent Nevi

Blum A, Hofmann-Wellenhof R, Marghoob AA, Argenziano G, Cabo H et al. Recurrent melanocytic nevi and melanomas in dermoscopy: results of a multicenter study of the International Dermoscopy Society. JAMA Dermatol. 2014 Feb; 150(2): 138–45.

Spitz Nevi

Bär M, Tschandl P, Kittler H. Differentiation of pigmented Spitz nevi and Reed nevi by integration of dermatopathologic and dermatoscopic findings. Dermatol Pract Concept. 2012 Jan 31; 2(1): 13–24.

Argenziano G, Scalvenzi M, Staibano S, Brunetti B, Piccolo D et al. Dermatoscopic pitfalls in differentiating pigmented Spitz naevi from cutaneous melanomas. Br J Dermatol. 1999 Nov; 141(5): 788–93.

Reed Nevi

Bär M, Tschandl P, Kittler H. Differentiation of pigmented Spitz nevi and Reed nevi by integration of dermatopathologic and dermatoscopic findings. Dermatol Pract Concept. 2012 Jan 31; 2(1): 13–24.

Marchell R, Marghoob AA, Braun RP, Argenziano G. Dermoscopy of pigmented Spitz and Reed nevi: the starburst pattern. Arch Dermatol. 2005 Aug; 141(8): 1060.

Blue Nevi

Di Cesare A, Sera F, Gulia A, Coletti G, Micantonio T et al. The spectrum of dermatoscopic patterns in blue nevi. J Am Acad Dermatol. 2012 Aug; 67(2): 199–205.

Unna and Miescher Nevi

Ackerman AB, Magana-Garcia M. Naming acquired melanocytic nevi. Unna's, Miescher's, Spitz's Clark's. Am J Dermatopathol. 1990 Apr; 12(2): 193–209.

Melanoma

Cancer Genome Atlas Network. Genomic Classification of Cutaneous Melanoma. Cell. 2015 Jun 18; 161(7): 1681–96.

Argenziano G, Cerroni L, Zalaudek I, Staibano S, Hofmann-Wellenhof R, et al. Accuracy in melanoma detection: a 10-year multicenter survey. J Am Acad Dermatol. 2012 Jul; 67(1): 54–9.

4 Metaphoric dermatoscopic terms and what they mean

The classical language of dermatoscopy consists of a large number of mainly metaphoric terms with no over-arching structure. It qualifies as a technical language or "jargon" in the sense that it has a specific vocabulary, which is incomprehensible outside its context. Although metaphors that are apt and colorful stick in the memory, their sheer number and the fact that many are ambiguous, redundant, or just bad analogies make them a potential barrier to learning, teaching and research. The metaphoric vocabulary of dermatoscopy has expanded so quickly that even experts find it difficult to oversee the plethora of terms (1).

In chapter 3 we introduced a simple descriptive terminology based on only five geometrically defined basic elements, which, like the letters of the alphabet, are the building blocks of any new descriptive term. Because of its simplicity and logic, this descriptive terminology is becoming increasingly popular. A survey of International Dermoscopy Society (IDS) members indicated that 23.5% prefer to use descriptive terminology while 20.1% prefer metaphoric terminology. Most participants, however, use both terminologies.

In 2015 the IDS initiated a new consensus conference with the primary aim of harmonizing metaphoric and descriptive terminology. Another goal was to rationalize metaphoric language by eliminating synonyms and terms that are poorly defined, of dubious significance, obscure, or otherwise unnecessary. The consensus conference expert panel proposed a standardized dictionary including both metaphoric and descriptive terms. (1) Although the authors of this book prefer descriptive terminology we think that teachers of dermatoscopy should be familiar with both languages and should be able to teach both terminologies. The aim of this chapter is to help those who are only familiar with metaphoric terminology. If you do prefer metaphoric terminology, we strongly encourage you to select metaphoric terms that are included in the standardized dictionary.

Descriptive terms are not the definitions of the metaphoric terms. The descriptive terms are used by those who prefer descriptive terminology over the metaphoric terms. The majority of the terms describe features, which, on their own, are not very specific, but become meaningful in the context of pattern and color. The method for assessment of patterns, colors and clues, the core of pattern analysis, is then described in chapter 5.

"Angulated lines (polygons)"
Strictly speaking the term "angulated lines" ("polygons") is not a metaphoric term. It is composed of two parts; one part is "line", which is a basic element, and the

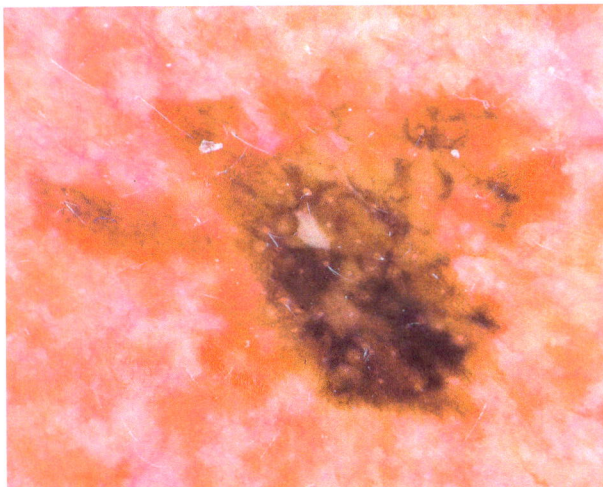

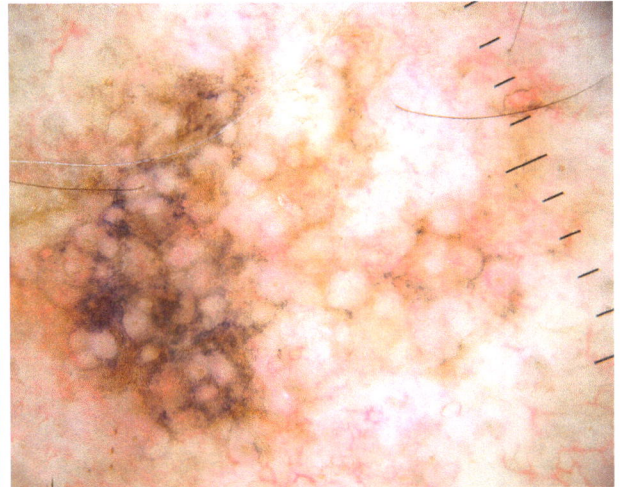

Figure 4.1: Angulated lines (polygons).
Angulated lines forming complete or incomplete "polygons" in two flat melanomas on chronically sun-damaged skin (non-facial skin).

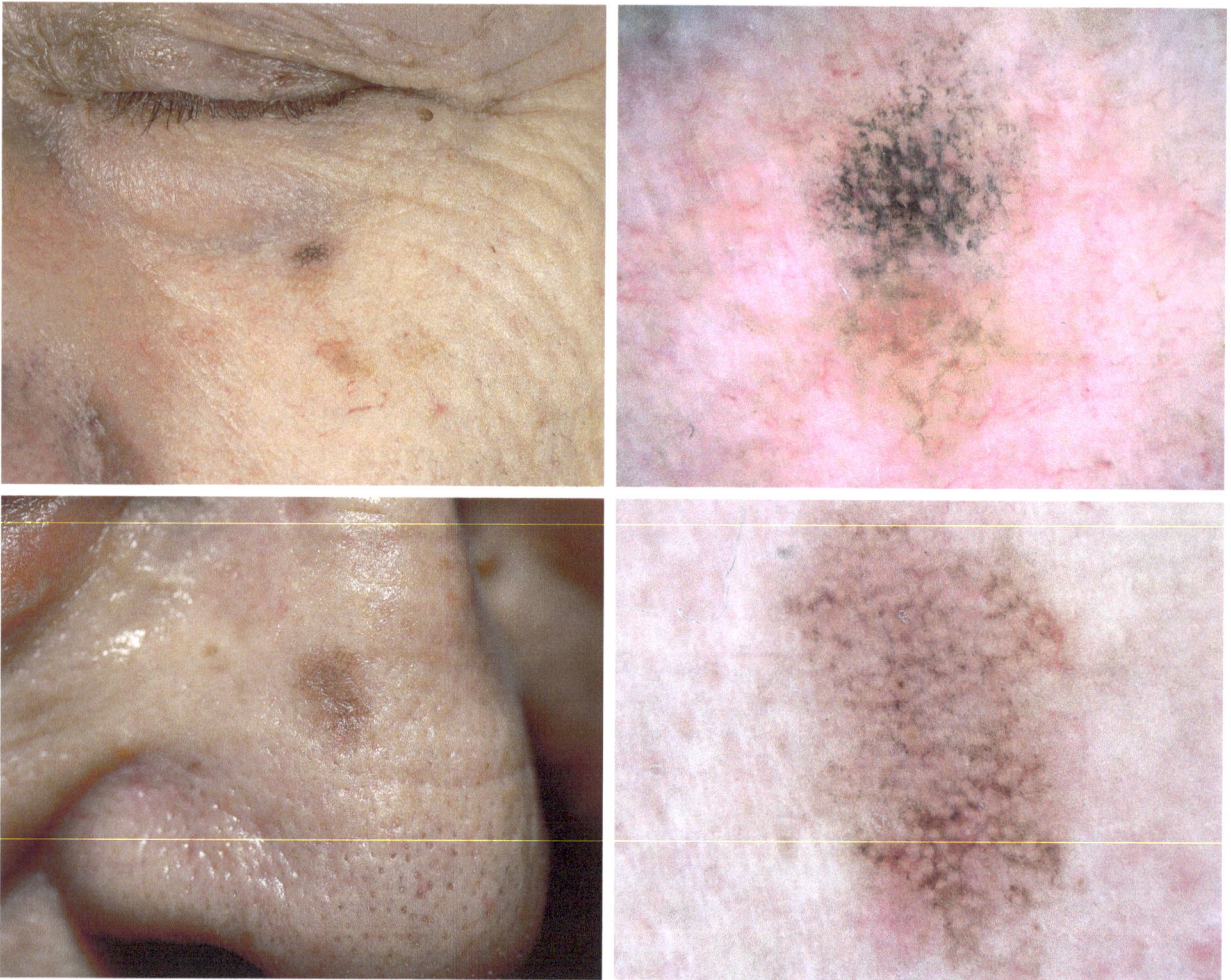

Figure 4.2: "Annular-granular" = gray dots arranged around follicular openings.
The appearance on dermatoscopy is shown in the **right column. Top row:** Gray dots around follicular openings **(right)** in a lichen planus-like keratosis (remnants of solar lentigo are seen in the lower region). **Bottom row:** Gray dots arranged around follicular openings **(right)** in an in situ melanoma (lentigo maligna). In this case the gray dots (and circles) of the in situ melanoma are much more subtle than those in the lichen planus-like keratosis seen in the upper row.

second part is "angulated", which describes the spatial arrangement. Originally, the term "polygon" was used to describe specific structures of flat melanomas on non-facial chronic sun damaged skin (2, 3). Polygons were defined as geometric polygonal shapes complete or incomplete, bounded by straight lines, or by a straight pigment interface, meeting at angles and larger than the holes caused by individual follicles and larger by far than the holes bounded by reticular lines (4.1). Throughout the book we use the term "angulated lines" or "polygon" in a broader sense. We use it for straight lines that do not intersect and which meet at angles in such a way that they form complete or incomplete polygonal shapes no matter if the skin involved is facial or non-facial. We summarize the terms "polygon",

"rhomboids" (4), and "zig-zag pattern" (5) under the umbrella term "angulated lines".

"Annular-granular pattern"

The "annular-granular" pattern is regarded as a characteristic feature of in situ melanoma (lentigo maligna) on the face (6). It describes the arrangement of gray or brown dots (granular) around follicular openings (annular). The major aspect of this feature is actually the gray color, but this is not part of the term. The feature is not particularly specific because it may occur in pigmented actinic keratoses (7) or lichen planus-like keratoses as well. The equivalent term in the descriptive terminology is "gray dots arranged around follicular openings" (4.2).

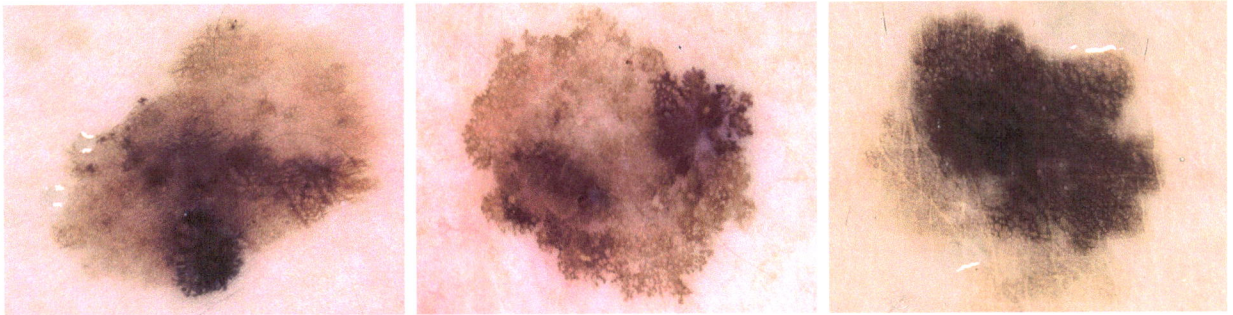

Figure 4.3: "Atypical" or "irregular" pigment network.
Dermatoscopic views of three melanomas, all with reticular lines ("pigment network"). In conventional terminology this "pigment network" would be termed "atypical" or "irregular". Such poorly defined and subjective terms are avoided in pattern analysis; elements termed "atypical" are incorporated in the description of pattern (reticular lines which are thicker than the spaces they enclose, over a significant part of the lesion, are termed "thick") and colors (more than one color, combined asymmetrically). In pattern analysis, thick reticular lines are a clue to melanoma.

"Atypical (or irregular) pigment network"

The terms "atypical" and "irregular" are subjective. According to the dictionary of standardized terms (8) an atypical network is defined as a network with increased variability in the color, thickness, and spacing of the lines of the network *(4.3)*. In pattern analysis, we make a distinction between structure and color. We speak of eccentric hyperpigmentation if the darker shade is seen at the periphery the lesion. We use the terms "speckled" or "variegate" if the pigmentation is distributed in such a way that areas of dark pigmentation alternate with areas of light pigmentation. If the network lines are broadened we call them thick reticular lines as opposed to thin reticular lines. Thick reticular lines are broader than or at least as broad as

the hypopigmented intermediary spaces. An atypical (or irregular) pigment network is a clue to melanoma and so are thick reticular lines.

"Blotch"

The original meaning of "blotch" was a darkly pigmented structureless area, but only used to describe melanocytic lesions. "Irregular blotches" are a criterion of melanoma in the 7-point checklist (9). "Irregular" means that several darkly pigmented structureless areas are irregularly distributed. In pattern analysis, we make a distinction between color and structure. Structureless areas may assume any color and are then termed brown, black, blue, gray, white, or red structureless zones. A "blotch" such as that shown in *figure 4.4* would therefore be

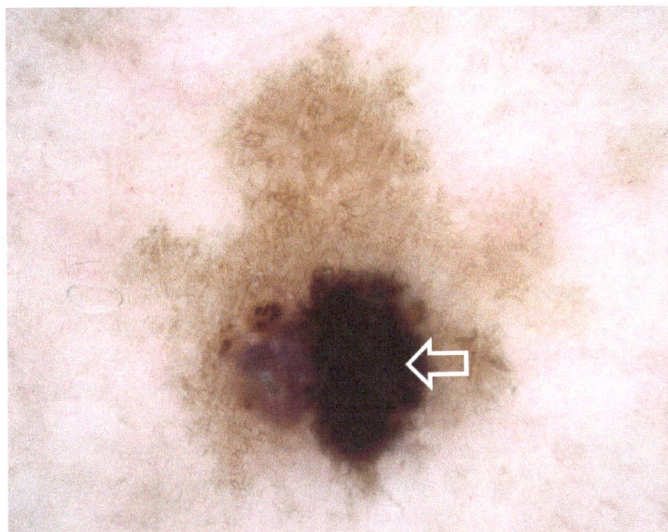

Figure 4.4: "Blotch".
In the language of pattern analysis, this "irregular blotch" (arrow) is described as an eccentric structureless (in this case black) zone. The pathological diagnosis is: melanoma in a preexisting Clark nevus.

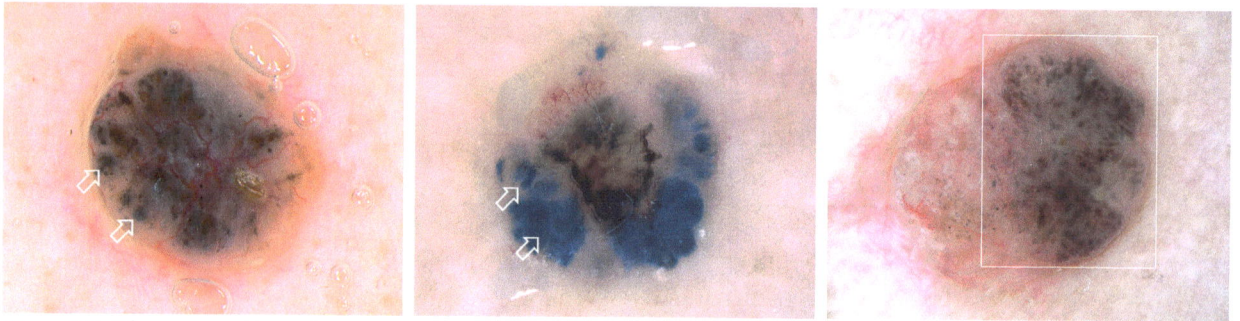

Figure 4.5: "Blue-gray ovoid nests".
On the left is a basal cell carcinoma with several round gray clods ("blue-gray ovoid nests"). In the **middle** (also a basal cell carcinoma) the clods are blue, but only slightly ovoid. Some clods are very large and polygonal, and bear no resemblance to ovoid nests. The basal-cell carcinoma on the right has several relatively small, round, gray and blue clods.

Figure 4.6: "Blue veil".
A very pronounced **(left)** and a less obvious **(middle)** "blue or blue-white veil" in two melanoma. This structure is occasionally found in seb-orrheic keratoses **(right)** as well as melanocytic lesions. In pattern analysis we use the term "blue structureless zone" instead of a "blue-white veil". This term is much more neutral than "blue-white veil" and is consistent with the simple and logical terminology of pattern analysis. All three lesions were photographed with non-polarized dermatoscopy. With polarized dermatoscopy the "blue-white veil" often appears as a blue structureless zone with white lines. The white lines are invisible in images taken with non-polarized dermatoscopy.

a black structureless zone in descriptive terminology. When this structureless zone is not central (eccentric structureless zone) or when several structureless zones are asymmetrically distributed, these probably best correspond to "irregular blotches". A "regular blotch" is best described as a central structureless, hyperpig-mented zone.

"Blue-gray ovoid nests"

"Blue-gray ovoid nests" are defined as an accumulation of blue or gray clods (8), of which some are supposed to be oval ("ovoid").

The clods are usually of different sizes and not regularly distributed over the lesion, but concentrated in groups (therefore nests). This is a relatively specific criterion of basal cell carcinoma *(4.5).* In the descriptive ter-minology we refer to blue (or gray) clods of various sizes and shapes. If desired, one may further describe the shape of clods in simple words, e.g. round, oval, or polygonal. However, this is rarely important for differential diagnosis.

"Blue-white veil", "blue veil"

The "blue-white veil" or "blue veil" is one of the most well known (8) and also most controversial terms in dermatoscopy. Originally it meant a structureless blue zone. The term "veil" probably referred to a translucent appearance, suggesting the superimposition of blue and white *(4.6).* When this superimposition is absent, the term "blue veil" is used. Nearly all algorithms for the diagnosis of melanoma, whether Argenziano's 7-point checklist (9) or Menzies' method (10), include this structure as an important criterion of melanoma. If one only considers melanocytic lesions, the criterion is also quite specific for melanoma, usually invasive. Obviously, blue structureless zones are also seen in blue nevi and combined congenital nevi. Apart from melanocytic lesions, this structure is occasionally found in seborrheic keratosis and rarely in pigmented basal cell carcinoma.

The specificity of a structure for a certain diagnosis depends on the diagnoses it is compared with. Com-pared to Clark nevi the "blue-white veil" is specific

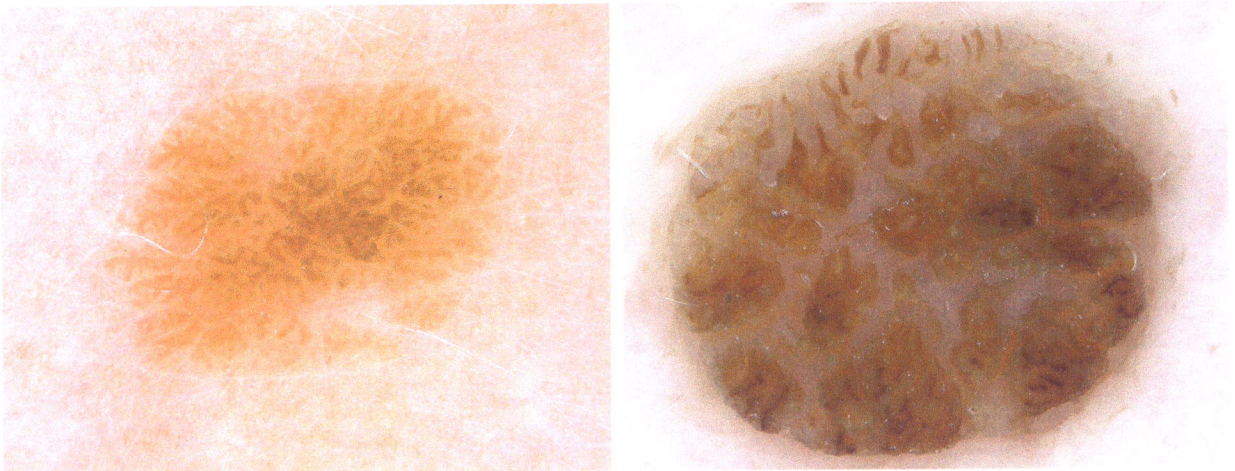

Figure 4.7: "Brain-like pattern".
A basic principle of pattern analysis is that (with few exceptions) pigment defines structures. In dermatoscopic images of these two seborrheic keratoses, we see brown (or orange) clods and (especially on the left) thick curved lines. The metaphoric term "brain-like pattern" is dispensable; the entity can be described in the simple terms of pattern analysis.

for melanoma; compared to seborrheic keratoses or blue nevi it is not. The disadvantages of metaphoric language become evident here. Associative metaphoric terms may be catchy and easy to remember, but they are also strongly linked to a specific diagnosis. The moment one refers to a blue-white veil, the association with the diagnosis of melanoma is so strong that all other differential diagnoses are not likely to be even considered. In pattern analysis, any structureless zone in an eccentric location, regardless of its color (except skin color), is a clue to melanoma. Thus, the term "blue-white veil" can be replaced by the descriptive term "blue structureless zone, eccentrically located".

"Brain-like pattern", "cerebriform pattern", "gyri and sulci"

These are archetypal metaphoric terms signifying a special arrangement of thick, curved, pigmented lines and clods and circles *(4.7)*. This pattern is vaguely reminiscent of the surface of a brain with its "gyri" (the hypopigmented spaces between the thick curved lines) and "sulci" (hyperpigmented curved lines, clods and circles) (11). As a rule, lesions with this pattern are raised and not flat.

When the lesion is flat and the curved lines are not thick but thin and the circles small, the pattern is referred to as "fingerprinting"(12) (see section on fingerprinting). Both patterns are regarded as being quite specific for seborrheic keratoses and their use generally causes other differential diagnoses to be discarded. In cases of "brain-like whorls" a seborrheic keratosis will be of the markedly acanthotic type and in cases of "fingerprint-

ing" they will be of the flat type, also known as solar lentigo . In pattern analysis the "brain-like pattern" can be simply described using descriptive terms. We refer to thick curved lines, clods and circles. Some "circles" may be distorted into ellipses.

"Branched streaks"

Branched streaks are considered to be specific to melanocytic lesions (13). However, they are also found in non-melanocytic lesions, such as ink-spot lentigo. In the language of pattern analysis, they are simply described as branched lines.

"Broadened pigment network"

A broadened pigment network (14) is found in the presence of melanoma, occasionally melanocytic nevi, seborrheic keratoses, and also ink-spot lentigo. In the descriptive terminology the synonymous term is "thick reticular lines". It is a useful clue for in situ melanomas and thin invasive melanomas *(4.3)*.

"Central white patch"

This is defined as a white structureless zone in the center of the lesion, which is quite specific for dermatofibroma (15, 16) *(4.8)*. This feature suggests the presence of a dermatofibroma, but not all dermatofibromas show this feature. The term "central white patch" actually denotes two things: the first characteristic is a symmetrical arrangement of two patterns (reticular peripheral and structureless "central"); the second characteristic is the center of the pattern showing a white structureless zone ("white patch").

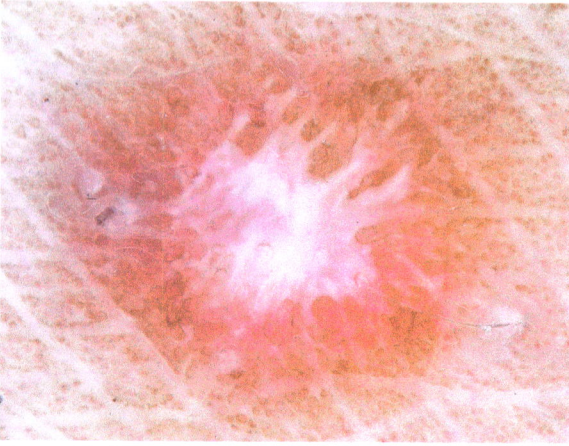

Figure 4.8: "*Central white patch*".
Structureless white zone ("central white patch") located in the center of a dermatofibroma.

"Chrysalis, Chrysalids, and Crystalline"

The term "chrysalis" was used to describe a pattern of straight white lines at right angles to each other seen only when a polarizing dermatoscope is used (17). Chrysalis is named after a vague resemblance of the structure to a wax moth infestation of a beehive. *Figure 4.9* shows an example of the structure of white lines in a thick melanoma which has grown rapidly. It can be seen that the white lines aligned at right angles are certainly brighter with polarized dermatoscopy. In the descriptive language these structures are referred to as "polarizing-specific white lines" or "perpendicular white lines". This pattern is seen in melanoma, Spitz nevus, basal cell carcinoma, and dermatofibroma. Sometimes the terms "chrysalids" and "crystalline"

were used instead of "chrysalis" (18). Because even the proponents of metaphoric language realized that the analogy of white lines and "chrysalis" or "crystalline" was weak, they decided to abandon all these terms and replace them with the term "shiny white streaks" or " shiny white lines" (19), which fortunately are both very similar to the descriptive term.

"Cobblestone pattern"

This is a metaphoric term (8) for a pattern of large, polygonal clods similar to cobblestones *(4.10)*. This pattern is supposed to evoke the impression of a primarily dermal nevus of the Unna or Miescher type. However, one may find it in the presence of other congenital nevi as well, and occasionally even in seborrheic keratoses. The metaphoric term "cobblestone pattern" may be simply substituted by a description of the pattern. These are large, polygonal, skin-colored or light-brown clods.

"Comedo-like openings"

This is not a descriptive term but an interpretation. Comedo-like openings are dilated, keratin-filled infundibula of a seborrheic keratosis *(4.11)*. As the keratin is usually contaminated by melanin or exogenous impurities and affected by oxygenation, colors seen are brown, yellow or orange. Comedo-like openings are usually seen as clods. Less often they appear as dots or – because the pigment is most dense at the margin of the keratin plug – as circles. As the term "comedo-like openings" already suggests a diagnosis (8), it is not used in pattern analysis. It is better to finish describing a lesion before moving on to interpret these findings and reach a diagnosis.

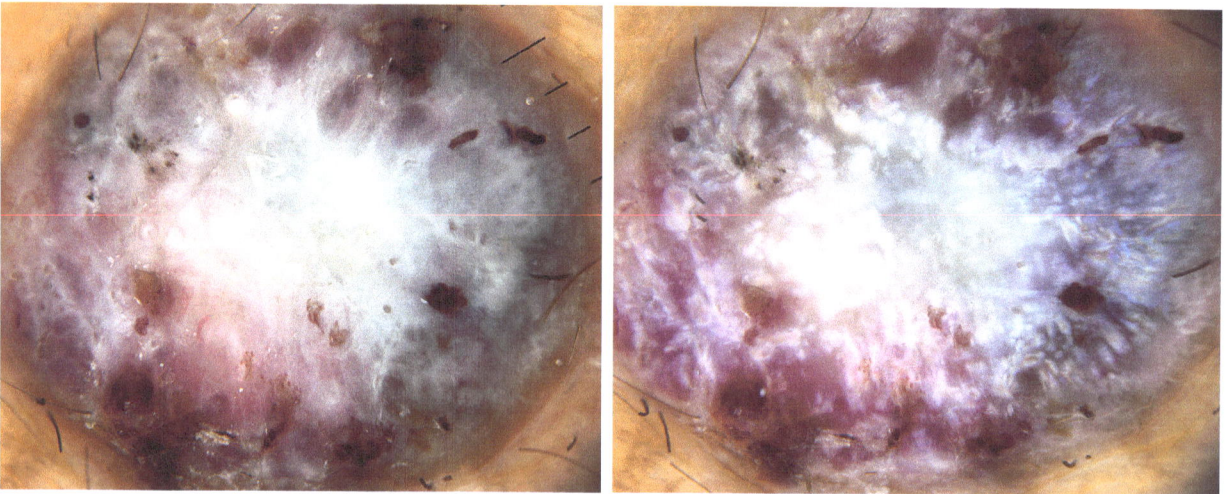

Figure 4.9: Non-polarized *(left)* and polarized *(right)* dermatoscopic view of an invasive melanoma (> 1 mm). White lines are seen as a clue to malignancy in both images but they are seen to be brighter, and perpendicular orientation is more evident, in the polarized image. One can also see so-called "shiny white blotches and strands" which correspond to white structureless zones and white clods.

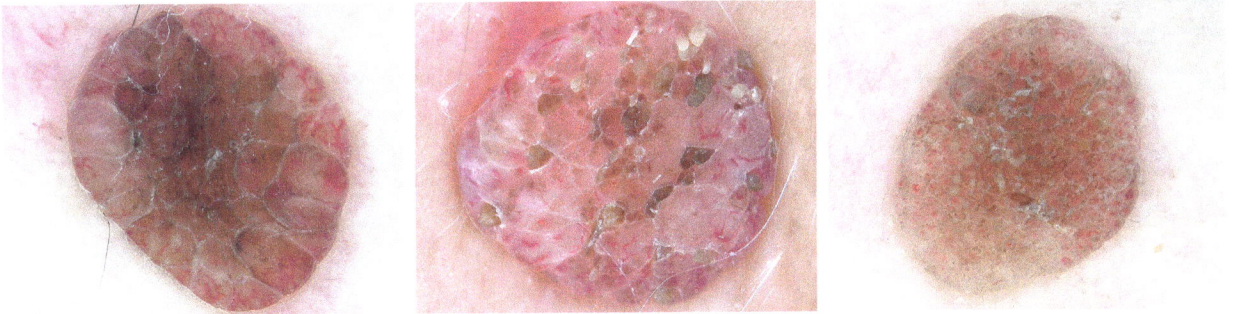

Figure 4.10: "Cobblestone pattern".
This pattern is described simply as large, polygonal clods. Their color may be skin-colored or light-brown. The metaphor "cobblestones" is not required. The figures in the **middle** and on the **right** show smaller yellow and orange clods between skin-colored clods. All three lesions are Unna nevi.

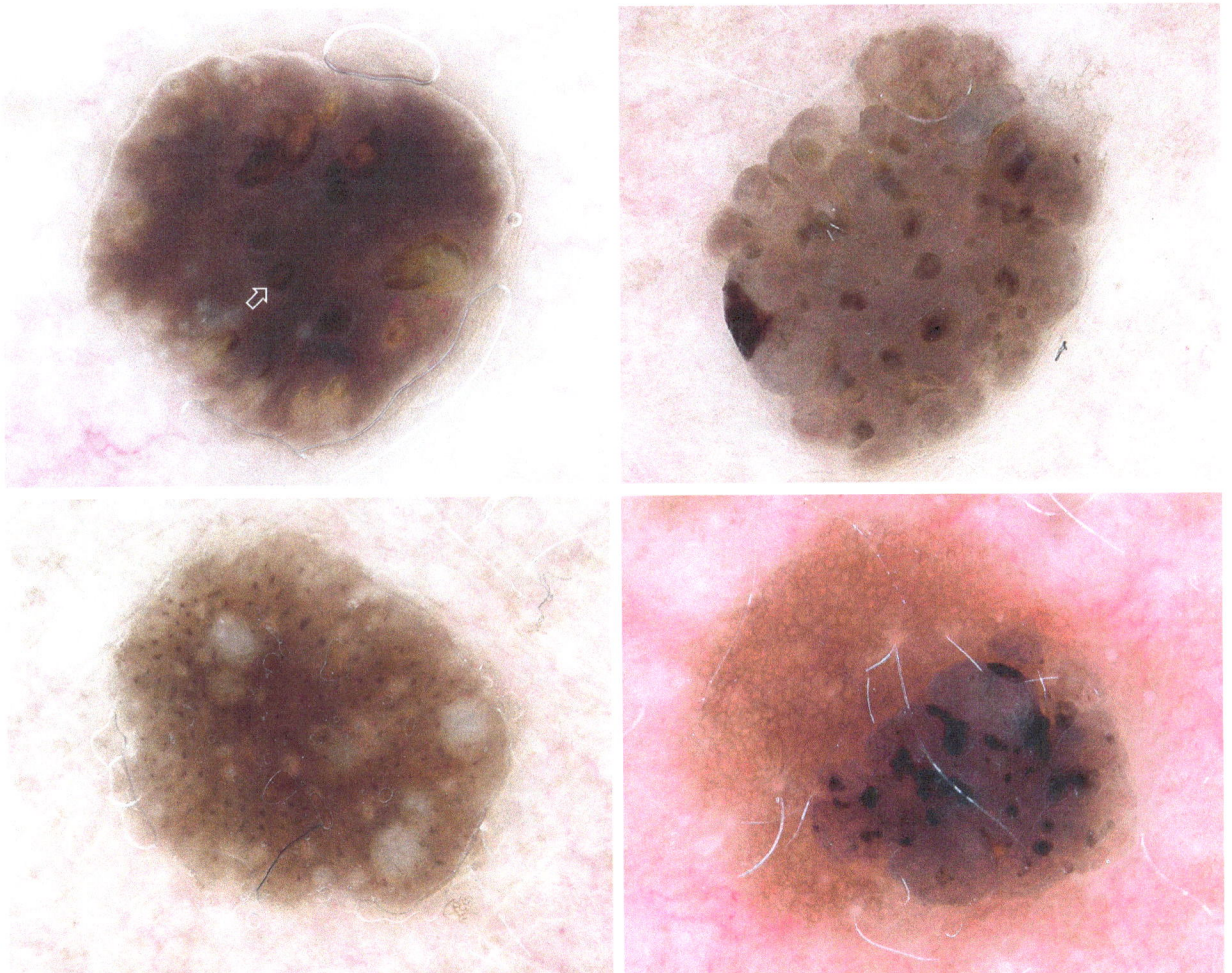

Figure 4.11: "Comedo-like openings".
"Comedo-like openings" may appear as orange or brown, very rarely as black clods, or as circles. **Top left:** "Comedo-like openings" seen as yellow and brown clods, and brown circles (arrow). **Top right:** "Comedo-like openings" seen as relatively large brown clods. **Bottom left:** "Comedo-like openings" seen as small brown clods and/or dots (in addition there are relatively large white clods). **Bottom right:** "Comedo-like openings" seen as black clods. This is a seborrheic keratosis colliding with a Clark nevus.

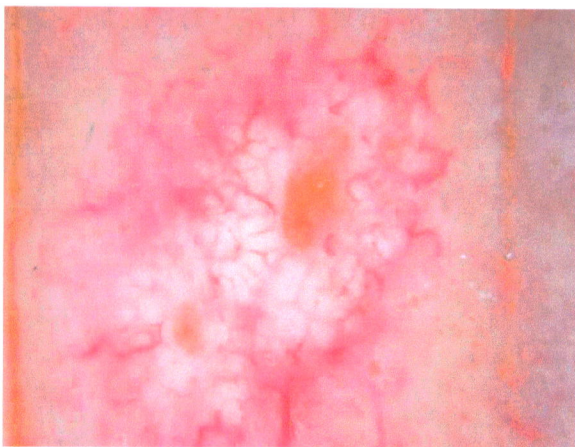

Figure 4.12: "Crown vessels".
Sebaceous gland hyperplasia with radial and peripheral branched vessels that do not cross the center ("crown vessels").

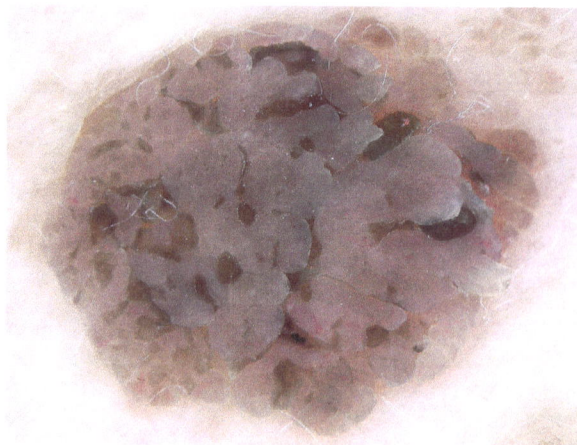

Figure 4.13: "Crypts".
Both the thick curved brown lines and the brown or orange clods of seborrheic keratoses are referred to as "crypts" in metaphoric language.

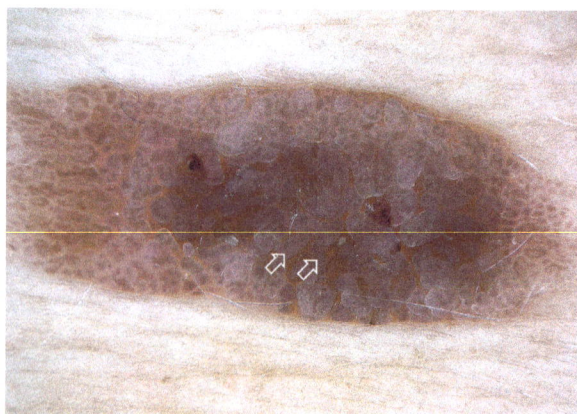

Figure 4.14: "Fat fingers".
"Fat fingers" (arrows) refer to the broad, hypopigmented intervening spaces between brown clods, or the thick curved lines of raised seborrheic keratoses.

"Crown vessels"

The metaphoric term "crown vessels" (20) is used for radial, serpentine or branched vessels at the periphery of the lesion that radiate towards the center but do not cross the midline of the lesion. It is a common finding of sebaceous hyperplasia and helps to differentiate it from basal cell carcinoma *(4.12)*.

"Crypts"

Crypts are defined in medicine as small pits or glandular cavities. In dermatoscopy this term is used to describe invaginations of the epidermis filled with keratin and melanin (8). It roughly corresponds to the "sulci" of the "brain-like pattern" (see the section on this term) of some seborrheic keratosis *(4.13)*. In descriptive terminology these structures are thick curved lines or elongated clods.

"Fat fingers"

"Fat fingers" are similar to "crypts", being another metaphoric term for thick curved lines *(4.14)*. However, the difference between this entity and "crypts" and "sulci" is that "fat fingers" does not refer to the pigmented curved lines themselves but the intervening hypopigmented spaces (12). Like "crypts" and "sulci", these structures are mainly found in seborrheic keratoses.

"Fibrillar pattern"

"Fibrillar"(21, 22) means "consisting of fibrils"; fibrils are very thin fibers. Regrettably, the term does not convey the principal characteristic of this pattern. According to the standardized dictionary it consists of "linear pigmented filamentous lines of similar length with one end at the furrows and oriented at a certain angle to the furrows and crossing the ridges" *(4.15)*. Because the spatial arrangement of the parallel lines is the characteristic feature of this pattern and not that it is composed of "fibrils", the descriptive term for this pattern is "parallel lines crossing the ridges".

"Fingerprinting"

The flat initial stage in the evolution of seborrheic keratoses, also known as solar lentigo, may (especially on the trunk) show a pattern consisting of long, thin, curved lines that are partly arranged in parallel fashion *(4.16)*. Together with a few interspersed circles these lines are vaguely reminiscent of dermatoglyphs; hence "fingerprinting". Describing this pattern as an accumulation of long curved lines serves the same purpose as using the metaphoric term "fingerprinting", without the obligatory inference that the lesion is a solar lentigo.

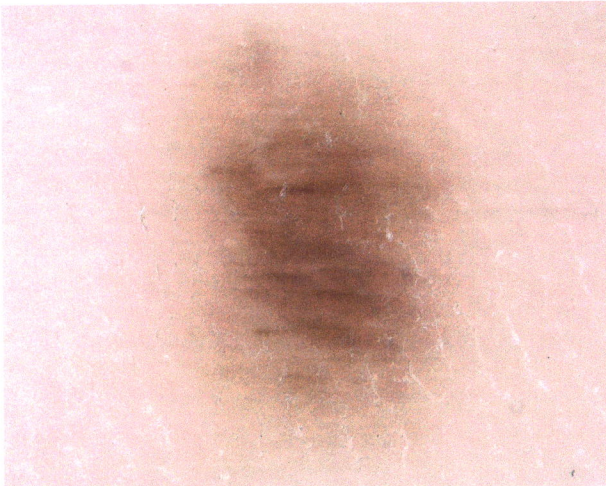

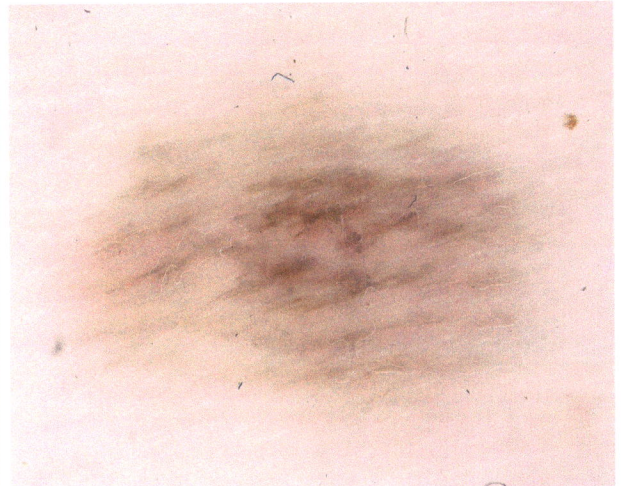

Figure 4.15: "Fibrillar pattern".
A linear pattern on acral skin in which the short pigmented lines cross the ridges is referred to as a "parallel lines, crossing the ridges" in the descriptive language and not as a "fibrillar pattern". Both cases are dermatoscopic views of classical acral nevi.

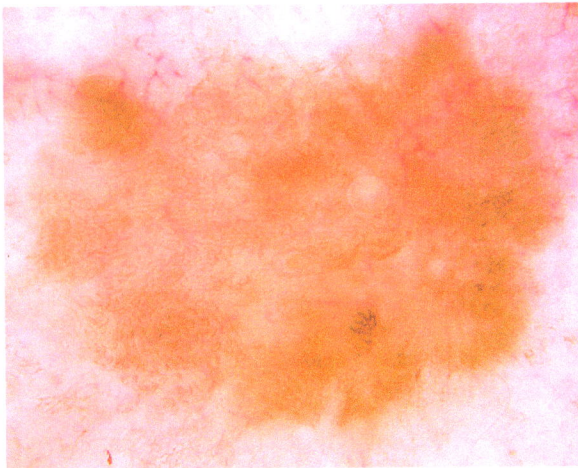

Figure 4.16: "Fingerprinting".
Solar lentigo with curved lines; vaguely similar to "fingerprints".

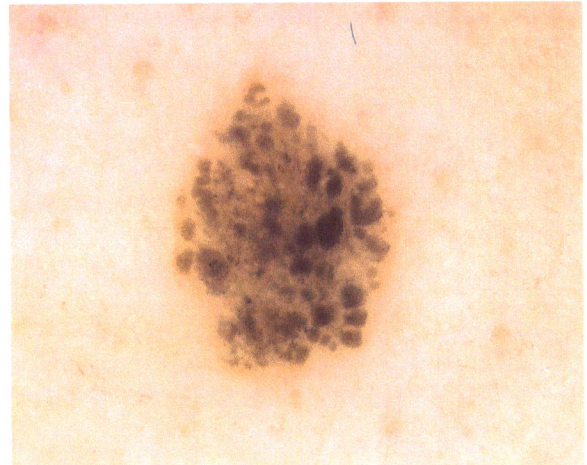

Figure 4.17: "Globules" (Clods).
"Globules" in pattern analysis are small to middle-sized, brown, round or oval clods – as in this nevus.

"Fissures and ridges"

"Fissures and ridges" (11) are merely other expressions of the previously mentioned "gyri" (i.e. ridges) and "sulci" (i.e. fissures).

"Globules"

"Globules" or "Globuli" in common terminology (8) are small to middle-sized, round or oval, brown clods (4.17). The term "clod" in pattern analysis is used to describe any round, oval or polygonal well circumscribed structure, of any color.

Thus, round or oval brown clods known as "globules" in metaphoric language are simply one small sub-group of clods. We consider it confusing to novice dermatosco-

pists that similarly shaped structures are given different names to describe their geometry, merely because they are a different color. Aggregated globules (aggregated brown clods) are, in most algorithms, taken to be indicative of a melanocytic lesion. However, this clue is not very specific as non-melanocytic lesions such as basal cell carcinoma or seborrheic keratoses may also have brown clods.

"Homogeneous pattern"

The term "homogenous" (8) is often used instead of structureless. We do not encourage that. Nothing in dermatoscopy is purely homogenous. Even blue nevi are not homogenously blue (4.18). Structureless is

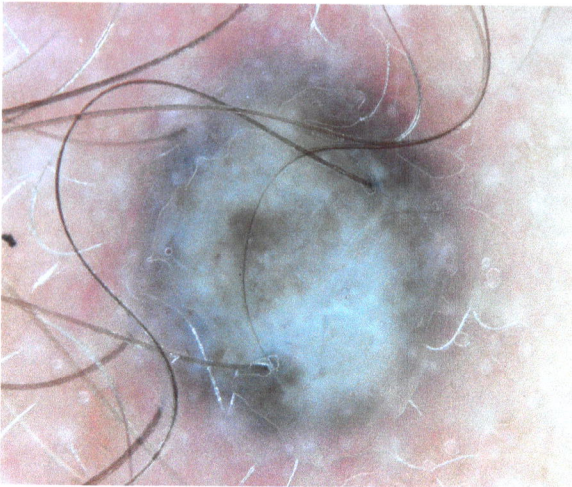

Figure 4.18: *"Homogenous pattern".*
We prefer the term "structureless" to "homogeneous ", because nothing in dermatoscopy is truly "homogeneous". This blue nevus has different shades of blue (it is not homogenous) but it lacks any discernable structure (it is structureless).

the better term because it indicates the lack of any discernable basic element.

Inverse or negative pigment network and reticular depigmentation

Normally, reticular lines (pigment network) are more pigmented than the spaces they enclose. When this relation is reversed, this is referred to as an inverse or negative pigment network (23). The term "reticular depigmentation" is used in a similar way. According to the standardized dictionary "negative network" or "reticular depigmentation" correspond to "serpiginous interconnecting broadened hypopigmented lines that surround elongated and curvilinear globules" (4.19). It is a clue to melanoma, but may also occur in Spitz nevi (24) and dermatofibroma. The difficulty with this term and the given definition is revealed by the following question: What is the foreground and what is the background? The "elongated and curvilinear globules" (clods in the descriptive language) are pigmented but the structure is named after the hypopigmented lines. In this case, therefore, the hyperpigmented portion is the background while the hypopigmented lines constitute the foreground. In the descriptive terminology we do not refer to reticular depigmentation or negative network but simply to hypopigmented or white reticular lines. The difficulty of the foreground and the background, however, is not entirely resolved by doing so. The solution is quite simple: If the reticular lines surrounding the clods are skin colored and not white we consider this not very specific. In this case we call it a pattern of clods. When the reticular lines are white (whiter than the surrounding skin) we consider it a clue to melanoma. Then the structure is named "white reticular lines" to point to the fact the white lines are more specific than the pigmented background.

"Lattice-like pattern"

This metaphoric term (8) applies only to lesions on volar skin. It describes volar pigmentation forming thin lines, parallel on the furrow and crossing perpendicular on the ridges. It is one of the benign patterns of volar skin and usually found in acral nevi (4.20).

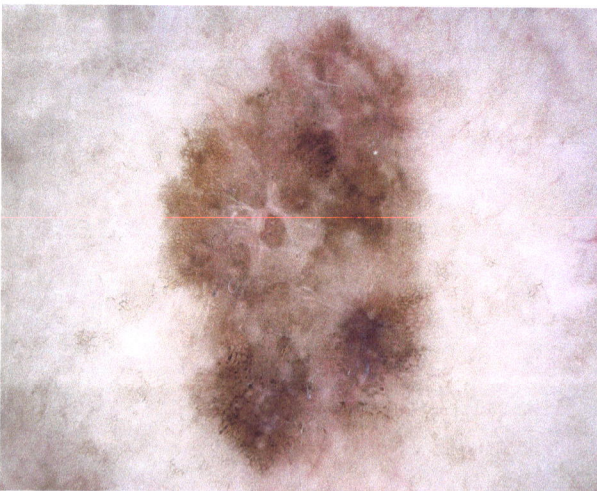

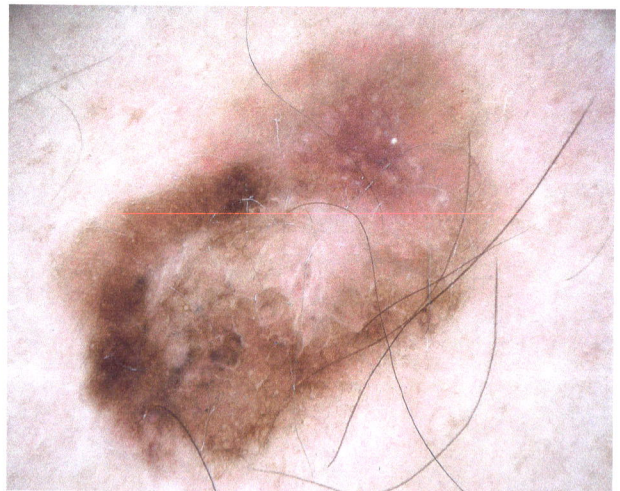

Figure 4.19: *"Inverse or negative pigment network" or "reticular depigmentation".*
Dermatoscopic view of reticular white lines in two melanomas. The melanoma on the left also has black dots in its periphery – a further clue to melanoma.

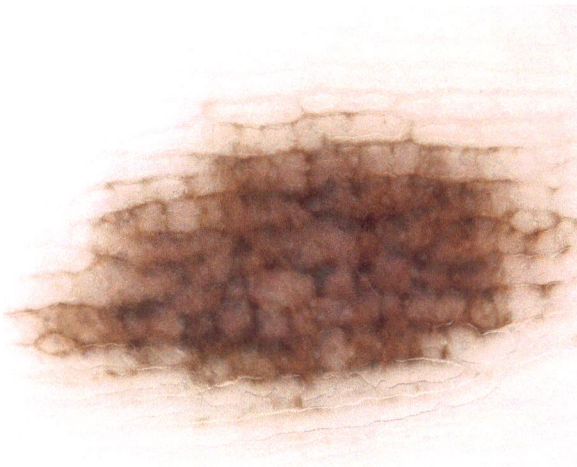

Figure 4.20: "Lattice-like pattern".
An acral nevus with a lattice-like pattern: Brown lines, parallel, on the furrows and crossing perpendicular on the ridges.

Figure 4.21: "Maple leaf-like areas".
The "maple leaves" of this basal cell carcinoma are radial lines at the periphery, which may be thin or thick. Their special feature is their common base. In rare cases they actually do look like "maple leaves", as they do here.

"Maple leaf-like areas"

"Maple leaves" are supposed to be visible at the periphery of some basal cell carcinomas (8) *(4.21)*. Maple leaves or leaf-like structures are formed by radial lines at the periphery of a lesion. According to the definition given in the consensus paper they correspond to "pigmented discrete linear or bulbous structures coalescing at a common off-center base, creating structures that resemble a leaf-like pattern" (1). This criterion is relatively specific for basal cell carcinoma, but they may sometimes be confused with the radial lines found in melanomas. Unfortunately, for most structures named "leaf-like", it takes imagination to see maple leaves. This description is therefore often post hoc, i.e. the description is chosen only after the

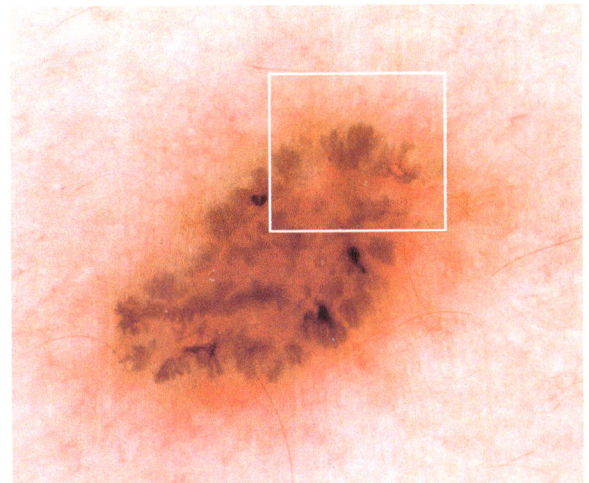

diagnosis has already been reached. Experts reach a diagnosis at a glance, and only then construct a description that fits this (usually accurate) diagnosis. However, outwardly it would appear as if the diagnosis were derived from maple leaves, although the opposite is the case. In descriptive terminology we call them radial lines converging to a common base.

"Milia-like cysts"

"Milia-like cysts" (8) is also not just a description, but also an interpretation. The term refers to small, epidermal inclusion cysts (milia) lined with an epithelium. They are typically found in seborrheic keratosis *(4.22)*. They are not as specific as is generally assumed and commonly

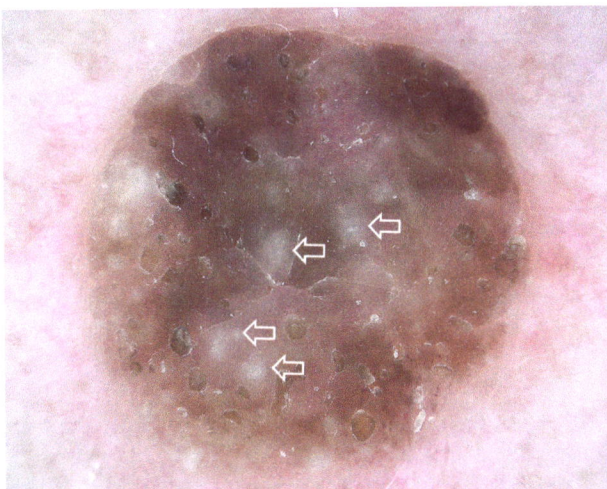

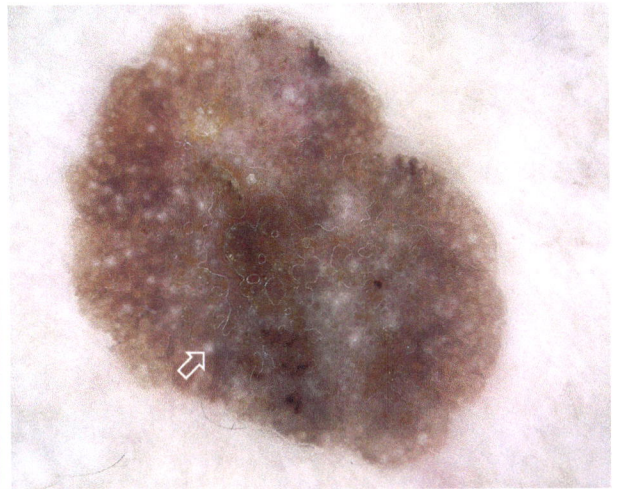

Figure 4.22: "Milia-like cysts".
*In these two seborrheic keratoses, "milia-like cysts" are seen on dermatoscopy as large white clods (**left**) or as white dots (**right**).*

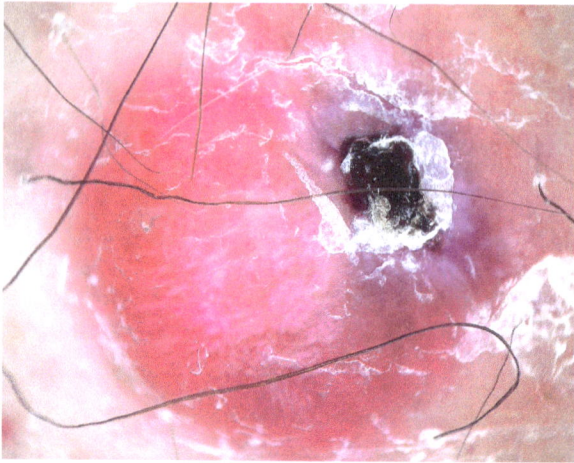

Figure 4.23: *"Milky red areas"*.
A melanoma with "milky red areas", which is called pink structureless zone in the descriptive terminology.

also occur in congenital nevi and basal cell carcinoma as well as less frequently in many other lesions, including melanoma. On dermatoscopy, milia-like cysts are seen as white or yellow dots and/or clods.

"Milky red areas"

According to the consensus paper (1) the term "milky red area" is used to characterize "a red vascular blush with no specific distinguishable vessels". In descriptive terms we simply call it a pink structureless area *(4.23)*. It is of some value for the diagnosis of hypo- or non-pigmented types of melanoma.

"Moth-eaten border"

The sharp border with concave or sharp punched-out invaginations that is frequently found in flat seborrheic keratoses and solar lentigines led investigators to make the comparison to a garment damaged by moths *(4.24)*.

"Peppering"

The pattern of gray dots on a white structureless background is known as peppering in metaphoric language (6) *(4.25)*. The white structureless zone corresponds to fibrosis of the dermis, interspersed with numerous melanophages (gray dots or small gray clods). Sometimes the term "regression" is used synonymously, but "peppering" is not always due to partial or complete regression of a pre-existing melanocytic lesion. Especially when the white structureless zone is absent, one should be cautious in interpreting the gray dots as regression. Like all metaphoric terms, this one is also replaceable with descriptive terminology (white structureless zone with gray dots and/or clods).

"Peripheral streaks" or "irregular peripheral extensions"

These terms refer to radial lines or pseudopods at a lesion's periphery, but only occupying part of the circumference *(4.26)*. This feature should cause one to suspect a melanoma. However, occasionally Reed nevi and recurrent nevi also have radial lines which are not distributed over the entire circumference, and basal cell carcinomas may also have radial lines.

Pigment network

The term "pigment network" refers to reticular lines. In contrast to the widespread view, the presence of a so-called pigment network is not unique to melanocytic lesions. Reticular lines are also found in solar lentigines, seborrheic keratoses, melanotic macules (especially

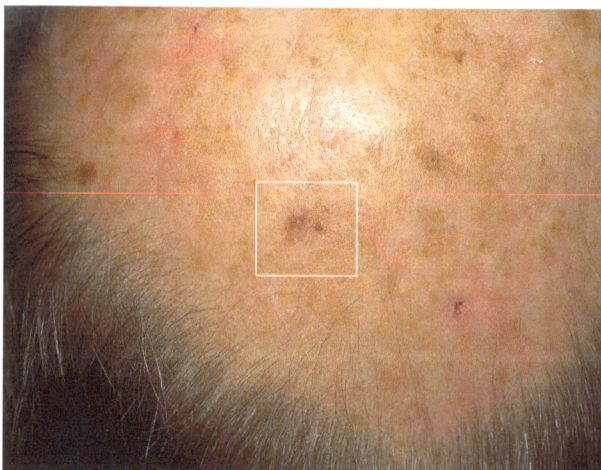

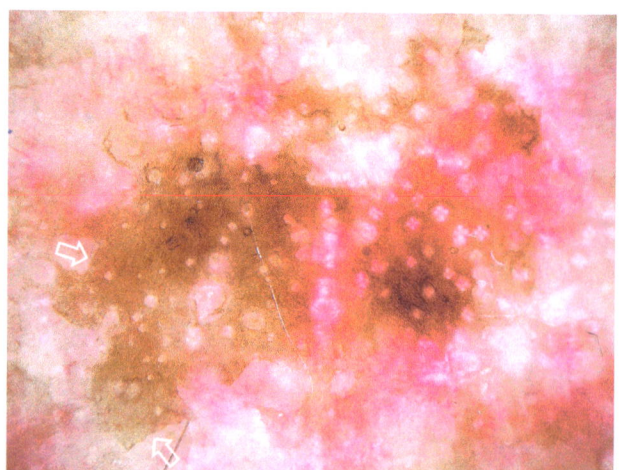

Figure 4.24: *"Moth-eaten border"*.
The well demarcated, scalloped margin (arrows) with sharp punched-out invaginations of a solar lentigo is known as a "moth-eaten border" in metaphoric language.

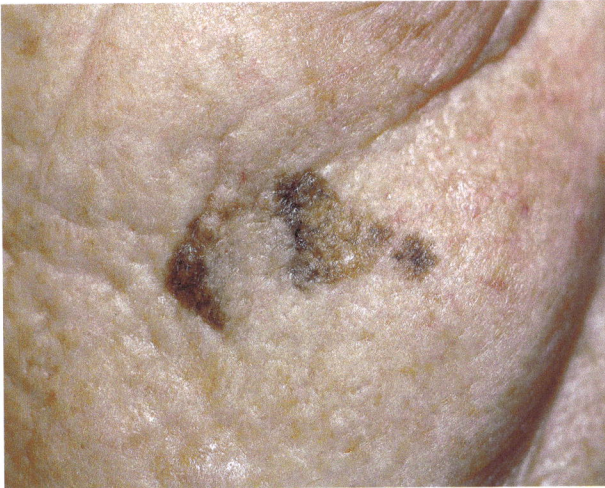

Figure 4.25: "Peppering".
A regressive melanoma with multiple gray dots ("peppering").

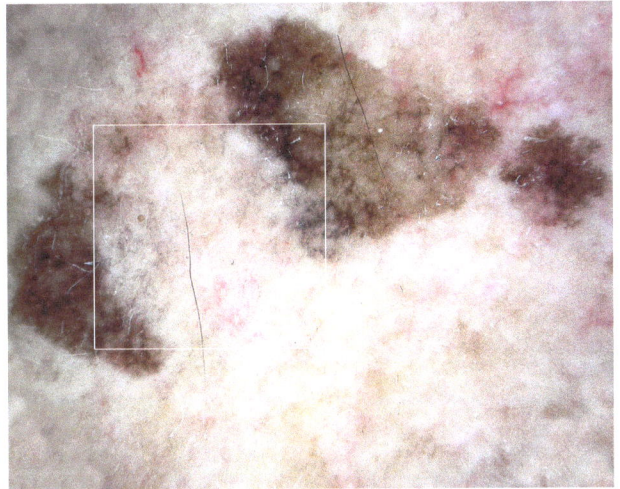

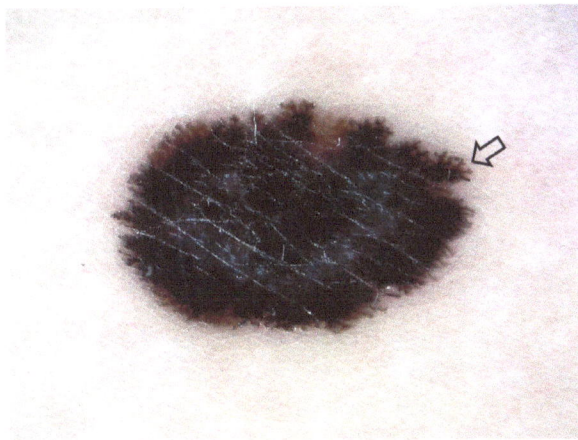

Figure 4.26: "Peripheral streaks" or "irregular peripheral extensions".
"Peripheral streaks" or "irregular peripheral extensions" at the periphery of a melanoma. In the language of pattern analysis one refers to peripheral radial lines or pseudopods, present segmentally (as opposed to occupying the entire circumference).

ink-spot lentigo), dermatofibroma, urticaria pigmentosa (a clinical variant of mastocytosis) and accessory nipple (25). In some skin types, pigment network is even seen on normal skin. Reticular lines are primarily due to hyperpigmentation of basal keratinocytes; the melanocytes are not necessarily increased in number.

"Pseudo-network"

Words with the prefix "pseudo" indicate that something is being mimicked. A pseudo-network looks like a pigment network (i.e. reticular lines) but is not one. This term is used to describe pigmented lesions on the face (4.27). In terms of anatomy, the epidermis of the face is usually (but not always) flattened in advanced age. In other words, the rete ridges are missing. However, rete ridges are a prerequisite if hyperpigmentation of basal keratinocytes is to be seen as reticular lines (i.e. pigment network) on dermatoscopy. A further special anatomic feature of facial skin is the presence of numerous follicular openings. As hyperpigmentation of the epidermis – regardless of whether it is caused by an increased number of melanocytes or not – spares the follicular openings, one gets the impression of thick reticular lines (pseudo-network). However, the pigmentation around the openings of the hair follicles may be structureless, it may consist of dots, or it may form circles. Therefore, this is more correctly and more specifically described as "structureless pattern", or "pattern of dots", or "pattern of circles" instead of "pseudo-network." It should be mentioned that, on the face, there may also be reticular lines (i.e. a "genuine" and not "pseudo"network) because the rete ridges are not always absent. However, the most common patterns on the face are the structureless pattern and the pattern of dots, which may occur in cases of in situ melanoma (lentigo maligna) as well as solar lentigo or pigmented actinic keratosis, and the pattern of circles that is rather specific for in situ melanoma (lentigo maligna) if some or all circles are gray.

"Radial streaming"

Interpreted literally this term makes no sense because dermatoscopy is a static and not a dynamic investigation; nothing can "flow" or "be streaming". It refers to peripheral radial lines, i.e. describes the same structures as "peripheral streaks" (refer to the section on this term).

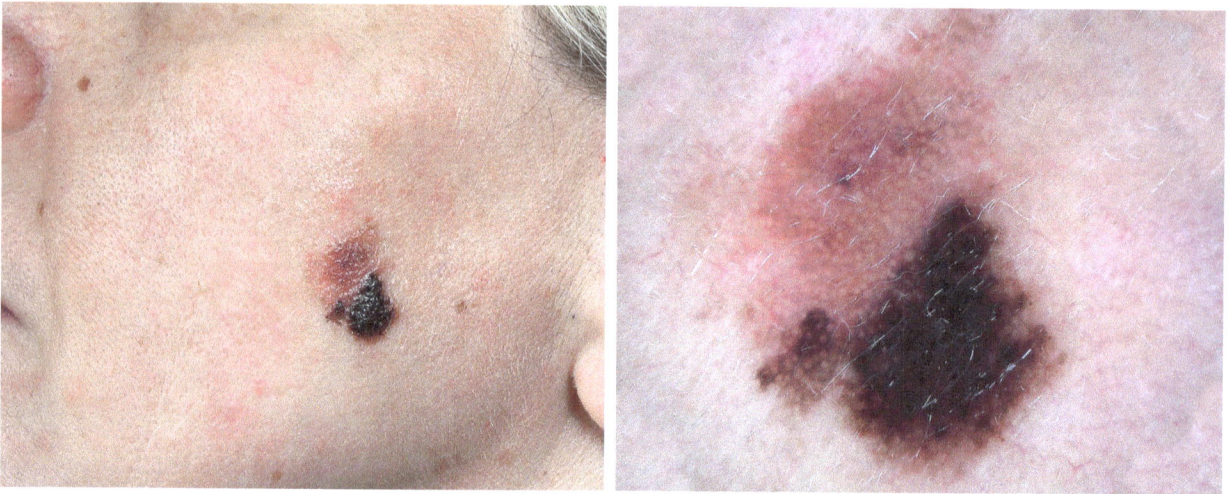

Figure 4.27: "Pseudo-pigment network".
A melanoma on the face in various stages of its development on dermatoscopy. In the upper portion there are only discrete circles (in situ portion of a melanoma). Between 6 o'clock and 9 o'clock the circles become confluent and form a so-called "pseudo-pigment network". Between 3 o'clock and 6 o'clock one finally finds only a structureless zone (invasive portion).

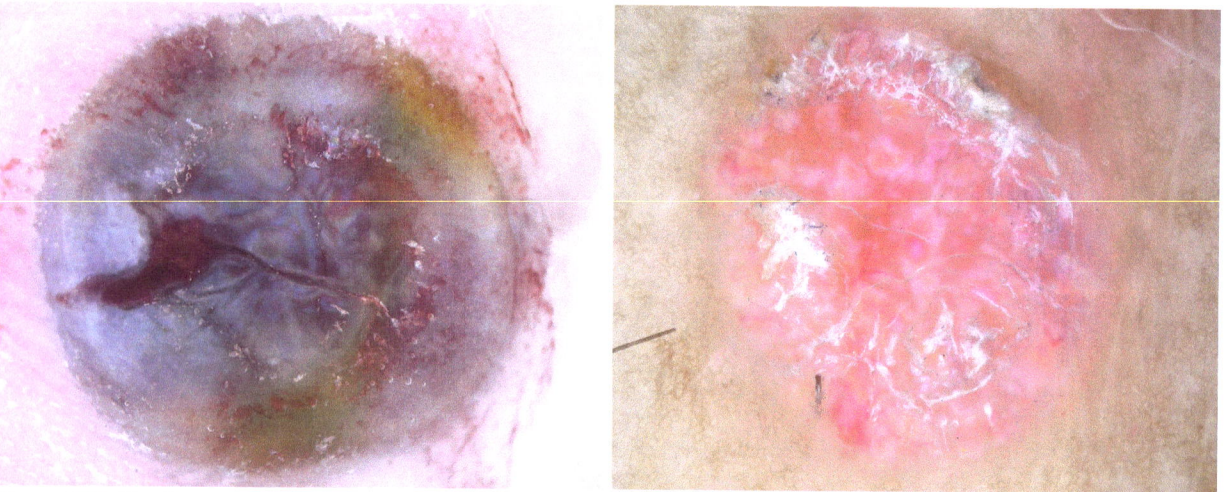

Figure 4.28: "Rainbow pattern".
Rainbow pattern in the center of a Kaposi sarcoma (left). In the descriptive terminology we call it polychromatic structureless zone. A similar structure can also be seen in some dermatofibromas (right), especially in the hemosiderotic subtype.

"Rainbow pattern"

The rainbow pattern is defined as "circumscribed structureless areas displaying colors of the whole spectrum of visible light". In the descriptive terminology we call it polychromatic structureless zone. Initially it was described as a specific clue to Kaposi sarcoma (26) but later it was found out that it can be found in other diagnosis too (for example in dermatofibroma or vascular lesions (4.28) (27).

"Red lacunes"

Lacunes (Latin, lacuna) are concavities or grooves, and "puddles" (Latin: lacus = the lake). Thus, "red lacunes"

are "red puddles". It is simpler to call them red clods (4.29). A collection of red clods is primarily found in vascular lesions, especially hemangiomas and recent hemorrhages.

However, red clods may rarely be found in melanoma – in which case the advocates of metaphoric language call them "milky red globules" rather than "red lacunes". This is a further instance of how the diagnosis can alter the description.

"Reticular depigmentation"

This term is discussed under the related term "inverse pigment network".

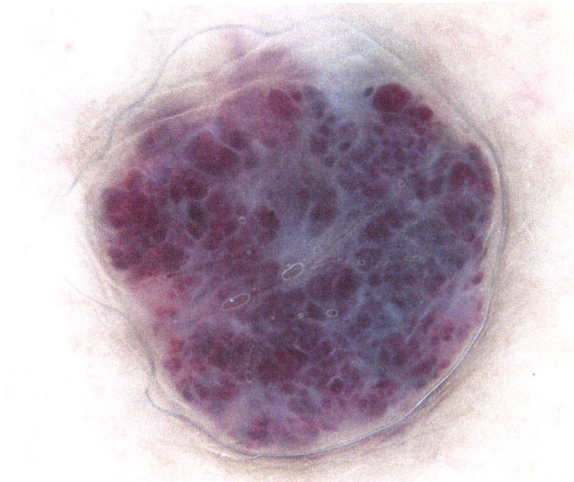

Figure 4.29: "Red lacunes".
The "red lacunes" seen in this hemangioma are simply called red clods in descriptive terminology.

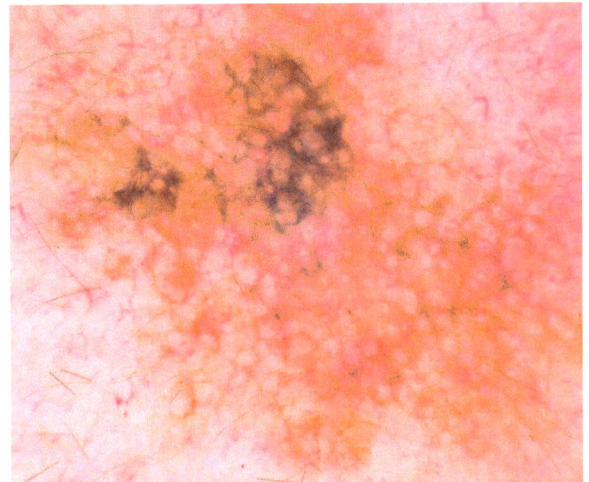

Figure 4.30: "Rhomboids".
Angulated lines around follicular openings of facial skin are called "rhomboids" in metaphoric language if they form complete polygons and "zig-zag" pattern if they form incomplete polygons.

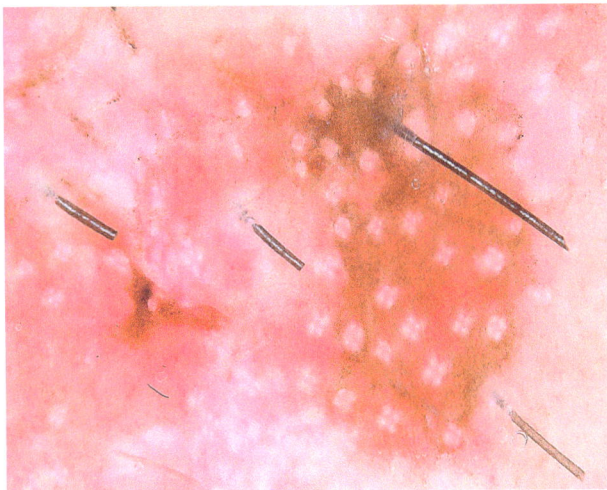

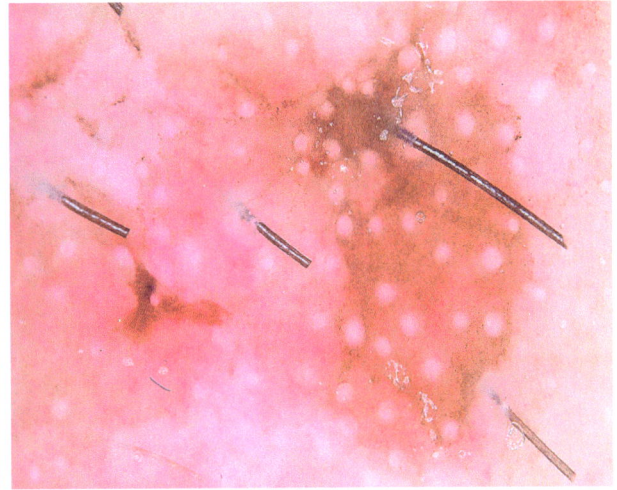

Figure 4.31: The structures known in metaphoric terminology as "rosettes" are clearly seen as 4 white dots arranged in a square (4 dot clod), but only on polarized dermatoscopy (**left**). With non-polarized dermatoscopy (**right**) they are simply seen as a white clod.

"Rhomboids"

Rhomboids are defined as "gray-brown angulated lines forming a polygonal shape around adnexal ostial openings". The term is reserved for facial lesions and it is a clue to melanoma in situ (4.30). It is similar but does not correspond to "polygons" on non-facial skin. In the descriptive terminology we call them "angulated lines".

"Rosettes"

This is an aggregation of four white dots arranged as a square or rhomboid. They are seen only when using a polarizing dermatoscope (4.31). In the language of pattern analysis we call this structure 4 white dots arranged in a square or 4-dot clod because when viewed with non-polarizing dermatoscopy the 4 dots appear as single white clod. This structure has been found in many different lesions (28) but most often in actinic keratosis.

"Scar-like depigmentation"

This is a term that constitutes an interpretation as well as a description. It describes a white structureless zone that is then interpreted as representing a scar or scar-like entity (4.32). The histological correlate of this area is a zone of fibrosis after complete or partial regression of a melanocytic lesion. Similar "scar-like" areas exist in basal-cell carcinoma, where they are known as "shiny white areas"; and in dermatofibromas, where they are

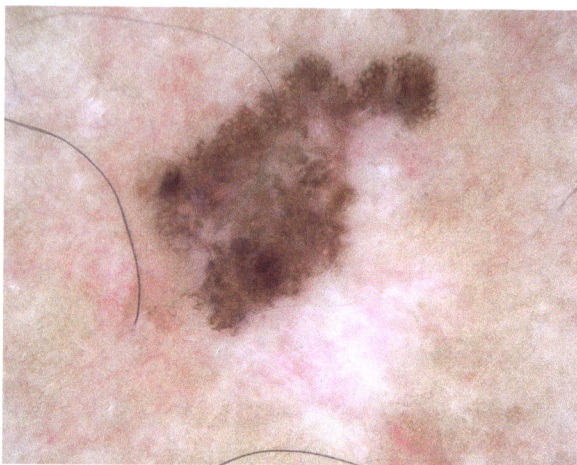

Figure 4.32: "Scar-like depigmentation".
"Scar-like depigmentation" in a melanoma. In the language of pattern analysis this is simply a white structureless zone.

Figure 4.33: "Spoke-wheel areas".
Dermatoscopic view of a basal cell carcinoma with a "spoke wheel" (arrow). In descriptive terminology this is described as radial lines converging at a central dot or a central clod.

known as a "central white patch" (see the respective sections). This is a further instance of the diagnosis influencing the description. In descriptive terminology we simply refer to either white structureless zones or white lines, as appropriate.

"Shiny white streaks, blotches and strands"

"Shiny white streaks" (19) correspond to perpendicular white lines in descriptive terminology. Former synonyms were chrysalis, chrysalids, or crystalline structures. The latter terms have been abandoned and should not be used even if you prefer metaphoric terminology. Shiny white blotches and strands correspond to white structureless areas, white clods, or thick white lines

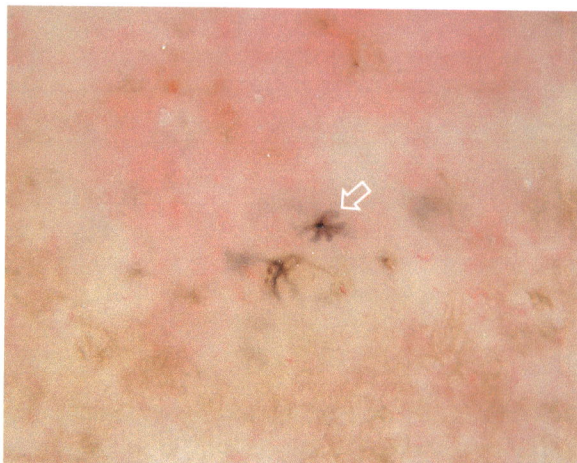

(4.9). If lines are present they are usually oriented perpendicular to each other. These structures are seen only under polarized dermatoscopy and can be found in melanoma, basal cell carcinoma, Spitz nevus and dermatofibroma.

"Spoke-wheel areas"

Structures consisting of radial lines that converge at a central point or a central clod are known as "spoke-wheel areas" (4.33). They are very specific to basal cell carcinoma and are not seen in other lesions. The variant consisting of radial lines with a dot or a clod as a common center shows some similarity with spoke wheels when the radial lines completely surround the

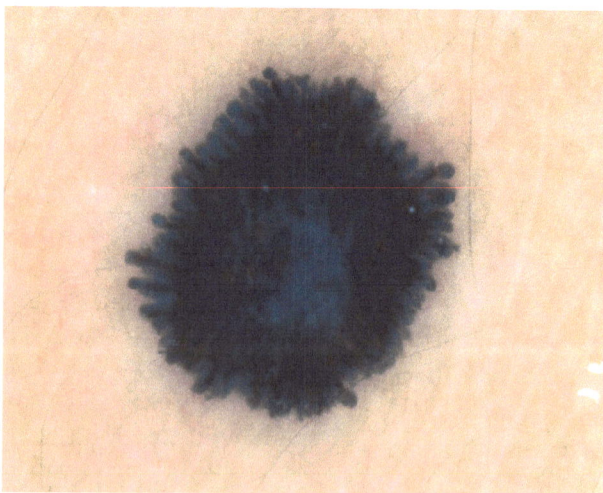

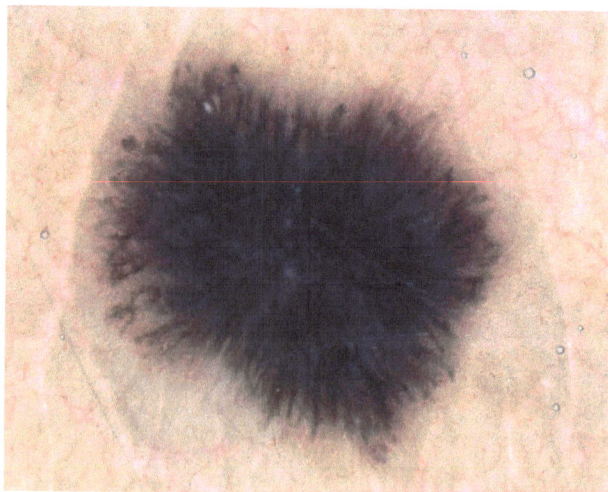

Figure 4.34: "Starburst pattern".
Two Reed nevi showing the "starburst pattern". Pseudopods (**left**) or radial lines (**right**) are seen around the entire circumference.

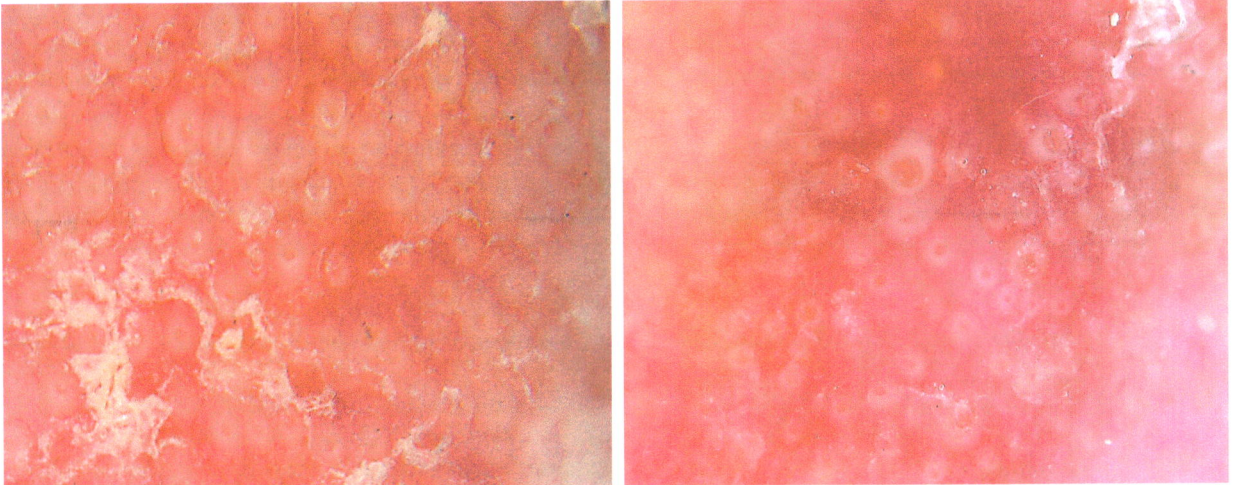

Figure 4.35: "*Strawberry pattern*".
High magnification of dermatoscopy images of two lesions which can be said to demonstrate the "strawberry pattern". This can be simply described as a pattern of white circles with background erythema (red structureless area). The pattern of white circles is seen in actinic keratosis and squamous cell carcinoma. The image on the **left** *is an actinic keratosis but the one on the* **right** *is a squamous cell carcinoma.*

central structure. Unfortunately, in many other cases they bear little similarity to spoke wheels. Usually the radial lines only partly surround the central structure. Another variant consists of a darkly pigmented dot in the center of a less heavily pigmented clod, reminiscent of a wheel, but without spokes. In any case the term "spoke wheel" is dispensable because these entities can also be described by the use of descriptive terminology.

"Starburst pattern"

The "starburst pattern" (8) is the combination of patterns consisting of a structureless zone centrally, with radial lines or pseudopods occupying the entire periphery

(4.34). This pattern is mainly found in Reed nevi and in those rare cases in which a melanoma mimics a Reed nevus. Occasionally the term "starburst pattern" is also used for a combination of clods at the periphery and a structureless hyperpigmented center. This pattern is more commonly found in the pigmented Spitz nevus. When two different patterns bear the same name, it is quite natural for the two different diagnoses – Reed nevus and pigmented Spitz nevus – to be lumped together.

"Strawberry pattern"

In metaphorical terminology this refers to a pattern which is sometimes seen in actinic keratoses in which

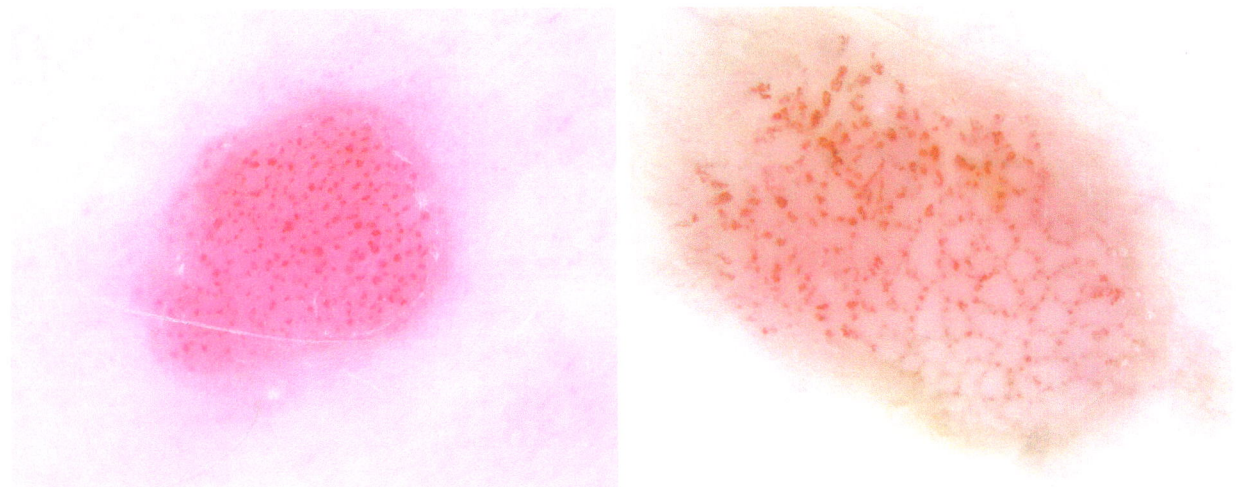

Figure 4.36: "*String of pearls*".
Two typical examples of clear cell acanthoma. The serpiginous arrangement of coiled vessels, which is relatively specific for this diagnosis, is called "string of pearls" in metaphoric language.

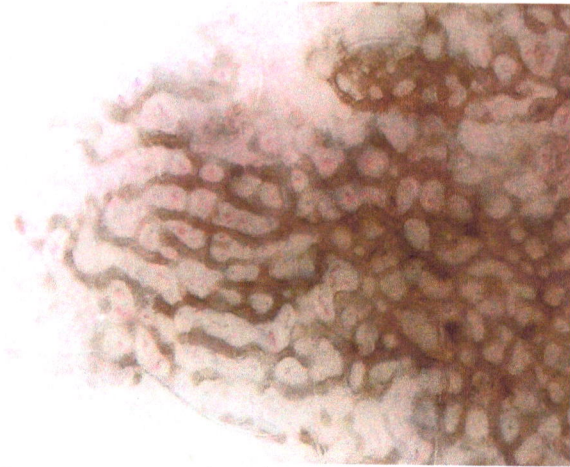

Figure 4.37: "Targetoid vessels".
Vessels as dots and coils in the hypopigmented area between reticular lines are sometimes called "targetoid vessels". Their significance is unclear.

the dermatoscopic appearance is said to resemble the surface of a strawberry (29). In figure 4.35 there is a red background due to vascular erythema with keratin clods in the infundibulae rimmed by white circles. The resulting pattern is called "strawberry pattern". The red background is not always seen. In the descriptive language we refer to this pattern as white circles against a red background.

"String of pearls"

The metaphor of "string of pearls" is used for coiled vessels that are arranged in serpentine lines (30). In the descriptive terminology we use the term "serpiginous" for this specific arrangement of vessels. It is rather specific for clear cell acanthoma although it has been described in other lesions too, most notably in prurigo or lichen simplex chronicus (4.36).

"Targetoid dots" and "targetoid vessels"

"Targetoid dots" and "targetoid vessels" refer to brown dots or red dots (vessels) in the center of hypopigmented space between reticular lines (4.37). These structures are found in some congenital nevi, especially larger ones, but their significance is unclear.

"Zig-zag pattern"

The term "zig-zag pattern" has been used for incomplete "rhomboids" on facial skin and corresponds to straight lines meeting at angles that form incomplete polygons around follicular openings (5) (4.30). They bear the same significance for facial melanoma in situ as "rhomboids". For this reason we make no difference in the descriptive terminology and simply call this pattern "angulated lines".

Tabelle 4.1: Translation of metaphoric language into simple terminology based on five simple geometric terms (five basic elements)

Metaphoric terminology	Descriptive terminology
Annular-granular pattern	Dots, gray and circles, gray
Atypical pigment network	Lines, reticular and thick or reticular lines that vary in color
Blotch	Structureless zone, brown or black
Blue-gray ovoid nests	Clods, blue, large, clustered
Blue-whitish veil, blue veil	Structureless zone, blue
Branched streaks	Lines, branched
Broadened network	Lines, reticular and thick
Central white patch	Structureless zone, white, central
Cerebriform pattern, fissures and ridges, gyri and sulci, fat fingers	Lines, curved and thick
Cobblestone pattern	Clods, brown or skin colored, large and polygonal
Comedo-like openings	Clods, brown, yellow, or orange (rarely black)
Crown vessels	Radial linear vessels, not crossing the center
Crypts	Lines, curved and thick, in combination with clods
Delicate network	Lines, reticular and thin
Fibrillar pattern	Lines, parallel, short, crossing ridges (volar skin)
Fingerprinting	Lines, brown, curved, parallel, thin
Globules	Clods, small, round or oval
Granularity or granules	Dots, any color
Homogenous pattern	Structureless, any color
Lattice-like pattern (volar skin)	Lines, parallel, thin, in the furrows and crossing the ridges
Leaf like areas	Lines, radial, connected to a common base (sometimes variously shaped clods have been called "leaf like areas")
Milia like cysts, cloudy or starry	Dots or clods, white, clustered or disseminated
Milky red areas	Structureless zone, pink
Milky red globules	Clods, pink and small
Moth eaten border	Sharply demarcated, scalloped border
Negative pigment network (synonyms: inverse network, reticular depigmentation)	Lines, reticular, hypopigmented, around brown clods
Peppering	Dots, gray
Pigment network	Lines, reticular
Pseudo-network	Structureless, brown, interrupted by follicular openings (facial-skin)
Radial streaming	Lines, radial, peripheral and segmental
Rainbow pattern	Structureless zone, polychromatic
Red lacunes	Clods, red or purple
Rhomboids	Lines, angulated (facial skin)
Rosettes	Dots, white, four arranged in a square, 4-dot clod
Scar-like depigmentation	Structureless zone, white
Shiny white blotches and strands	Clods, white
Shiny white streaks (synonyms: chrysalis, chrysalids, crystalline structure)	Lines, white, perpendicular
Spoke wheel area	Lines, radial, converging to a central dot or clod
Starburst pattern	Pseudopods, circumferential or lines, radial, circumferential
Strawberry pattern	Structureless, red, interrupted by follicular openings
Streaks	Lines, radial (always at periphery)
String of pearls	Coiled vessels arranged in serpentine lines
Targetoid dots	Dots, brown, central (in the center of hypopigmented spaces between reticular lines)
Zig-zag pattern	Lines, angulated (facial skin)

References

1   Kittler H, Marghoob AA, Argenziano G, et al. Standardization of terminology in dermoscopy/dermatoscopy: Results of the third consensus conference of the International Society of Dermoscopy. J Am Acad Dermatol. 2016; 74(6): 1093–106.

2   Jaimes N, Marghoob AA, Rabinovitz H, et al. Clinical and dermoscopic characteristics of melanomas on nonfacial chronically sun-damaged skin. J Am Acad Dermatol. Jun 2015; 72(6): 1027–1035.

3   Keir J. Dermatoscopic features of cutaneous non-facial non-acral lentiginous growth pattern melanomas. Dermatol Pract Concept. Jan 2014; 4(1): 77–82.

4   Schiffner R, Schiffner-Rohe J, Vogt T, et al. Improvement of early recognition of lentigo maligna using dermatoscopy. J Am Acad Dermatol. Jan 2000; 42(1 Pt 1): 25–32.

5   Slutsky JB, Marghoob AA. The zig-zag pattern of lentigo maligna. Arch Dermatol. Dec 2010; 146(12): 1444.

6   Stolz W, Schiffner R, Burgdorf WH. Dermatoscopy for facial pigmented skin lesions. Clin Dermatol. May-Jun 2002; 20(3): 276–278.

7   Tschandl P, Rosendahl C, Kittler H. Dermatoscopy of flat pigmented facial lesions. J Eur Acad Dermatol Venereol. Jan 2015; 29(1): 120–127.

8   Argenziano G, Soyer HP, Chimenti S, et al. Dermoscopy of pigmented skin lesions: results of a consensus meeting via the Internet. J Am Acad Dermatol. May 2003; 48(5): 679–693.

9   Argenziano G, Fabbrocini G, Carli P, De Giorgi V, Sammarco E, Delfino M. Epiluminescence microscopy for the diagnosis of doubtful melanocytic skin lesions. Comparison of the ABCD rule of dermatoscopy and a new 7-point checklist based on pattern analysis. Arch Dermatol. Dec 1998; 134(12): 1563–1570.

10 Menzies SW, Ingvar C, McCarthy WH. A sensitivity and specificity analysis of the surface microscopy features of invasive melanoma. Melanoma Res. Feb 1996; 6(1): 55–62.

11 Braun RP, Rabinovitz HS, Krischer J, et al. Dermoscopy of pigmented seborrheic keratosis: a morphological study. Arch Dermatol. Dec 2002; 138(12): 1556–1560.

12 Kopf AW, Rabinovitz H, Marghoob A, et al. "Fat fingers:" a clue in the dermoscopic diagnosis of seborrheic keratoses. J Am Acad Dermatol. Dec 2006; 55(6): 1089–1091.

13 Pizzichetta MA, Argenziano G, Talamini R, et al. Dermoscopic criteria for melanoma in situ are similar to those for early invasive melanoma. Cancer. Mar 1 2001; 91(5): 992–997.

14 Soyer HP, Kenet RO, Wolf IH, Kenet BJ, Cerroni L. Clinicopathological correlation of pigmented skin lesions using dermoscopy. Eur J Dermatol. Jan-Feb 2000; 10(1): 22–28.

15 Agero AL, Taliercio S, Dusza SW, Salaro C, Chu P, Marghoob AA. Conventional and polarized dermoscopy features of dermatofibroma. Arch Dermatol. Nov 2006; 142(11): 1431–1437.

16 Zaballos P, Puig S, Llambrich A, Malvehy J. Dermoscopy of dermatofibromas: a prospective morphological study of 412 cases. Arch Dermatol. Jan 2008; 144(1): 75–83.

17 Marghoob AA, Cowell L, Kopf AW, Scope A. Observation of chrysalis structures with polarized dermoscopy. Arch Dermatol. May 2009; 145(5): 618.

18 Balagula Y, Braun RP, Rabinovitz HS, et al. The significance of crystalline/chrysalis structures in the diagnosis of melanocytic and nonmelanocytic lesions. J Am Acad Dermatol. Aug 2012; 67(2): 194 e191–198.

19 Di Stefani A, Campbell TM, Malvehy J, Massone C, Soyer HP, Hofmann-Wellenhof R. Shiny white streaks: An additional dermoscopic finding in melanomas viewed using contact polarised dermoscopy. Australas J Dermatol. Nov 2010; 51(4): 295–298.

20 Argenziano G, Zalaudek I, Corona R, et al. Vascular structures in skin tumors: a dermoscopy study. Arch Dermatol. Dec 2004; 140(12): 1485–1489.

21 Malvehy J, Puig S. Dermoscopic patterns of benign volar melanocytic lesions in patients with atypical mole syndrome. Arch Dermatol. May 2004; 140(5): 538–544.

22 Saida T, Oguchi S, Ishihara Y. In vivo observation of magnified features of pigmented lesions on volar skin using video macroscope. Usefulness of epiluminescence techniques in clinical diagnosis. Arch Dermatol. Mar 1995; 131(3): 298–304.

23. Pizzichetta MA, Talamini R, Marghoob AA, et al. Negative pigment network: an additional dermoscopic feature for the diagnosis of melanoma. J Am Acad Dermatol. Apr 2013; 68(4): 552–559.

24 Botella-Estrada R, Requena C, Traves V, Nagore E, Guillen C. Chrysalis and negative pigment network in Spitz nevi. Am J Dermatopathol. Apr 2012; 34(2): 188–191.

25 Tschandl P, Rosendahl C, Kittler H. Accuracy of the first step of the dermatoscopic 2-step algorithm for pigmented skin lesions. Dermatol Pract Concept. Jul 2012; 2(3): 203a208.

26 Cheng ST, Ke CL, Lee CH, Wu CS, Chen GS, Hu SC. Rainbow pattern in Kaposi's sarcoma under polarized dermoscopy: a dermoscopic pathological study. Br J Dermatol. Apr 2009; 160(4): 801–809.

27 Vazquez-Lopez F, Garcia-Garcia B, Rajadhyaksha M, Marghoob AA. Dermoscopic rainbow pattern in non-Kaposi sarcoma lesions. Br J Dermatol. Aug 2009; 161(2): 474–475.

28 Liebman TN, Scope A, Rabinovitz H, Braun RP, Marghoob AA. Rosettes may be observed in a range of conditions. Arch Dermatol. Dec 2011; 147(12): 1468.

29 Zalaudek I, Giacomel J, Argenziano G, et al. Dermoscopy of facial nonpigmented actinic keratosis. Br J Dermatol. Nov 2006; 155(5): 951–956.

30 Miyake T, Minagawa A, Koga H, Fukuzawa M, Okuyama R. Histopathological correlation to the dermoscopic feature of "string of pearls" in clear cell acanthoma. Eur J Dermatol. Jul-Aug 2014; 24(4): 498–499.

5 An algorithmic method for the diagnosis of pigmented lesions

We now come to the core of the method, making a specific diagnosis. Pigmented skin lesions can be described very clearly and reliably using the method (patterns, colors and clues) described in the previous chapters. An exact morphological description is like a thread winding through a labyrinth; the thread leads a wandering or disoriented clinician safely to the outcome or exit. The essence of pattern analysis is a structured description formulated using a clearly defined algorithmic method. The diagnostic method is structured in such a way that one starts by describing the most general of features, then proceeds progressively to finish with the most specific features. Rules prescribe, at each turn, the direction one should take so that the clinician is not misled, as happens easily when using a method where descriptive terms are subjective, poorly defined, or dependent on diagnosis. Only after a comprehensive description and after all observable data have been taken into account are the findings interpreted and a specific diagnosis established.

The algorithm always takes the general form:

Pattern + Color + Clues = Diagnosis

The algorithmic method will be presented here in a stepwise manner. When you are confronted with an unknown pigmented lesion you may use the following pages as a classification reference guide. Using patterns, colors and clues, the number of potential diagnoses is progressively minimized. Finally just one or a few diagnoses remain. In those cases in which it is not possible to reach a confident specific diagnosis, the degree of doubt and the type of possible diagnoses will determine whether histopathology is required.

Pattern analysis is not an algorithm carved in stone, it is a method by which algorithms are constructed.

With experience, every investigator will develop their own individual algorithm. Only then does one become an expert. General criteria, guidelines and concepts are certainly required, but personal experience is also crucial. Beginners must rely on recipes, but experts personalize the recipe, refine and develop it further,

and so create their own style. Pattern analysis is the framework for developing this personal algorithm.

In every algorithmic method one makes decisions, which progressively reduce the number of differential diagnoses. In formulating the algorithmic method of pattern analysis, we attempted to fulfill the following basic principles: The criteria used to make decisions must be clearly and unambiguously defined. The criteria should be exclusive, i.e. the properties being assessed do not overlap, so unequivocal classification is possible. Decisions should be so simple that even beginners are able to perform the task. Decisions should show a high degree of concordance when judged by a range of clinicians. This decision process should be carried as far as possible – but no further!

The first step is to decide whether a pigmented lesion is composed of one or more than one pattern.

5.1 One pattern

The first step in pattern analysis of a pigmented lesion is to decide: is there one pattern or more than one pattern? This decision is nearly always both simple and unequivocal. When a pigmented lesion consists of just one pattern, then of course the next question is, which pattern? As we know, a pattern is formed by an aggregation of one of the five basic elements (lines, pseudopods, circles, clods and dots, *5.1*). When basic elements are not seen or there are too few basic elements to constitute a pattern, the "pattern" is termed structureless. When evaluating patterns, individual dots or clods are not important; at this stage the general impression takes precedence. Once this decision is made, we progress through the algorithm in a stepwise manner, which divides into smaller and smaller branches with a progressively smaller differential diagnosis.

5.1.1 Lines

Lines may form six different patterns, created by differences both in the form of individual lines, and the arrangement of the lines relative to one another. These

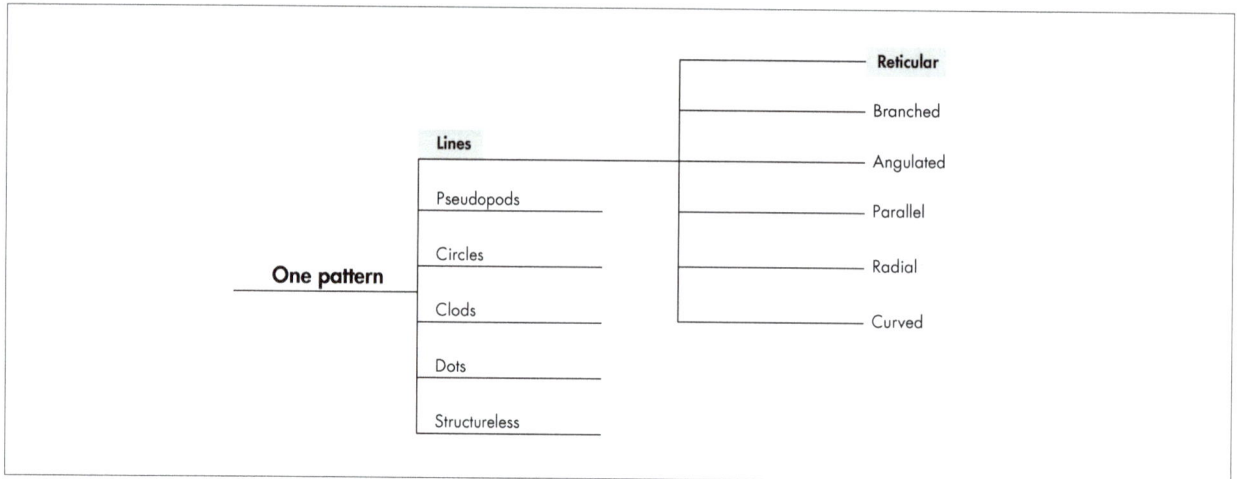

Figure 5.1: Decision tree for one pattern, branch: Lines

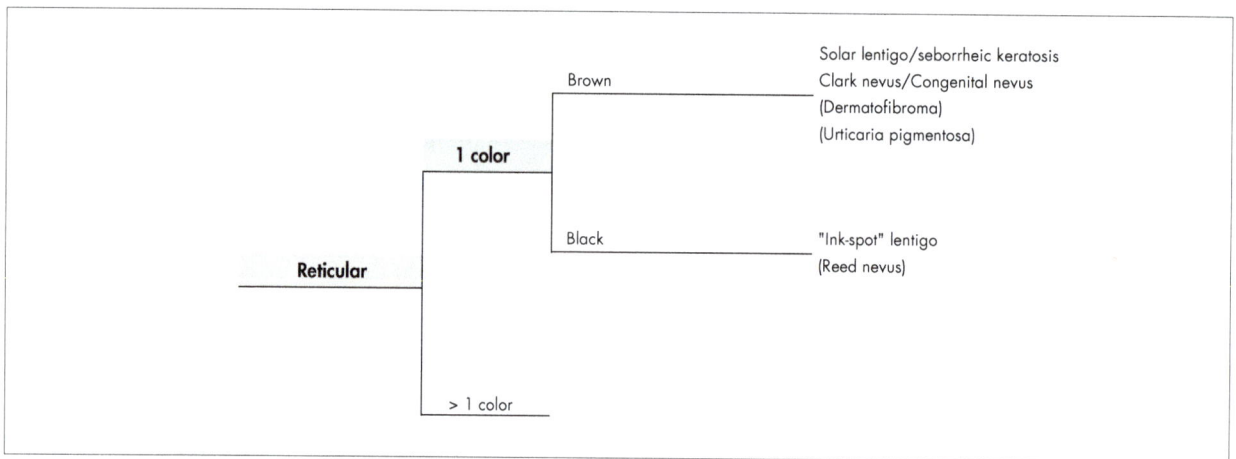

Figure 5.2: Continuation of the decision tree for lines, reticular

patterns are reticular, branched, angulated, parallel, radial, and curved.

Reticular lines

Lesions that consist exclusively of reticular lines are extremely common. Although many algorithms use reticular lines as a criterion to diagnose lesions as melanocytic (1), lesions with reticular lines are not always melanocytic (2). In most cases the histological correlate of reticular lines is hyperpigmentation of basal keratinocytes on rete ridges, which may or may not be created by an increase in the numbers of melanocytes. As the next step the investigator assesses color *(5.2)*. As melanin appears brown in the epidermis, reticular lines are usually light-brown or dark-brown. If the pigment is very dense, the lines are black. Rarely reticular lines are gray. Beginners are often too strict in assessing color and therefore tend to see too many colors. Not

every shade of brown is to be interpreted as a separate color. One or two black lines do not render the lesion multicolored. The normal hypopigmentation around follicular openings does not create an extra color. Nearly all pigmented lesions are somewhat lighter at the periphery than in the center; again this does not constitute an additional color.

If there is only one color, namely light-brown, and the lesion consists of thin reticular lines, the diagnosis is either junctional Clark nevus or solar lentigo *(5.3)*. A Clark nevus is round or oval and the pigmentation does not end abruptly at the periphery. In contrast, the border of a solar lentigo is usually sharply demarcated and scalloped. A few brown dots may be found in both diagnoses, but more frequently in Clark nevus. It is not always possible to make a reliable distinction on dermatoscopy, but as both lesions are benign this is seldom crucial. Rare differential diagnoses for thin,

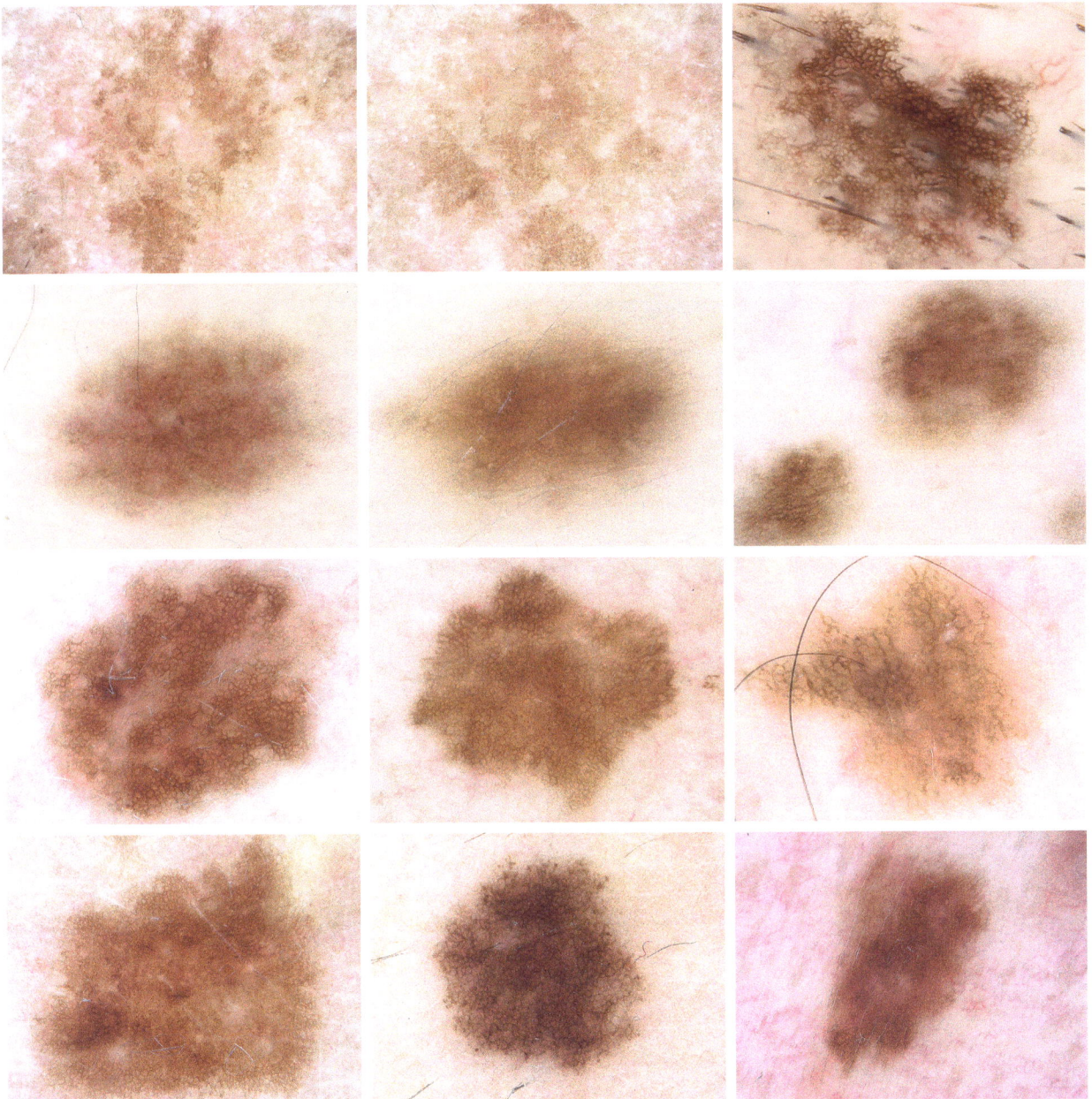

Figure 5.3: *One pattern, lines, reticular, brown and thin.*
Dermatoscopy of lesions composed exclusively of thin, brown reticular lines. The differential diagnosis for this pattern and color combination is solar lentigo or Clark nevus. **First row:** Solar lentigines. **Second, third and fourth row:** Clark nevi. The presence of a dot or two should not be counted as a separate pattern. The hypopigmented spaces between the lines constitute the background and not a pattern. This is an example of the general rule that structure (pattern) is defined by pigment.

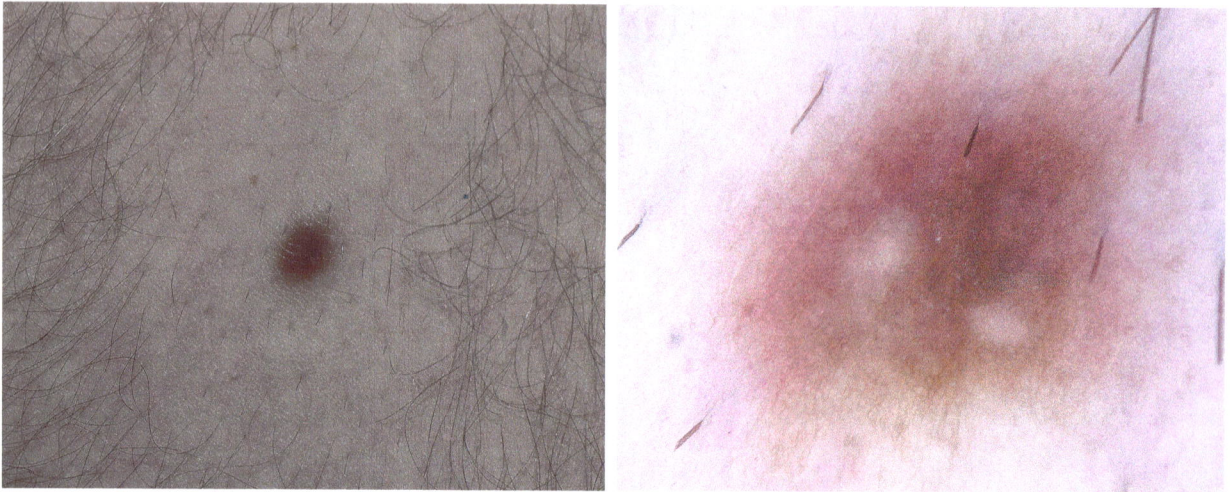

Figure 5.4: A variant of dermatofibroma with a reticular pattern only.
On dermatoscopy (right) one finds only light brown reticular lines. The typical white structureless zone in the center is missing. This is one of the many variants of dermatofibroma.

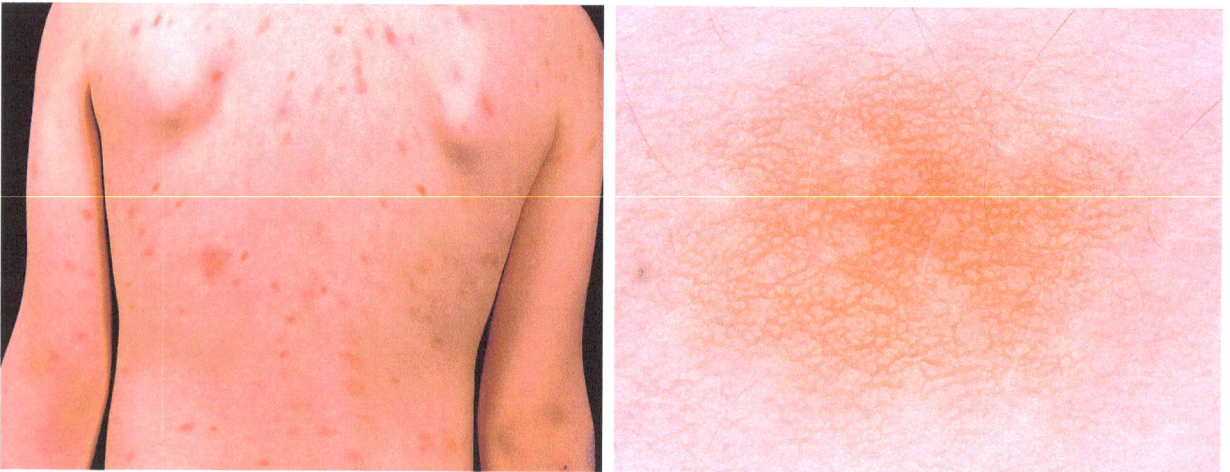

Figure 5.5: Urticaria pigmentosa with a reticular pattern.
This variant of mastocytosis is typified by a rash composed of light brown macules and papules. Dermatoscopy (right) of an individual lesion shows reticular pattern. For reasons unknown a proliferation of mast cells in the papillary dermis induces hyperpigmentation of basal keratinocytes which gives rise to the light brown reticular lines seen on dermatoscopy.

light-brown reticular lines on dermatoscopy are a variant of dermatofibroma (3) with reticular lines only *(5.4)* and urticaria pigmentosa (4), a type of mastocytosis *(5.5)*. When brown reticular lines are thick and not thin, one should first consider a Clark nevus or less often a superficial congenital nevus *(5.6)*. A solar lentigo is very unlikely. A seborrheic keratosis may present with thick, brown, reticular lines, but in this case one nearly always sees reticular lines in combination with other characteristic features of seborrheic keratosis.

Black or at least very dark-brown reticular lines are a clue to the diagnosis of ink-spot lentigo *(5.7)*. Additional clues are abrupt ending of lines within the lesion and a sharply demarcated border. Normally no differential diagnosis needs to be considered. Very rarely a Reed nevus may demonstrate this pattern and color combination, but without the additional clues to "ink-spot lentigo". For a lesion with only reticular lines but more than one color, one first should exclude a solar lentigo or seborrheic keratosis. This is done best by considering the clues to solar lentigo (well-demarcated, scalloped border) and seborrheic keratosis (white dots or clods, orange or yellow clods, well-demarcated border, circles, thick curved lines, vessels as loops or coils). Once a

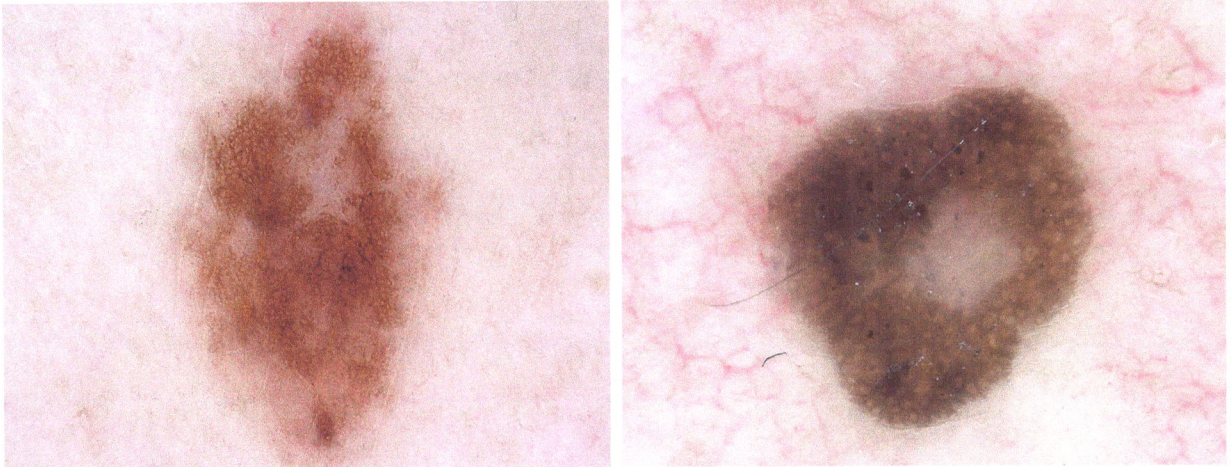

Figure 5.6: One pattern, lines, reticular, brown and thick.
Thick reticular lines are found in some Clark nevi **(left)** or in reticular seborrheic keratoses **(right).** The right lesion shows – in addition to thick reticular lines – a few clods ("comedo-like openings") and a small structureless area. In this case the clods and the structureless area were not interpreted as separate patterns because they do not occupy a significant part of the lesion.

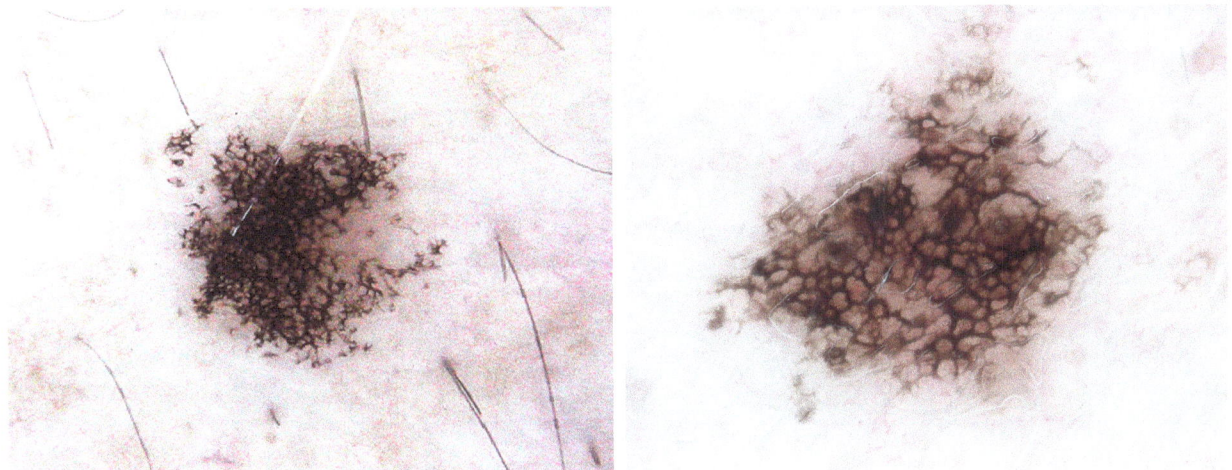

Figure 5.7: One pattern, lines, reticular, black.
This pattern and color combination is typical of "ink-spot lentigo".

solar lentigo or a seborrheic keratosis has been ruled out, three differential diagnoses should be considered: a) Clark nevus, b) "superficial" or "superficial and deep" congenital nevus, and c) in situ melanoma (5.8). One proceeds in the usual stepwise manner. The colors and their distribution are assessed before the final step, resolving the differential diagnosis using clues. For a pattern of reticular lines, only the colors light-brown, dark-brown, black and very rarely gray will be seen. In practice, there are only three ways that two colors combine in reticular lesions (in theory, of course, there is an infinite number of combinations). The first possibility

is central hyperpigmentation, i.e. light-brown reticular lines peripherally and dark-brown or even black lines in the center (5.9). This pattern is typical of a Clark nevus. All other diagnoses may be safely ruled out. When dark-brown or black and light-brown areas are present alternately so that one obtains the impression of a speckled lesion, this type of color distribution is termed variegate. The differential diagnosis for a variegate reticular lesion is: Clark nevus, "superficial" or "superficial and deep" congenital nevus, or an in situ melanoma (5.10). While the distinction between a Clark nevus and a congenital nevus is purely of academic

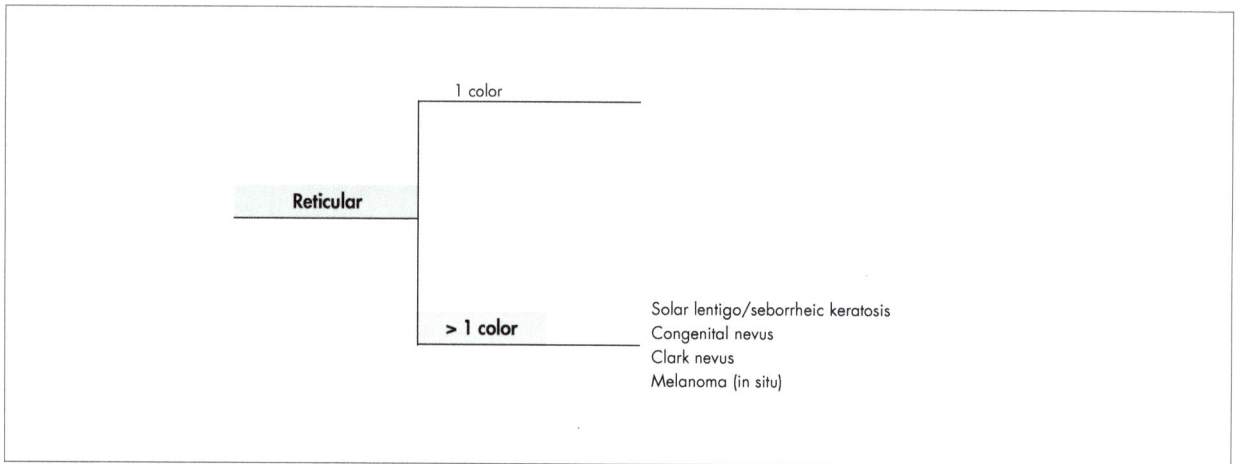

Figure 5.8: *Continuation of the algorithm for the reticular pattern, when more than one color is present*

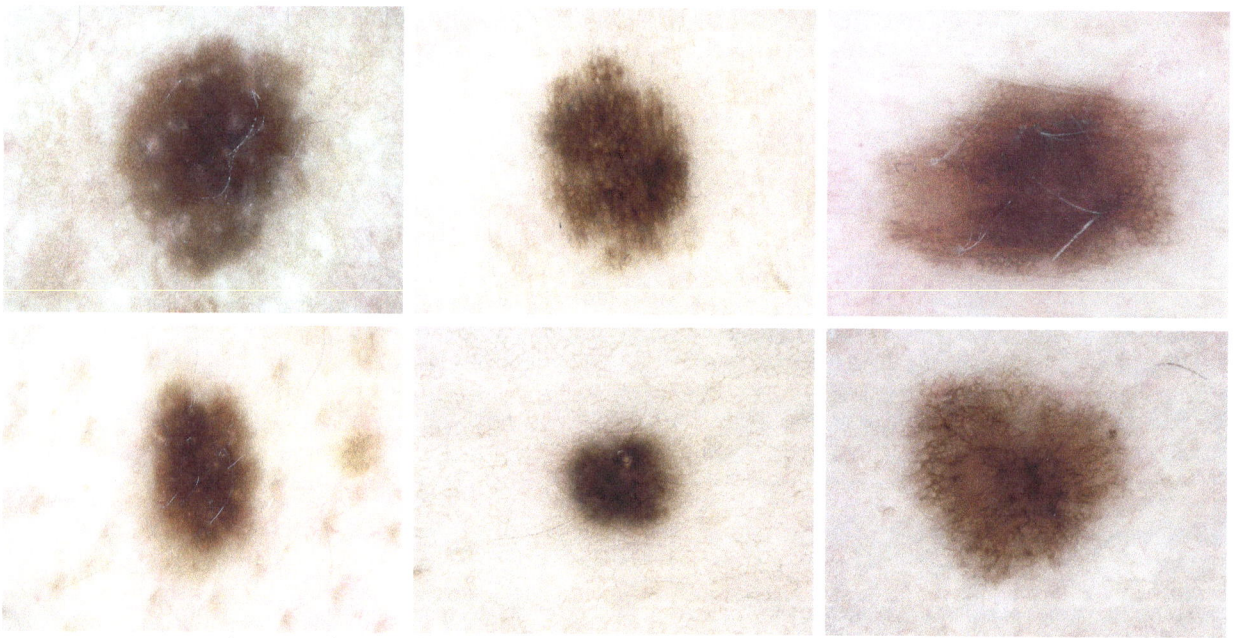

Figure 5.9: *One pattern, lines, reticular, more than one color, central hyperpigmentation.*
This pattern and color combination is the typical dermatoscopic appearance of the Clark nevus. The six Clark nevi seen here are all variations on this pattern.

interest, the differentiation between these and an in situ melanoma is of course very significant, and is based on the presence or absence of the clues to melanoma outlined in chapter 3. Only 5 of the 9 clues to melanoma are seen in reticular pattern lesions: a) gray dots, clods, circles or lines; b) radial lines or pseudopods seen only in some segments of the periphery; c) black dots or clods at the periphery d) thick reticular lines and e) angulated lines (polygons). When one of these clues is present, the diagnosis of melanoma should be seriously considered.

The third and last color combination seen in reticular pattern lesions is eccentric hyperpigmentation, i.e. the more heavily pigmented area is peripheral, not central. This color combination is found in both Clark nevi and in situ melanomas *(5.11)*, but only rarely in congenital nevi. As in the case of variegate pigmentation, the differential diagnosis is resolved by assessing the lesion for clues to melanoma. When no clue to melanoma is present, a Clark nevus is the most likely diagnosis. A common difficulty is how one should proceed when the overall assessment shows a symmetrical pattern and

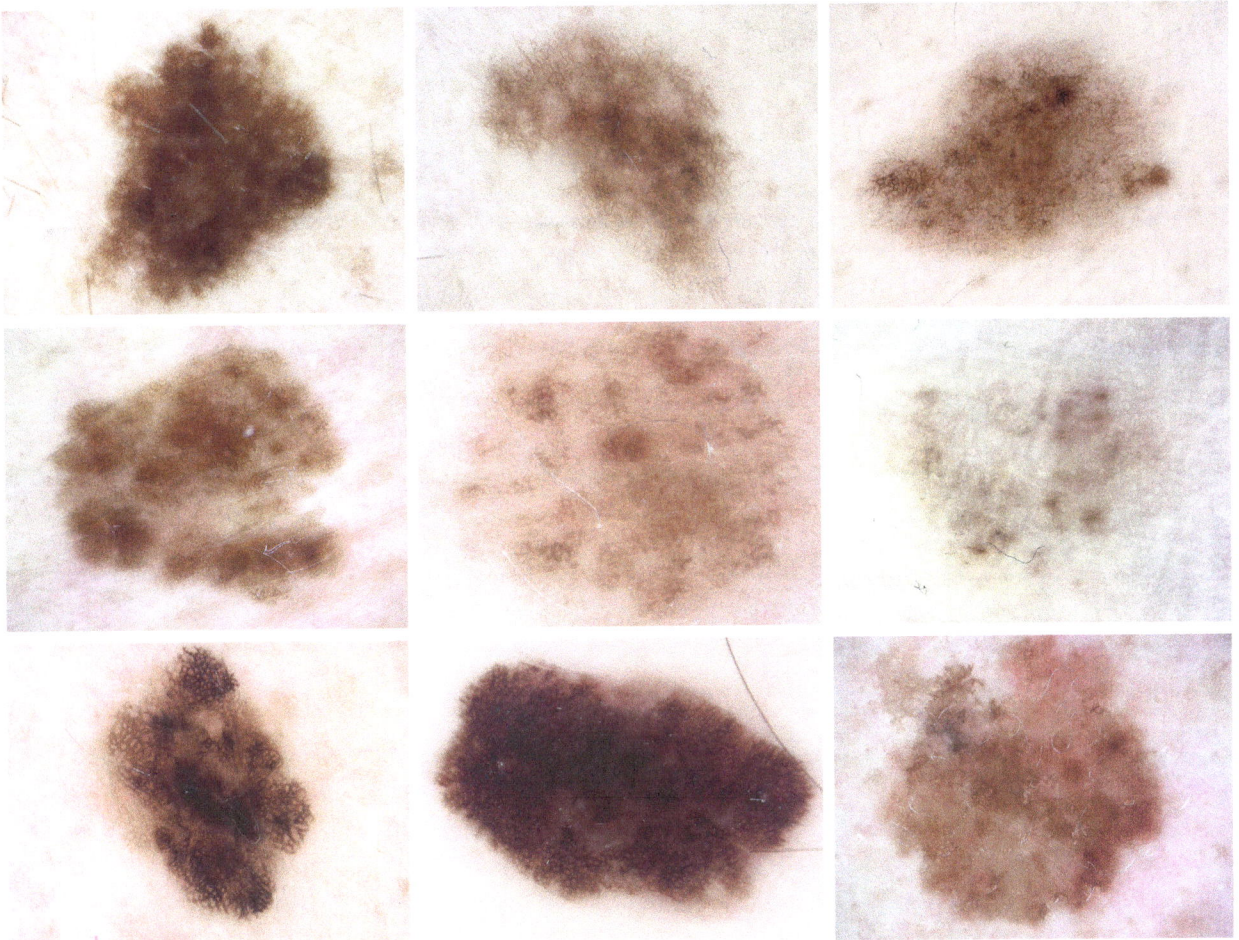

Figure 5.10: One pattern, lines, reticular, more than one color, variegate.
The **first and the second row** show Clark nevi and "superficial" or "superficial and deep" congenital nevi with a reticular pattern and variegate pigmentation. These two types of nevus can be distinguished from each other only on histopathology; the distinction is purely of academic interest. Clues to melanoma are not seen in any of these lesions. The lesions shown in the third row are in situ melanomas with thick reticular lines **(left and middle)** or gray dots and small gray clods **(right,** at 11 o'clock position) as clues to melanoma.

color combination, but a clue to melanoma is present, e.g. gray dots. This is a situation where experts will make better decisions than beginners, as the strength of the clue must be weighed against one's level of certainty that the lesion is in fact symmetrical. As a general principle, symmetry of pattern and color should be given greater weight than the clue; in short, "pattern trumps clues". Nevertheless, some of these lesions must be submitted for histopathology to confidently exclude malignancy. A clue should also be weighed differently depending on the number of lesions with similar features in the same patient. For example, some patients have multiple reticular lesions with gray dots or gray lines. In this context, gray structures have a lower weight as a clue to malignancy. This "comparative approach" (5) helps to increase specificity (to reduce the number of excisions of

nevi). If, on the other hand, there is only a single reticular lesion with gray structures the clue should be given more weight. This helps to increase sensitivity (to detect more melanomas). The management of patients with multiple nevi will be discussed in more detail in chapter 9.

Branched lines
Branched lines and reticular lines are closely related and often occur together. Sometimes they are difficult to distinguish, in which case one should analyze according to the much more common reticular pattern. There are, however, lesions that are exclusively composed of branched lines. In practice, these lesions are either black or brown, and they are all benign. Lesions that have only brown branched lines are either a Clark nevus or a "superficial" or "superficial and deep" congenital

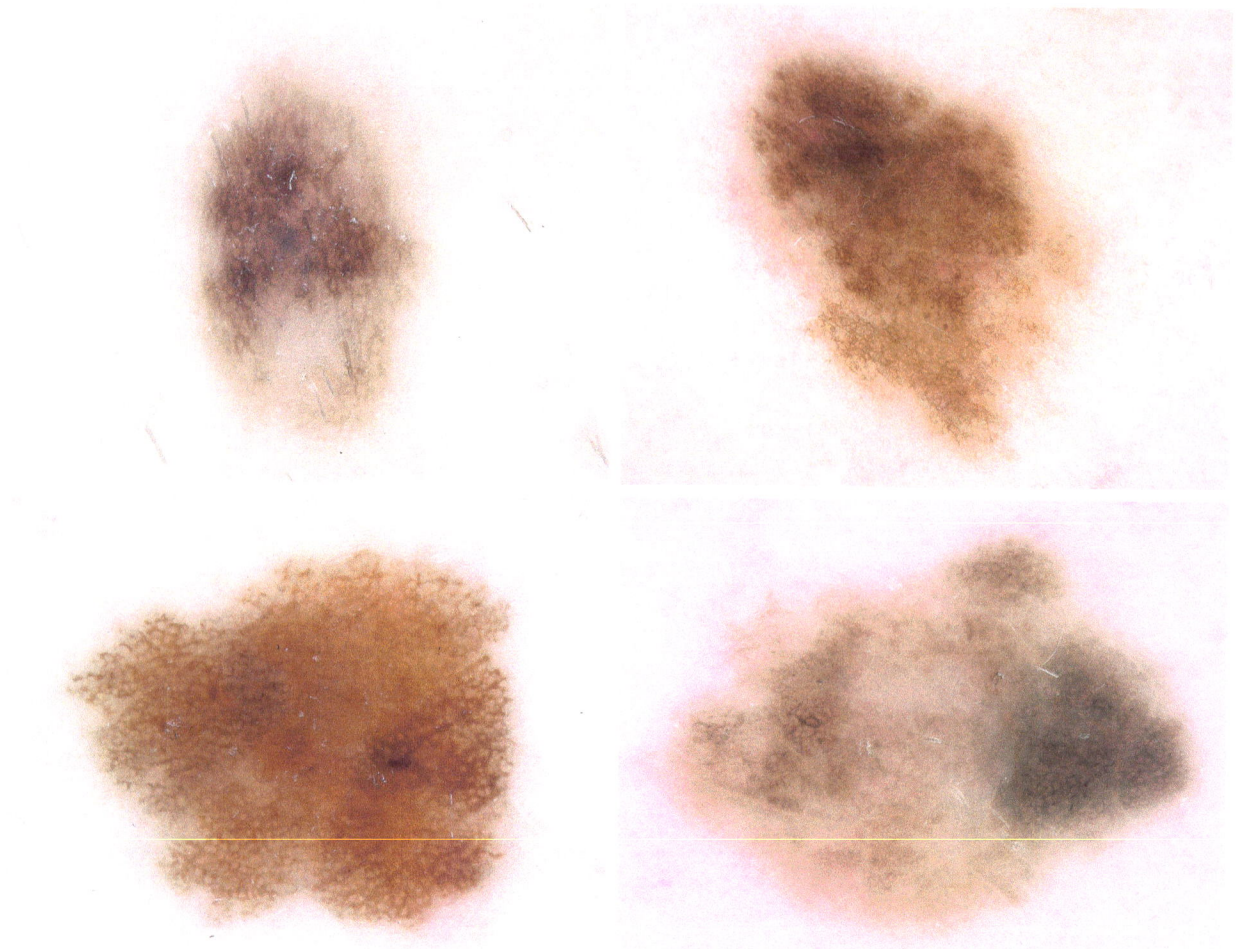

Figure 5.11: One pattern, lines, reticular, more than one color, peripheral hyperpigmentation.
*This color and pattern combination is found in Clark nevi (**top row**) and in situ melanomas (**bottom row**). Clark nevi usually have no clues to melanoma. The melanoma **bottom left** has thick reticular lines; the melanoma **bottom right** has peripheral black dots (at 3 o'clock position) as clues to melanoma.*

nevus. The branched lines are probably columns of melanocytes at the base of rete ridges, which appear as nests in the vertical plane of the histopathological specimen. Black (or very dark-brown) branched lines indicate an "ink-spot" lentigo. Here again the pigmentation is at the base of the rete ridges but it is in basal keratinocytes, not in melanocytes as in Clark nevus or in superficial congenital nevus.

Angulated lines
Angulated lines are the hallmark of flat melanomas on skin with chronic sun damage, on both facial and non-facial skin (6, 7) *(5.12).* They often appear in conjunction with another pattern, most often with the reticular pattern on non-facial skin and with circles on facial skin. On non-facial skin, a pattern of angulated

lines is one of the most specific clues to the diagnosis of melanoma. On facial skin, however, angulated lines are also seen in pigmented actinic keratoses (8, 9). Most melanomas with angulated lines are in situ (not invasive). The lines are usually brown or gray. Many melanomas with angulated lines also have gray dots, but usually too few to be called a pattern. Close inspection of angulated lines may show them to be formed by densely packed gray dots.

Parallel lines
The pattern of parallel lines is the typical pigment pattern of acral skin. Parallel lines may be arranged in one of three ways; on the ridges (ridge pattern), in the furrows (furrow pattern), or crossing ridges and furrows (crossing pattern). Acral lesions that only show

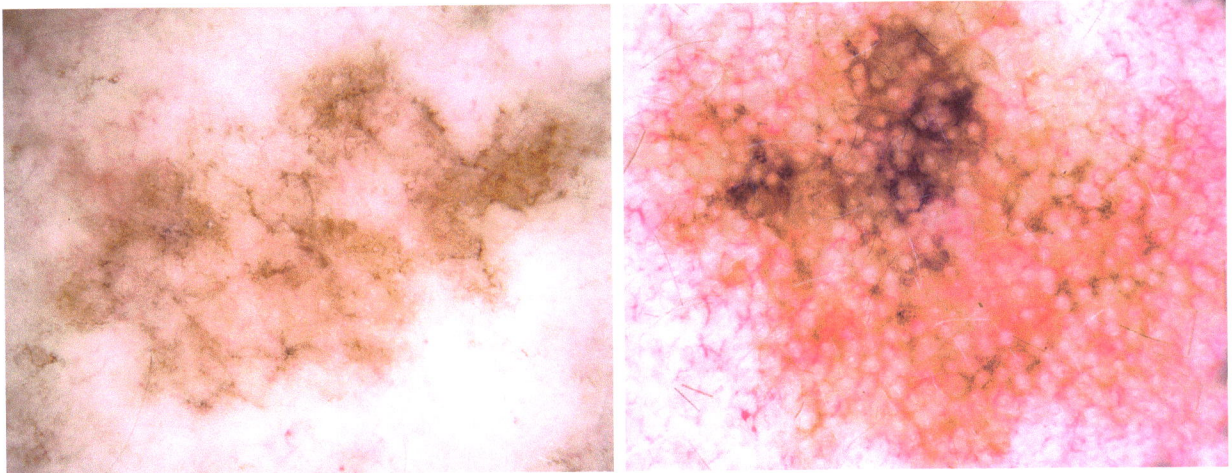

Figure 5.12: Angulated lines.
Angulated lines form the typical pattern seen in flat melanomas on chronic sun-damaged skin. They appear in melanomas on non-facial (**left**) *and facial* (**right**) *skin.*

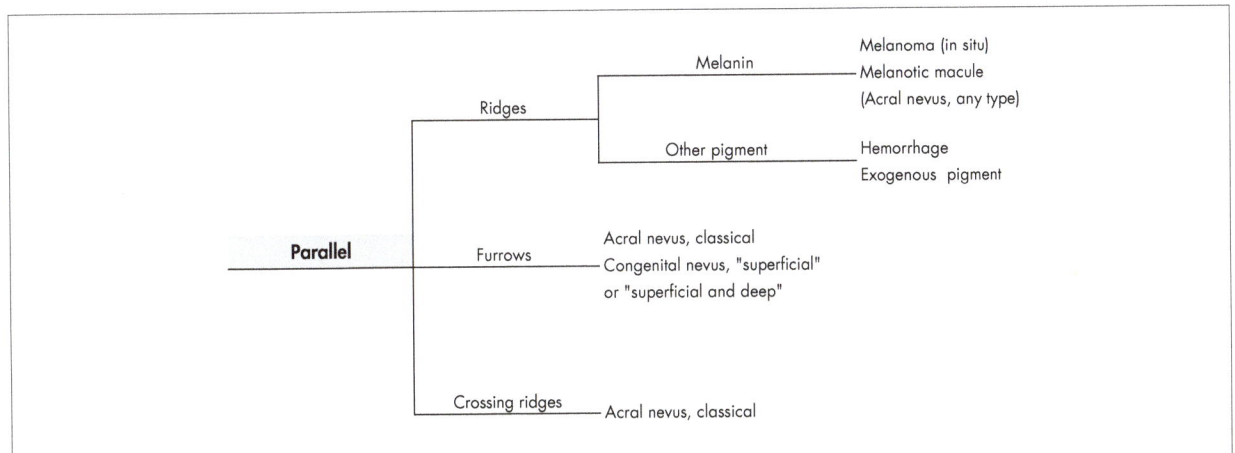

Figure 5.13: Continuation of the decision tree for lines, parallel

a furrow pattern or a crossing pattern, and without any of the clues to melanoma, may be safely considered to be benign (10). These are either classical acral nevi or small "superficial" or "superficial and deep" congenital nevi *(5.13)*.

Assessment of a lesion showing the ridge pattern proceeds in the normal stepwise fashion by evaluating color. If it is brown, in situ melanoma must be considered. Occasionally, acral nevi may also have a ridge pattern; the same is true for acral lentigines or melanotic macules related to the person's ethnic origin or found as part of rare diseases such as the Laugier-Hunziker syndrome (11). However, a biopsy is usually required to confirm such a benign diagnosis.

Black, red or purple parallel lines on the ridges indicate either hemorrhage or exogenous pigmentation *(5.14*

bottom right). Satellite clods are a strong clue to the diagnosis of hemorrhage. As both hemorrhage and exogenous pigmentation are found in the stratum corneum (i.e. superficially) one can remove the pigmentation by careful paring with a scalpel. This is, of course, not possible with a melanocytic lesion.

Radial lines
As radial lines always occur in combination with another pattern, they are discussed in the section dedicated to lesions with more than one pattern.

Curved lines
Curved lines usually occur in combination with other patterns. However, some solar lentigines or seborrheic keratoses may have only curved lines *(5.15)*. In these

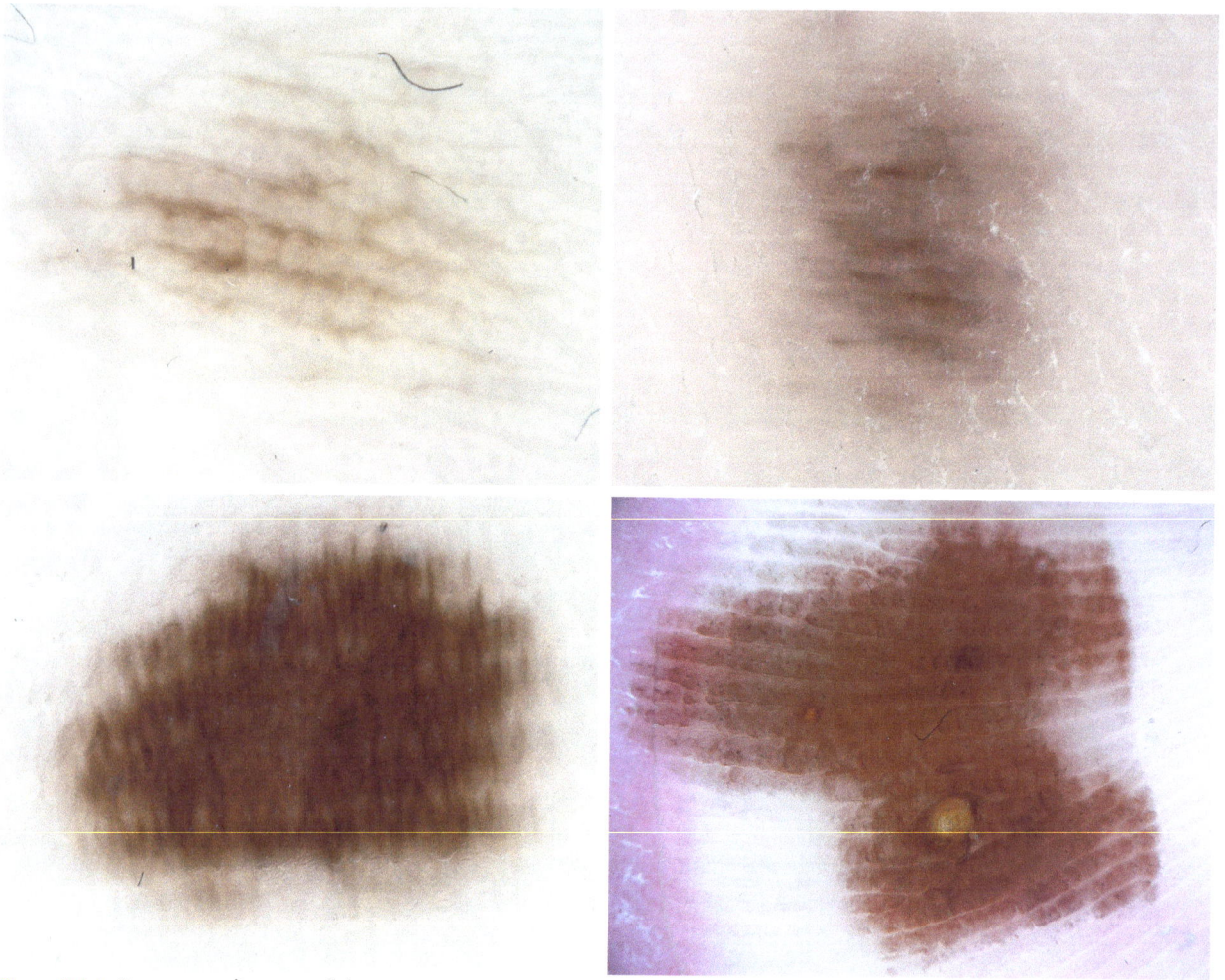

Figure 5.14: One pattern, lines, parallel.
Top left: *Parallel lines in the furrows form the most common pattern of benign melanocytic lesions on acral skin, as in this classical acral nevus.* ***Top right:*** *Thin, short parallel lines crossing the ridges are typical of acral nevi located on the weight bearing parts of the sole.* ***Bottom left:*** *Occasionally parallel crossing lines may be thick rather than thin, as in this lesion which is presumably a congenital nevus.* ***Bottom right:*** *Parallel lines on the ridges are found in melanoma, melanotic macules, hemorrhage and, as in this case, exogenous pigmentation. Here the pigmentation was caused by a silver nitrate cautery pen, used to treat warts.*

cases one often finds clues like a curved, sharply demarcated border, or a few circles, to support the diagnosis of solar lentigo or seborrheic keratosis.

5.1.2 Pseudopods
Like radial lines, pseudopods occur only in combination with other patterns and are also discussed in the section dedicated to lesions with more than one pattern.

5.1.3 Circles
Just as the pattern of parallel lines is the pattern of acral skin, the pattern of circles is the pattern of facial skin. In contrast to parallel lines, the pattern of circles is not unusual at other locations on the body. On the face,

circles are formed by melanin pigment arranged either around the openings of the crater-like infundibula or in infundibular epithelium. The center of the infundibulum appears hypopigmented. If infundibula contain keratinized material rather than a hair-shaft, (which is not unusual) the hypopigmented center is seen as yellow or orange clods. Facial circles, especially when they are broad and confluent, are often seen on close inspection to be small dots arranged as circles around the openings of the infundibula. On facial skin it is crucial to differentiate between a pattern of circles (or dots arranged as circles) formed by pigment, and gaps in other patterns created by the infundibula, as this is of great diagnostic significance. This is most commonly

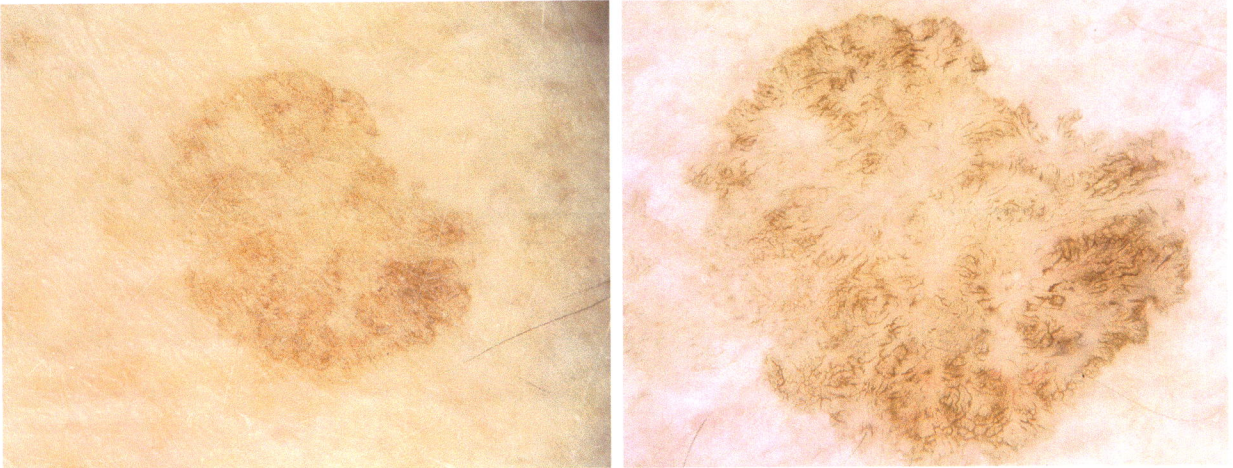

Figure 5.15: *Curved lines.*
*A solar lentigo with curved lines on dermatoscopy **(right)**. The **left** image shows the lesion as seen without dermatoscopy.*

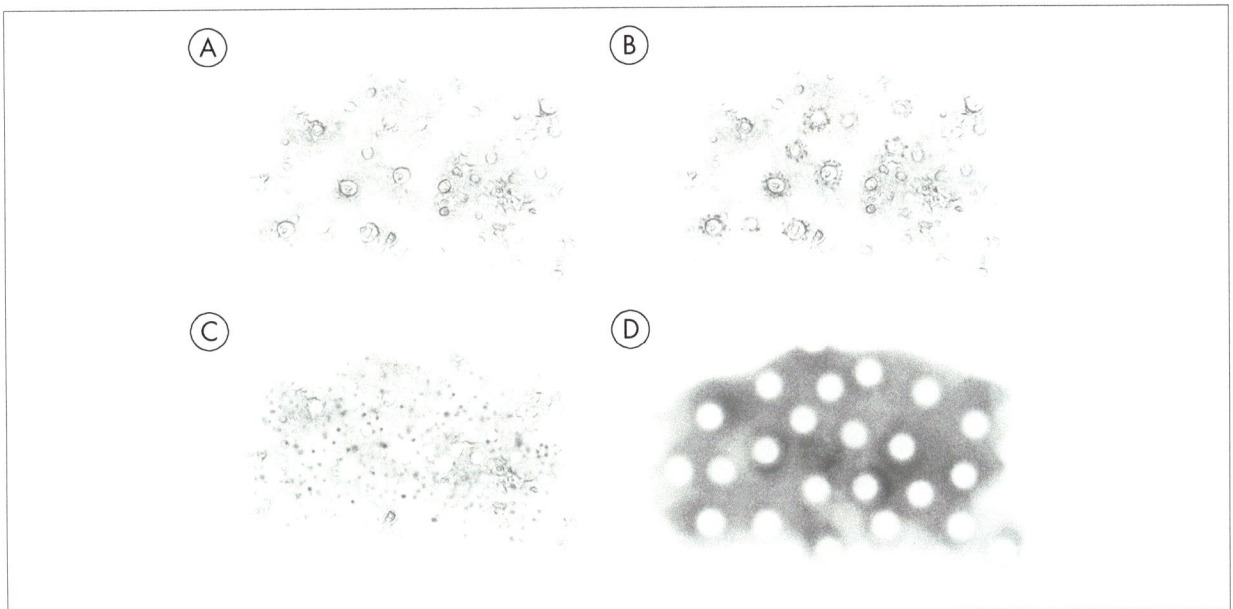

Figure 5.16: *Circles on facial skin.*
*Only A and B show a pattern of circles on facial skin. In **A** circles consist of thin fine lines around follicular openings and in **B** circles are composed of dots arranged in circles around follicular openings. There are no circles in **C**, where the dots are evenly dispersed between the follicular openings but not arranged in circles. In **D** the pattern is structureless. The structureless pattern is interrupted by the hypopigmented follicular openings.*

an issue with the pattern of dots and the structureless pattern (5.16).
Circles (or dots arranged as circles) may be brown or gray (5.17). Brown circles not associated with hair follicles are usually signs of solar lentigo or flat seborrheic keratosis. Brown circles associated with hair follicles can also be seen in solar lentigo and flat seborrheic keratosis. Occasionally, brown circles are present in

facial melanoma in situ but usually there is also another clue present. Gray circles on facial lesions indicate melanoma in situ. Gray dots arranged in circles, even when the gray color is only present in some parts of the lesion, give rise to the differential diagnosis of lichen planus-like keratosis, pigmented actinic keratosis and in situ melanoma. Clues that favor pigmented actinic keratosis (in addition to the non-dermatoscopic clue of

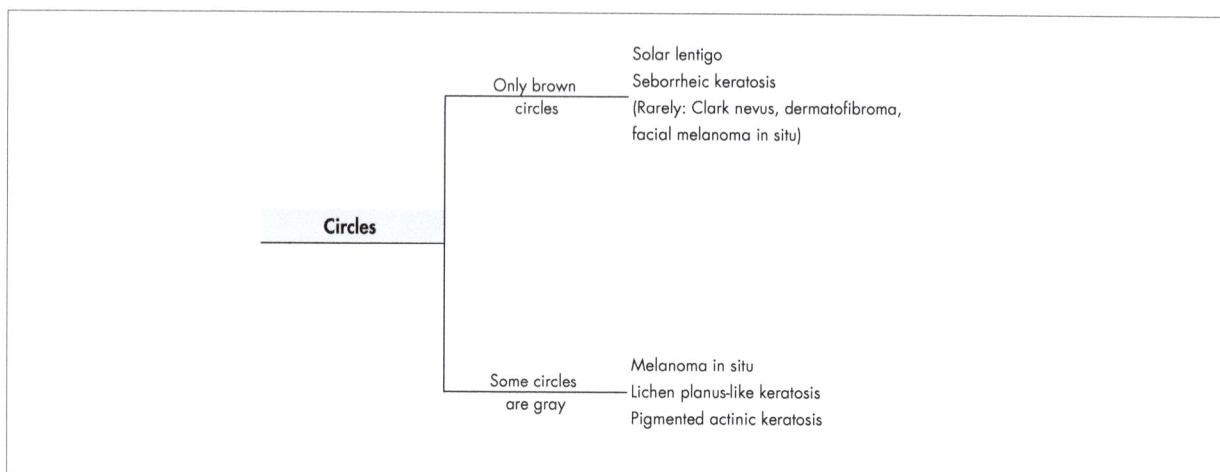

Figure 5.17: Decision tree for circles

palpable roughness) are white circles, scale, and 4-white dots in a square (the latter visible only with polarized dermatoscopy). In lichen planus-like keratosis one can usually see remnants of a solar lentigo. The differential diagnosis of facial lesions with grey circles can be challenging (8) and is discussed further in chapter 8. In *figure 5.18* we show a potpourri of facial lesions with circles or dots arranged as circles.

A biopsy is often needed to diagnose facial lesions with gray circles, as dermatoscopy cannot always differentiate between melanoma in situ, lichen planus-like keratosis and pigmented actinic keratosis. Confocal laser scanning microscopy may prove useful in this special case.

The pattern of circles is not confined to facial skin. On the trunk or the extremities, the pattern of thin brown circles has the same differential diagnoses as thin reticular lines, i.e. the pattern of circles may be a variant of the reticular pattern. In both cases there is melanin hyperpigmentation in the basal keratinocytes. In the reticular pattern, the rete ridges are narrow so that the lines touch each other, thus creating the impression of a network pattern. In a pattern of circles, however, the rete ridges are broad so that the lines arranged as circles around the papillae do not touch each other and on dermatoscopy one sees discrete circles *(5.19)*. For both brown circles and brown reticular lines, the differential diagnosis includes a junctional Clark nevus and a solar lentigo. Dermatofibroma is an additional diagnosis for the pattern of circles *(5.20)*. Rarely, a dermatofibroma may consist of just one pattern, i.e. thin brown circles.

5.1.4 Clods

After reticular lines, the pattern of clods is the second most common. Proceeding according to the method, color is assessed next.

One color predominates

When a lesion consists exclusively of clods, the color of the clods determines the diagnosis *(5.21)*. When white and/or yellow clods predominate, seborrheic keratosis is the most common diagnosis. Dilated infundibula and inclusion cysts ("milia") filled with keratin are clearly seen as yellow or white clods *(5.22)*. It is important to remember that the white clods of seborrheic keratosis may not be accurately appreciated when using polarized dermatoscopy, only becoming clearly visible when a non-polarized instrument is used (12).

White and/or yellow clods are also found in cases of sebaceous gland hyperplasia. These clods are located centrally and are all of similar size and shape. Radial vessels, which do not cross the center of the lesion, are a strong clue to sebaceous gland hyperplasia. The central clods are subtle and easily overlooked if one is distracted by the more obvious peripheral vessels. The color of clods in a seborrheic keratosis depends on the quantity of the melanin mixed with keratin and may range from white or yellow to orange, brown or black. While orange clods are a sign of seborrheic keratosis, one should include basal cell carcinoma in the differential diagnosis because orange clods may also be due to ulceration (serum crust). Whereas multiple orange clods are seen in seborrheic keratosis

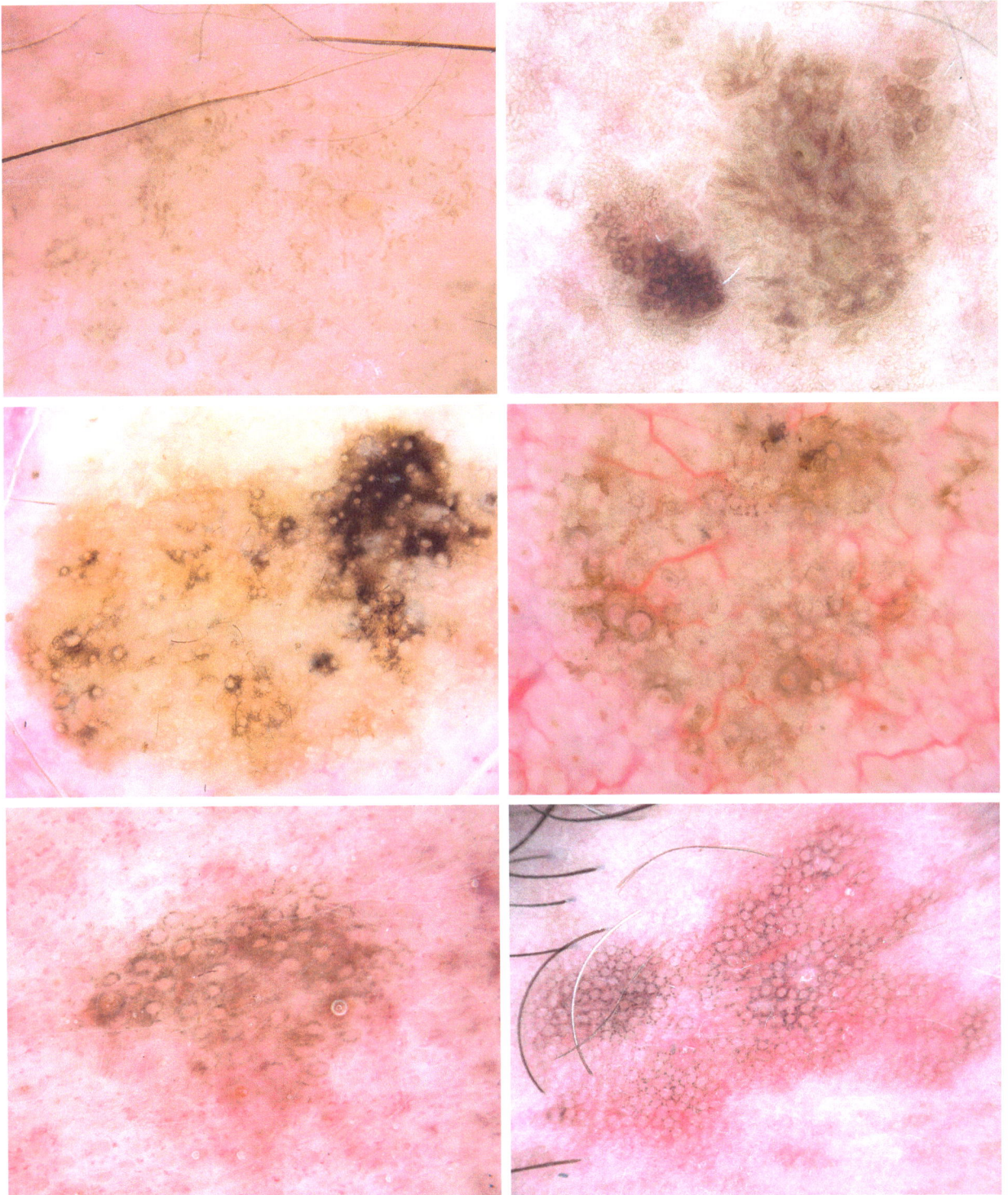

Figure 5.18: One pattern, circles, facial lesions.
Top left: Solar lentigo. On dermatoscopy one sees a single pattern, brown circles. **Top right:** A solar lentigo/seborrheic keratosis with a pattern of circles. There are also curved lines, some of which are arranged as parallel pairs, and some yellow clods as clues to seborrheic keratosis. **Middle left:** Melanoma in situ with thin brown, gray, and black circles on a tan background. **Middle right:** Melanoma in situ with thin brown and gray circles. **Bottom left:** Melanoma in situ with gray circles. **Bottom right:** A nearly completely regressed lichen planus-like keratosis (solar lentigo in regression) consisting solely of gray dots arranged as circles.

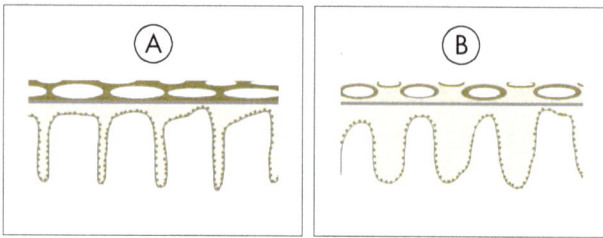

Figure 5.19: Histopathologic correlates of the pattern of circles (non-facial lesions with circles not correlated to follicles) and the reticular pattern.
In the reticular pattern, the rete ridges are narrow so that the lines touch each other (A). In a pattern of circles (non-facial lesions with circles not correlated to follicles) the rete ridges are broad so that the lines do not touch each other and on dermatoscopy one sees discrete circles (B).

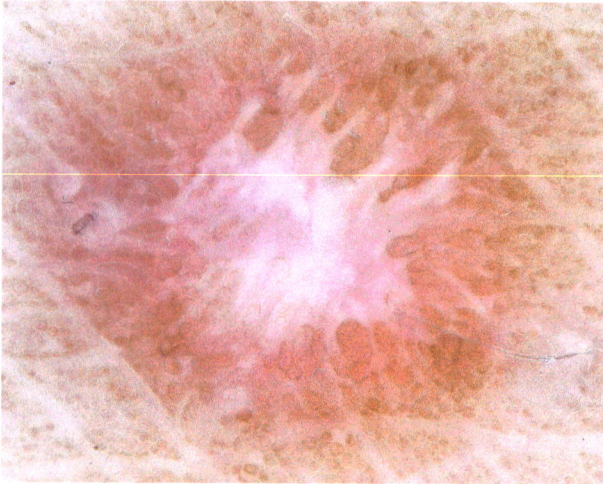

Figure 5.20: Circles non-facial skin.
Dermatoscopy of a dermatofibroma with brown circles of various sizes. The small white structureless zone in the center is the clue to the correct diagnosis.

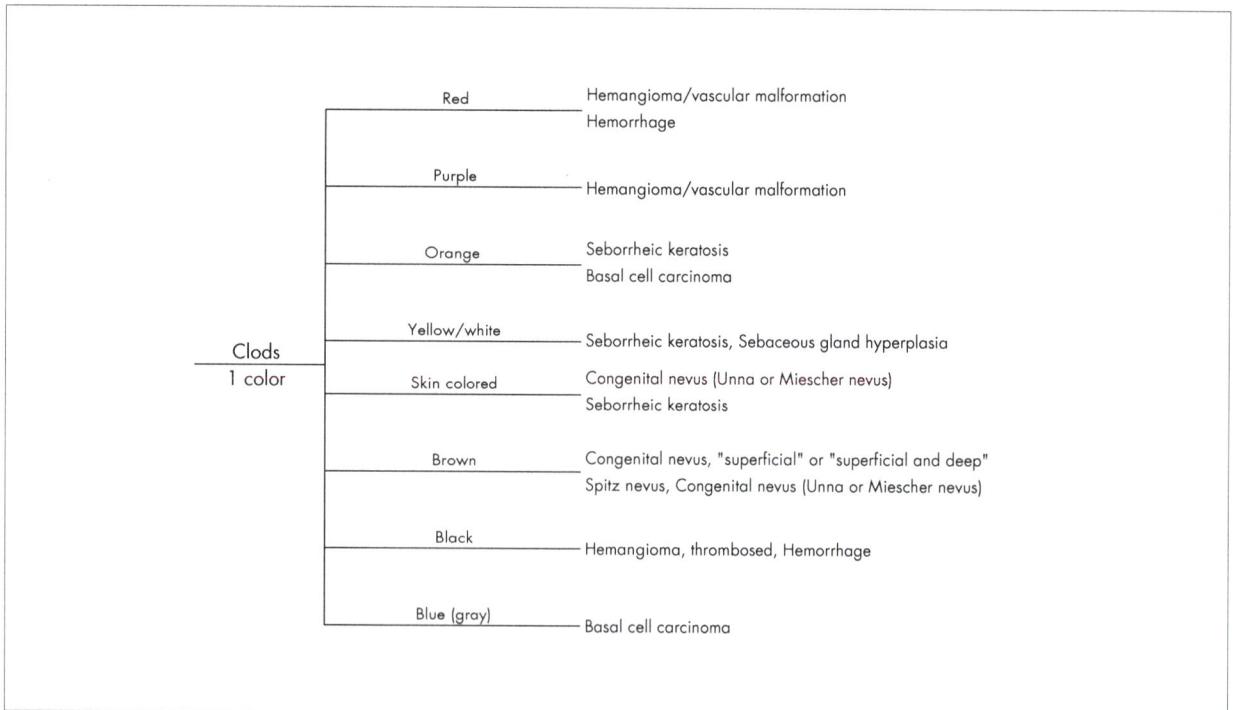

	Red	Hemangioma/vascular malformation
		Hemorrhage
	Purple	Hemangioma/vascular malformation
	Orange	Seborrheic keratosis
		Basal cell carcinoma
	Yellow/white	Seborrheic keratosis, Sebaceous gland hyperplasia
Clods	Skin colored	Congenital nevus (Unna or Miescher nevus)
1 color		Seborrheic keratosis
	Brown	Congenital nevus, "superficial" or "superficial and deep"
		Spitz nevus, Congenital nevus (Unna or Miescher nevus)
	Black	Hemangioma, thrombosed, Hemorrhage
	Blue (gray)	Basal cell carcinoma

Figure 5.21: Continuation of the decision tree for one pattern, clods, one color

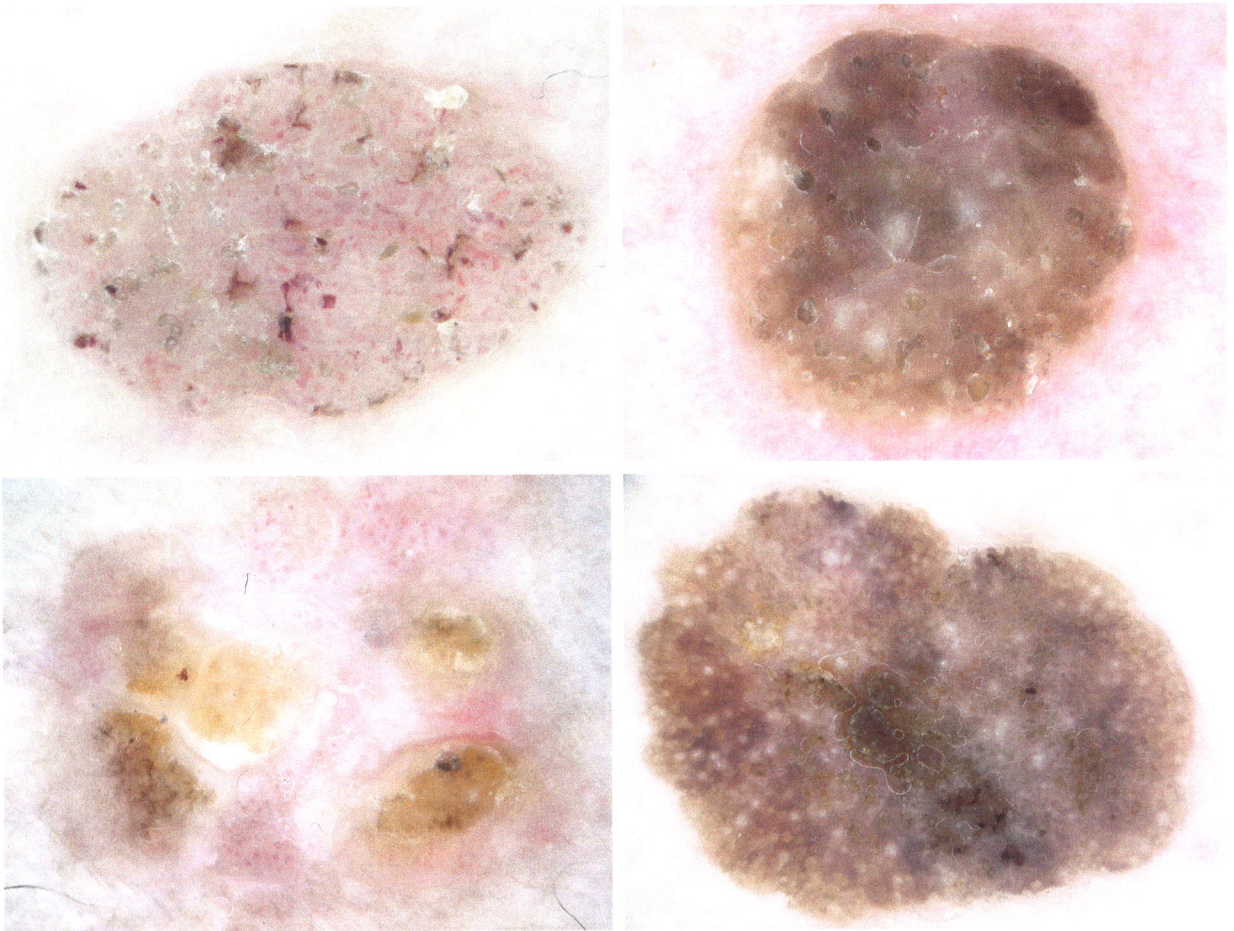

Figure 5.22: White and/or yellow clods.
*When white and/or yellow clods predominate, as seen in these four lesions, the diagnosis is seborrheic keratosis. White structures – as in the two lesions in the **right column** – are the only exceptions to the general rule that structure is defined by pigment while the hypopigmented portion constitutes the background. White clods are nearly always seen on a structureless brown background. In the two lesions in the **left column** one also sees the characteristic vessels of seborrheic keratosis, i.e. looped vessels (**top left**) and coiled vessels (**bottom left**).*

(5.23), in basal cell carcinoma one usually finds one or two orange clods with traces of red due to red blood cells in the serum crust. A further clue is the pattern of vessels: in basal cell carcinoma serpentine vessels, often branched; in seborrheic keratosis, looped or coiled vessels (only rarely serpentine). White dots or clods may be found in both diagnoses.

Unconscious rules often affect how patterns and morphology are perceived. Understanding these unconscious rules is important in all of dermatoscopy, but it is particularly relevant to the interpretation of white structures. In familiar settings one has no difficulty in establishing which features constitute foreground and which constitute background, but this is not always the case in unfamiliar settings, for example when one is learning dermatoscopy. The unconscious tendency is to interpret what one perceives to be the most prominent features

as the foreground and hence constituting structure. In practice this assumption usually works, but it is incorrect and is a common cause of errors in dermatoscopy.

The correct general principle is that structure is defined by pigment. For example, the spaces between reticular lines are not clods because the (more heavily pigmented) lines represent the structure and the (less pigmented) spaces are merely the background against which the lines are defined. It takes experience and deliberate training of the eye to (when necessary) override unconscious rules and correctly make this distinction between foreground and background.

By definition, a structure is called "white" only when it is clearly lighter than the normal perilesional skin. White structures (lines, circles, dots or clods) are exceptions to the general principle that pigment defines structure. That is, when white structures are seen one should

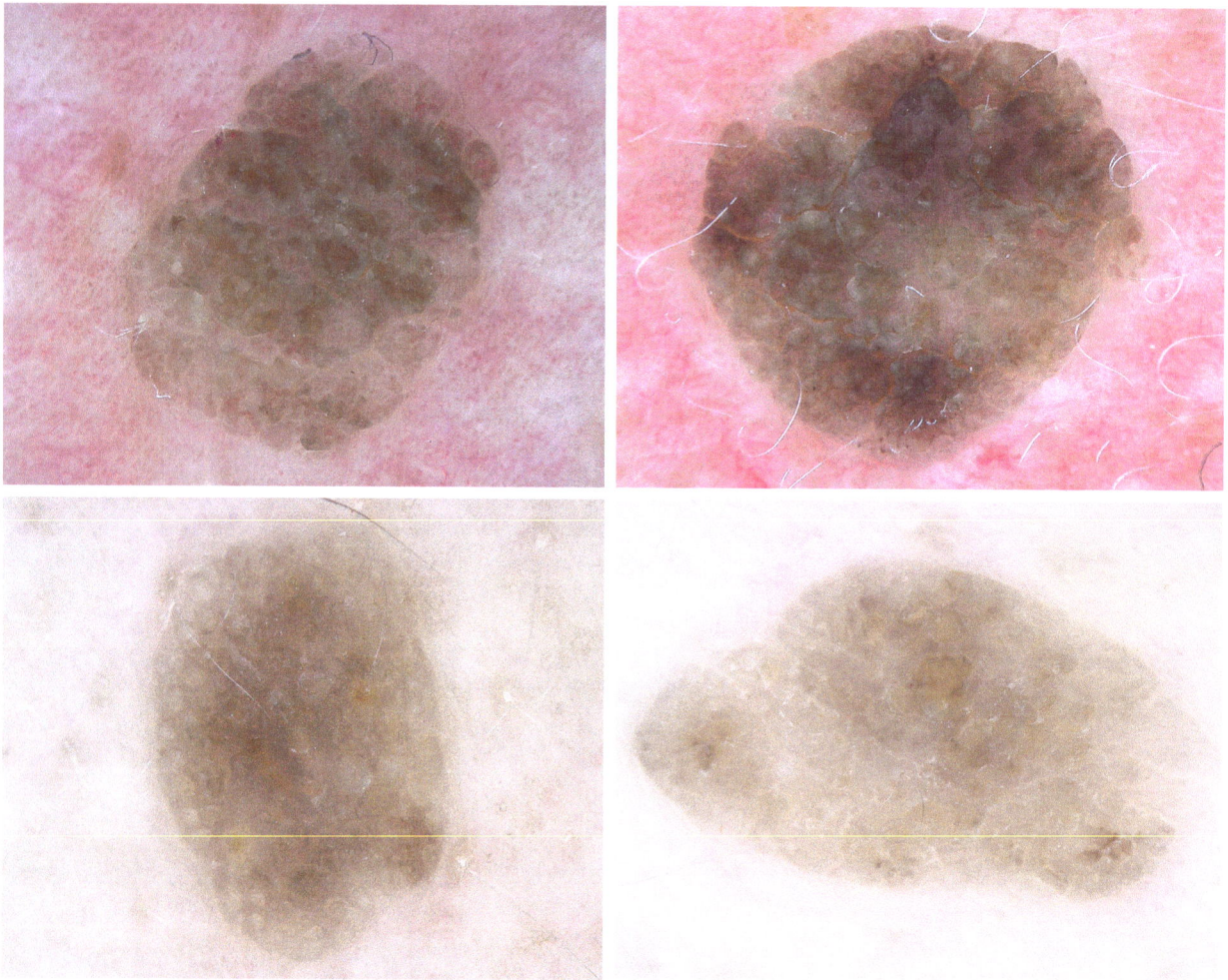

Figure 5.23: Orange clods.
Orange clods are a typical pattern of seborrheic keratosis.

reverse normal practice and interpret the more heavily pigmented structures as constituting the background against which the hypopigmented white structures are defined.

For the sake of completeness it should be mentioned that, in rare cases, Bowen's disease (especially when it occurs in conjunction with a seborrheic keratosis) may have only white, yellow and/or orange clods. Invasive squamous cell carcinomas are usually non-pigmented but may have white circles or clods as a clue to the correct diagnosis (13). The diagnosis of non-pigmented lesions is discussed in greater detail in chapter 6.

Red or purple clods are characteristic of hemangioma or vascular malformations *(5.24)*. Thrombosed vessels are seen as black clods. Hemorrhage may be seen as red clods. The differential diagnosis of blue clods is quite different from that of purple or black clods, so this distinction must be made carefully.

Large, polygonal skin-colored clods are usually found in exophytic congenital nevi with a papillomatous surface, such as Unna nevus or Miescher nevus, and also occasionally in verrucous seborrheic keratosis *(5.25)*. In all of these lesions one may also find smaller orange clods interspersed between the skin-colored clods.

When a pigmented lesion consists exclusively of brown clods, various types of melanocytic nevi must be considered in the diagnosis *(5.26)*. Large, polygonal light-brown clods are primarily signs of an Unna nevus or Miescher nevus, especially when the clinical appearance is papillomatous. Quite often typical curved vessels are found in the center of the clods, but the vascular morphology of these nevi may be highly polymorphous. In general, pigmented lesions should be diagnosed on the basis of their structure and color. A diagnosis made on the basis of the pattern and color should not be discarded because the corresponding pattern of

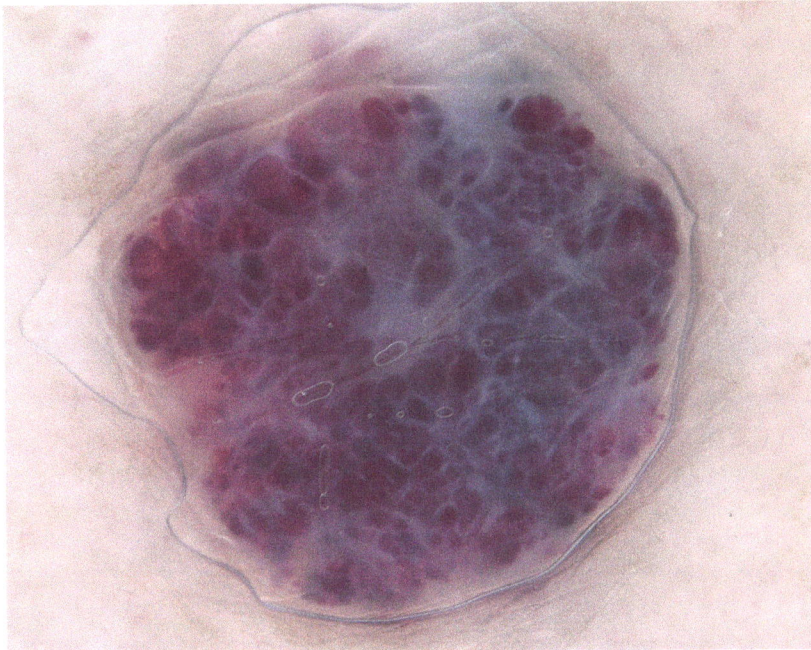

Figure 5.24: *Red clods.*
Red or purple clods of an hemangioma.

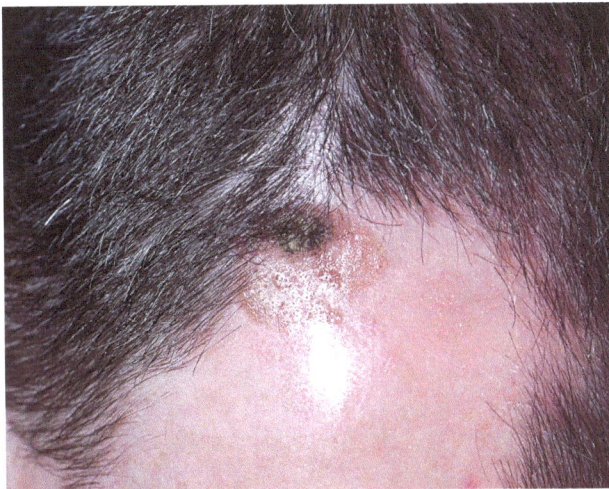

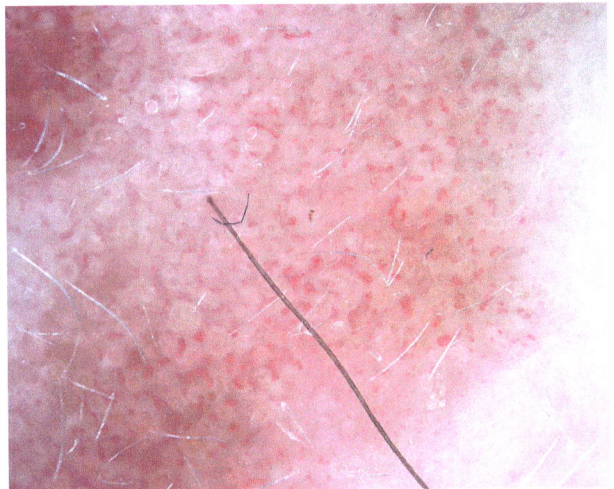

Figure 5.25: *Seborrheic keratosis with skin-colored clods.*
On dermatoscopy (right) one finds skin-colored clods with a looped vessel in the center.

vessels is absent. The pattern of vessels should, at most, be used to confirm the diagnosis.

Small to medium-sized, round and oval brown clods are characteristic features of small congenital nevi, of both the "superficial" and "superficial and deep" types. Some pigmented Spitz nevi may also have only brown clods, or brown clods peripherally may combine with gray clods or lines centrally (5.27). Central hyperpigmentation is also common in pigmented Spitz nevi, and peripheral clods are usually smaller than those in the center. However, these clues are not sufficiently specific to always distinguish Spitz nevi from small congenital nevi. Blue clods are characteristic of pigmented basal cell carcinoma (5.28). While melanoma and combined congenital nevus may also show a pattern of blue clods, they nearly always also have clods of other colors, or another pattern in addition to blue clods. Therefore, when confronted with only blue clods one should first look for clues to support or refute a diagnosis of basal cell carcinoma.

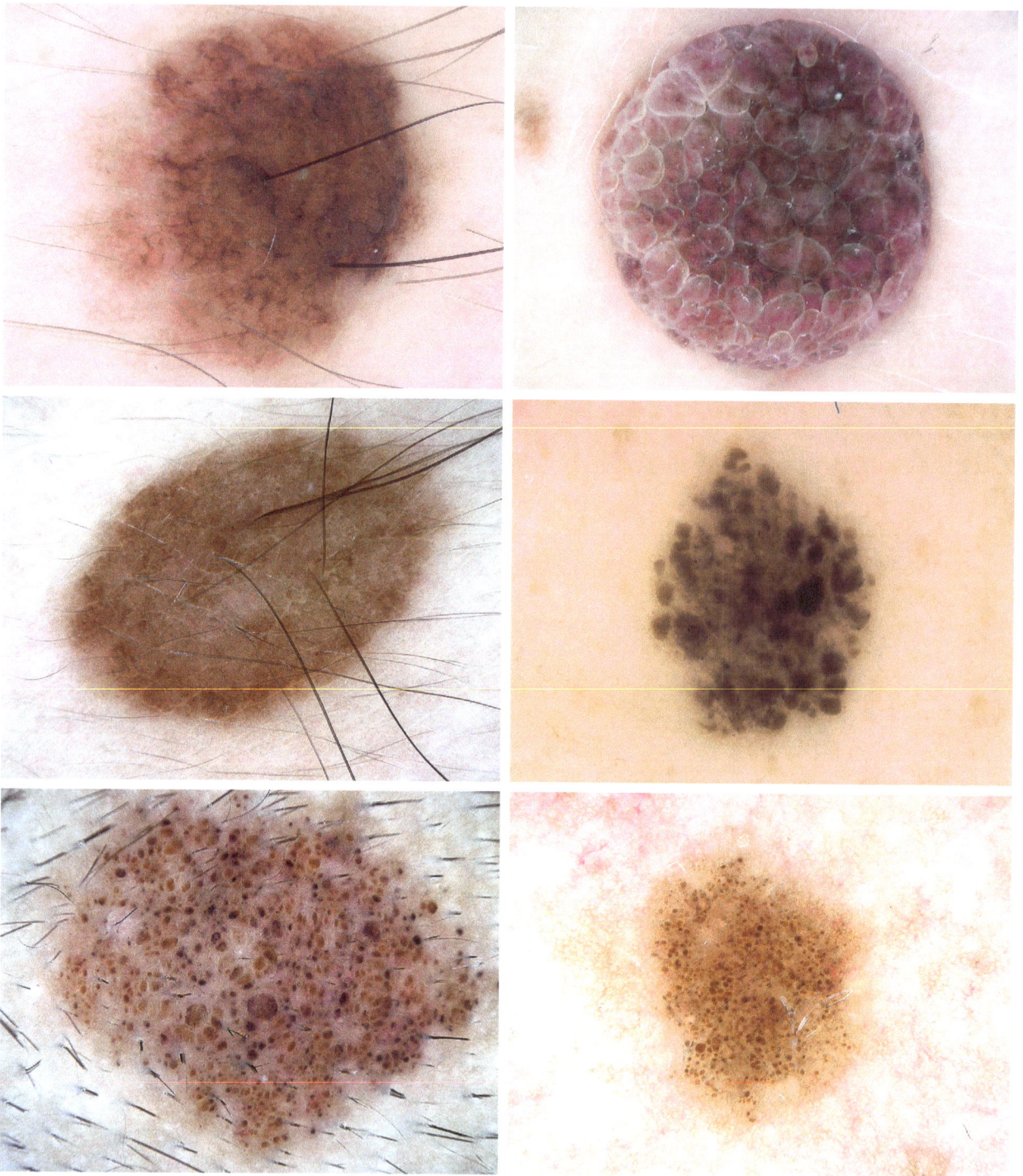

Figure 5.26: *One pattern, skin-colored and brown clods.*
Top left: *An Unna nevus composed of large polygonal brown clods, interspersed with a few small yellow clods.* **Top right:** *Unna nevus with large and polygonal, mostly skin-colored clods and a few brown clods.* **Middle:** *"Superficial and deep" congenital nevi with relatively large brown clods.* **Bottom:** *"Superficial and deep" congenital nevi with smaller brown clods.*

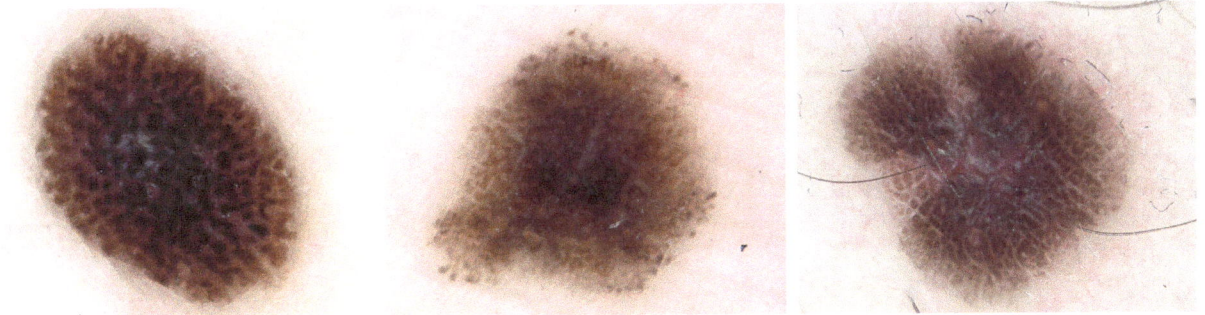

Figure 5.27: *Brown clods in Spitz nevi.*
*Three Spitz nevi with brown clods. Pigmented Spitz nevi are commonly hyperpigmented in the center. Peripheral clods are usually smaller than those in the center. Quite often one finds gray clods or lines in the center (especially evident on the photograph on the **right**).*

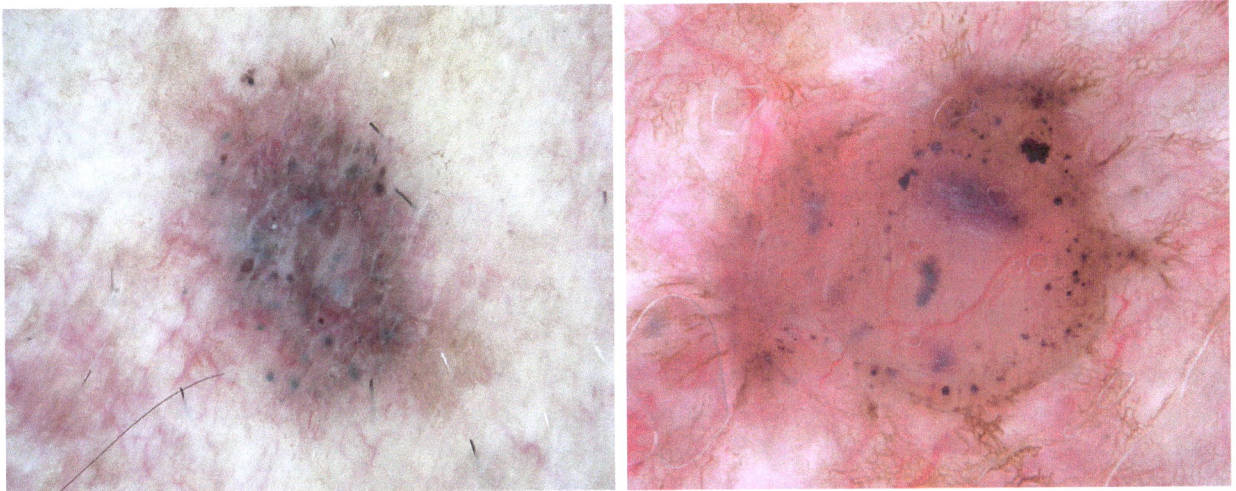

Figure 5.28: *Blue clods in basal cell carcinoma.*
*If one finds only blue clods the diagnosis is nearly always basal cell carcinoma, as in these two examples. The lesion on the **right** also has branched serpentine vessels, another strong clue to basal cell carcinoma.*

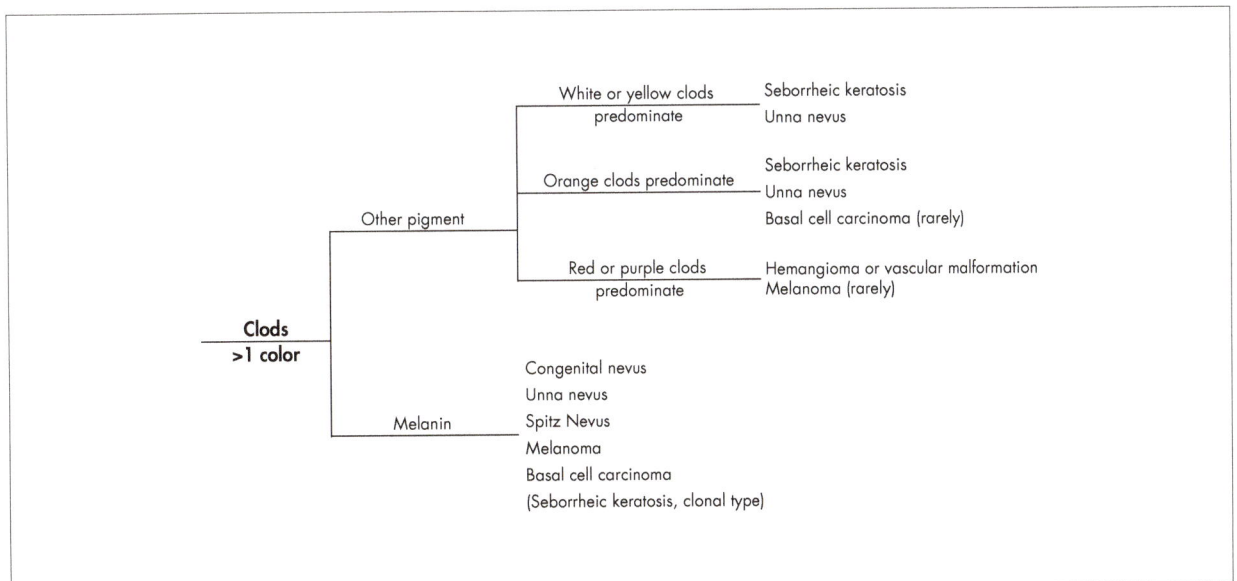

Figure 5.29: *Continuation of the decision tree for one pattern, clods, more than one color*

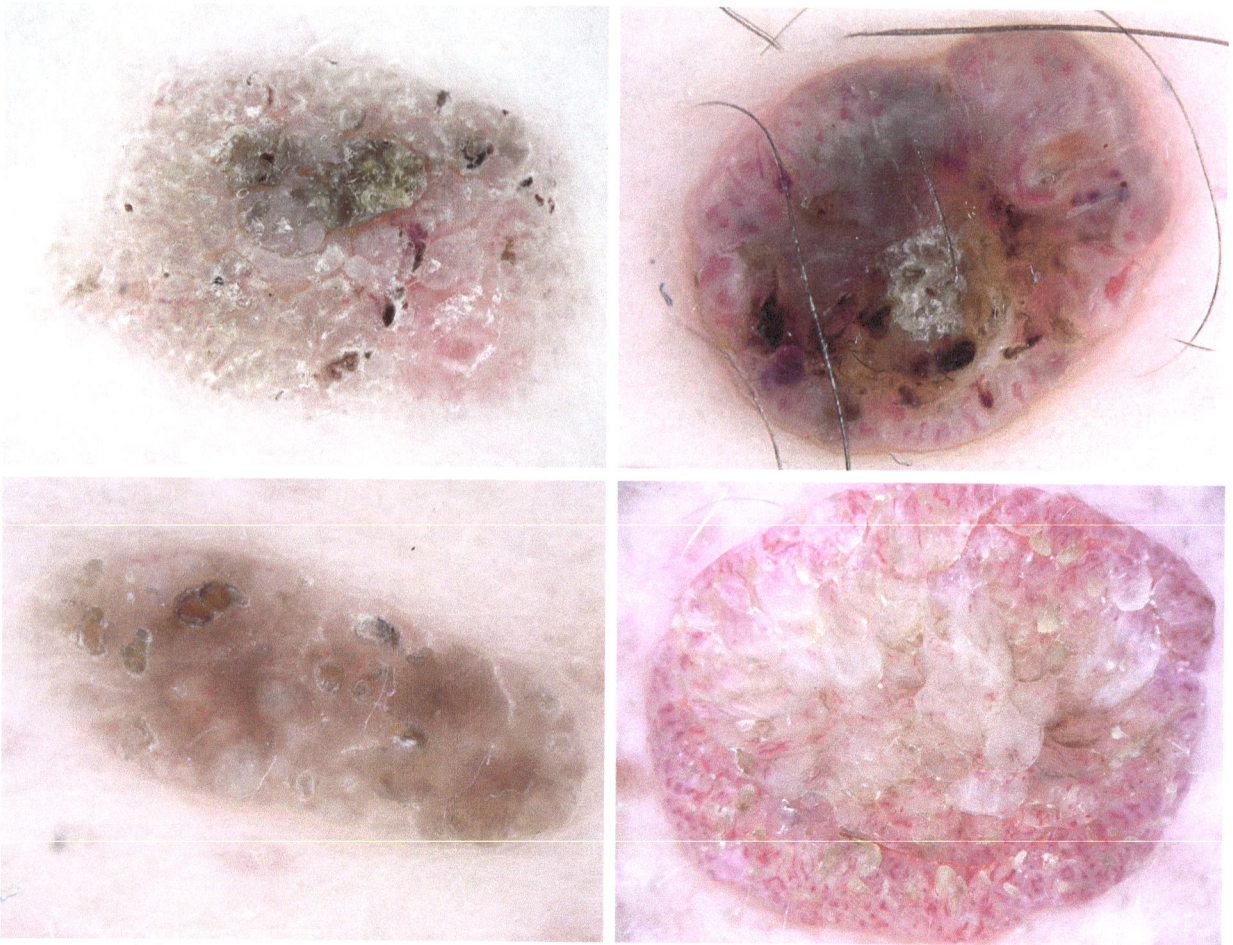

Figure 5.30: Clods, more than one color, no melanin.
Top left: *Large skin-colored and yellow clods in a seborrheic keratosis.* **Top right:** *Skin-colored, yellow and orange clods, and a few small black clods (coagulated blood) in an irritated seborrheic keratosis. Note the typical looped and coiled vessels.* **Bottom left:** *White, yellow and orange clods in a seborrheic keratosis.* **Bottom right:** *Large skin-colored and small yellow clods in an Unna nevus. Note the short, curved linear vessels.*

More than one color

When one finds clods of different colors it is helpful to distinguish between the colors of melanin and the colors of other pigments *(5.29)*. Clods whose pigmentation is due to melanin are brown, blue or gray. Although melanin may also appear black on dermatoscopy, a pattern of black clods is nearly always a sign of the blood pigment hemoglobin. Accumulations of melanin appear black in the stratum corneum but usually appear as dots rather than as clods. When one finds black melanin clods, there are almost never enough to form a pattern. To differentiate between melanin and hemoglobin one may also consider the other colors present in the lesion. If black clods appear together with red or purple clods it is almost always hemoglobin. If black clods appear together with brown clods it is likely that the pigmentation is due to melanin.

White, yellow or orange clods signify keratin with (orange) or without (white or yellow) inclusions of melanin. However, orange clods may also result from ulceration (serum crust). White or yellow clods are mainly found in seborrheic keratoses and less often in Unna nevi *(5.30)*. Orange clods in large numbers also indicate a seborrheic keratosis or less often an Unna nevus. In addition, just a few orange clods can be produced by ulceration in a basal cell carcinoma. When any combination of red, purple or black clods is seen, the differential diagnoses are the same as for a pattern of clods with only one of these colors; hemangioma, vascular malformation or hemorrhage.

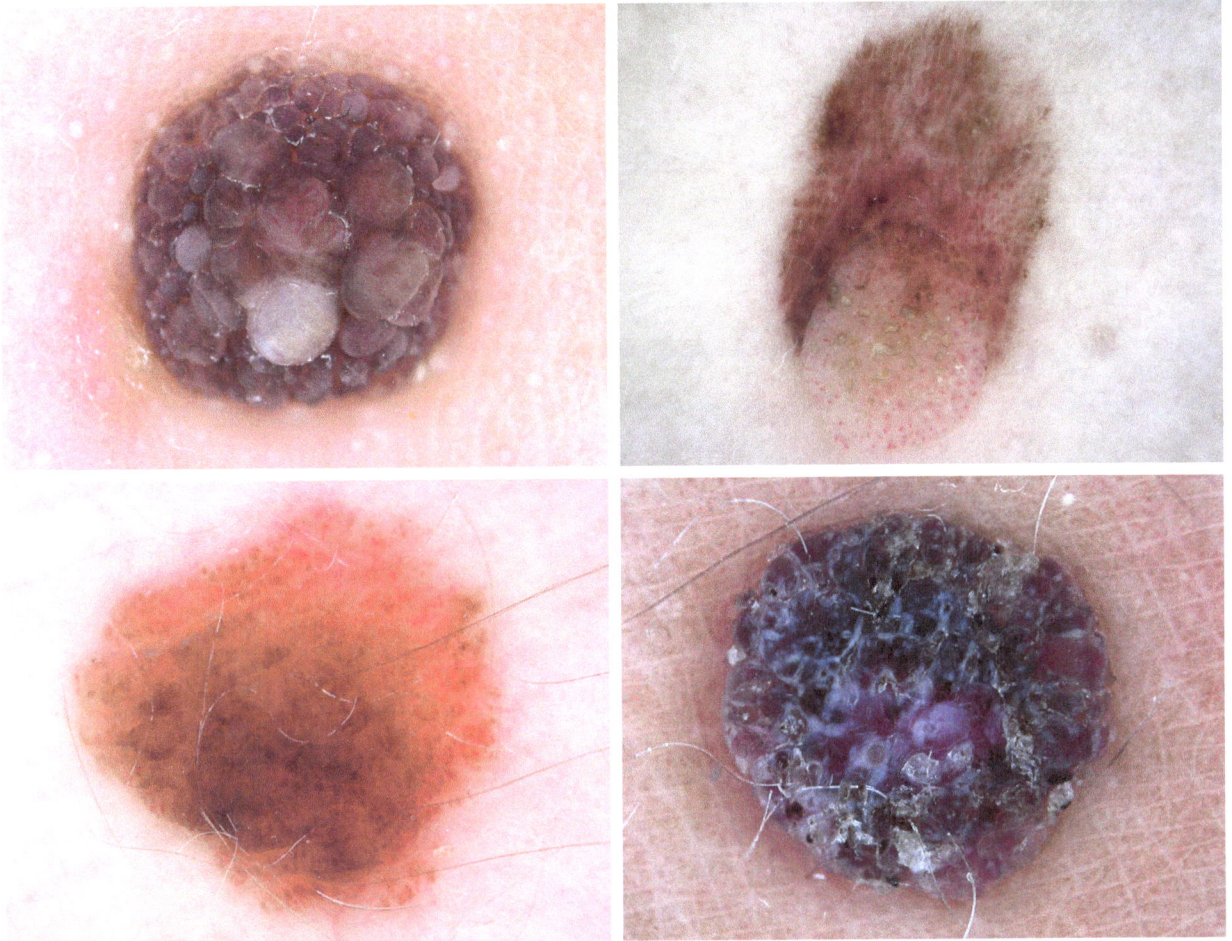

Figure 5.31: Clods, more than one color, melanin.
Top left: *Large brown and skin-colored clods in an Unna nevus. There are even some grey clods but the overall pattern suggests Unna nevus.*
Top right: *Skin-colored yellow and brown clods in a superficial and deep congenital nevus. The distribution of colors is asymmetric but there are no clues to melanoma or basal carcinoma.* **Bottom left:** *Light-brown and dark-brown clods in a superficial and deep congenital nevus. The distribution of colors is asymmetric but there are no clues to melanoma or basal carcinoma.* **Bottom right:** *Blue, red and gray clods in a melanoma (Breslow thickness > 1 mm). The white lines seen under polarized dermatoscopy are a clue to melanoma. Note the few vessels within the clods (e.g. at 3 o'clock position), which rule out a hemangioma.*

As emphasized in chapter 3, hemangioma must not be diagnosed if vessels are seen as dots or lines. Ignoring discrete vessels in this situation could lead to the grave error of misdiagnosing a non-pigmented nodular melanoma.

When the pattern is clods and the colors of melanin (brown, blue or gray) predominate, the possible differential diagnoses includes congenital nevi (all types including Unna nevi), pigmented Spitz nevi, basal cell carcinoma, and melanoma *(5.31)*. The distinction between nevi and these two malignant diagnoses can usually be made on the basis of the presence or absence of additional clues. Rarely a seborrheic keratosis, especially the so-called "clonal" type can present with a pattern of brown and gray clods *(5.32)*.

5.1.5 Dots

The pattern of dots usually occurs in combination with other patterns. When a pattern of dots does occur in isolation, diagnosis proceeds as usual, by assessing color. In practice, only gray or brown dots are found in lesions without another pattern. When only red dots are found, i.e. vessels as dots, the lesion is assessed as a non-pigmented lesion (chapter 6). When gray dots are predominant, the differential diagnosis includes lichen planus-like keratosis (solar lentigo in regression), pigmented actinic keratosis or pigmented Bowen's disease, and melanoma *(5.33)*. Differentiating between these diagnoses on the basis of additional clues may be quite challenging, and is sometimes impossible *(5.34)*. In cases of lichen planus-like keratosis one

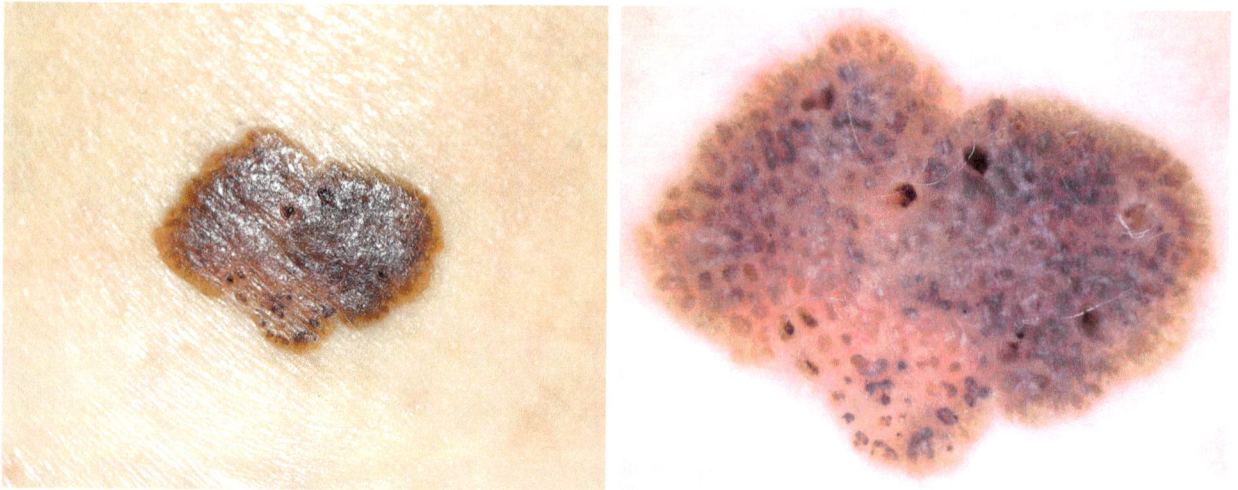

Figure 5.32: Seborrheic keratosis (clonal type) with brown and gray clods

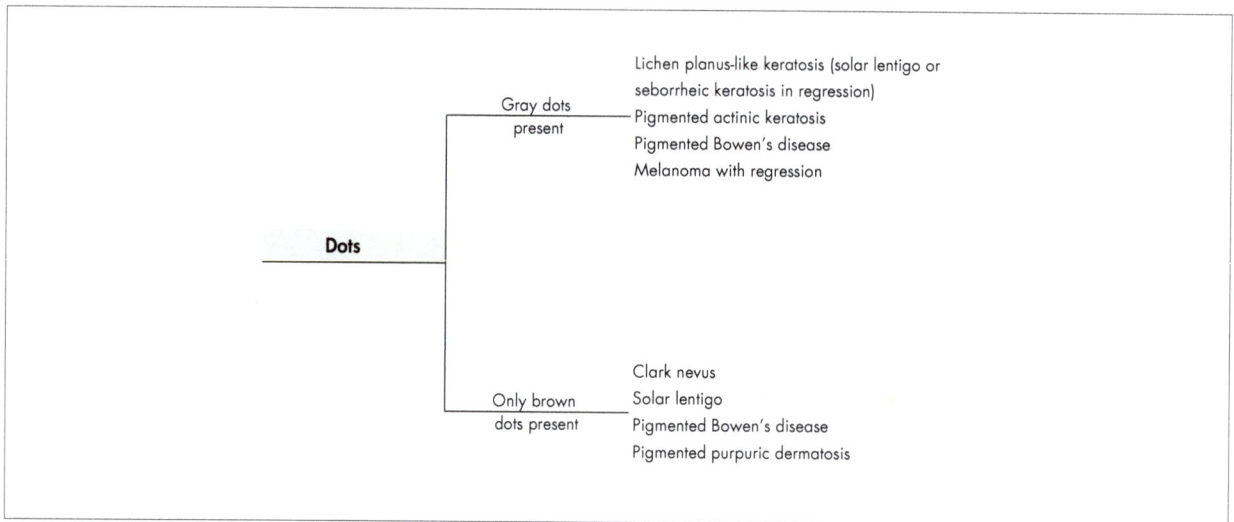

Figure 5.33: Continuation of the decision tree for one pattern, dots

may find residual features of the original solar lentigo or seborrheic keratosis e.g. curved lines or the typical sharply defined and scalloped border. Lichen planus-like keratosis occurs usually – but not exclusively – on chronic UV-exposed sites such as the face or the dorsum of the hand, surrounded by other solar lentigines and other signs of UV-related aging of the skin. Quite often one may find several lesions simultaneously.

Pigmented actinic keratoses occur predominantly on the face whereas pigmented Bowen's disease preferentially occurs on the trunk and the extremities. Pigmented Bowen's disease is notorious for mimicking other lesions, but usually the clues of coiled vessels and dots arranged as lines lead to the correct diagnosis (14). Finally, in situ melanomas may also have gray dots, usually mixed with

brown dots. Distribution may be random, or (mainly on the face) dots may be arranged as circles or as angulated lines around the openings of the infundibula (15). On the trunk or the extremities, the gray and brown dots of an in situ melanoma may also form angulated lines (polygons). These angulated lines on non-facial skin are much larger than structures formed around infundibular openings (7).

Finally it should be mentioned that some inflammatory skin diseases are associated with melanophages in the dermis and so may also have gray dots. In most such cases, one must rely on the clinical signs to reach the correct diagnosis.

The exclusive presence of brown dots usually indicates a Clark nevus. Rarely a solar lentigo or pigmented

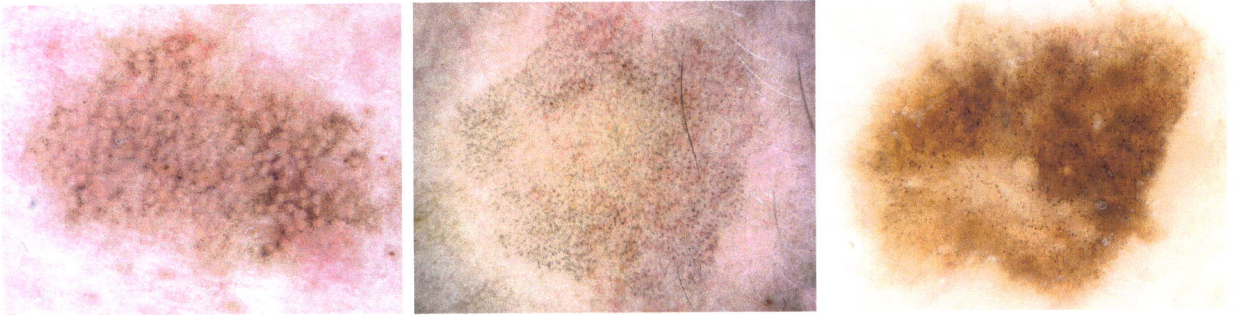

Figure 5.34: Pattern of dots.
Left: *Brown and gray dots between hypopigmented follicular openings are a characteristic feature of lesions on the face – in this case an in situ melanoma (lentigo maligna). In some parts the dots are arranged in angulated lines, which is a clue to flat melanomas on chronic sun damaged skin.* **Middle:** *The differential diagnosis for lesions composed exclusively of gray dots includes an almost completely regressed lichen planus-like keratosis, a pigmented actinic keratosis and pigmented Bowen's disease, a regressed melanoma and even healed inflammatory lesions. When (as in this case) the only finding on histopathology is melanophages in the dermis, an exact diagnosis is not possible.* **Right:** *Brown dots in pigmented Bowen's disease. Following the general principle that pigment defines structure, although the background in this lesion is structureless brown, it is not assessed as a pattern because it is entirely covered with (more heavily pigmented) brown dots.*

Bowen's disease may also have only brown dots. The combination of brown and red dots may also occur in inflammatory skin diseases associated with extravasation of red blood cells, such as various forms of pigmented purpuric dermatosis. As in other inflammatory skin diseases, clinical signs rather than dermatoscopy lead to the correct diagnosis.

5.1.6 Structureless

When no basic elements are seen, or there are too few to constitute a pattern, or the visible structures cannot be reliably assigned to just one of the five basic elements, this is termed a structureless pattern. However, "structureless" does not mean "featureless" – whether due to different shades of color within the lesion or a type of "granularity". One should therefore avoid the term "homogeneous". The structureless pattern is the least specific pattern, thus giving rise to a long list of differential diagnoses. In the absence of structure, color may be the only clue. Even clues are often absent because most clues are based on some kind of "structure". In summary, lesions that only have a structureless pattern are difficult to diagnose using dermatoscopy and therefore often require histopathology.

One color predominates over all others

The colors black, blue, brown and red are of practical relevance *(5.35)*. Black and structureless usually indicates the presence of hemoglobin (not melanin) and its degradation products. Hemorrhagic crusts, hemorrhages in the epidermis in general, and thrombosed vessels all appear black and structureless. In exceptional cases, melanin in the stratum corneum can entirely cover all other structures and colors. The differential diagnosis then includes heavily pigmented melanocytic lesions like Reed nevus, Clark nevus or melanoma.

A blue structureless pattern is quite specific for blue nevi of all types. One should keep in mind the fact that a blue nevus may – in addition to blue structureless zones – have gray or even brown areas which make the nevus appear variegate. Within blue or dark-gray structureless zones one may also find light-gray areas that could be interpreted as structures – usually lines or clods. In accordance with general principle that structures are defined by pigment, these light-gray lines or clods should be ignored, as they have less (not more) pigment than the surrounding area and so should not be considered to be structures.

In exceptional cases, melanomas and metastases of melanomas may be blue and structureless. However, even in these exceptional cases one finds additional clues to the correct diagnosis. These clues include black dots and gray lines, which should not be present in a blue nevus. Unlike blue nevus, there will be a history of progressive growth. Metastases of melanoma can usually be diagnosed on the basis of their clinical features in combination with the past history of melanoma. Apocrine hidrocystomas and exogenous pigmentation (for example tattoos) can be structureless blue. Structureless blue pigmented basal cell carcinomas have also been reported, but these are excessively rare. A history of progressive growth or the presence of clues to basal cell carcinoma may alert the clinician to this possibility. The brown and structureless pattern indicates solar lentigo, flat seborrheic keratosis, pigmented Bowen's disease, or melanocytic nevus, usually of the "superficial" or "superficial and deep" congenital type. A red structureless lesion is created by a recent hemorrhage

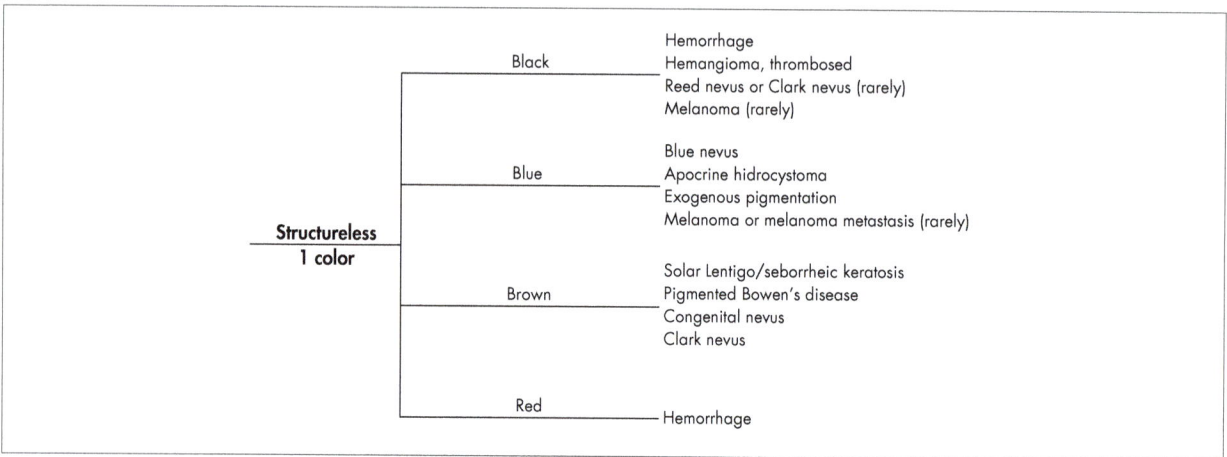

```
                                          Hemorrhage
                           Black          Hemangioma, thrombosed
                                          Reed nevus or Clark nevus (rarely)
                                          Melanoma (rarely)

                                          Blue nevus
                           Blue           Apocrine hidrocystoma
                                          Exogenous pigmentation
         Structureless                    Melanoma or melanoma metastasis (rarely)
         1 color
                                          Solar Lentigo/seborrheic keratosis
                           Brown          Pigmented Bowen's disease
                                          Congenital nevus
                                          Clark nevus

                           Red
                                          Hemorrhage
```

Figure 5.35: *Continuation of the decision tree for one pattern, structureless, one color*

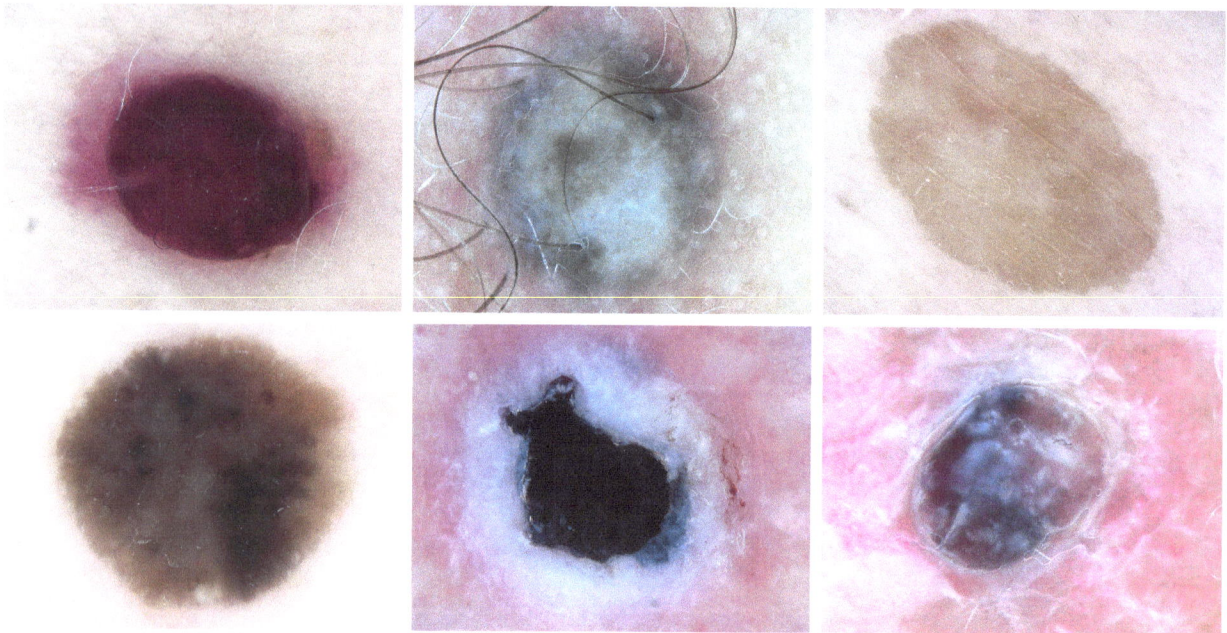

Figure 5.36: *Structureless lesions.*
Top: *Structureless, one color.* **Left:** *Recent hemorrhage in a nevus (red).* **Middle:** *Blue nevus (blue).* **Right:** *Solar lentigo (brown).* **Bottom:** *Structureless, more than one color.* **Left:** *Various shades of brown in a seborrheic keratosis. The few white clods are a clue to the diagnosis.* **Middle:** *The black structureless area in the center is a hemorrhagic crust in a traumatized angioma.* **Right:** *A structureless melanoma with brown, blue and gray areas and white lines as a clue to melanoma.*

in the stratum corneum. This will become a black structureless lesion as the hemoglobin degrades, before it entirely disappears due to transepidermal elimination.

More than one color
Sometimes for lesions with more than one color it is difficult to decide whether the pattern is one of clods or structureless. The difference is that clods are well circumscribed, and always occur in numbers. When

only one large contiguous area is seen, the lesion should be interpreted as structureless and not as a large clod. Skin color and white are not regarded as pigment. Lesions consisting only of these two "colors" are discussed in chapter 6 as non-pigmented lesions. When the colors of keratin, namely yellow and orange are predominant, one should first consider keratinizing lesions such as seborrheic keratosis. Structureless lesions that are only yellow or orange are rare. Occasionally a

Stepwise Procedure

1. Lines+

2. Pseudopods+

> 1 Pattern   3. Circles+

4. Clods+

5. Dots+

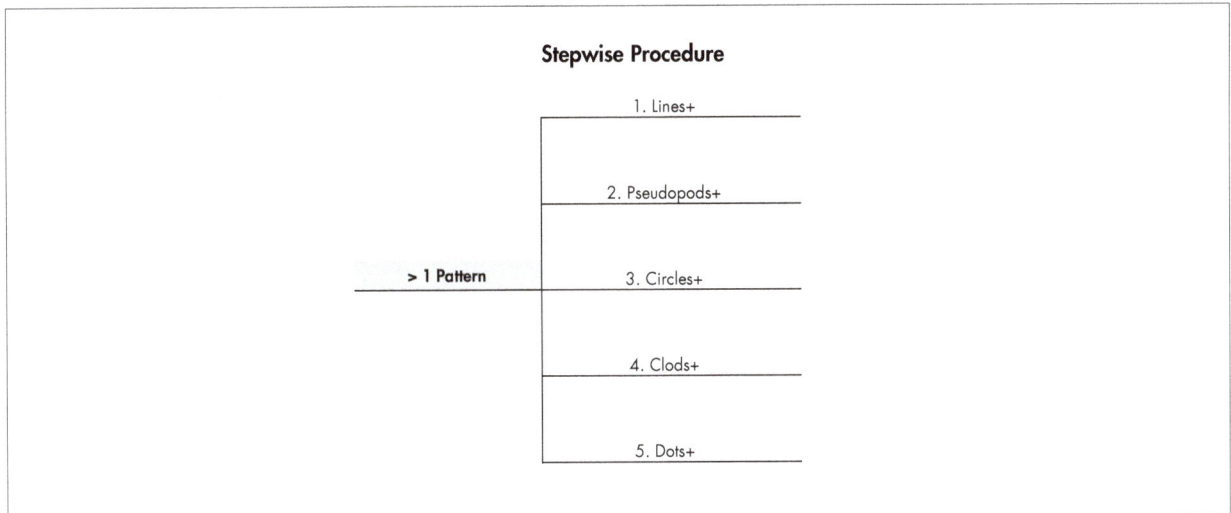

Figure 5.37: Continuation of the algorithm for more than one pattern

basal cell carcinoma may have a large, orange structureless area, corresponding to an erosion. When the colors of hemoglobin, namely red and purple predominate, the only diagnoses to consider are hemorrhage, or hemorrhage in a pre-existing lesion such as a nevus. Structureless lesions whose pigmentation is primarily due to melanin may have black, brown, gray or blue areas *[5.36]*. Black zones in a structureless lesion can also result from thrombosis. As a rule of thumb, black should be attributed to blood when it appears together with red or purple and attributed to melanin when it appears together with brown, blue or gray.

When the colors of melanin are symmetrically distributed in a structureless lesion, this is most likely a nevus but it could be practically any type of nevus. A specific classification is usually not possible by dermatoscopy. When the colors of melanin are distributed asymmetrically in a structureless lesion, one should consider melanoma, a metastasis of a melanoma, and seborrheic keratosis. The distinction is made on the basis of specific clues. In nodular structureless lesions that are blue and black a melanoma should be ruled out (16). The color black, which usually indicates melanin in the stratum corneum, is not expected in blue nevi. Exceptionally, a pigmented basal cell carcinoma or a dermatofibroma may show a structureless pattern with blue, brown, or grey areas.

5.2 More than one pattern

Although it is true that the majority of pigmented lesions have more than one pattern, beginners tend to classify far too many lesions as having more than one pattern. To constitute a pattern, multiple repetitions of a given basic element must be found, in an area occupying a significant part of a lesion. Two or more such areas must be found before a lesion can be classified as having more than one pattern. A few isolated lines, dots, clods, circles or pseudopods in a pattern of another basic element does not mean there is more than one pattern, and such isolated basic elements should be ignored at this stage. When appropriate, they can be taken into account when one is weighing clues.

The exact number of patterns is unimportant; no more diagnostic accuracy is achieved by counting patterns than by simply distinguishing between one and more than one pattern. Requiring only this simple judgment improves agreement between observers.

As lesions become more complex, it becomes increasingly likely that more than one interpretation could reasonably be considered by the investigator. In part this reflects the skill of the investigator, but it also reflects (often poorly understood) variations in basic perception between observers. Two features of the algorithm reduce errors in diagnosis due to differing interpretations. Firstly, as will be detailed below, descriptions are generated in a defined stepwise fashion. Secondly, the algorithm is constructed in such a way that various interpretations, as long as they are plausible, lead to the same diagnosis. The result is that the algorithmic method generally leads to the same conclusion regardless of which algorithmic pathway is followed. Of course, this redundancy in the algorithm is not infallible, so when the investiga-

Stepwise Procedure

1. Reticular or branched

2. Angulated

Lines+   3. Parallel

4. Radial

5. Curved

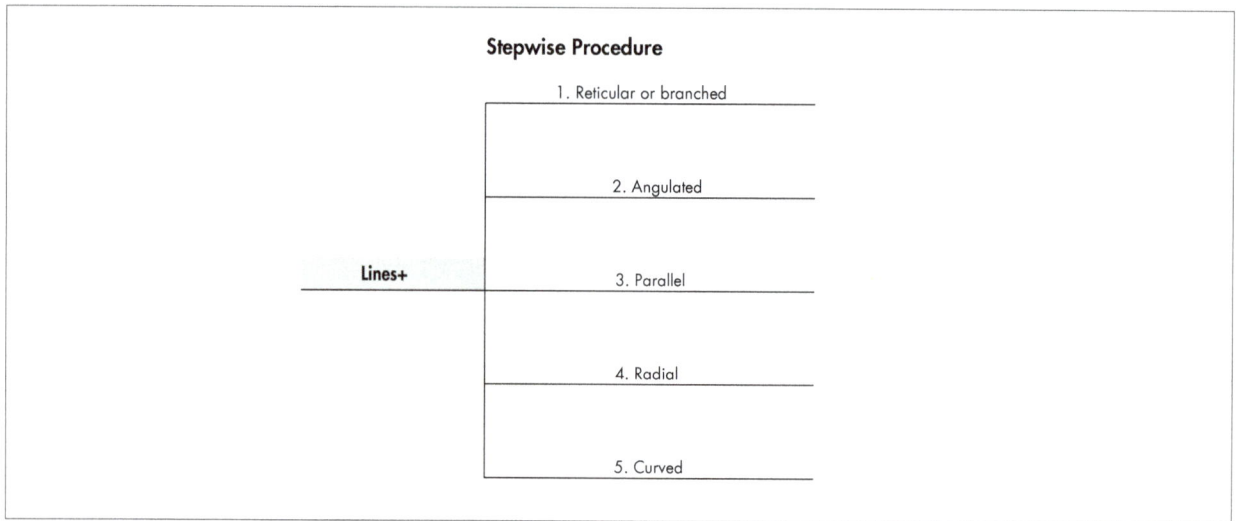

Figure 5.38: Continuation of the algorithm for more than one pattern, lines

tor is uncertain which pathway to follow, it is good practice to follow all the plausible pathways and consider all the differential diagnoses that the different pathways offer.

In contrast to lesions with only one pattern, for which all patterns are regarded as being equally important, the algorithm for pigmented lesions with more than one pattern is constructed in a hierarchical manner. If there is more than one pattern, one looks for the individual patterns in a stepwise manner, following a sequence established on the basis of pattern specificity [5.37]. The sequence starts with the pattern of lines, the most specific pattern in dermatoscopy, and ends with the structureless pattern, which is the least specific. Thus the description begins not with the most prominent pattern present, but with the most specific.

When a lesion consists of more than one pattern the investigator first determines whether a pattern of lines is present or not. When a pattern of lines is present, one follows the algorithm for patterns of lines. When no pattern of lines is present, one looks next for pseudopods, then for circles, then clods, and finally for dots. When none of these patterns of basic elements are seen, the lesion logically must consist of only one pattern, namely structureless, and the analysis is performed in accordance with the known rules for this pattern.

The most important decision in the analysis of pigmented lesions with more than one pattern is the presence or absence of structural symmetry. Symmetry in lesions with one pattern is judged on the distribution of colors within the lesion. In lesions with more than one pattern, the distribution of color is not assessed,

and symmetry is judged purely on arrangement of patterns. The more patterns there are, the less is the likelihood of symmetry.

Structural symmetry has been defined in chapter 3. In theory there are an infinite number of ways that two patterns can combine symmetrically. In practice, there are only three symmetrical arrangements of two patterns in pigmented skin lesions: a) One pattern is in the center and the other at the periphery, b) the opposite is the case, and c) the basic elements of one pattern (e.g. dots) are regularly spread over a second pattern (e.g. reticular lines). All other combinations of two patterns are, by definition, considered asymmetrical.

When assessing symmetry we should keep in mind that we are dealing with biological structures. Assessment of symmetry is therefore a matter of judgment as to the type and degree of variation that is expected in nature, rather than a strict application of the propositions of geometry. At times there will be uncertainty as to whether a lesion should be judged symmetrical or asymmetrical.

This is an important role of experience in dermatoscopy; experts can confidently call more lesions symmetrical than beginners, reducing the need for exhaustive assessment to exclude malignancy. In cases of uncertainty, it is prudent to consider all the differential diagnoses at the ends of both applicable branches of the algorithm. Considering all applicable branches of the algorithm is appropriate in any situation when one reaches a decision point and is uncertain of the correct pathway. This ensures that no potential diagnosis is discarded prematurely.

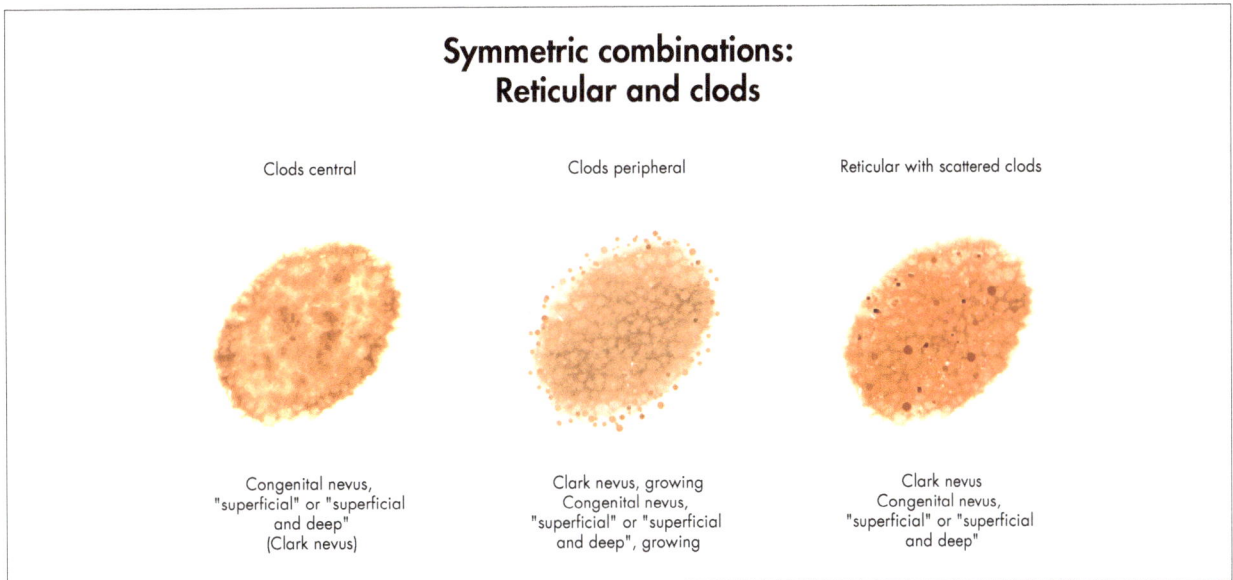

Symmetric combinations:
Reticular and clods

Clods central

Clods peripheral

Reticular with scattered clods

Congenital nevus,
"superficial" or "superficial
and deep"
(Clark nevus)

Clark nevus, growing
Congenital nevus,
"superficial" or "superficial
and deep", growing

Clark nevus
Congenital nevus,
"superficial" or "superficial
and deep"

Figure 5.39: Symmetrical combinations of the two patterns – reticular and clods

5.2.1 Lines

When analyzing a lesion with more than one pattern, lines are the first of the basic elements the investigator should look for. When a pattern of lines is found, again one proceeds in a stepwise manner (in order of specificity of pattern) through the various types of lines: first look for a reticular or branched pattern of lines, then a pattern of angulated lines, then a parallel line pattern, followed by a radial and finally a curved pattern of lines *(5.38)*.

Reticular and/or branched lines

As in lesions with one pattern, it is sometimes difficult to distinguish between reticular and branched lines. Unlike lesions with one pattern, this distinction has no diagnostic significance when assessing lesions with more than one pattern and so is not assessed. When a lesion contains both these patterns of lines, they are interpreted jointly as one pattern. Reticular lines are much more common than branched lines.

The first step in assessing lesions with reticular or branched lines is to rule out unequivocal cases of solar lentigo, seborrheic keratosis and their regressing variant, the lichen planus-like keratosis. The exclusion of these diagnoses is made on the basis of clues, such as a sharply demarcated scalloped border and curved lines in cases of solar lentigo or lichen planus-like keratosis; or a sharply demarcated border, white dots or clods, yellow or orange clods, and thick curved lines and a few circles in cases of seborrheic

keratosis. When enough of these clues are present to make an unequivocal diagnosis, the analysis stops. When there are no such clues, or too few to make an unequivocal diagnosis, the analysis proceeds.

Once these unequivocally benign lesions have been ruled out, the next step is to assess symmetry. If the patterns are arranged symmetrically the investigator will usually be able to establish a specific diagnosis, depending on the type of combination.

There are three combinations of the reticular (or branched) pattern with dots or clods that are symmetrical *(5.39, 5.40)*: The first combination is clods in the center and reticular lines at the periphery. Most of these lesions are "superficial" or "superficial and deep" congenital nevus, some are Clark nevi. As mentioned earlier, many dermatopathologists (regrettably) make no distinction between the two entities and refer to both as "dysplastic" or "compound" nevi. The second combination is reticular lines in the center and clods (or dots) peripherally. These lesions are usually a Clark nevus in its phase of growth, or a growing superficial or superficial and deep congenital nevus. Peripheral brown dots or clods are seen in growing melanocytic nevi of all types. The third combination is reticular lines with uniformly distributed clods (or dots). These are equally likely to be Clark nevi or "superficial" or "superficial and deep" congenital nevi.

In practice, only one symmetrical combination of reticular or branched lines and a structureless zone is seen, with the lines seen peripherally and the struc-

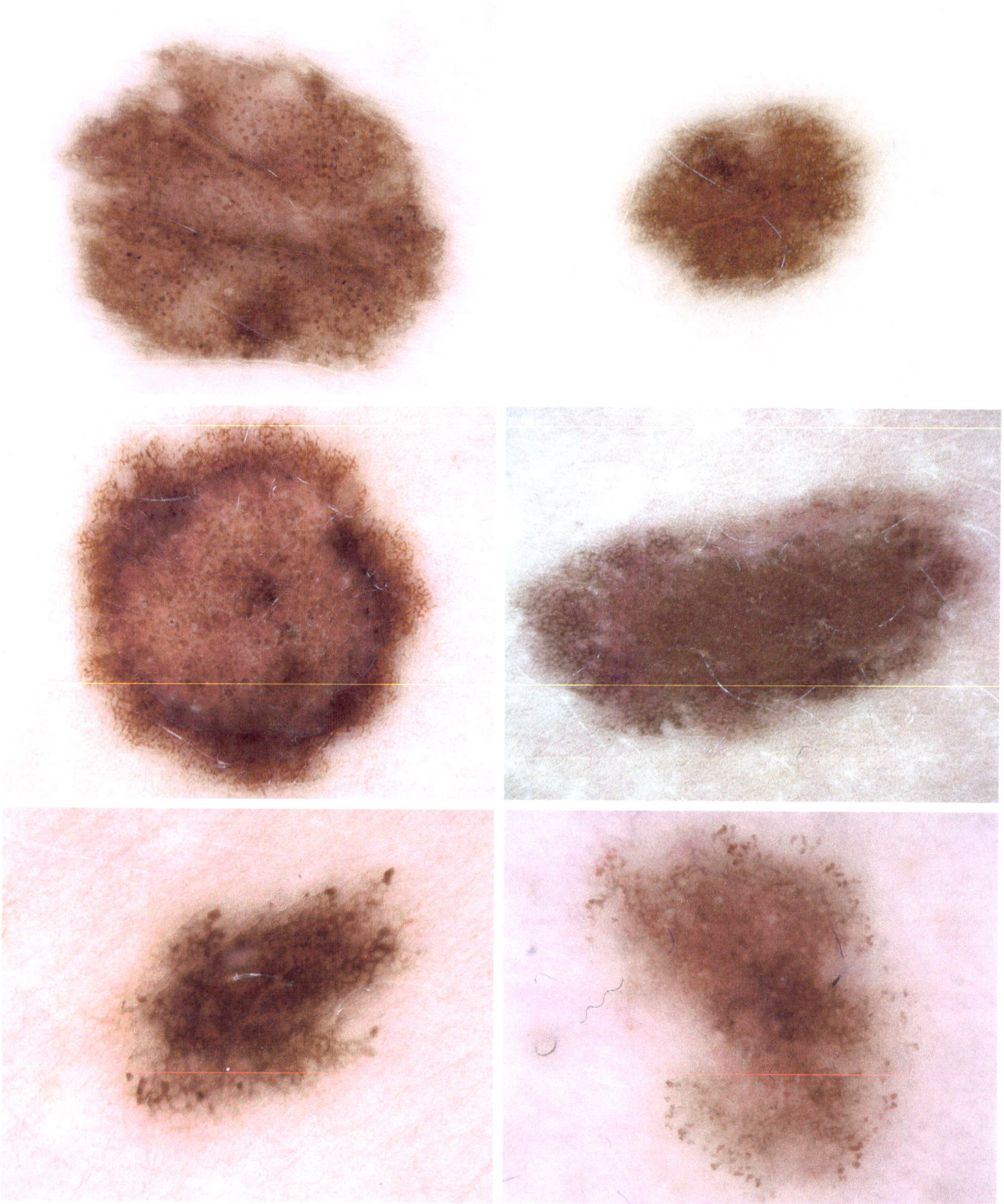

Figure 5.40: *Symmetrical combinations of patterns – reticular and clods.*
Top left: *Reticular lines and uniformly distributed clods in a Clark nevus.* **Top right:** *Reticular lines peripherally and small brown clods in the center, in a Clark nevus.* **Middle:** *Two "superficial and deep" congenital nevi with peripheral reticular lines and brown clods in the center.* **Bottom:** *Two growing Clark nevi with peripheral clods and reticular lines in the center.*

Symmetric combinations:
Reticular and structureless

Structureless skin colored or light brown in the center

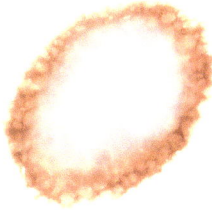

Structureless black or dark brown in the center

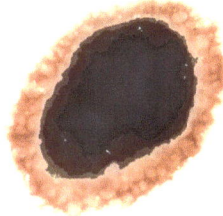

Structureless blue in the center

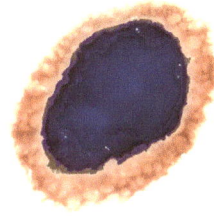

Congenital nevus, "superficial" or "superficial and deep", Clark nevus

Clark nevus (Reed nevus)

Combined congenital nevus

Figure 5.41: Symmetrical combinations of patterns: reticular and structureless

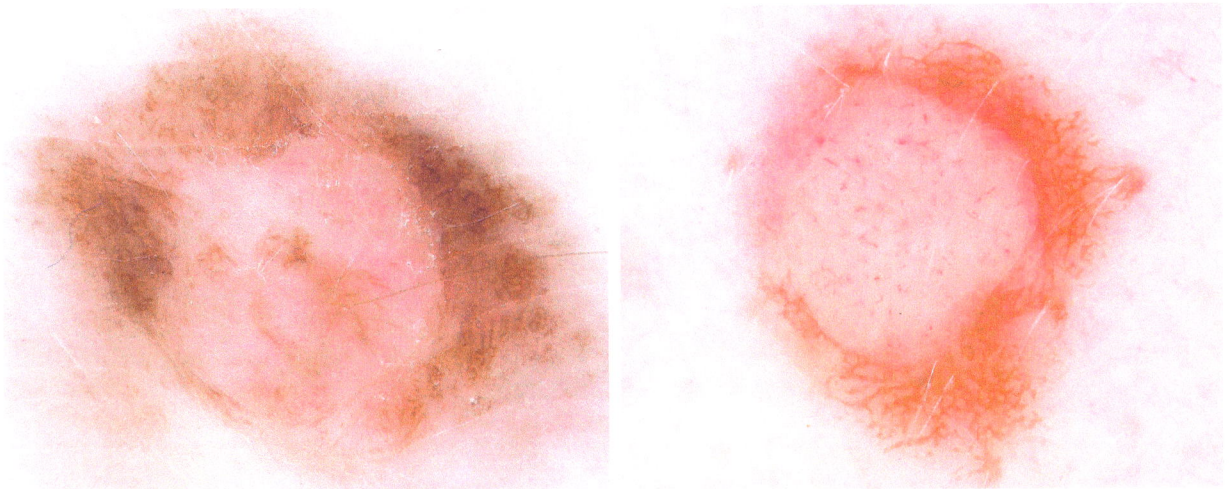

Figure 5.42: Symmetrical combinations of reticular at the periphery and structureless skin-colored in the center. Two congenital nevi with reticular lines at the periphery and a structureless skin colored zone in the center.

tureless zone centrally (5.41). The central structureless zone may be skin-colored or light brown. If the central structureless zone is skin-colored and raised or papillomatous, the diagnosis is most commonly a "superficial and deep" congenital nevus (5.42). If the central structureless zone is light brown and flat it could be a superficial or superficial and deep congenital nevus or a Clark nevus (5.43). An accessory nipple may also have this pattern.

If the central structureless area is black, the diagnosis is nearly always Clark nevus, or rarely a Reed nevus (5.43). One should not be misled by the histopathological finding of a "dysplastic junctional nevus" because this is just a different name for Clark nevus. When the center is structureless blue, this is usually a combined congenital nevus (5.44). If the center is white, i.e. lighter than the surrounding skin, and the adjacent reticular lines are light-brown and thin, the most likely diagnosis is dermatofibroma (5.45).

A symmetrical combination of pseudopods and/or radial lines with the reticular pattern (i.e. the pseudopods/radial lines are seen occupying the entire

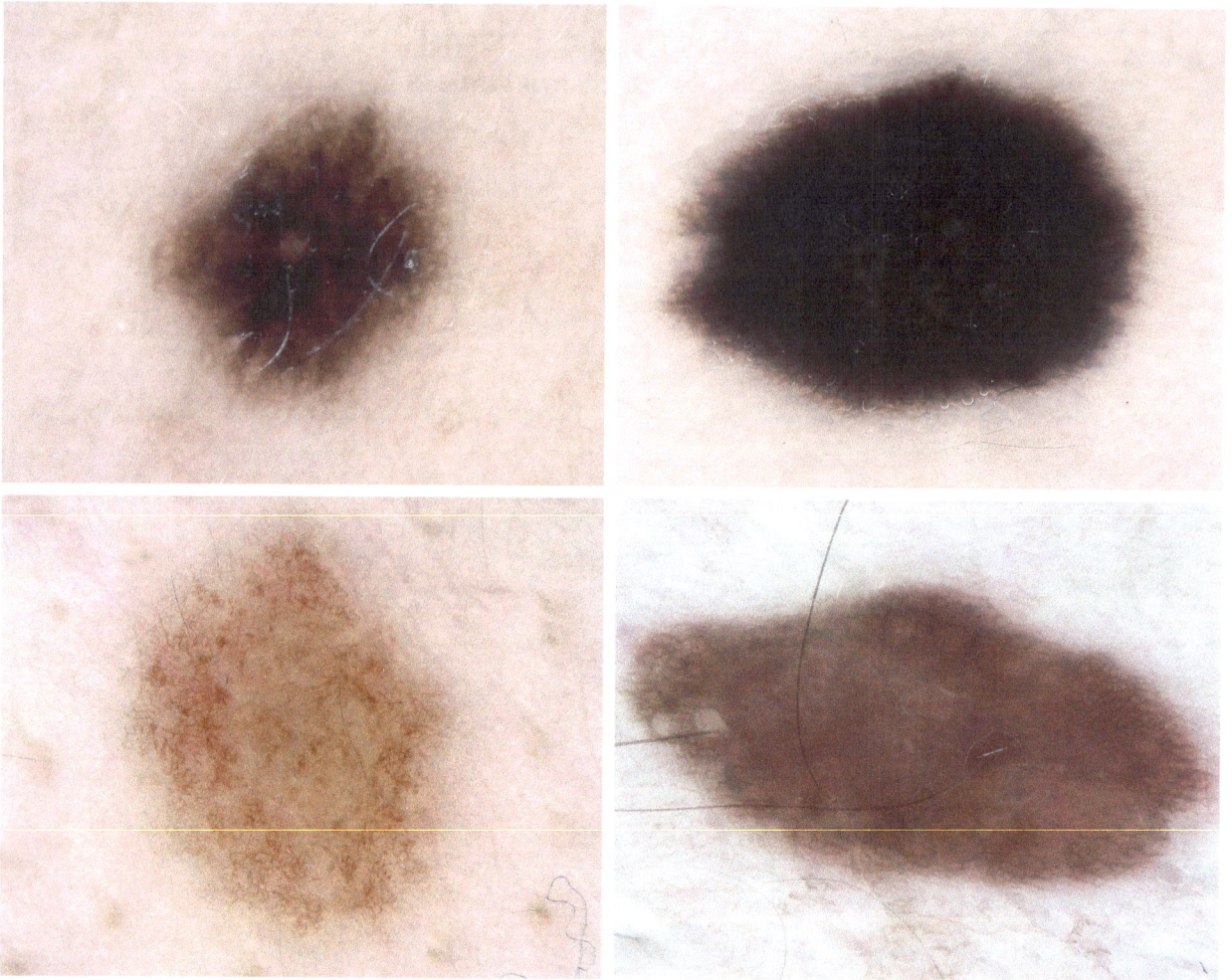

Figure 5.43: *Reticular and structureless.*
Top left: *Structureless black or dark-brown in the center and reticular at the periphery – a Clark nevus.* **Top right:** *Structureless black in the center and reticular at the periphery – a Reed nevus.* **Bottom left and right:** *Reticular at the periphery and structureless light-brown in the center – "superficial and deep" congenital nevi.*

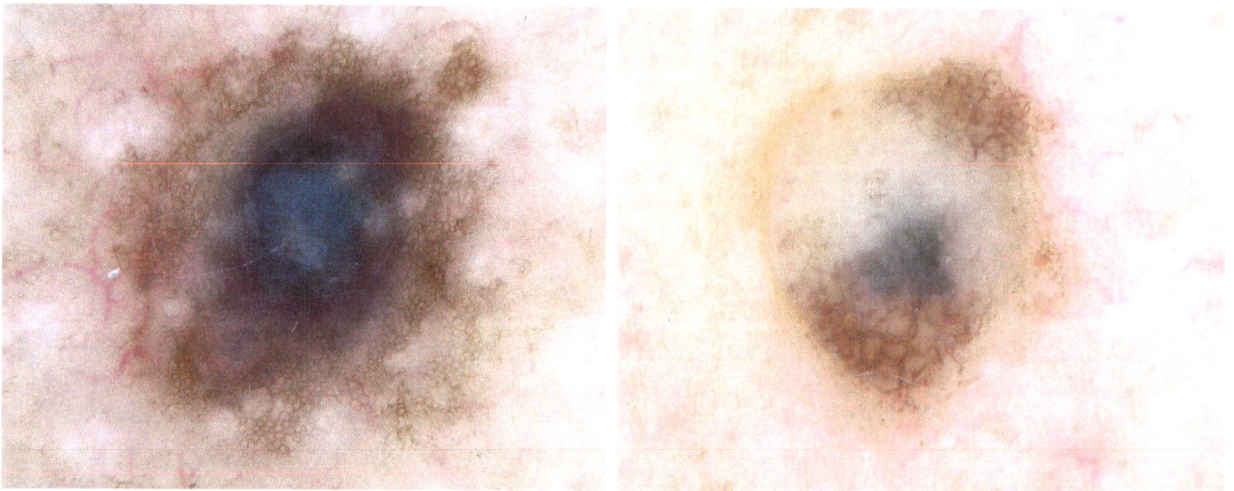

Figure 5.44: *Reticular and structureless.*
Two combined congenital nevi with a structureless blue center and reticular lines at the periphery.

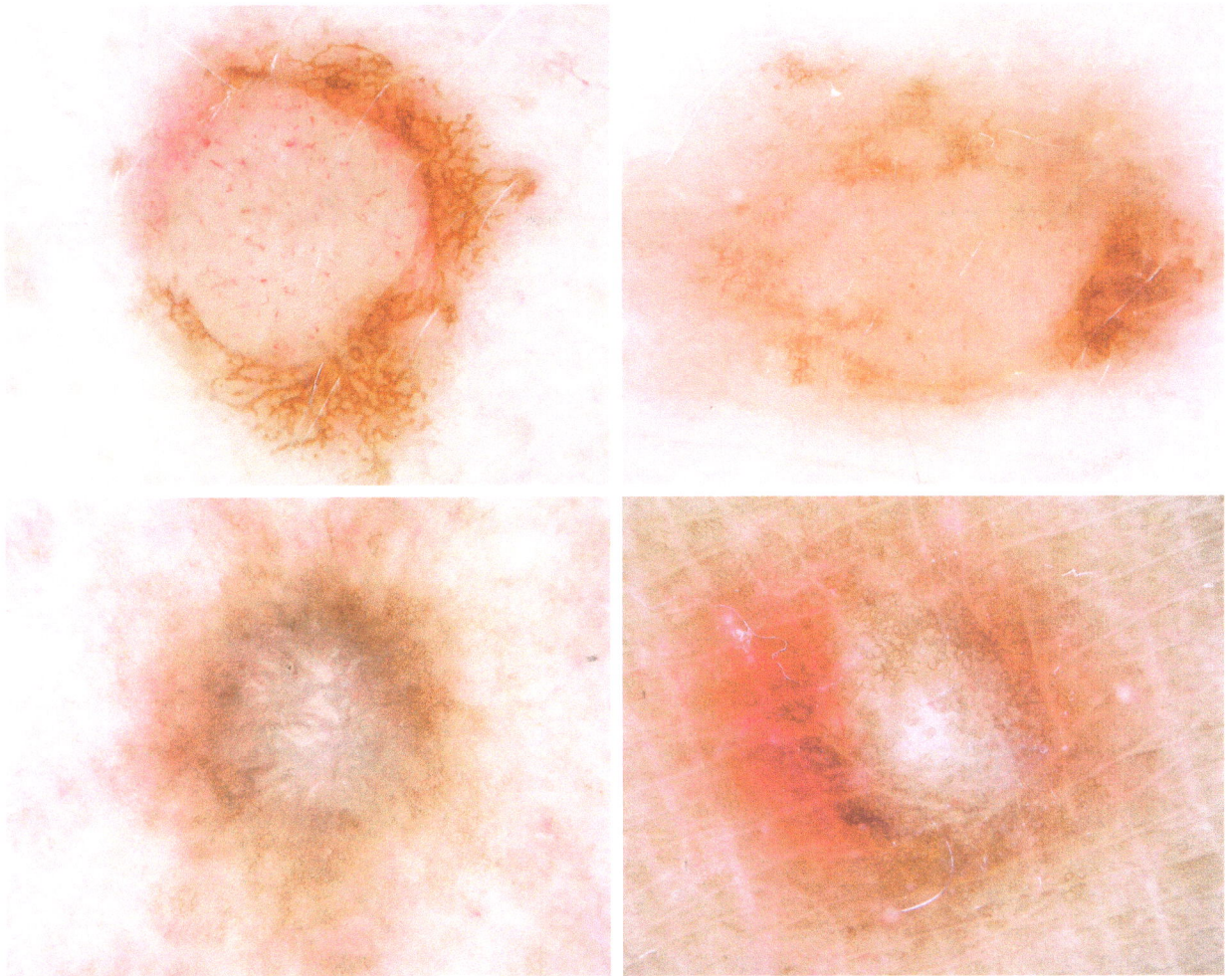

Figure 5.45: Difference between structureless skin-colored and structureless white.
Top: Reticular at the periphery and structureless skin-colored in the center – "superficial and deep" congenital nevi. **Bottom:** Reticular at the periphery and structureless white in the center – dermatofibromas. The structureless center of both these dermatofibromas is lighter than the surrounding skin and therefore correctly called white.

circumference) indicates a Reed nevus. A symmetrical combination of peripheral radial lines with a reticular pattern in the center is also rarely seen with a Clark nevus. In practice, when any of these patterns are seen it is difficult to reliably exclude melanoma, so such lesions (in adults at least) should be submitted for histopathology.

Symmetrical combinations of three patterns are seen, though less often than symmetrical combinations of two patterns. One example would be structureless in the center and a combination of reticular lines and dots or clods at the periphery. These three-fold combinations are usually found in "superficial" and "superficial and deep" congenital nevi.

Any lesion with an asymmetrical combination of patterns that includes reticular or branched lines needs careful assessment and should specifically be assessed for clues to melanoma (5.46). As a general rule when assessing a lesion for clues, a clue is only considered to be present when it is clearly present. Imagination and fantasy have no place in the search for clues. The diagnosis is nevus (Clark nevus, combined congenital nevus, "superficial" or "superficial and deep" congenital nevus) only when there are no clues to melanoma (5.47). The diagnosis is melanoma when (by these standards) at least one clue to melanoma is present (5.48).

Angulated lines

The main differential diagnosis of lesions with angulated lines is flat melanoma on chronic sun-damaged skin (including facial and non-facial skin). Many

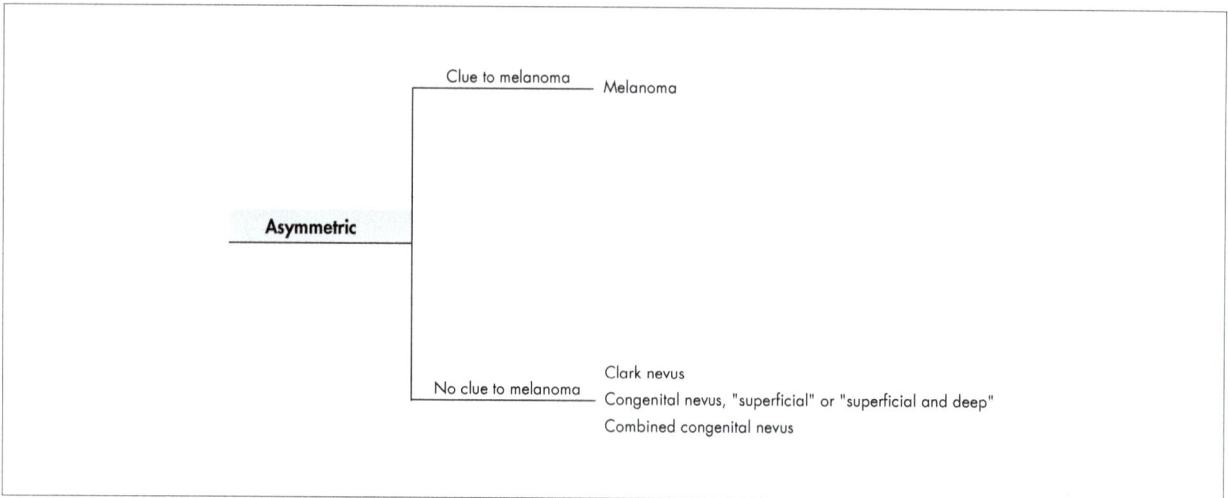

Figure 5.46: *Continuation of the algorithm for more than one pattern, reticular, with asymmetrical combination of patterns*

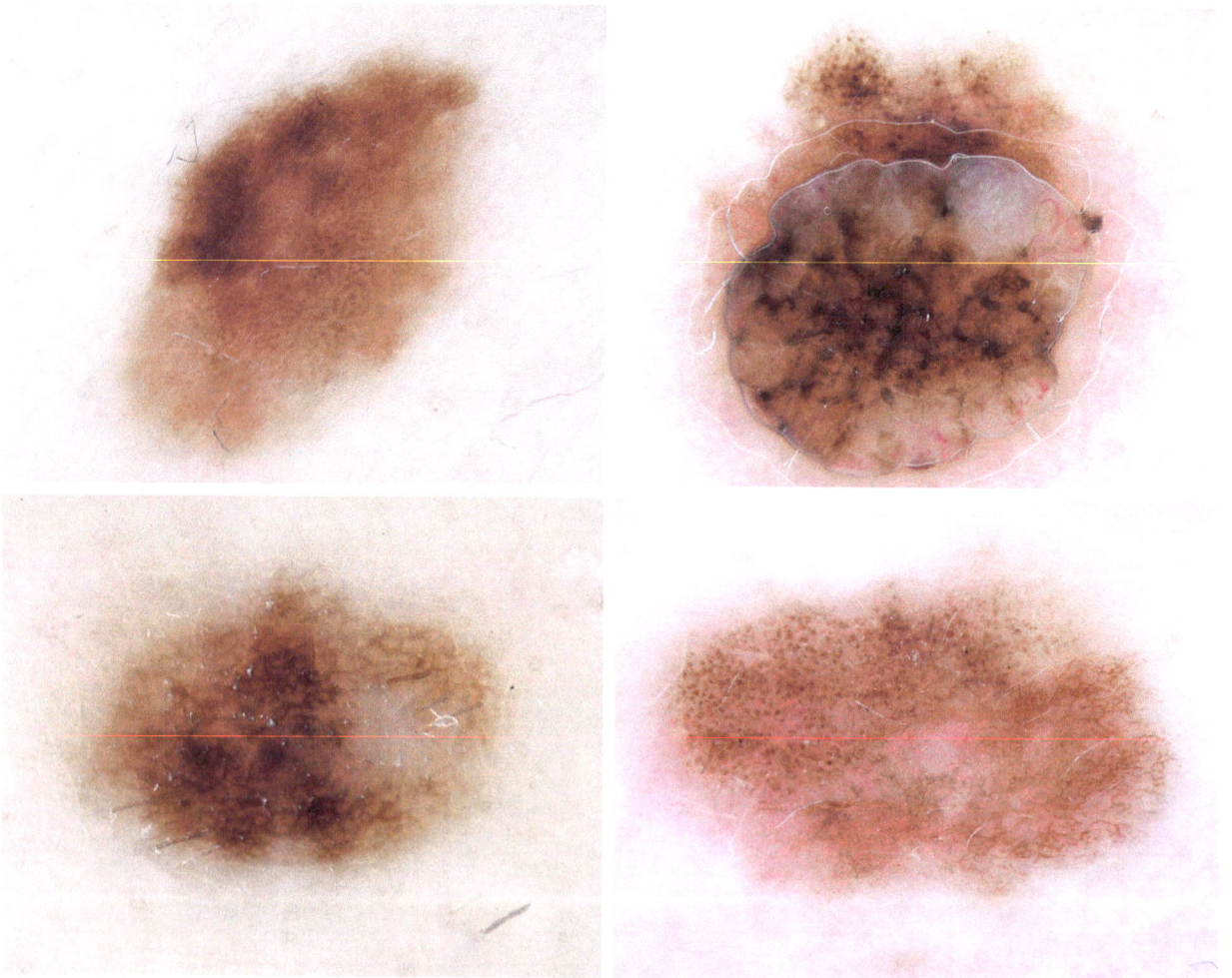

Figure 5.47: *More than one pattern, reticular, asymmetrical, without clue to melanoma.*
Top: *More than one pattern, reticular and clods, combined asymmetrically, more than one color (light-brown and dark-brown), but no clue to melanoma – "superficial and deep" congenital nevi.* **Bottom left:** *More than one pattern, reticular and structureless, combined asymmetrically, more than one color (light-brown and dark-brown), but no clue to melanoma (the eccentric structureless area is skin-colored and therefore not a clue) – a Clark nevus.* **Bottom right:** *More than one pattern, reticular and clods, combined asymmetrically, one color (brown) and no clue to melanoma – a "superficial and deep" congenital nevus.*

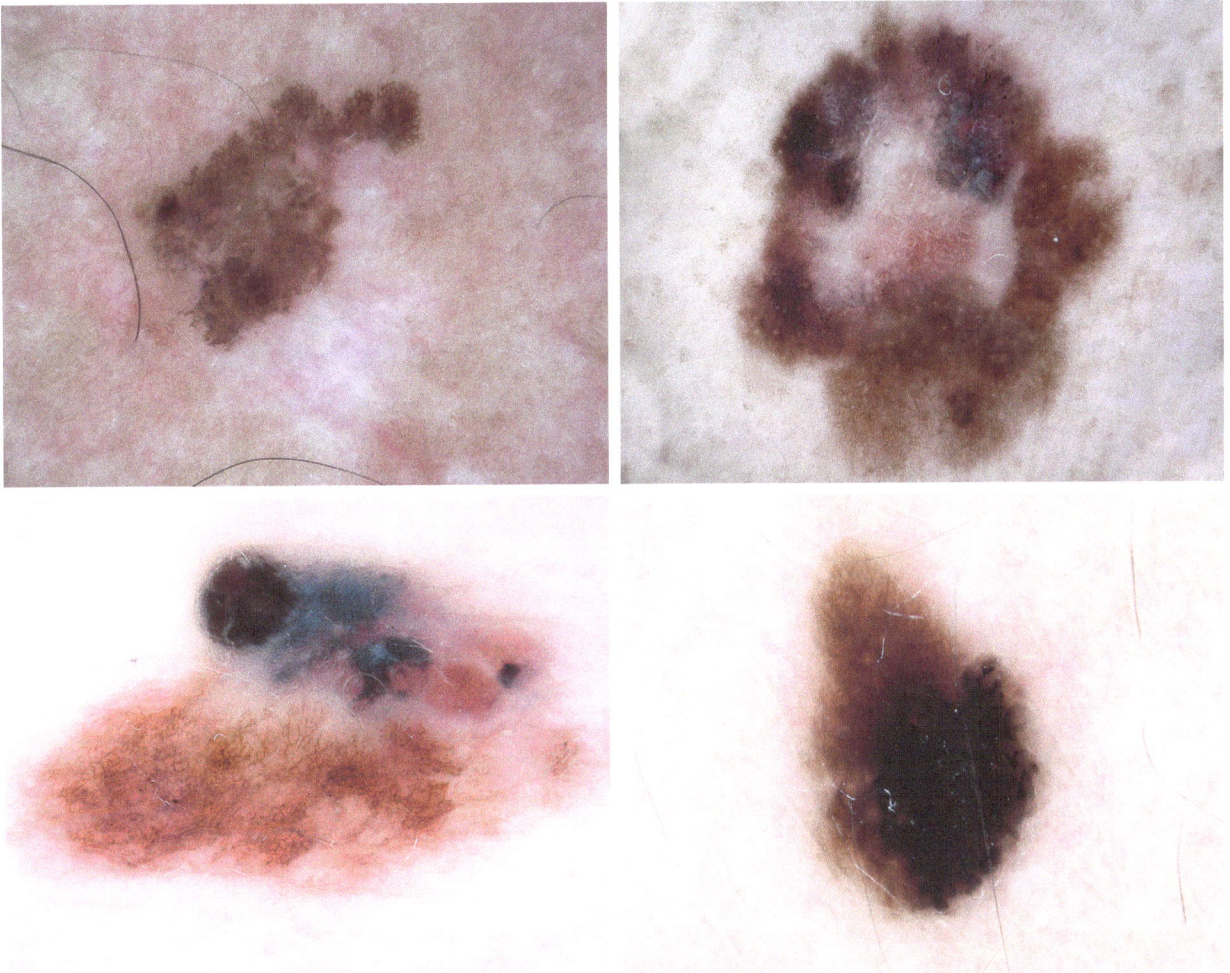

Figure 5.48: More than one pattern, reticular, asymmetrical, with clues to melanoma.
Top left: *More than one pattern, reticular and structureless, combined asymmetrically, more than one color, white eccentric structureless zone as a clue to melanoma – a melanoma.* ***Top right:*** *More than one pattern, reticular and structureless, combined asymmetrically, more than one color, white eccentric structureless zone and gray structures and black dots as clues to melanoma – a melanoma.* ***Bottom left:*** *More than one pattern, reticular and structureless, combined asymmetrically, more than one color, and an eccentric structureless zone with multiple colors as a clue to melanoma – a melanoma.* ***Bottom right:*** *More than one pattern, reticular, structureless and pseudopods, combined asymmetrically, more than one color, with pseudopods occupying only some segments of the periphery as a clue to melanoma. Histopathology shows this is actually a Reed nevus and not a melanoma; nevertheless, melanoma was still the best diagnosis on the dermatoscopy.*

flat melanomas on chronic sun-damaged non-facial skin have a lentigo-like reticular pattern and will be assessed according to the algorithm for lesions with a reticular pattern. Some flat melanomas, however, have angulated lines but no reticular lines *(5.49)*. On facial skin reticular lines are rare and therefore facial flat melanomas usually have other combination of patterns including combinations with angulated lines. A lesion with angulated lines on facial skin could also be a pigmented actinic keratosis, which is the main differential diagnosis of facial lesions with angulated lines *(5.50)*.

Parallel lines

Parallel lines are commonly seen in acral pigmented lesions with more than one pattern. Assessment proceeds as for one pattern lesions; first one determines whether the lines are on the ridges, in the furrows, or crossing ridges and furrows *(5.51)*. The ridge pattern takes precedence if more than one parallel line pattern is seen.

Further assessment of the ridge pattern is also similar to that for one pattern lesions, with the color of the ridge pigmentation taking precedence over the symmetry of pattern combination. If pigmentation on

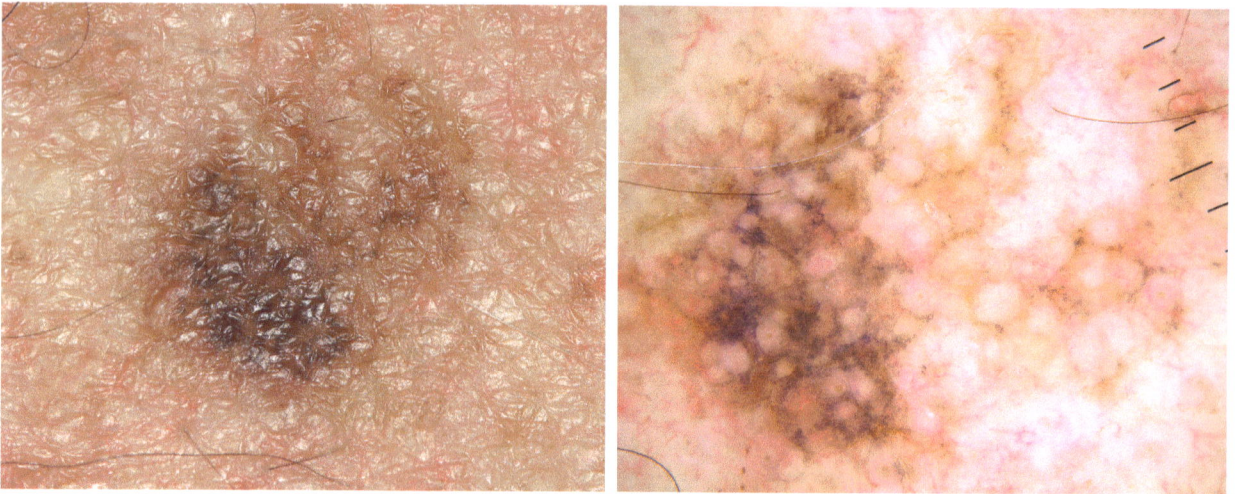

Figure 5.49: A flat melanoma on chronic sun damaged skin with angulated lines

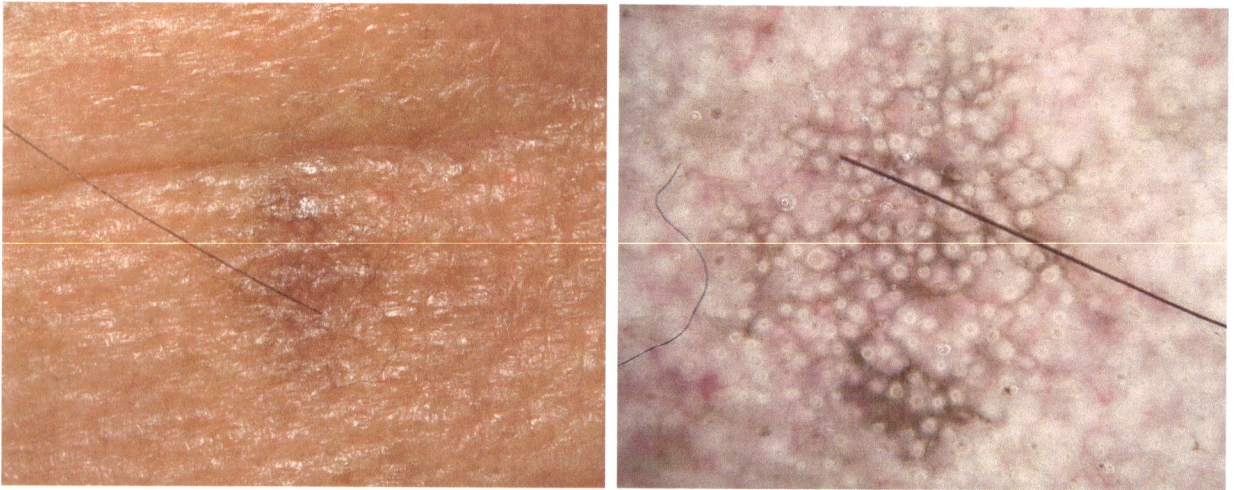

Figure 5.50: Pigmented actinic keratosis on facial skin with angulated lines and white circles

the ridges is in the colors of melanin, the diagnosis of melanoma must be considered, even in the absence of other clues to melanoma. Hemorrhage or exogenous pigmentation are the likely diagnoses when colors other than those of melanin are seen.

When the pattern is the furrow- or crossing-pattern, a distinction is made between symmetrical and asymmetrical combinations of patterns. Symmetrical combinations are found in classical acral nevi and all other nevi, such as Reed nevi or "superficial" and "superficial and deep" congenital nevi *(5.52 left)*. Not all melanomas on acral skin have a parallel ridge pattern. In asymmetrical combinations involving the pattern of furrows or the crossing pattern, the clues to melanoma are the same at acral locations as those

seen at other sites *(5.52 right)*. As a general rule, the thicker a melanoma at an acral site, the more it resembles melanoma at other locations.

It may be difficult to distinguish between the structureless pattern and the parallel ridge pattern, when the lines in the ridge pattern are wide enough to almost occupy the furrows. When the distinction cannot be made with certainty, both possibilities should be followed in the algorithm.

Radial lines

Radial lines always occur in combination with other patterns. When the radial lines occupy the entire circumference of the lesion the combination of patterns is symmetrical. When assessing symmetry, pseudopods

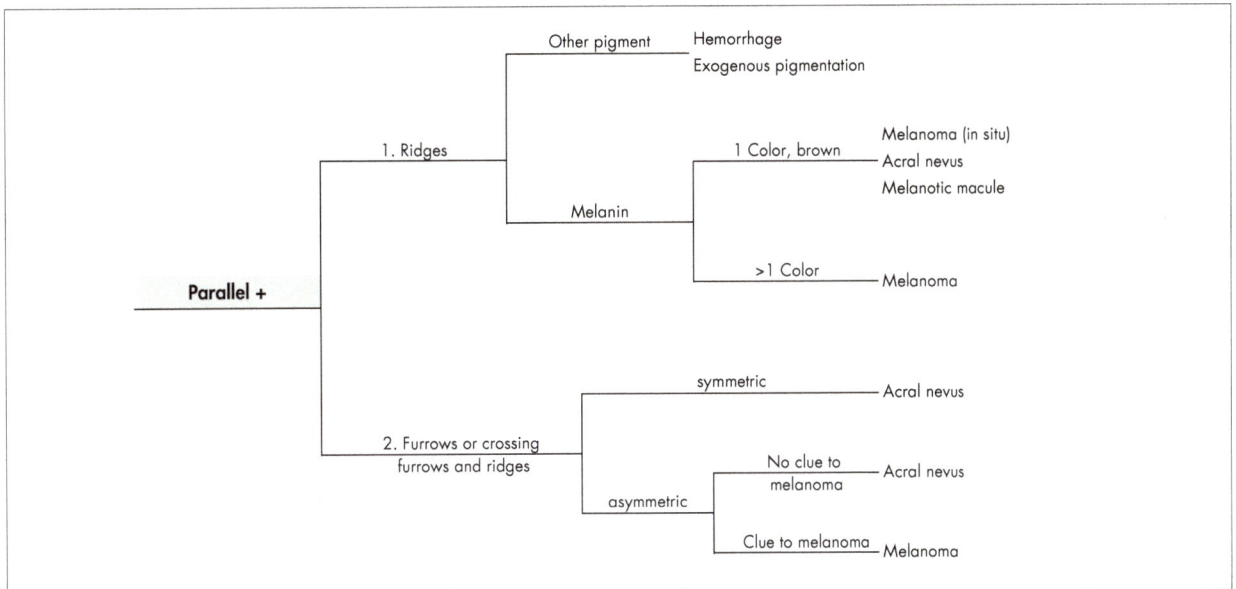

Figure 5.51: *Continuation of the algorithm for more than one pattern, lines, parallel*

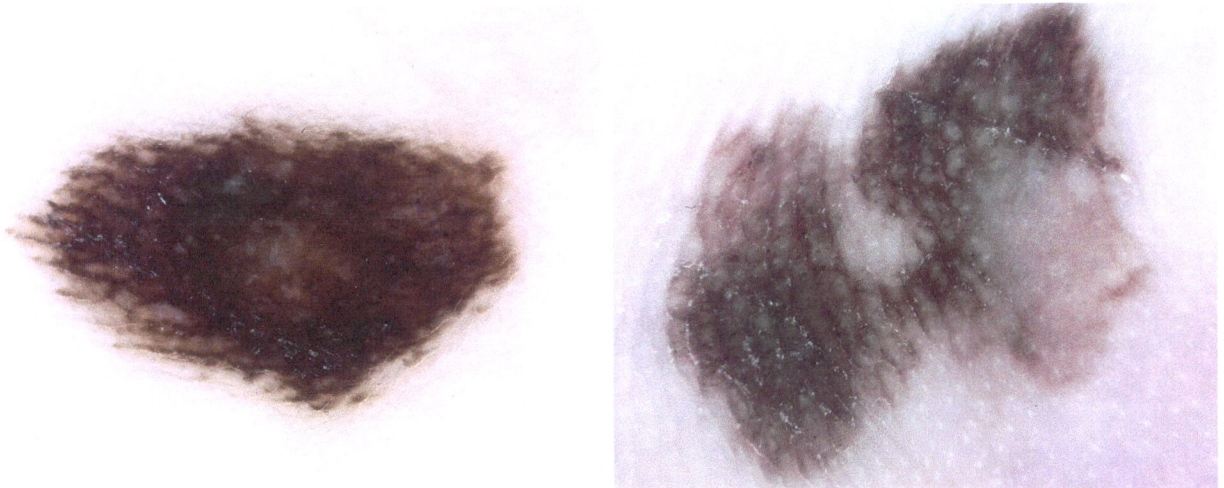

Figure 5.52: *More than one pattern, parallel lines.*
Left: *Parallel lines in the furrows peripherally, and structureless in the center combine symmetrically in a "superficial and deep" congenital nevus in acral location.* **Right:** *An asymmetrical combination of patterns consisting of parallel lines (mostly) in the furrows and an eccentric structureless zone. Here the eccentric structureless zone constitutes both a pattern and a clue to melanoma. Peripheral black dots are an additional clue. Histopathology confirmed an invasive melanoma, < 1 mm Breslow thickness, arising in a pre-existing "superficial and deep" congenital nevus (which could not be reliably identified on dermatoscopy).*

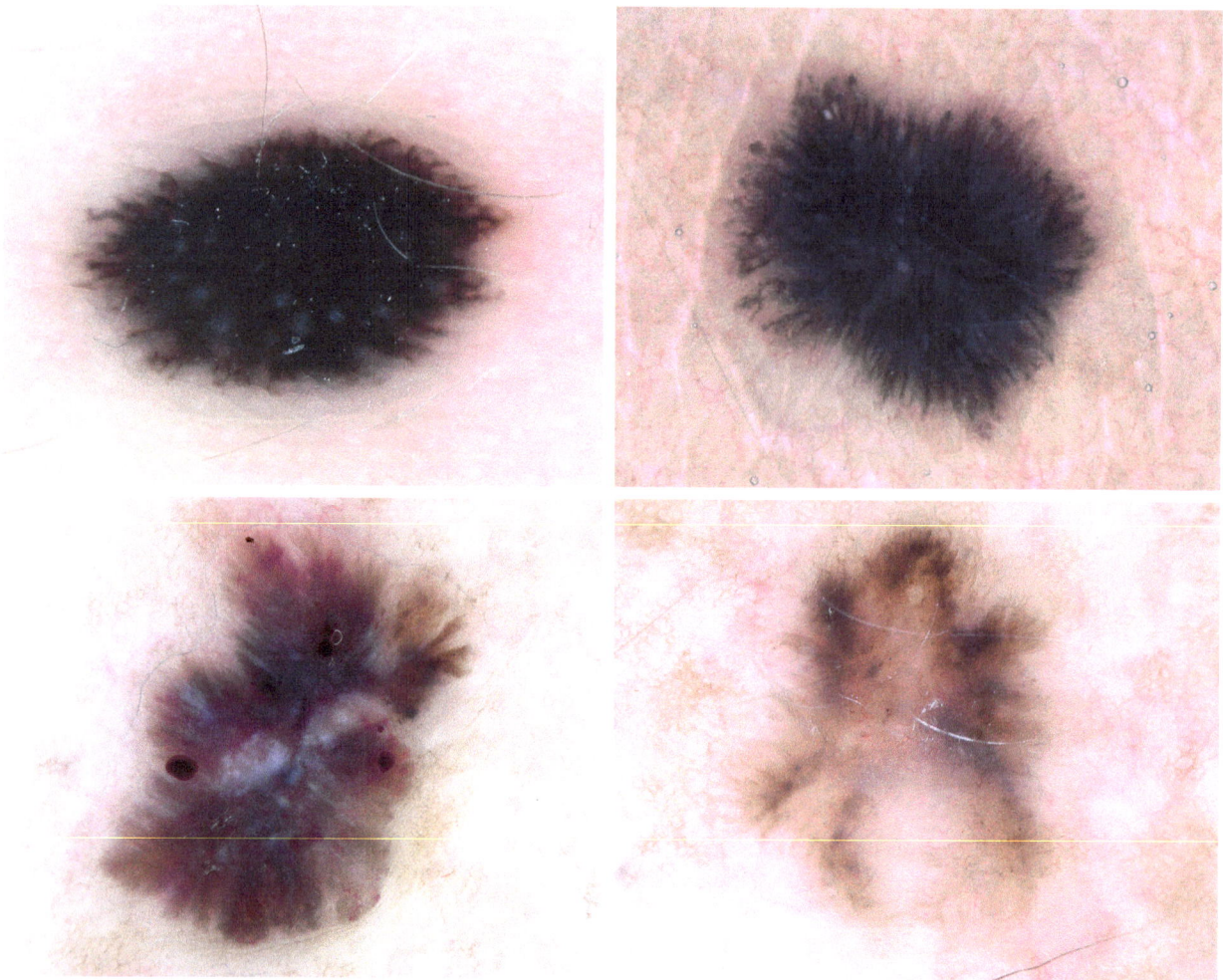

Figure 5.53: *More than one pattern, radial lines at the periphery.*
Top: *Radial lines at the periphery, distributed over the entire circumference, are typical of Reed nevi.* **Bottom:** *The peripheral radial lines are not regularly distributed over the entire circumference, but are present only in some segments. This is an asymmetrical combination of patterns. This pattern is seen in basal cell carcinoma and melanoma. The absence of reticular lines, a few blue clods* **(left)** *and serpentine vessels* **(right)** *are more indicative of basal cell carcinoma than melanoma. Histopathology confirmed basal cell carcinoma in both cases.*

and radial lines are considered equivalent. In practice, radial lines peripherally are found in combination with only two different patterns in the center; clods and structureless. When the center is structureless and white, the lesion is usually a dermatofibroma. When the center is structureless and brown, black or gray, the lesion is usually a Reed nevus *(5.53, top row)*. In the latter case one may find brown or gray clods instead of the structureless center.

Asymmetry is necessarily created when peripheral radial lines do not occupy the entire circumference of a lesion but are present only in some segments. The primary differential diagnosis is then melanoma versus basal cell carcinoma *(5.53 bottom row)*. The distinction

between these diagnoses is made on the basis of clues. Two arrangements of radial lines are strong clues to basal cell carcinoma. Peripheral radial lines in basal cell carcinoma usually have a common base, which is not usually the case in melanoma. Also, in basal cell carcinoma, radial lines are not only seen at the periphery, as in melanoma, but also within the lesion. In this case the radial lines do not just converge at the center but do so at a dot or a clod. These structures are usually multiple, and are possibly the most specific clue in dermatoscopy. Another feature often seen in basal cell carcinoma but only rarely in melanoma is radial lines extending from a hypopigmented structureless area *(5.53 bottom right)*. Usually in melanoma radial

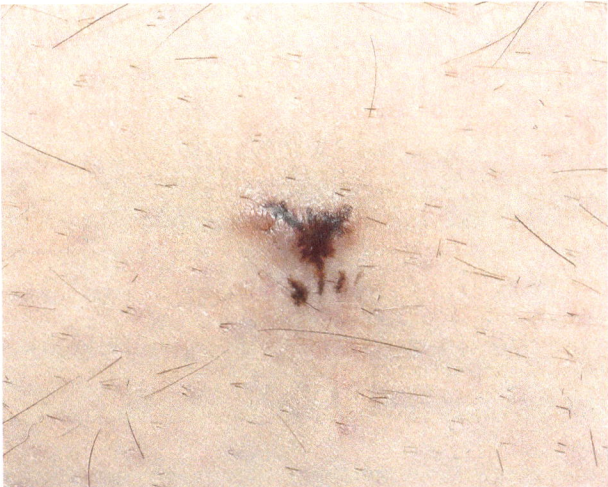

Figure 5.54: Recurrent nevus with radial lines.
Radial lines at the periphery of a recurrent nevus.

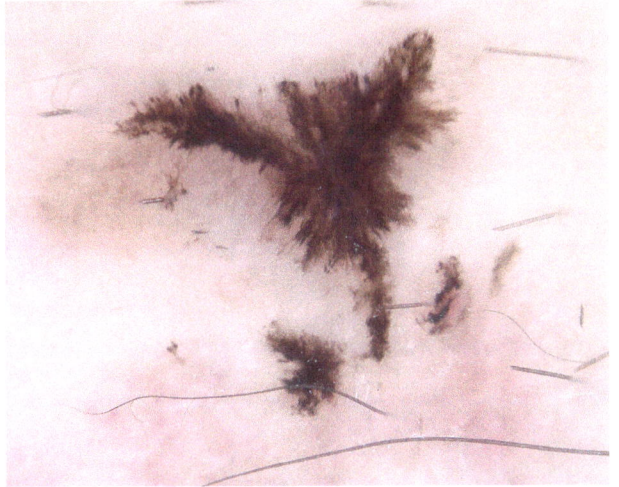

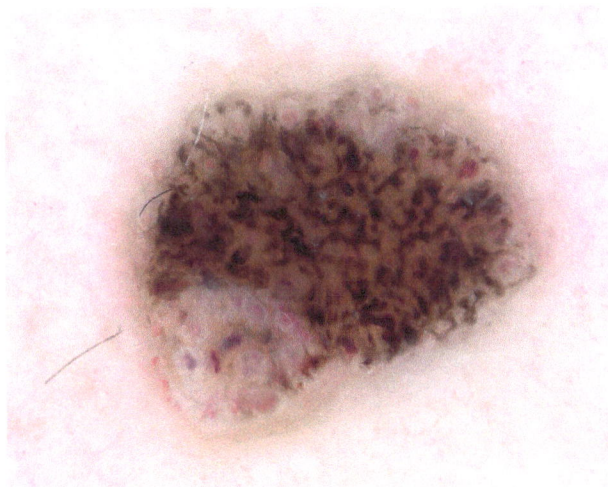

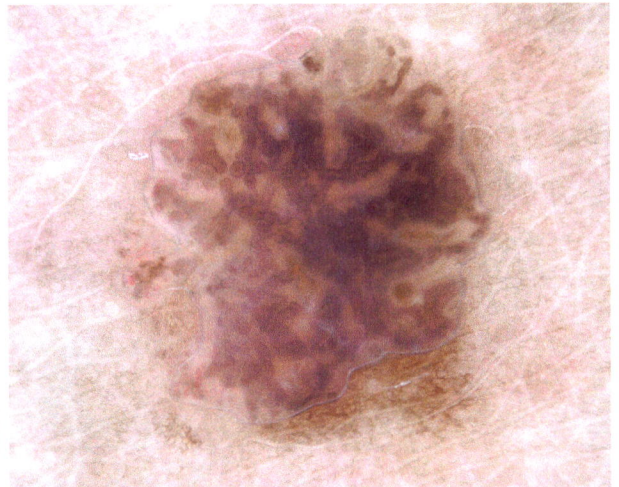

*Figure 5.55: **More than one pattern, curved lines.***
Left: *Curved lines and skin-colored clods in a seborrheic keratosis. A few brown and red clods do not rule out this diagnosis.* **Right:** *Curved lines arranged as parallel pairs, and circles in a seborrheic keratosis. The small zone with reticular lines at the lower margin does not exclude this diagnosis.*

lines or pseudopods extend from pigmented reticular lines or from pigmented areas just as darkly pigmented as the radial lines/pseudopods.

Radial lines or pseudopods can also be seen in recurrent nevi *(5.54)*. As a rule radial lines in recurrent nevi are arranged asymmetrically. They cover the entire circumference only rarely. As a general rule the pigmentation in recurrent nevi does not extend beyond the scar. The radial lines that are occasionally seen in pigmented Bowen's disease are usually composed of brown or gray dots or coiled vessels in linear arrangement (14).

Curved lines

Once all other patterns of lines have been excluded, only curved lines remain. The pattern of curved lines is the least specific and therefore the last assessed of the patterns formed by lines. A combination of patterns that includes curved lines is almost always asymmetrical. When the color is only brown, the most likely diagnosis is solar lentigo or seborrheic keratosis *(5.55)*. However, when any of the other colors of melanin (gray, blue or black) are present, melanoma must be ruled out before diagnosing either seborrheic keratosis or lichen planus-like keratosis.

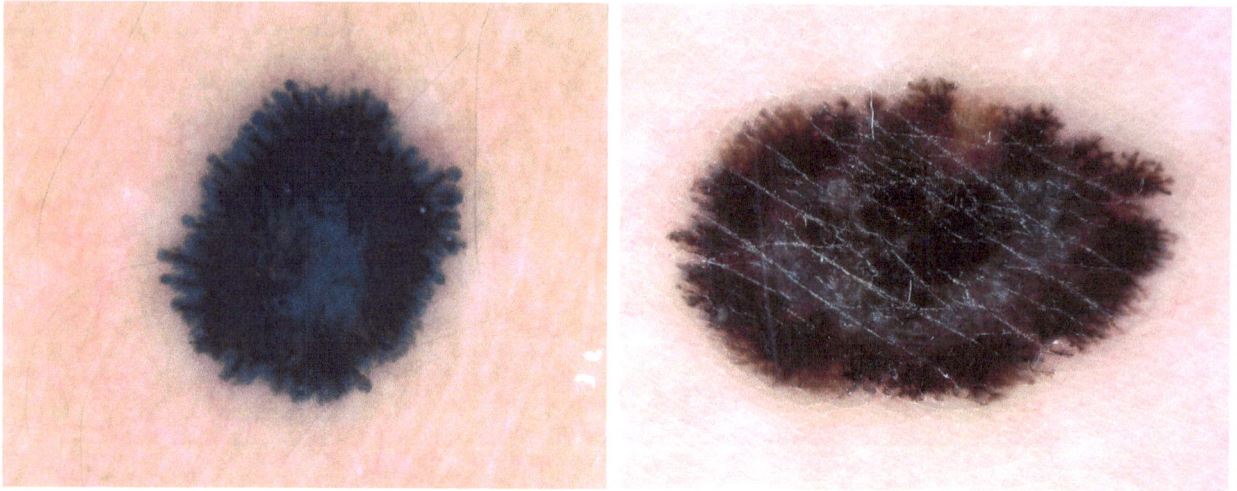

Figure 5.56: More than one pattern, pseudopods.
Left: *More than one pattern, pseudopods peripherally and structureless in the center, arranged symmetrically, add up to the diagnosis of Reed nevus.* **Right:** *More than one pattern, pseudopods peripherally (in some segments only) and structureless in the center, arranged asymmetrically, yield the diagnosis of melanoma.*

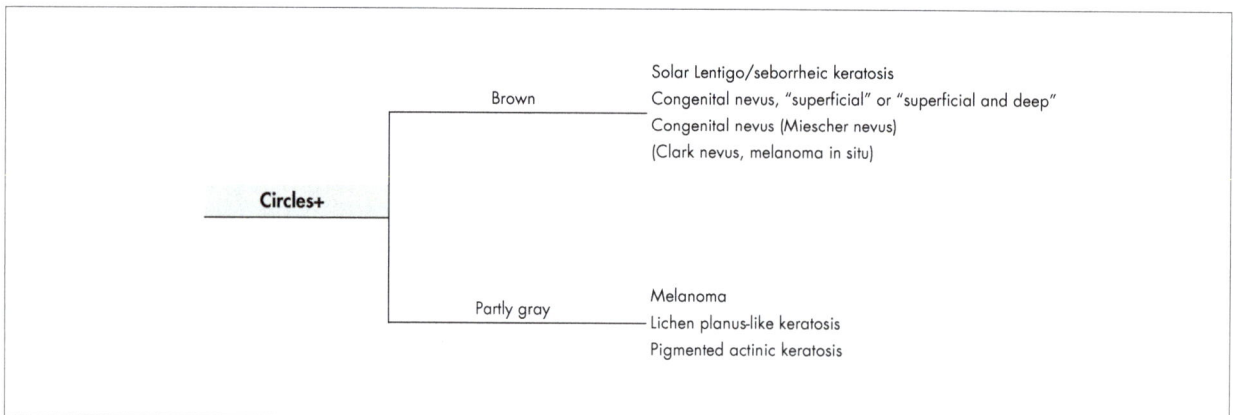

Figure 5.57: Continuation of the algorithm: more than one pattern, circles

5.2.2 Pseudopods

Pseudopods, like radial lines, are only seen in combination with another pattern. The only arrangement seen is with the pseudopods at the periphery and the other pattern in the center of the lesion. The pattern in the center is usually structureless, occasionally clods, and least often reticular lines. The distribution of the pseudopods at the periphery is far more important than the type of pattern in the center. Once again, when assessing symmetry, pseudopods and radial lines are considered equivalent. When the pseudopods are regularly distributed over the entire circumference (symmetrically) the lesion usually is a Reed nevus *(5.56 left)*. However, when the pseudopods are only present in some segments of the periphery (asymmetrically), the diagnosis of melanoma must be considered *(5.56 right)*.

Recurrent nevi sometimes have pseudopods at the periphery but usually they can be diagnosed easily based on the history and the presence of a scar (17, 18). When diagnosing lesions with pseudopods, variables other than dermatoscopy must be considered. Factors such as the patient's age, skin type, number of nevi, their distribution and clinical appearance, and history of change, are all relevant to the diagnosis. While these factors may influence the diagnosis, they should not influence the dermatoscopic description. In other words, the same dermatoscopic pattern may lead to different conclusions in different situations. When one finds a pattern of pseudopods in a child, the diagnosis is almost certainly Reed nevus, regardless of whether the pattern is symmetrical or asymmetrical. In an adult, on the other hand, the diagnostician would be inclined to

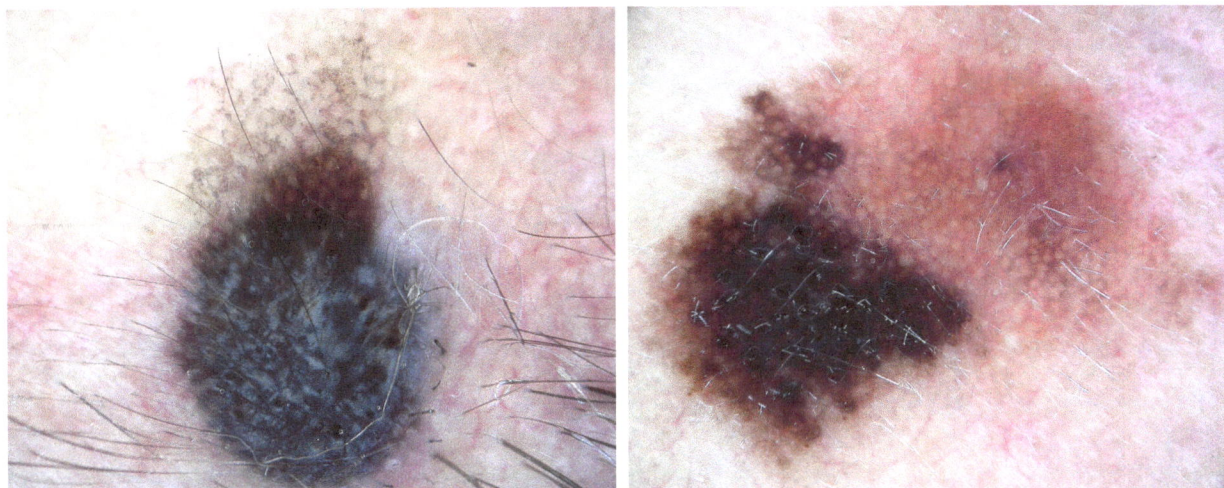

Figure 5.58: More than one pattern, circles.
Melanomas on the face frequently show a combination of gray circles (or dots arranged in circles) and another pattern – in this case structureless. The structureless portion constitutes the invasive part of both melanomas (Breslow thickness > 1 mm). In both of these lesions, circles are visible in the thin areas of the tumor, but moving towards the thicker parts of the lesion, the circles first merge with adjacent circles and the pattern becomes structureless.

favor melanoma and would be inclined to submit even symmetrical lesions for histopathology. There is nothing wrong with this, provided factors such as age do not influence the process of formulating a dermatoscopic description; there is ample opportunity to take these factors into account later in the diagnostic process. Our eyes are quite easily tempted and misled to see what we want to see, and preconceptions increase the chance that such errors of perception will occur.

Objectivity and independence from extraneous influences are essential aspects of pattern analysis. While this must be strictly applied in formulating descriptions, there is leeway in weighing the clues afterwards, such as described above for the assessment of pseudopods. Another example would be weighing the significance of gray dots as a clue to melanoma, which is of much greater significance in lesions on the face than at other locations on the body. This flexibility in weighing the clues is responsible for much of the power of pattern analysis, and learning the judicious application of this flexibility is one of the major roles of experience in dermatoscopy. On the other hand, this flexibility can generate difficulties for beginners, so in general beginners should be more strict than experts in their application of pattern analysis. Flexibility in weighing clues does not mean that one may twist and turn all of one's observations until one reaches the diagnosis formed in the first second. The art lies in knowing how far one can go in the process of interpretation, and then stopping.

5.2.3 Circles

Once lines and pseudopods have been excluded, the pattern of circles is the next most specific pattern. The pattern of circles is the typical pattern of facial skin, but it may be found at any location. Sometimes it may be difficult to distinguish between a pattern of closely adjacent circles and reticular lines; in fact, the two patterns are often seen together, both on the face (reticular lines may be seen on the face) and elsewhere. When these patterns co-exist, the lesion should be analyzed by reticular lines, the more specific pattern. The only common symmetrical combination of circles with another pattern is that of peripheral brown circles combined with a structureless zone (or less often white lines) centrally, seen in dermatofibroma. Other combinations that include the pattern of circles but no lines are nearly all asymmetrical, so the color of the circles becomes more important than assessment of symmetry. If the color is only brown, one must consider a solar lentigo or a seborrheic keratosis on the one hand, and a "superficial" or "superficial and deep" congenital nevus or a Clark nevus on the other. Occasionally a Miescher nevus may also have brown circles. If any of the circles are gray, the differential diagnosis includes melanoma *(5.57, 5.58)*, lichen planus-like keratosis and, especially on facial skin pigmented actinic keratosis. Occasionally facial melanomas will present with brown circles, without any grey color. This means that melanoma is always in the differential diagnosis of pigmented circles on the face, regardless of their color (8).

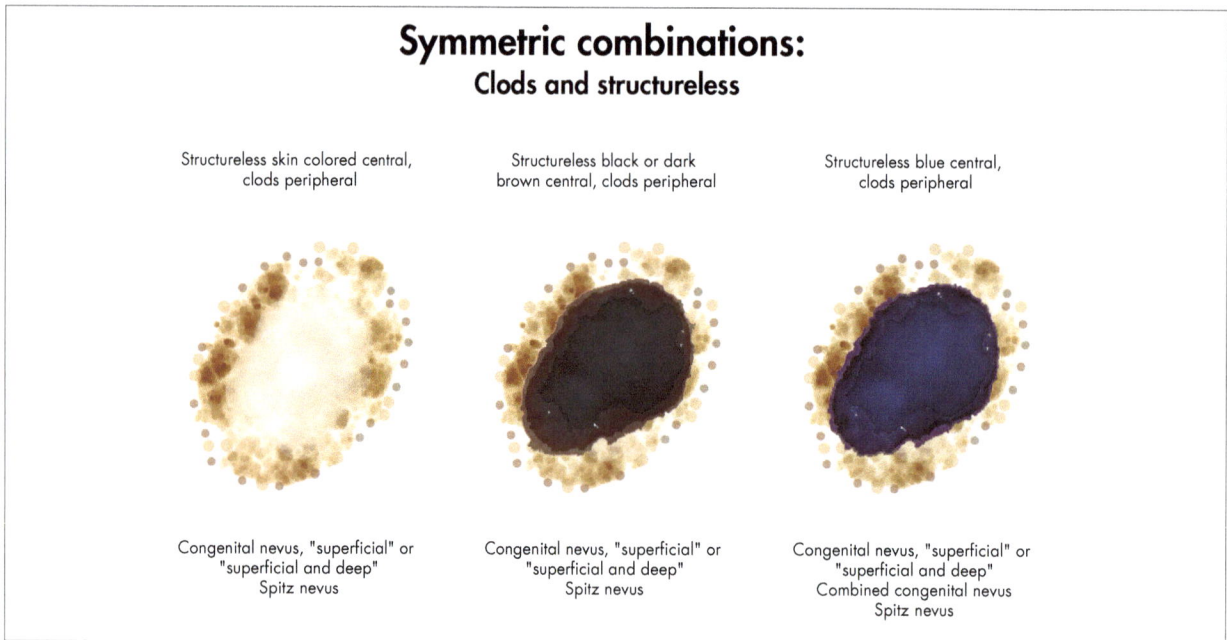

Figure 5.59: *More than one pattern, clods, symmetrical combination*

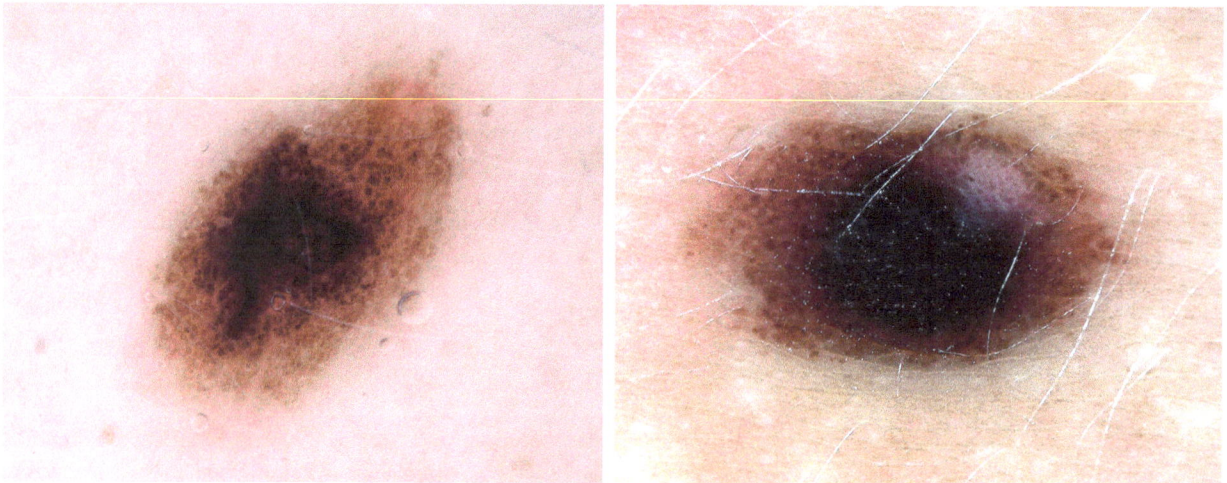

Figure 5.60: *Symmetrical combinations with clods.*
Left: *Structureless dark-brown in the center and brown clods at the periphery, in a "superficial and deep" congenital nevus.* **Right:** *Structureless blue in the center and brown clods at the periphery, in a combined congenital nevus.*

5.2.4 Clods

The next pattern in order is clods. Because lesions to be analyzed by the pattern of clods lack lines, pseudopods and circles (otherwise the lesion would be analyzed by these more specific patterns), the only combinations to be considered are clods plus dots and clods plus structureless. Clods and structureless may be combined with each other symmetrically or asymmetrically. In cases of a symmetrical combination the structureless zone is in the center of the lesion while the clods (which are usually brown) are seen at the periphery (5.59).

When the center is skin-colored the lesion is most probably a "superficial and deep" congenital nevus, more rarely a Spitz nevus. When the structureless center is brown or black, the diagnostician should first consider a growing "superficial and deep" congenital nevus (commonly in children) or a pigmented Spitz

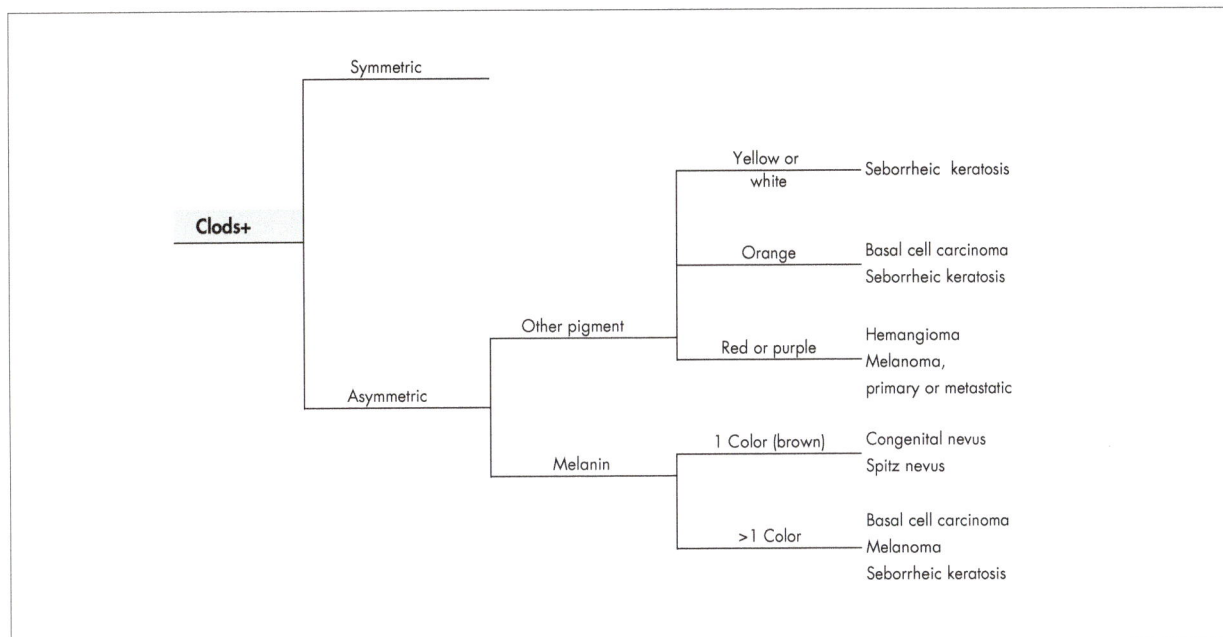

Figure 5.61: *Continuation of the algorithm for more than one pattern, clods, asymmetrical*

nevus. In cases of a blue structureless center, the first entity to be considered is a combined congenital nevus *(5.60 right)*.

Asymmetrical combinations of patterns containing clods but no lines, pseudopods or circles are analyzed differently depending on whether the colors are predominantly those of melanin, or those of another pigment *(5.61)*.

Lesions pigmented by melanin are predominantly black, brown, gray or blue. Black pigmentation can be caused by coagulated blood as well as melanin, so the interpretation of the color black depends on what other colors are present. When the colors brown, blue or gray are predominant in the remainder of the lesion, the color black is best interpreted as melanin in the stratum corneum. However, when red or purple is predominant, the color black is best interpreted as coagulated blood.

Lesions with no pigment, or with pigments other than melanin predominant, are assessed based on the color of the clods, and not on the color of the rest of the lesion. A predominance of white or yellow clods is indicative of a seborrheic keratosis. Orange clods in large numbers also indicate a seborrheic keratosis but when only a very few are present, basal cell carcinoma must also be considered. The orange clods of basal cell carcinoma are simply serum crusts arising from erosion or ulceration, so red inclusions (representing blood) within the clods are common. As serum crusts are sticky, fibers of clothing may become adherent to them and serve as an indirect sign of ulceration. Red or purple clods usually indicate a hemangioma or a vascular malformation, but may also signify a melanoma or metastasis of melanoma when occurring in combination with another pattern. In particular, hemangioma should not be diagnosed when vessels as lines or dots are seen within the red clods.

When melanin is the predominant pigment, the color of the whole lesion is assessed, and not just the clods. When the lesion is one color, brown, the diagnostician should consider a "superficial and deep" congenital nevus or a Spitz nevus. When other colors are also present the diagnostician should consider a basal cell carcinoma or a melanoma in addition to a seborrheic keratosis and its variants *(5.62)*. The distinction between these three differential diagnoses is made, as mentioned earlier, on the basis of additional clues.

5.2.5 Dots

When all other patterns have been excluded, only dots remain *(5.63)*. In the algorithm we are currently in the category of "more than one pattern". Thus, all lesions that now follow consist of dots and a structureless zone. As structureless is the least specific pattern, the diagnostic process is mainly based on the color of dots, meaning that the algorithm for "dots and structureless" differs only slightly from the algorithm for "dots".

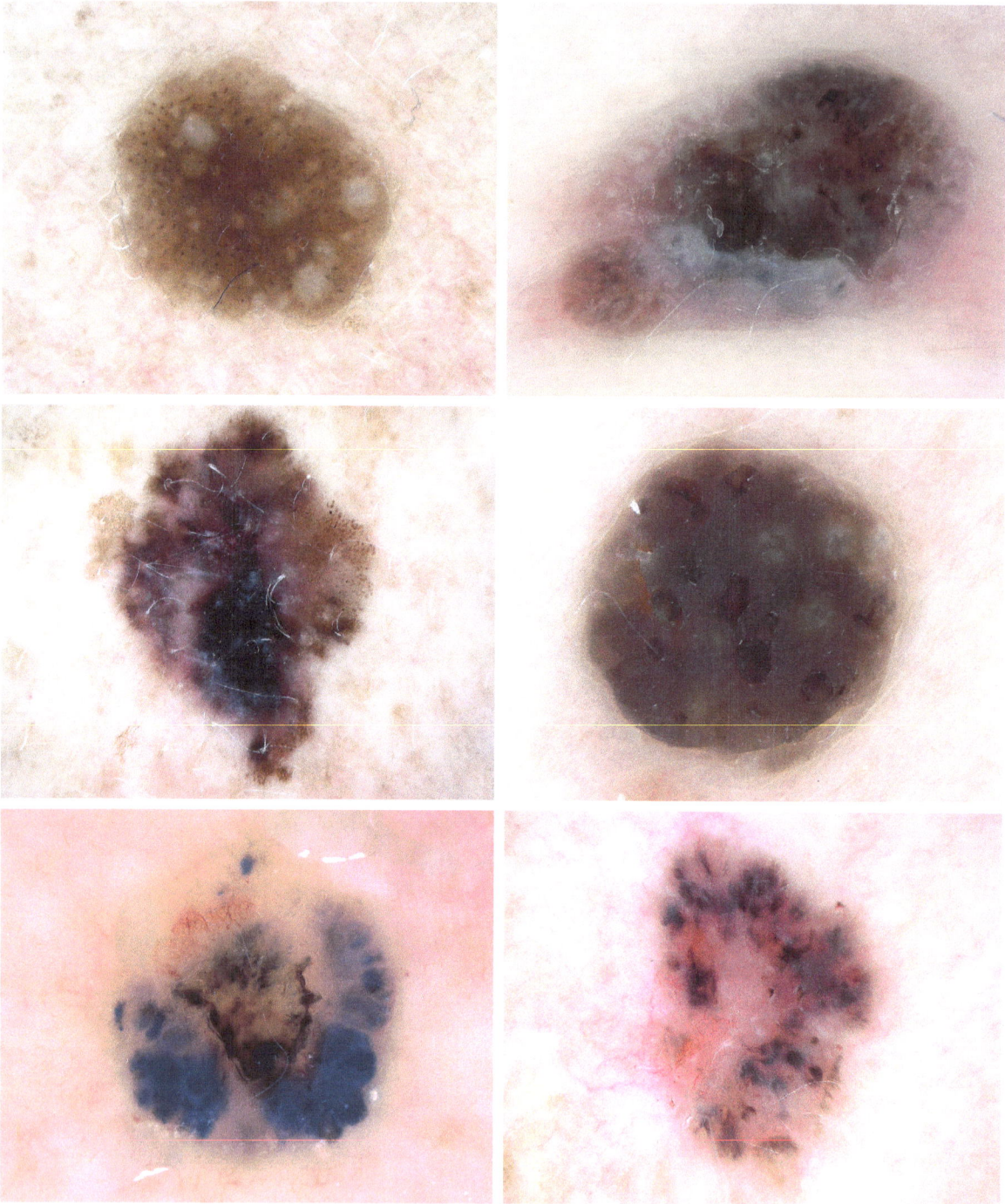

Figure 5.62: *More than one pattern, clods, asymmetrical.*
Top left: *More than one pattern, clods and dots; the clods are white and yellow – seborrheic keratosis.* **Top right:** *More than one pattern, clods and structureless, more than one color (brown, blue and gray). Of the three differential diagnoses (basal cell carcinoma, seborrheic keratosis, melanoma) this lesion is most likely a melanoma. Histopathological diagnosis: Melanoma (> 1 mm).* **Middle left:** *More than one pattern, clods and structureless, more than one color (brown, blue and gray). Of the three differential diagnoses (basal cell carcinoma, seborrheic keratosis, melanoma), this lesion is most likely a melanoma. Histopathological diagnosis: Melanoma (< 1 mm).* **Middle right:** *More than one pattern, clods and structureless, more than one color (light-brown, dark-brown). Of the three differential diagnoses (basal cell carcinoma, seborrheic keratosis, melanoma), the most likely diagnosis is seborrheic keratosis – due to the white and yellow clods. Histopathological diagnosis: Seborrheic keratosis.* **Bottom left and right:** *More than one pattern, clods and structureless, more than one color (melanin). Of the three differential diagnoses (basal cell carcinoma, seborrheic keratosis, melanoma), the most likely diagnosis is basal cell carcinoma because of the blue clods, the serpentine vessels and solitary orange clod (left). Histopathological diagnosis: Two basal cell carcinomas.*

Stepwise procedure

- 1. Gray dots
  - Lichen planus-like keratosis
  - Pigmented actinic keratosis
  - Pigmented Bowen's disease
  - Melanoma, regressive
  - Basal cell carcinoma
- 2. Blue dots
  - Basal cell carcinoma
- 3. Black dots
  - Melanoma
  - Clark nevus
- 4. Brown dots
  - Clark nevus
  - Congenital nevus
  - Solar lentigo
  - Pigmented Bowen's disease

Dots+

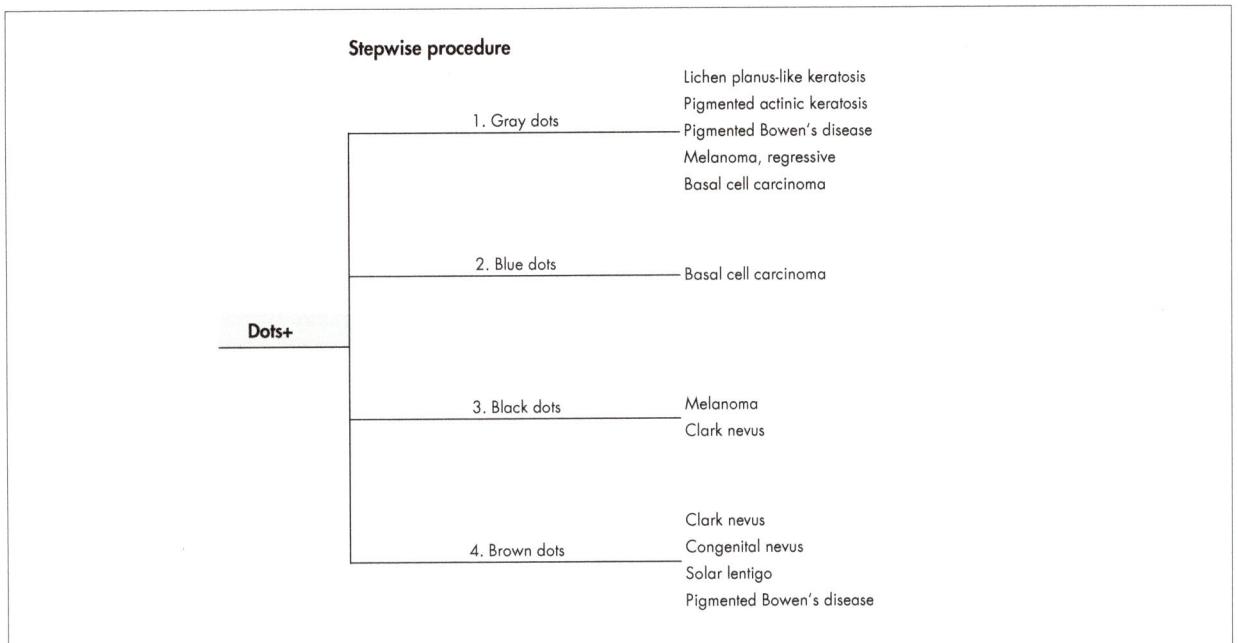

Figure 5.63: Continuation of the algorithm for more than one pattern, dots

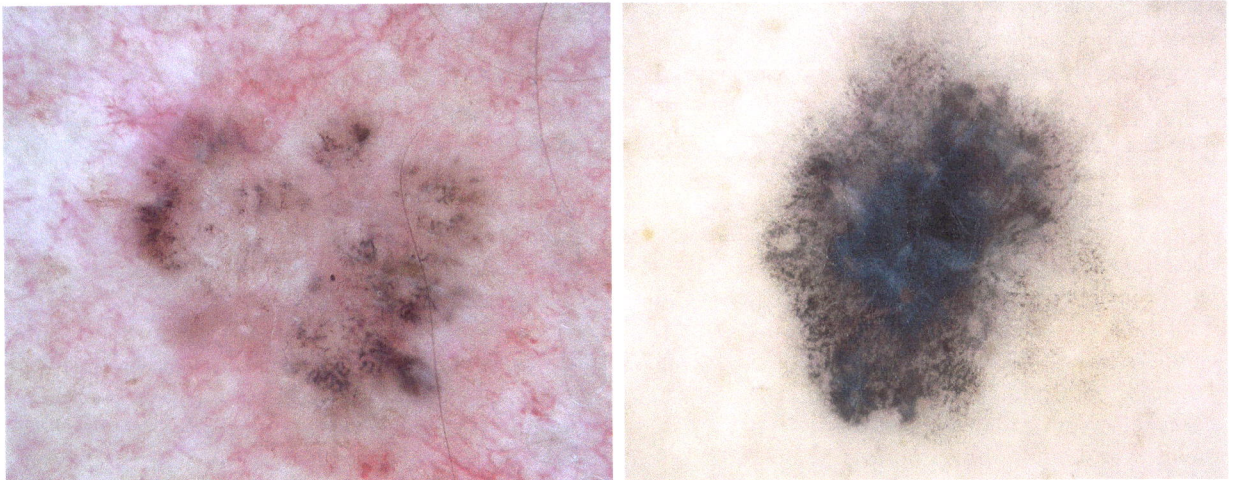

Figure 5.64: More than one pattern, dots.
Left: *More than one pattern, dots and structureless. The dots are gray and blue. Of the possible differential diagnoses, this lesion is most likely a basal cell carcinoma because of its serpentine vessels. Histopathological diagnosis: Basal cell carcinoma.* **Right:** *More than one pattern, dots and structureless: The dots are gray. Of the possible differential diagnoses, this lesion is most likely a melanoma. Histopathological diagnosis: Melanoma with signs of regression.*

Gray dots may signify a melanoma *(5.64 right)*, a lichen planus-like keratosis, a pigmented superficial squamous cell carcinoma (actinic keratosis or Bowen's disease) or a basal cell carcinoma. Of these differential diagnoses, the basal cell carcinoma can be differentiated most easily from the others on the basis of additional clues. Blue dots are quite specific for basal cell carcinoma *(5.64 left)*. Usually there also will be additional clues to support this diagnosis. Black dots are uncommon but should cause the investigator to think of melanoma, and prompt a search for other clues to this diagnosis. Brown dots are found in solar lentigo and pigmented Bowen's disease. Very rarely a Clark nevus may have just brown dots and a structureless area. The distinction between solar lentigo and pigmented Bowen's disease can be made quite easily when the pattern is brown dots plus structureless. In pigmented Bowen's disease, the dots are usually arranged as lines. These lines are often radial, and may include coiled vessels. Coiled vessels are also common in the structureless zone.

5.3 Applying pattern analysis to clinical practice

The basics of pattern analysis are easy to learn, but its application is sometimes complex and needs experience. Gaining experience requires time and the opportunity to work regularly with dermatoscopy; i.e. regular use in one's medical practice. The spectrum of pigmented skin lesions is not very large yet to personally examine the full gamut of pigmented lesions of the skin, including rare diagnoses and unusual appearances of common diagnoses, takes some time even at specialized centers, and proportionately longer in small practices. Fortunately, seeing photographs of unusual or rare lesions in dermatoscopy atlases or on various internet websites can speed up this process. Familiarity with the spectrum of common diagnoses is at least as important as knowing about rare diagnoses. It is absolutely essential to be aware of the morphological spectrum of the Clark nevus and the seborrheic keratosis. This knowledge is best acquired by first-hand experience gained in the course of regular – ideally everyday – application of dermatoscopy to one's own patients. The use of the algorithmic method will become quite natural over time.

The algorithm need not be learned by heart, but it must be explored. After all, one of the roles of experience is to discover one's own pathway while traversing the road to expertise. With time, experts become so familiar with the pathway that they do not require a map, appearing to arrive at their goal blind – i.e. without an algorithm. In actual fact they make decisions so rapidly that it can appear that they follow no method other than their own intuition. This illusion is so strong that some experts do actually believe in their own intuition. The disadvantage of intuitive diagnosis is that the method cannot be taught. A method that cannot be taught is barely a method at all. Beginners should beware of intuitive diagnoses: without experience they are frequently incorrect.

5.4 Chaos and Clues

No diagnostic system will detect every pigmented skin malignancy. Melanomas, pigmented basal cell carcinomas, and pigmented squamous cell carcinomas including pigmented Bowen's disease, must all start as minute lesions at which time dermatoscopic features of malignancy may not be recognizable. Unlike benign lesions, however, malignant lesions will grow continuously, and with increasing size clues to malignancy can be expected to become visible to the dermatoscopist.

Several diagnostic methods have been developed for pigmented skin lesions based on dermatoscopic analysis. Classical pattern analysis was the original method published by Pehamberger, Steiner and Wolff in 1987 (19) and it is still widely used by experienced dermatoscopists. The method we present in this book is nothing but pattern analysis presented using an objective, geometric language and with a clear, stepwise path to generate descriptions and reach a diagnosis. Not every clinician has the time or the desire to become an expert in dermatoscopy. Many simply wish to have uncomplicated and easily assimilated guidelines for daily use. The ABCD rule was designed specifically for melanocytic lesions for the detection of melanomas (20). The 7-point checklist (21), Menzies' method (22), and the CASH algorithm (23) involve a 2-step process where the first step attempts to determine whether a lesion is melanocytic before an algorithm is applied to determine whether it should be biopsied to exclude melanoma. Finally, the 3-point checklist was developed in 2000 to detect pigmented malignancy (24).

These algorithms may be easy to learn but, with the exception of Menzies' method, they are not easy to apply. No one actually calculates scores for all lesions assessed, because it takes too long to fit into normal clinical routine.

In structure, Menzies' method can be seen to be a simplified version of the algorithms of pattern analysis as it assesses in sequence pattern, color and clues. Unlike pattern analysis, Menzies' method is limited to melanocytic lesions.

Fortunately, simple and easily learned rules of thumb based on pattern analysis can be formulated, that fulfill the demand for a rapid and uncomplicated algorithm, but without this restriction to melanocytic lesions. We now present one such method.

"Chaos and Clues" is designed to be applied to any pigmented skin lesion (25) to detect any type of malignancy and to achieve this rapidly in the setting of a busy practice (26). In essence lesions are examined

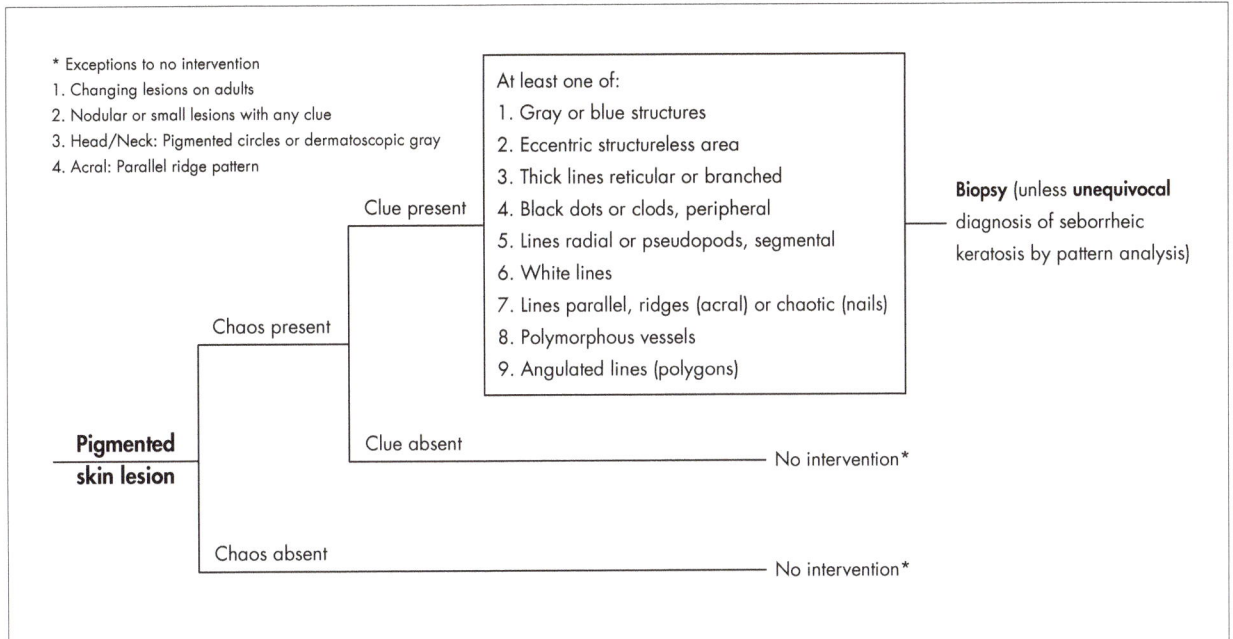

Figure 5.65: "Chaos and Clues" algorithm.
If a pigmented skin lesion exhibits dermatoscopic chaos it is carefully examined for one of nine clues to malignancy and if a clue is discovered the lesion is carefully considered for excision biopsy. The clue of gray structures is present in most malignancies but is the least specific clue. An additional clue increases specificity for malignancy. The four exceptions listed are situations in which non-chaotic lesions should be carefully assessed.

clinically and dermatoscopically for chaos (defined as asymmetry of pattern or color) and only when this is discovered does the clinician pause to search for one of nine clues to malignancy. If there are both chaos and at least one clue to malignancy then (excision) biopsy is indicated *(5.65)*. Lesion descriptions in the chaos and clues algorithm are formulated using the same method and language as for pattern analysis. "Chaos and Clues" is designed to detect malignancy rather than to make a specific diagnosis. In other words, it guides the clinician in the decision whether or not to submit a lesion for histopathology. We do not believe that attempting to determine melanocytic status is a useful part of this process (2).
Sometimes this may be obvious but we believe this is rightly the domain of the pathologist, who is actually able to see melanocytes. The exact diagnosis is also left to the pathologist. Of course, with increasing experience and expertise, the clinician may attempt to reach a specific diagnosis by applying pattern analysis.
Unlike previously proposed "simplified" algorithms, "Chaos and Clues" has been evaluated in the normal clinical situation which requires the detection of all pigmented malignancies and not just melanoma. This

study was based on 463 consecutive pigmented skin lesions from a primary care skin cancer practice (25). This included 29 melanomas (20 in situ), 72 pigmented basal cell carcinomas and 37 pigmented squamous cell carcinomas (including pigmented Bowen's disease and pigmented actinic keratosis). Diagnostic sensitivity was 90.6 % and specificity was 62.7 % for the diagnosis of malignancy and significantly better than with the unaided eye. The specificity increased to 77 % when solar lentigines/seborrheic keratoses were diagnosed by pattern analysis.

Chaos
Chaos is defined as asymmetry of pattern and/or color within a lesion, the shape of a lesion is not relevant *(5.66)*. By definition a lesion with one pattern and one color, regardless of its shape, is symmetrical and therefore does not exhibit chaos. If any line drawn through the center of a lesion has different colors or patterns on opposite sides it is asymmetrical and exhibits chaos. Any color other than skin color at the edge of a lesion (such as white) should be regarded as part of the lesion.
Lesions without chaos, subject to four exceptions, are not analyzed any further.

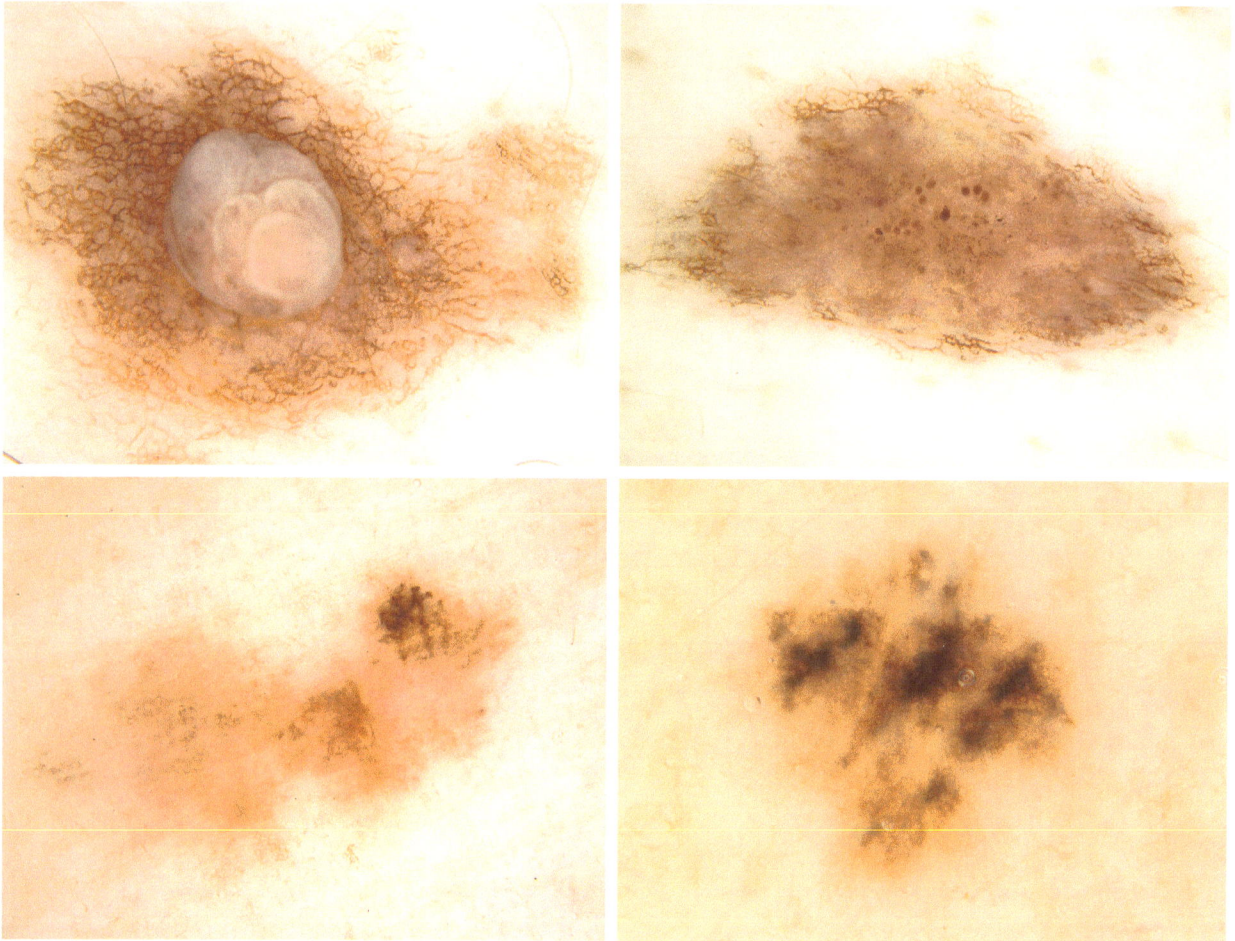

Figure 5.66: Chaos as a screening tool.
Dermatoscopic images of four lesions on the same patient taken on the same day. Lesions in the top row are symmetrical with respect to both color and structure. The lesion in the bottom row on the right is also symmetrical when the shape of the lesion is disregarded. The lesion in the bottom row on the left exhibits asymmetry both with respect to pattern and color (although only one of these variables needs to be asymmetrical to constitute chaos). Excision biopsy confirmed it to be a melanoma in situ.

While natural laws such as gravity, surface tension, electromagnetic forces and biological feedback mechanisms favor symmetry, malignant tissue tends to not be restrained by feedback mechanisms and this is a plausible explanation for dermatopathologic and therefore dermatoscopic chaos.

While natural laws do favor symmetry it is very rare to find perfect symmetry in nature, and so judgement is required in deciding whether deviations from geometrically perfect symmetry fall within normal biological variation. It can be useful when assessing equivocal chaos to consider whether what is observed is consistent with the chaotic behavior of malignant tissue. If a decision cannot be made the lesion should be assessed as exhibiting chaos and fully assessed. There are four exceptions where a lesion without chaos

should be assessed further. These include changing lesions on adults, nodular or small lesions with any clue, dermatoscopic pigmented circles or gray structures on the head or neck and a parallel ridge pattern on palms or soles. The beginning dermatoscopist can reasonably be expected to assess more lesions as asymmetrical than experts. By refining this judgement with accumulated experience, one reduces the number of lesions requiring full assessment.

Clues to Malignancy
In pattern analysis, a clue is a feature which favors one diagnosis over another, when analysis of patterns and colors has not led to a specific diagnosis. In the chaos and clues algorithm, a clue is simply a feature which, when present, indicates that a lesion

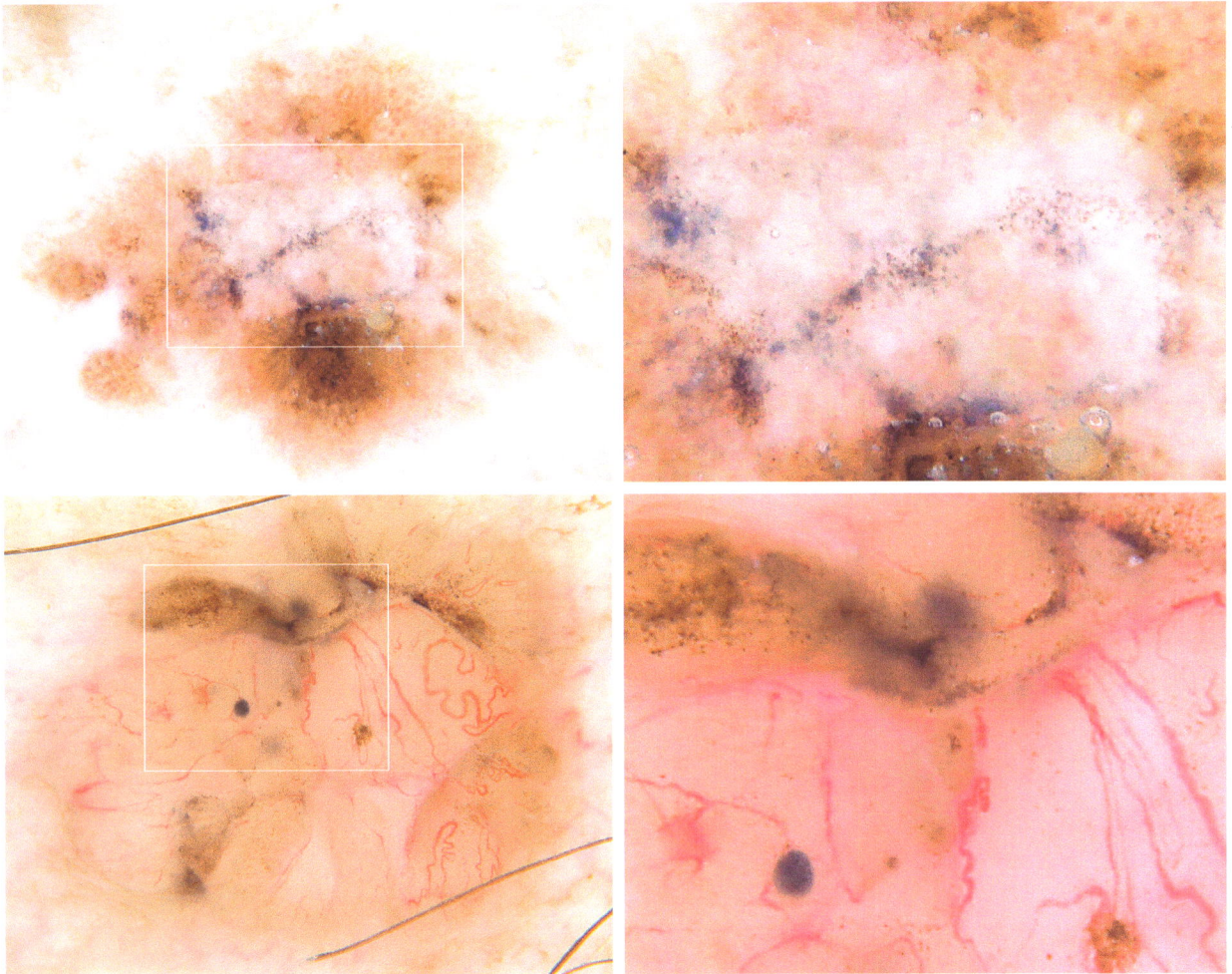

Figure 5.67: Gray structures as a clue to malignancy.
*Dermatoscopic images of a pigmented Bowen's disease (**top row**) and a basal cell carcinoma (**bottom row**). The overview is shown on the left and the detail on the **right**. Both lesions exhibit a high degree of chaos with gray dots (Bowen's disease) and gray clods and dots (basal cell carcinoma).*

requires a biopsy to exclude malignancy. One clue is sufficient. Both chaos and clue can be produced by the same feature.

Because some clues depend on the colors gray, blue and white it is important to recognize that the type of dermatoscope used can influence the way these colors are observed. As a general rule, gray and blue structures in all skin lesions and the white dots and clods in seborrheic keratoses are seen more vividly with non-polarized light. Certain white structures are only seen when using polarized light. Polarizing-specific white lines — bright white lines at right angles to each other (but not crossing each other) — can be seen in certain lesions, most notably melanomas, Spitz nevi, basal cell carcinomas and dermatofibromas. These structures vary in intensity as the dermatoscope is rotated. Both types of light are suitable for dermatoscopy, but the dermatoscopist should be aware of the different information each can give. Unless otherwise specified, dermatoscopic images in this chapter were taken with non-polarized dermatoscopes.

The Nine Clues

1. Gray or blue structures (*dots, clods, circles, or lines, 5.67*):
   Gray dots may be seen in pigmented basal cell carcinoma, in pigmented Bowen's disease or pigmented actinic keratosis, as well as in melanoma. Gray circles occur in facial in situ melanomas. Dense deposition of melanin in the dermis causes blue clods in pigmented basal cell carcinomas and invasive melanomas. Gray lines occur in melanomas.

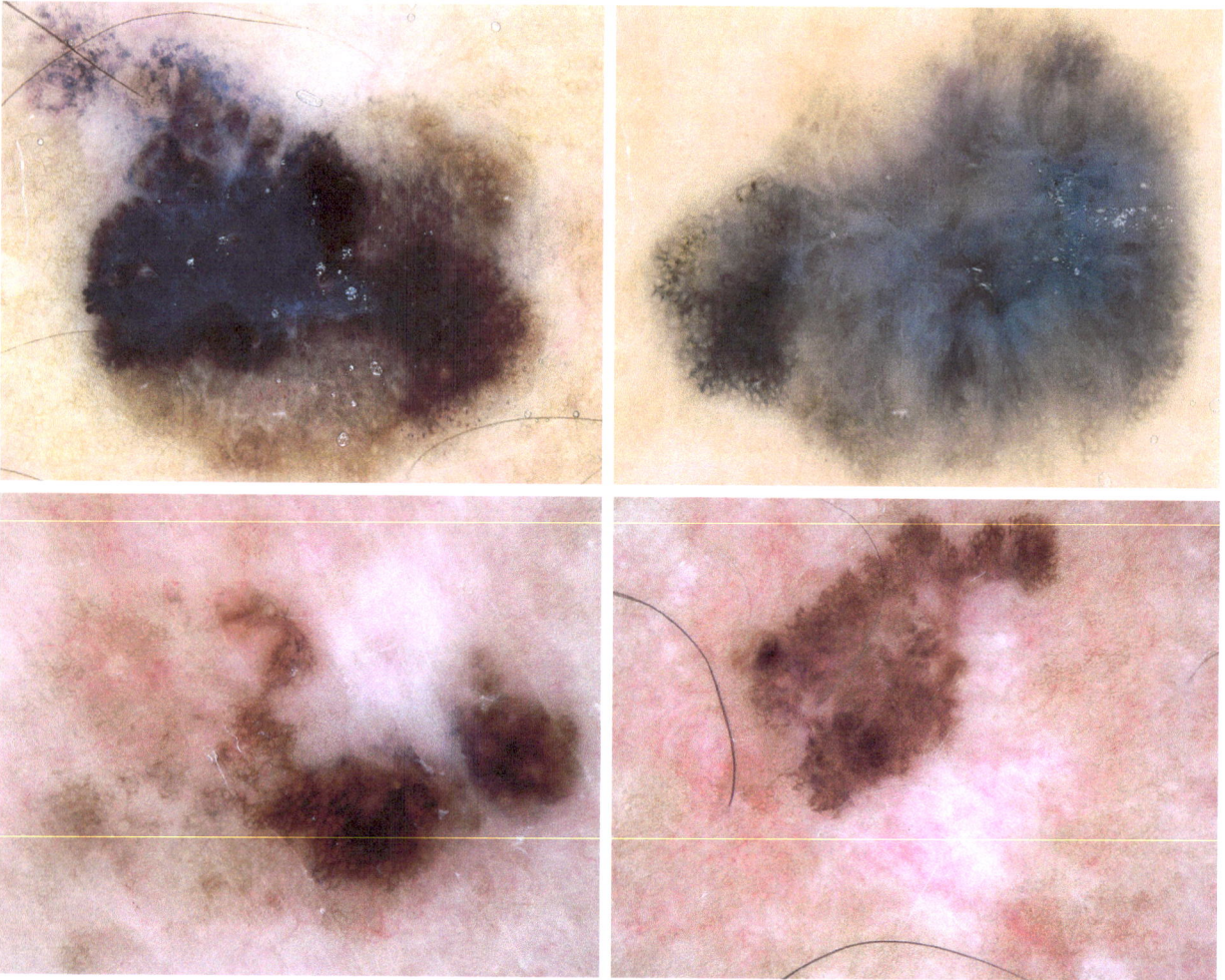

Figure 5.68: *Eccentric structureless area as a clue to malignancy.*
*Dermatoscopic images of 4 melanomas. All are chaotic, with an eccentric structureless area. These eccentric structureless areas are variously black (**top left**), blue (**top right**), or white (**bottom left and right**).*

2. Eccentric structureless area *(any color except skin color, 5.68)*:
    This may be any of the colors of melanin (black, brown, gray, or blue), white, (if pigment is lacking but fibrosis or sclerosis is present), or pink (if pigment is lacking but hyperemia is present). Eccentric blue or black structureless areas are frequently seen in melanomas and occasionally in basal cell carcinoma, but are not expected in squamous cell carcinoma in-situ. Eccentric structureless brown, white and pink can occur in all pigmented malignancies. To rate as a clue the structureless area must not be skin colored, it must be eccentric, it must cover a sufficient area to rate as a pattern and it must exist in contrast to a structured pattern.

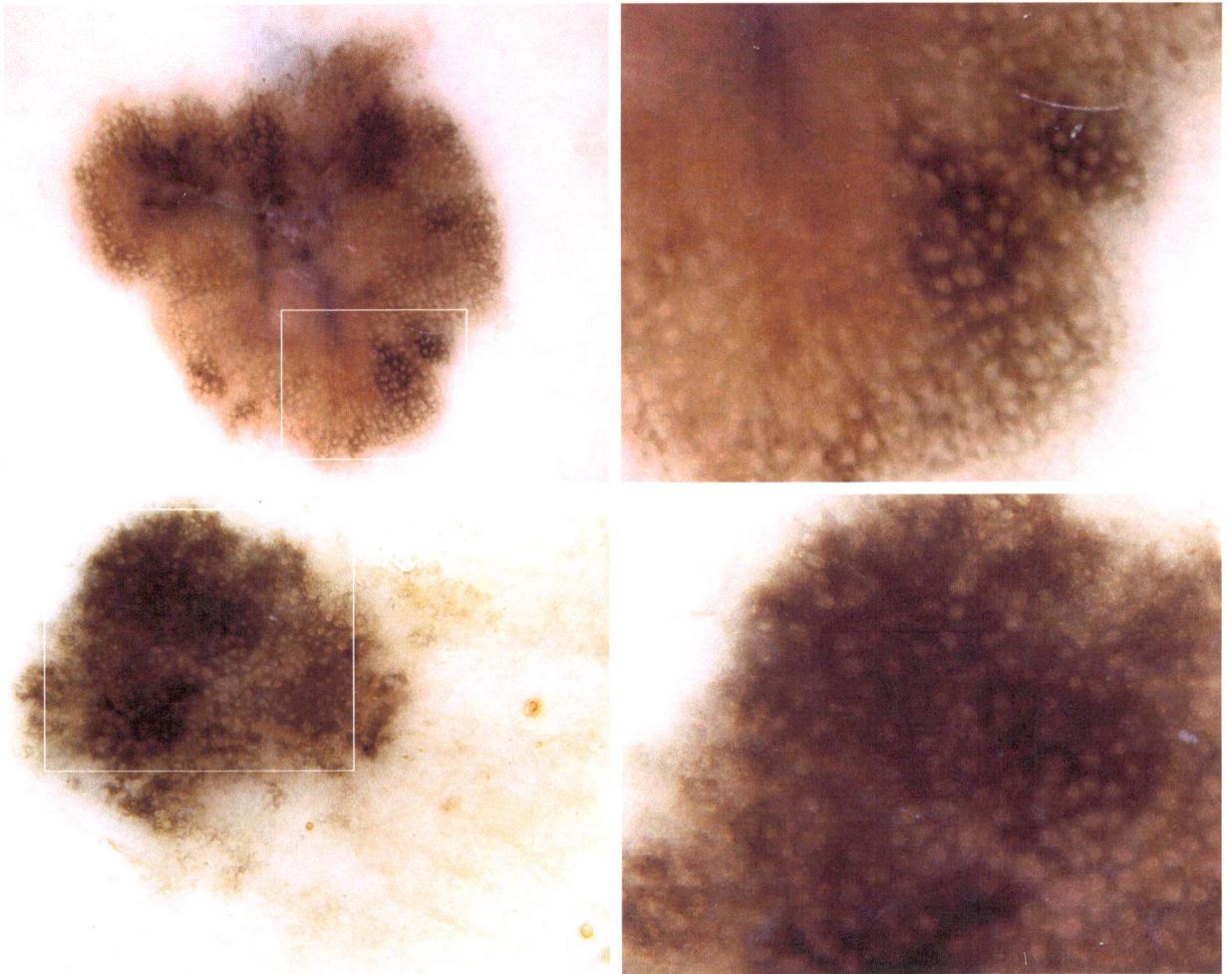

Figure 5.69: Thick reticular lines as a clue to melanoma.
*Dermatosopic images of two in situ melanomas (overview on the **left** and detail on the **right**). Both melanomas are chaotic with thick reticular lines present in a significant part.*

3. Lines reticular or branched, thick *(5.69)*:
To be called thick, the lines must be thicker than the spaces they surround and must cover a significant part of the lesion (one or two thick lines are not sufficient to call it a clue). This pattern is produced by melanoma cells proliferating in the rete ridges and therefore in melanocytic lesions it is only seen in melanoma. Thick lines reticular in seborrheic keratoses are due to acanthosis of pigmented rete ridges and other clues to that diagnosis will be present.

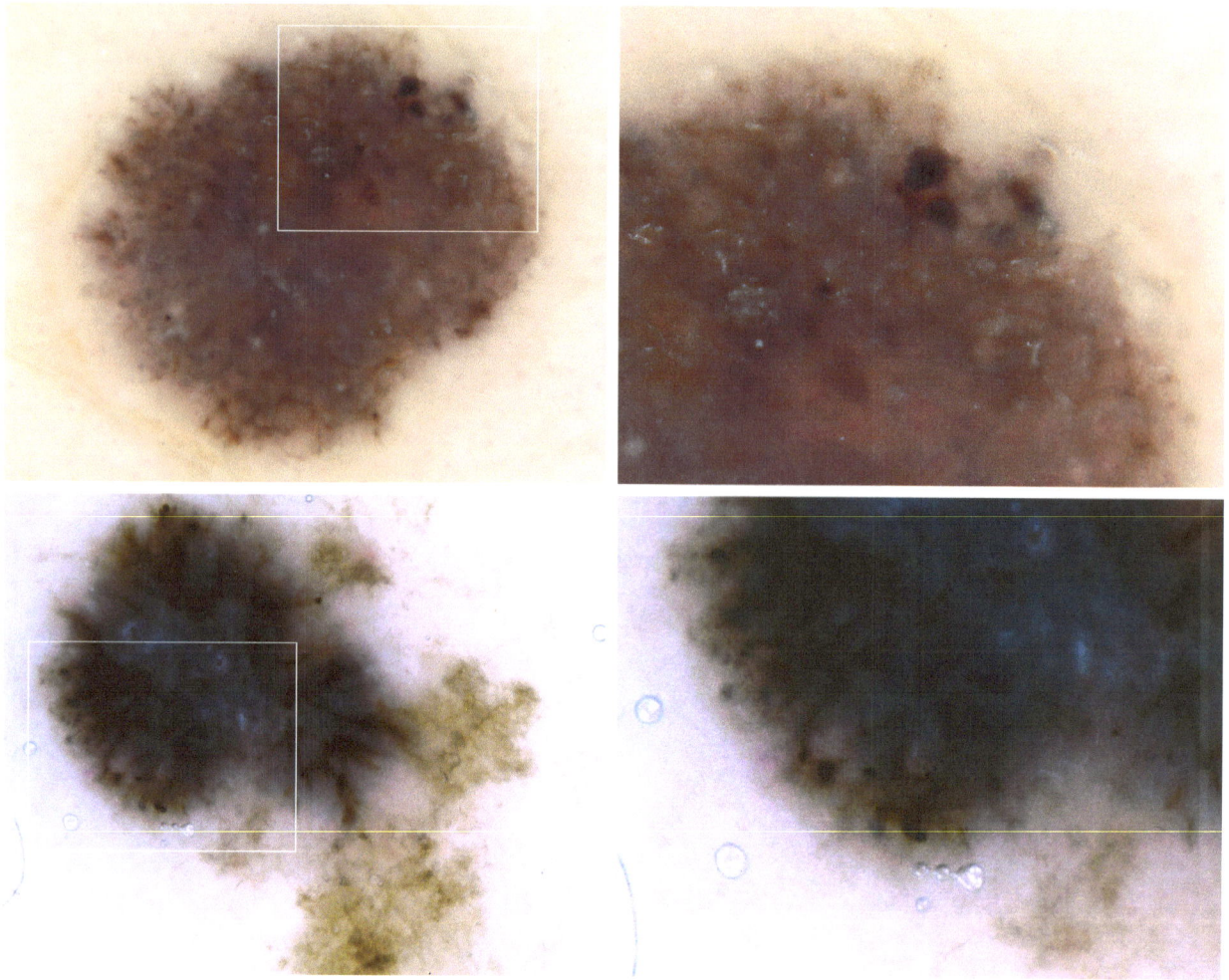

Figure 5.70: Peripheral black dots or clods as a clue to malignancy.
*The overview is shown on the **left** and the detail on the **right**. These two melanomas are chaotic and exhibit black clods (**top row**) or black dots (**bottom row**) as a clue to malignancy.*

4. Black dots or clods, peripheral *(5.70)*:
    Black dots and clods are generally produced by melanin in keratinocytes or pigmented melanocytes close to, or at the level of, the stratum corneum. Central black dots frequently occur in Clark nevi, but when they are peripheral and not located on reticular lines, they are a clue to malignancy.

5. Lines radial or pseudopods, segmental *(5.71)*:
    Peripheral pseudopods or radial lines are a feature of Reed nevus when they occupy the entire periphery ("circumferential"), but when only seen in part of the periphery ("segmental") they are a clue to malignancy. When radial lines converge to a central dot or clod they are highly specific for pigmented basal cell carcinoma. Radial lines which converge also occur in pigmented SCC in-situ; these lines are often formed by dots in linear arrangement. Radial lines (and pseudopods) in melanomas are expected to be connected to either a pattern of reticular lines or to a pigmented structureless area whereas in basal cell carcinoma they frequently extend from a hypopigmented area.

6. White lines *(5.72, 5.73)*: To be considered "white" and therefore a clue to malignancy, lines must be clearly whiter than normal perilesional skin. This clue is not restricted to lines in a reticular pattern, any pattern of white lines seen with either polarized or non-polarized dermatoscopy constitutes a clue. As polarizing-specific white lines may occasionally be the only clue to malignancy in melanomas, we believe that examination with polarized dermatoscopy should be routine.

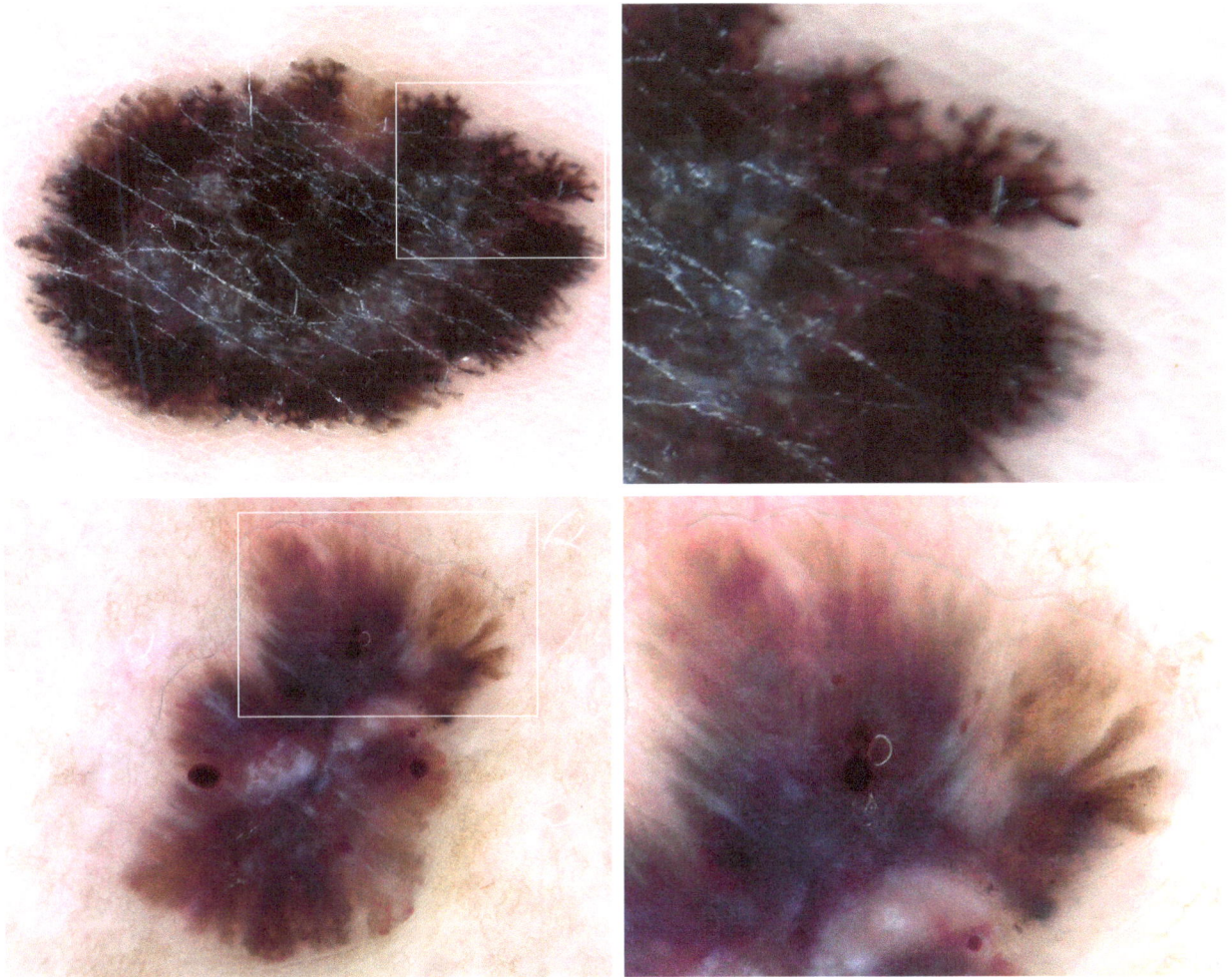

Figure 5.71: *Pseudopods or radial lines as a clue to malignancy.*
*The overview is shown on the **left** and the detail on the **right. Top row:** A melanoma that is chaotic and has segmental peripheral pseudo-pods. **Bottom row:** A basal cell carcinoma that exhibits chaos and peripheral segmental radial lines.*

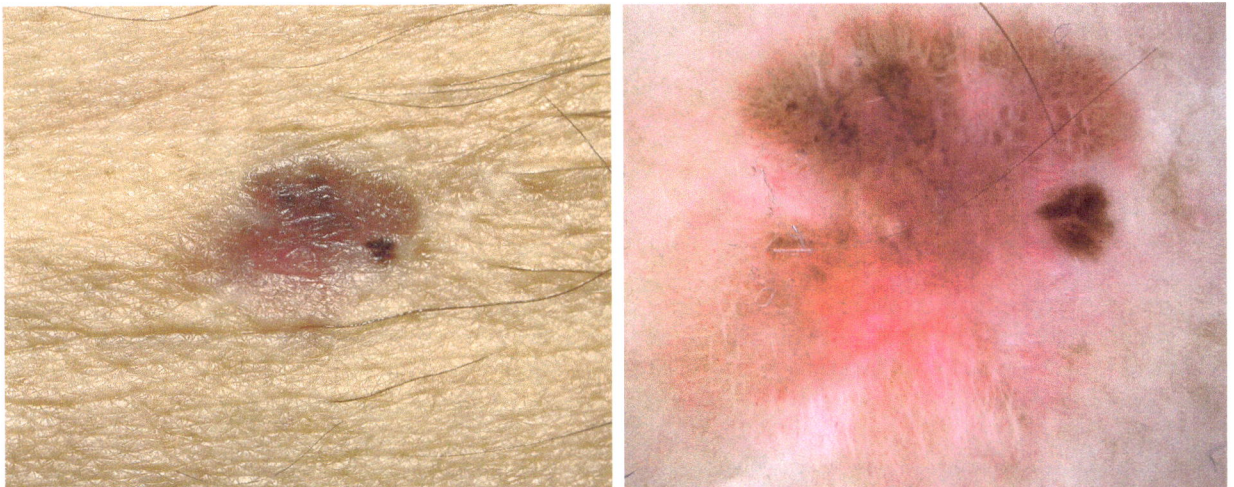

Figure 5.72: *Reticular white lines as a clue to malignancy.*
*This melanoma shows reticular white lines on dermatoscopy **(right image).** Reticular white lines can be seen with and without polarization.*

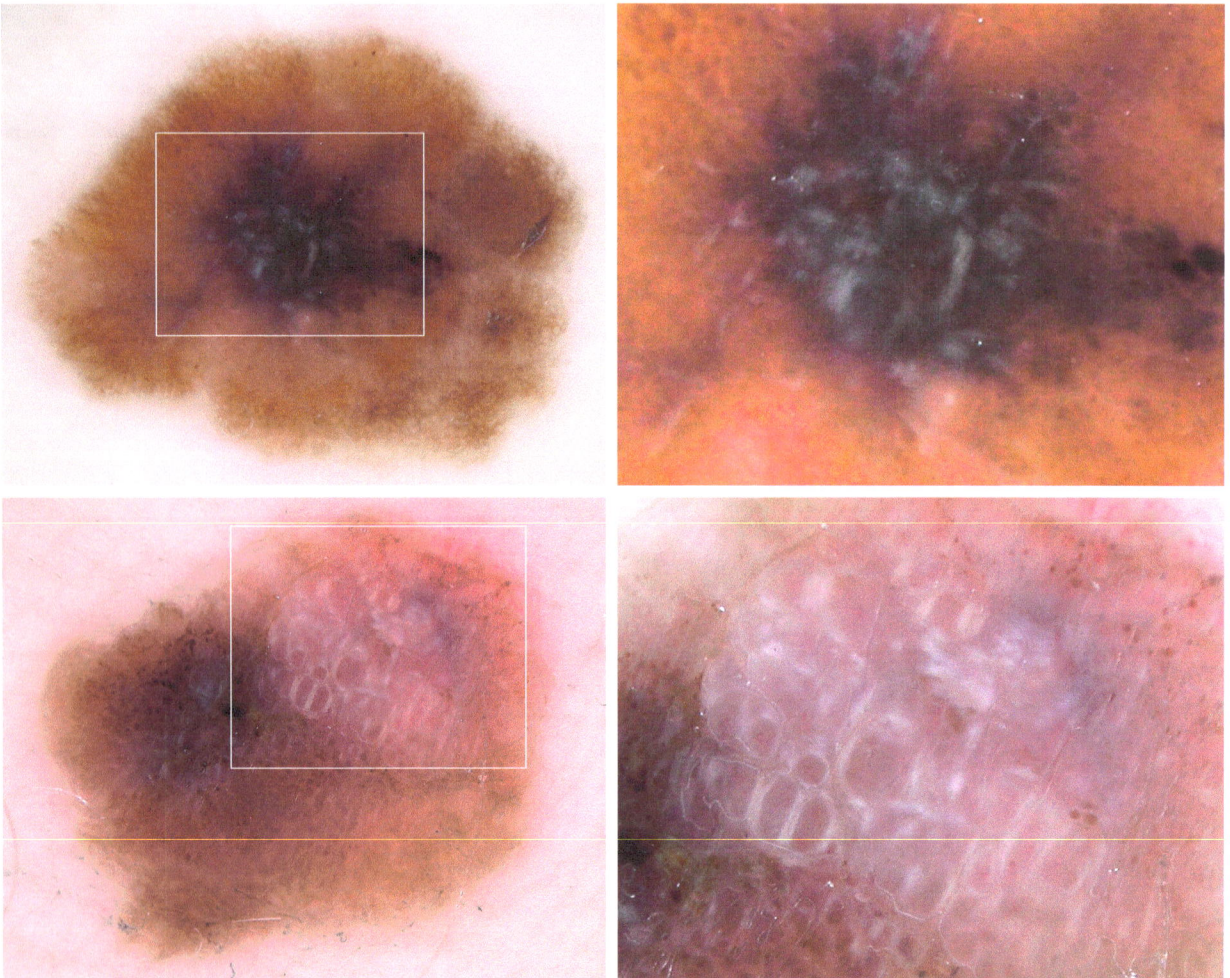

Figure 5.73: Polarization-specific white lines as a clue to malignancy.
*The overview is shown on the **left** and the detail on the **right**. Two invasive melanomas exhibit chaos and short white lines that are arranged perpendicular to each other. These white lines are only visible with polarized dermatoscopy.*

7. Lines parallel, ridges *(acral skin, 5.74)*:
    This is a clue to malignancy even in the absence of chaos. Whether pigmented lines are on ridges or in furrows is often easier to assess at the edges of a lesion. Pigment may be present in both ridges and furrows, but it is the location of the lines that decides whether the pattern is a ridge pattern or a furrow pattern. It must be remembered that melanoma can arise within a furrow-pattern acral nevus, so all of the other clues to malignancy remain clues to malignancy at acral sites, even in parallel furrow pattern lesions. A parallel ridge pattern can occasionally occur in congenital nevi so the clinical context should always be considered. Sub-corneal hemorrhage and exogenous pigmentation can also produce this pattern.

8. Polymorphous vessels *(5.75)*:
    Vessels are called polymorphous when more than one type of vessel pattern is seen. One or two vessels do not constitute a pattern. Polymorphous vessels are commonly seen in both basal cell carcinomas and melanomas but are not expected in pigmented Bowen's disease, which are most likely to have monomorphic coiled vessels. If polymorphous vessels include a pattern of dots, then melanoma is more likely than basal cell carcinoma.

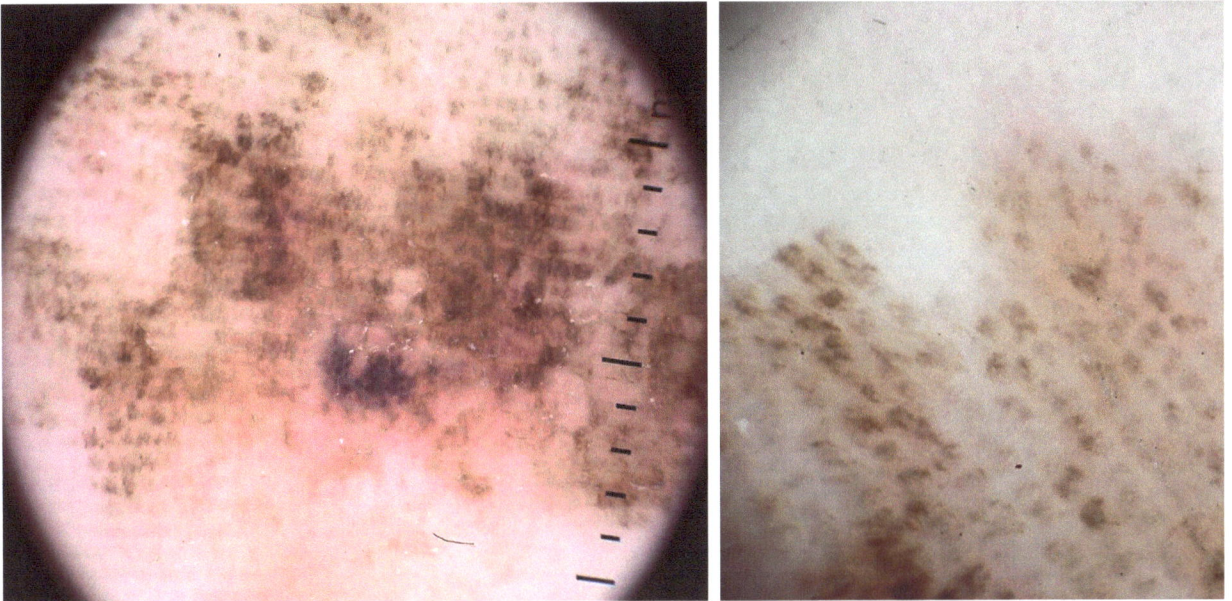

Figure 5.74: *Parallel lines on the ridges as a clue to acral melanoma.*
The overview is shown on the **left** *and the detail on the* **right.** *This acral melanoma has pigmentation on the ridges.*

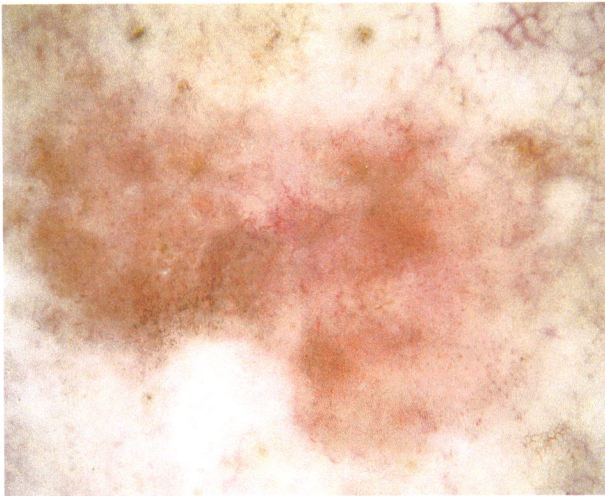

Figure 5.75: *Polymorphous vascular pattern as a clue to malignancy.*
A lightly pigmented skin lesion exhibits chaos and this is substantial when the extensive peripheral white area is considered. Because the main pattern is lightly pigmented structureless, vessels are clearly seen. The vessels are polymorphous being present as dots in combination with both serpentine and coiled lines.

9. Angulated lines (Polygons) *(5.76)*

Angulated lines or polygons were first described by Keir in flat melanomas on non-facial skin with chronic sun-damage (7). Angulated lines on non-facial skin form complete or incomplete polygonal shapes which are larger than the holes caused by individual follicles and larger by far than the holes bounded by reticular lines. These lines meet but do not cross.

Angulated lines may also appear in flat facial melanomas. Angulated lines of facial skin are situated around follicular openings and therefore border a smaller zone than angulated lines on non-facial skin. While angulated lines can be seen in some benign lesions and particularly in facial pigmented actinic keratosis, we have found it to be a valuable clue to melanoma. The sensitivity and specificity have not yet been formally assessed but author CR has found it to be present in 20 % of consecutively excised melanomas (unpublished data). The clue of angulated lines (polygons) is usually, but not always, associated with dermatoscopic grey color.

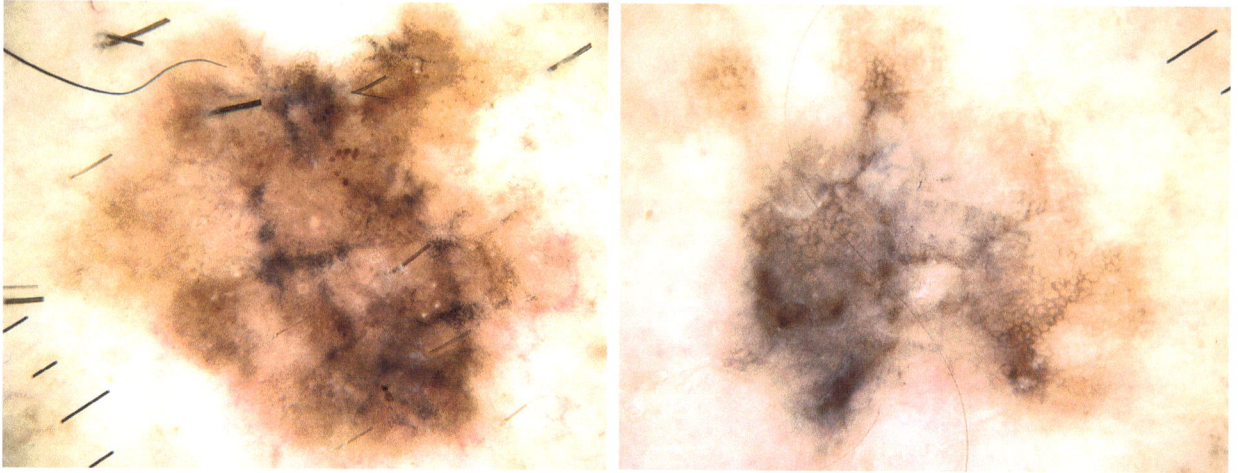

Figure 5.76: Angulated lines (polygons) as a clue to flat melanomas on chronic sun-damaged skin.
Polygons bounded by straight, angulated lines in two flat melanomas on non-facial chronic sun damaged skin. In both cases there are geometric shapes, some complete and some incomplete, formed by lines meeting at angles and larger than the holes caused by individual follicles and larger by far than the holes bounded by reticular lines.

Exclusion of unequivocal seborrheic keratoses from biopsy

The specificity of this algorithm is increased if unequivocal seborrheic keratoses are diagnosed by applying pattern analysis, and excluded from biopsy (see chapter 3 for specific clues to seborrheic keratosis). Only when the diagnosis of seborrheic keratosis is unequivocal can biopsy be avoided. Melanomas can mimic seborrheic keratoses. Squamous cell carcinomas can arise in seborrheic keratoses, and all malignancies can occur in collision with them. A single criterion for seborrheic keratosis should only be used to make a diagnosis when the lesion has no clues to malignancy, and even then with considerable caution. Despite these caveats, the diagnosis of seborrheic keratosis can be made quickly and unequivocally in most cases.

Summary

Examining for chaos is a screening procedure and with practice requires minimal cognition and time. If chaos is encountered, clues are searched for. This search for clues requires more time and cognition, but as there are no calculations required this is still practical in a busy practice setting. The experienced dermatoscopist may then choose to apply pattern analysis to resolve the differential diagnosis, but the prior application of "Chaos and Clues" will have reduced this workload.

References

1 Marghoob AA, Braun R. Proposal for a revised 2-step algorithm for the classification of lesions of the skin using dermoscopy. Archives of dermatology 2010; 146: 426–8.

2 Tschandl P, Rosendahl C, Kittler H. Accuracy of the first step of the dermatoscopic 2-step algorithm for pigmented skin lesions. Dermatology practical & conceptual 2012; 2: 203a08.

3 Zaballos P, Puig S, Llambrich A, Malvehy J. Dermoscopy of dermatofibromas: a prospective morphological study of 412 cases. Archives of dermatology 2008; 144: 75–83.

4 Akay BN, Kittler H, Sanli H, Harmankaya K, Anadolu R. Dermatoscopic findings of cutaneous mastocytosis. Dermatology 2009; 218: 226–30.

5 Argenziano G, Catricala C, Ardigo M, Buccini P, De Simone P, Eibenschutz L et al. Dermoscopy of patients with multiple nevi: Improved management recommendations using a comparative diagnostic approach. Archives of dermatology 2011; 147: 46–9.

6 Jaimes N, Marghoob AA, Rabinovitz H, Braun RP, Cameron A, Rosendahl C et al. Clinical and dermoscopic characteristics of melanomas on nonfacial chronically sun-damaged skin. Journal of the American Academy of Dermatology 2015; 72: 1027–35.

7 Keir J. Dermatoscopic features of cutaneous non-facial non-acral lentiginous growth pattern melanomas. Dermatology practical & conceptual 2014; 4: 77–82.

8 Tschandl P, Rosendahl C, Kittler H. Dermatoscopy of flat pigmented facial lesions. Journal of the European Academy of Dermatology and Venereology: JEADV 2015; 29: 120–7.

9 Akay BN, Kocyigit P, Heper AO, Erdem C. Dermatoscopy of flat pigmented facial lesions: diagnostic challenge between pigmented actinic keratosis and lentigo maligna. The British journal of dermatology 2010; 163: 1212–7.

10 Saida T, Miyazaki A, Oguchi S, Ishihara Y, Yamazaki Y, Murase S et al. Significance of dermoscopic patterns in detecting malignant melanoma on acral volar skin: results of a multicenter study in Japan. Archives of dermatology 2004; 140: 1233–8.

11 Sendagorta E, Feito M, Ramirez P, Gonzalez-Beato M, Saida T, Pizarro A. Dermoscopic findings and histological correlation of the acral volar pigmented maculae in Laugier-Hunziker syndrome. The Journal of dermatology 2010; 37: 980–4.

12 Benvenuto-Andrade C, Dusza SW, Agero AL, Scope A, Rajadhyaksha M, Halpern AC et al. Differences between polarized light dermoscopy and immersion contact dermoscopy for the evaluation of skin lesions. Archives of dermatology 2007; 143: 329–38.

13 Rosendahl C, Cameron A, Tschandl P, Bulinska A, Zalaudek I, Kittler H. Prediction without Pigment: a decision algorithm for non-pigmented skin malignancy. Dermatology practical & conceptual 2014; 4: 59–66.

14 Cameron A, Rosendahl C, Tschandl P, Riedl E, Kittler H. Dermatoscopy of pigmented Bowen's disease. Journal of the American Academy of Dermatology 2010; 62: 597–604.

15 Stolz W, Schiffner R, Burgdorf WH. Dermatoscopy for facial pigmented skin lesions. Clin Dermatol 2002; 20: 276–8.

16 Argenziano G, Longo C, Cameron A, Cavicchini S, Gourhant JY, Lallas A et al. Blue-black rule: a simple dermoscopic clue to recognize pigmented nodular melanoma. The British journal of dermatology 2011; 165: 1251–5.

17 Blum A, Hofmann-Wellenhof R, Marghoob AA, Argenziano G, Cabo H, Carrera C et al. Recurrent melanocytic nevi and melanomas in dermoscopy: results of a multicenter study of the International Dermoscopy Society. JAMA dermatology 2014; 150: 138–45.

18 Tschandl P. Recurrent nevi: report of three cases with dermatoscopic-dermatopathologic correlation. Dermatology practical & conceptual 2013; 3: 29–32.

19 Pehamberger H, Steiner A, Wolff K. In vivo epiluminescence microscopy of pigmented skin lesions. I. Pattern analysis of pigmented skin lesions. Journal of the American Academy of Dermatology 1987; 17: 571–83.

20 Nachbar F, Stolz W, Merkle T, Cognetta AB, Vogt T, Landthaler M et al. The ABCD rule of dermatoscopy. High prospective value in the diagnosis of doubtful melanocytic skin lesions. Journal of the American Academy of Dermatology 1994; 30: 551–9.

21 Argenziano G, Fabbrocini G, Carli P, De Giorgi V, Sammarco E, Delfino M. Epiluminescence microscopy for the diagnosis of doubtful melanocytic skin lesions. Comparison of the ABCD rule of dermatoscopy and a new 7-point checklist based on pattern analysis. Archives of dermatology 1998; 134: 1563–70.

22 Menzies SW, Ingvar C, McCarthy WH. A sensitivity and specificity analysis of the surface microscopy features of invasive melanoma. Melanoma research 1996; 6: 55–62.

23 Henning JS, Dusza SW, Wang SQ, Marghoob AA, Rabinovitz HS, Polsky D et al. The CASH (color, architecture, symmetry, and homogeneity) algorithm for dermoscopy. Journal of the American Academy of Dermatology 2007; 56: 45–52.

24 Soyer HP, Argenziano G, Zalaudek I, Corona R, Sera F, Talamini R et al. Three-point checklist of dermoscopy. A new screening method for early detection of melanoma. Dermatology 2004; 208: 27–31.

25 Rosendahl C, Tschandl P, Cameron A, Kittler H. Diagnostic accuracy of dermatoscopy for melanocytic and nonmelanocytic pigmented lesions. Journal of the American Academy of Dermatology 2011; 64: 1068–73.

26 Rosendahl C, Cameron A, McColl I, Wilkinson D. Dermatoscopy in routine practice – 'chaos and clues'. Aust Fam Physician 2012; 41: 482–7.

6 Non-pigmented (amelanotic) lesions

As originally described, pattern analysis is a method for assessing pigmented lesions. This restriction to pigmented lesions is not an accident: patterns formed by melanin pigment are more prominent and more specific diagnostically than other features seen at dermatoscopy. The absence of melanin structures in non-pigmented lesions restricts the range of features available for diagnosis. Furthermore, because structures pigmented by melanin are the building blocks of current diagnostic algorithms, alternative methods are required to diagnose non-pigmented lesions.

For the purposes of this chapter, we have defined as "pigmented" any lesion containing any area at all pigmented by melanin (i.e. black, brown, gray, or blue). While a "non-pigmented" lesion lacks these colors, white, yellow, orange, pink, or red may be seen, either singly or in combination. As these lesions only lack melanin pigment, "amelanotic" is a more accurate term than "non-pigmented". The latter term, although less precise, remains more popular. In this chapter we use both terms interchangeably.

The assessment of amelanotic lesions is challenging and a specific diagnosis is not always possible even when dermatoscopy is added to clinical examination. For some non-pigmented lesions, diagnosis with the unaided eye is easier than with dermatoscopy. Other non-pigmented lesions that are difficult to diagnose with the unaided eye have specific dermatoscopy features. However, in most cases a satisfactory level of diagnostic accuracy is only achieved by supplementing dermatoscopic features with clinical findings.

Because many inflammatory diseases have to be included in the list of differential diagnoses, the number of possible diagnoses is higher than for pigmented lesions. In this chapter we focus on neoplastic non-pigmented lesions and discuss inflammatory diseases only as differential diagnoses. The dermatoscopy of inflammatory diseases is dealt with in more detail in chapter 8.

6.1 Clues used in the diagnosis of non-pigmented (amelanotic) lesions

In the absence of melanin pigment, other clues must be used in the diagnosis of non-pigmented lesions. In general, these clues may also be seen in pigmented lesions, but being less specific, they are of less significance when diagnosis can proceed on the basis of structures pigmented by melanin.

The pattern of non-pigmented lesions is usually structureless. However, non-pigmented lesions may show patterns of white, yellow, orange, pink, skin colored, or red clods; and white lines, circles or dots. Lesions with orange or red clods, which have been addressed in detail in the section on pigmented lesions, may be analyzed as either pigmented or non-pigmented.

Ulceration
Ulceration is not a strong clue to a specific diagnosis, but in the absence of a clear history of trauma it is a good clue to malignancy. As an over-riding principle, in the absence of a clear and convincing history of trauma, any solitary ulcerated non-pigmented lesion should be submitted for histopathology. Ulceration is usually manifested dermatoscopically as an orange or yellow structureless area, which represents dried serum crust (6.1). Bleeding due to ulceration will be seen at dermatoscopy as either red clods or red structureless zones (6.2). Sometimes ulceration appears together with necrosis. Necrosis can be white, yellow or black (6.3). Especially when a contact fluid is used, ulceration may not be apparent dermatoscopically with the appearance of ulceration often mimicking compacted keratin. However, adherent fiber, either clothing fabric or loose hair, is an indirect dermatoscopic clue to ulceration. Fibers adhere to ulcerated surfaces because of the sticky consistency of the serum.

Surface scale
The multiple air-tissue interfaces created by scale means that more of the light incident on the skin surface is reflected, making scale appear white. Like ulceration, scale is usually better assessed clinically. Dermatoscopes are designed to make surface scale more transparent,

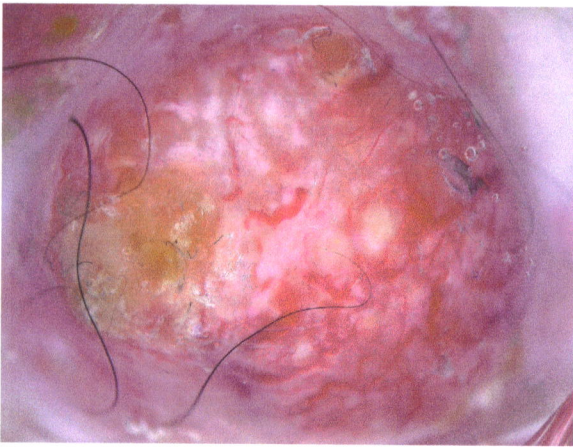

Figure 6.1: Ulceration with serum crusts and adherent fibers.
A basal cell carcinoma with ulceration (yellow structureless area representing a serum crust) and adherent fibers. The adherent fibers are thinner and shorter than the adjacent hairs.

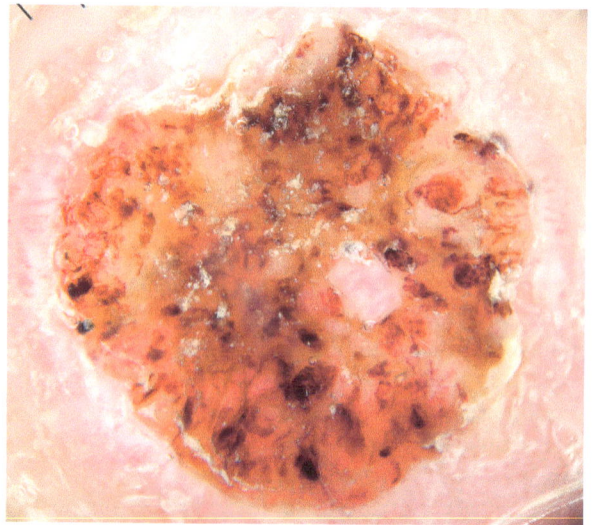

Figure 6.2: Ulceration with bleeding.
As in figure 6.1, a yellow structureless zone indicates ulceration (serum crust). In addition one can see black and red clods which correspond to blood spots due to bleeding (hemorrhagic crust) in a poorly differentiated squamous cell carcinoma.

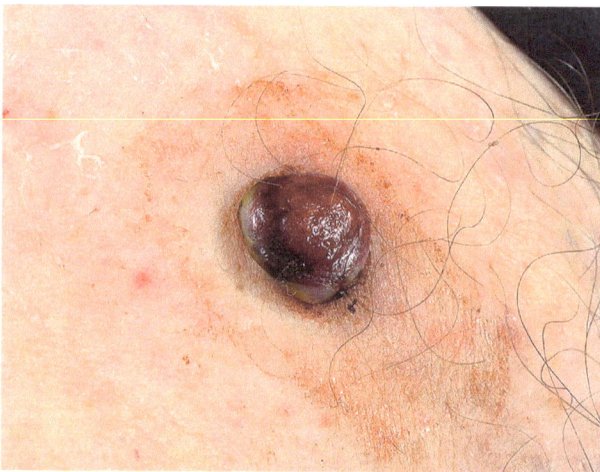

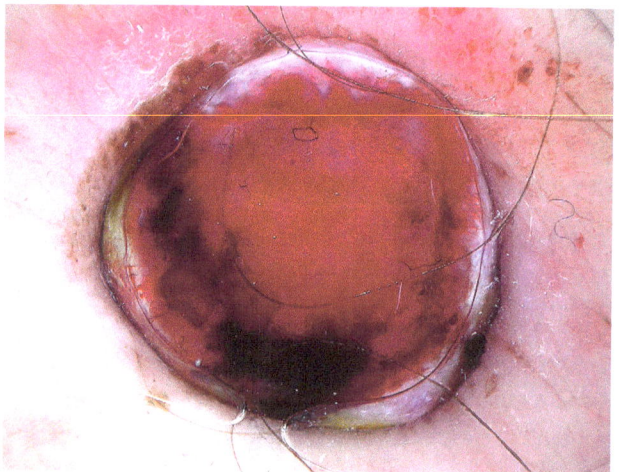

Figure 6.3: Ulceration and necrosis.
A pyogenic granuloma with bleeding and necrosis. The zone of necrosis at the periphery appears yellow and black.

i.e. invisible, to allow better visualization of pigment structures and vessels.

If serum is present in the stratum corneum (e.g. in a spongiotic dermatitis), scale appears yellow and not white. Scale may be present both in inflammatory diseases (e.g. psoriasis) and in neoplasms (e.g. Bowen's disease). In both cases, scale is produced by hyper- and parakeratosis of the stratum corneum, with conglomerates of corneocytes (keratinocytes that form the stratum corneum) with preserved nuclei remaining adherent to the skin surface because of incomplete desquamation.

When visible, scale is seen on dermatoscopy as white or silvery polygonal clods that are not entirely homogeneous (6.4).

Keratin
While scale indicates mild hyper- and parakeratosis, keratin corresponds to prominent hyperkeratosis. Subsurface keratin (e.g. in the "milia-like cysts" of seborrheic keratosis) has no contact with air and usually appears white on dermatoscopy. Surface keratin that has contact with air usually appears yellow or orange (6.5).

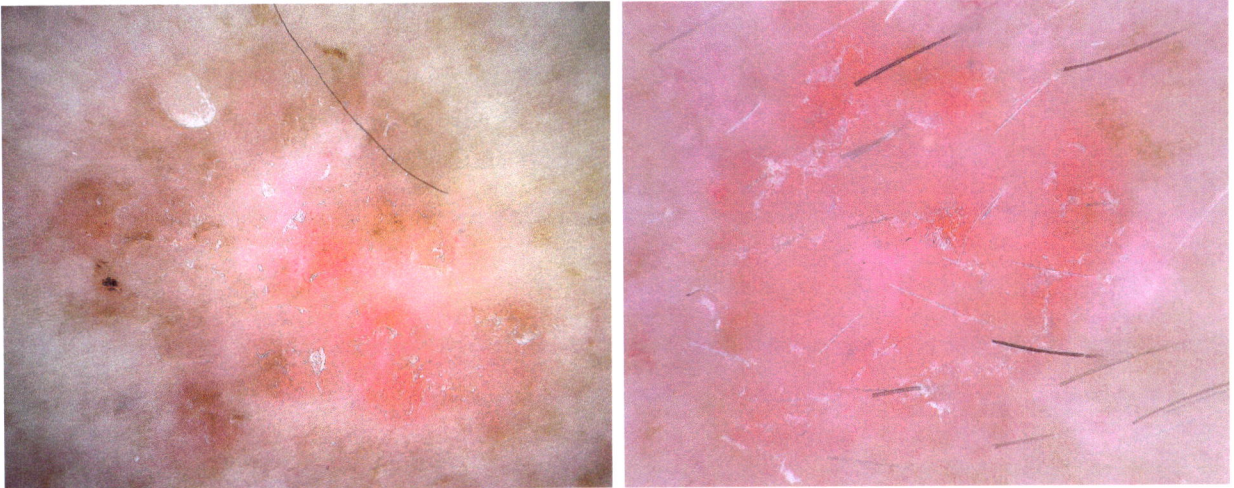

Figure 6.4: Scale in Bowen's disease.
*Dermatoscopic images of two cases of Bowen's disease (intraepidermal carcinoma). The lesion on the **left** is lightly pigmented (structureless brown) the lesion on the **right** is non-pigmented (amelanotic). In both cases one can see scales and coiled vessels. In low magnification it is difficult to differentiate vessels as dots from coiled vessels.*

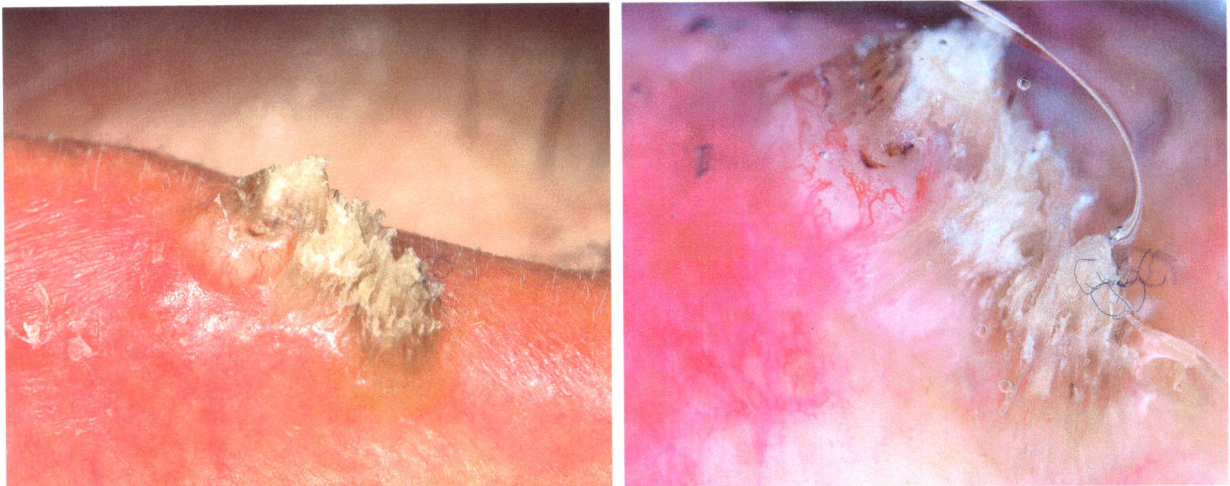

Figure 6.5: Keratin.
Surface keratin in a well differentiated squamous cell carcinoma that appears white, yellow or orange on dermatoscopy.

This color is emphasized by any serum inclusions. In non-pigmented (amelanotic) seborrheic keratoses the infundibular keratin plugs ("comedo-like openings") are usually yellow. If melanin is admixed with keratin, keratin plugs can be even brown or black as in some hyperpigmented seborrheic keratoses.

White clues

In dermatoscopy, "white" is defined as lighter than surrounding normal skin. All basic elements except pseudopods have a white variant. The various white structures are listed in *table 6.1,* and their role in the

differential diagnosis of amelanotic lesions is further discussed in section 6.3.

There are two types of white lines. One is seen only with polarizing dermatoscopes; the other is seen regardless of instrument type. Polarizing-specific white lines are arranged as two groups of parallel lines at right angles to each other *(6.7).* These lines may be short or long, but do not cross each other. They are most commonly found in melanoma, Spitz nevus, basal cell carcinoma, and dermatofibroma (1–5), but can also occasionally be seen in a wide range of other lesions including scar

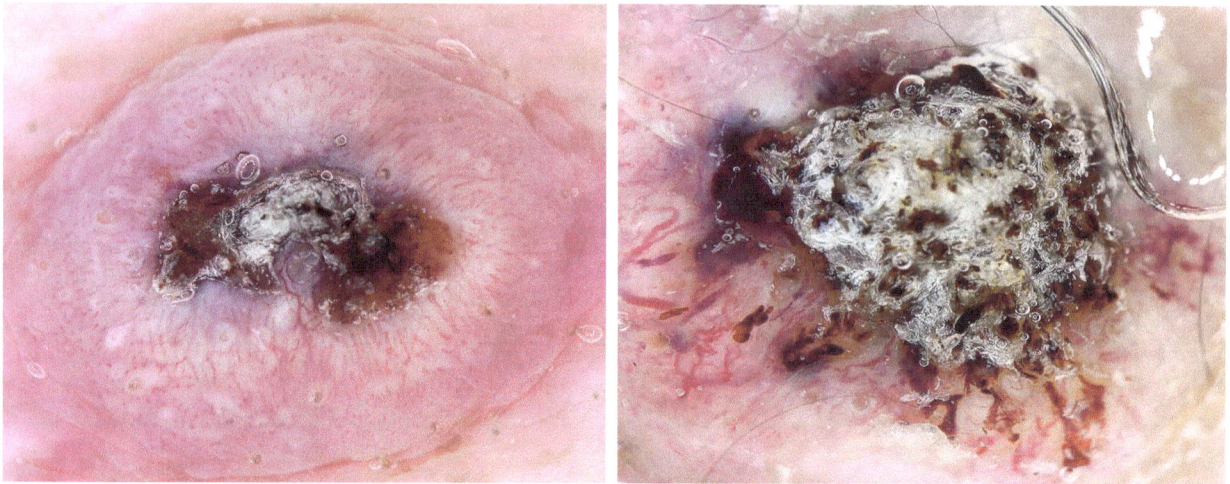

Figure 6.6: *Keratin with blood spots.*
Dermatoscopic image of two keratoacanthomas. Both lesions show blood spots in the central keratin plug.

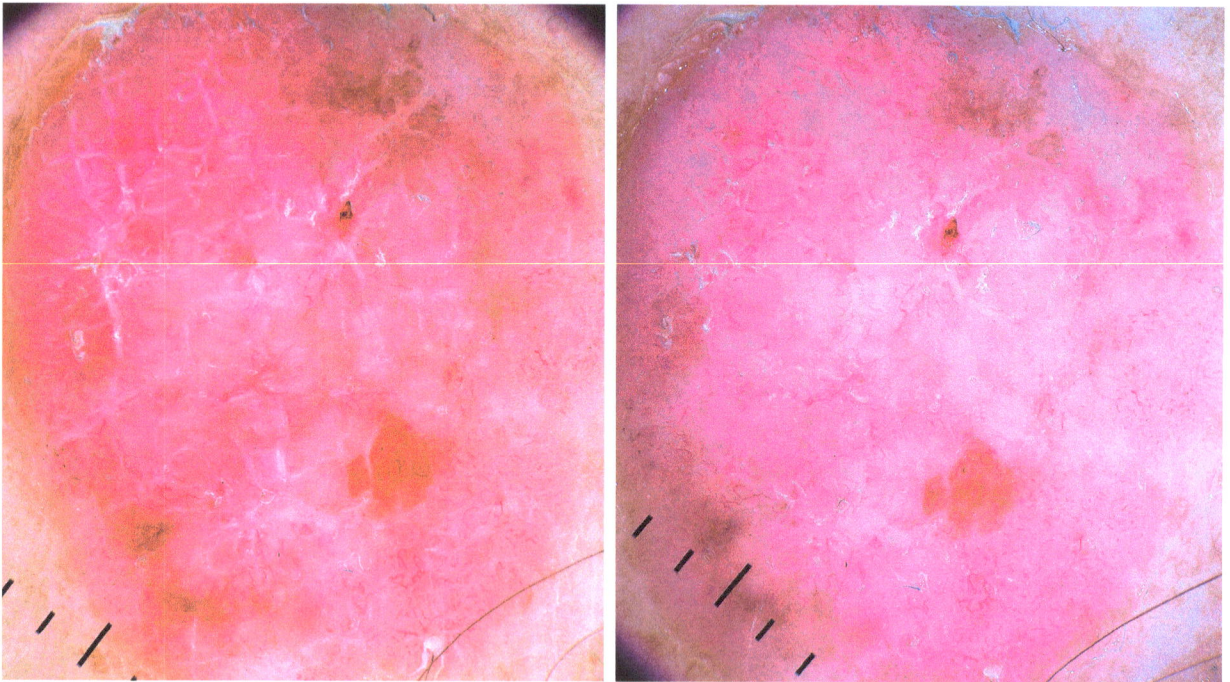

Figure 6.7: *Polarizing specific white lines.*
Perpendicular white lines in a nodular non-pigmented lesion are seen with polarized dermatoscopy (left) but not non-polarized dermatoscopy (right).

tissue (6). Polarizing-specific white lines correspond to fibrosis and sclerosis in the dermis. Usually the overlying epidermis is devoid of rete ridges (i.e. flat).

White lines are also produced by fibrosis of the papillary dermis when the rete ridges are intact. These white lines often (but not always) form the reticular pattern (7), and are seen regardless of the type of dermatoscope used. They are most often seen in melanomas, nevi,

and dermatofibromas but they are absent in basal cell carcinomas.

While they can be seen in benign lesions, white lines of any type in amelanotic lesions should be regarded as a clue to malignancy (7).

White circles are the most specific clue to actinic keratoses (flat lesions) (8) and well-differentiated squamous cell carcinomas/keratoacanthomas (raised lesions) (9)

Table 6.1: White structures

White structures	Polarized dermatoscopy	Non-polarized dermatoscopy	Pathologic correlation	Significance
Perpendicular white lines	Visible	Invisible	Dermal fibrosis and sclerosis, epidermis usually devoid of rete ridges	BCC, melanoma, Spitz nevus, dermatofibroma
Reticular white lines	Visible	Visible	Fibrosis of papillary dermis, rete ridges preserved	Melanoma, Spitz nevus, Clark nevus, dermatofibroma
White dots and clods (multiple)	Barely visibly	Visible	Milia (superficial epidermal inclusion cysts)	Seborrheic keratosis
White clods of sebaceous gland hyperplasia	Visible	Visible	Sebaceous glands	Sebaceous gland hyperplasia
Pus (central white dot surrounded by erythema)	Visible	Visible	Pus	Folliculitis, furuncle, myiasis
Polarizing specific white clods (nearly always appear together with perpendicular white lines)	Visible	Invisible	Mid-dermal fibrosis and sclerosis, epidermis usually devoid of rete ridges	BCC, melanoma, Spitz nevus, dermatofibroma
Four white dots in a square (four-dot clod)	Visible	Invisible	Keratin plug in follicular opening, fibrosis surrounding infundibular epidermis	Actinic keratosis but can be found in many lesions and on normal skin
White circles	Visible	Visible	Acanthosis of infundibular epidermis with hypergranulosis	Actinic keratosis, keratoacanthoma/SCC, well differentiated
Structureless white (flat lesion)	Visible	Visible	Dermal fibrosis and sclerosis, epidermis usually devoid of rete ridges	Regressive melanoma, dermatofibroma, BCC, scar, lupus erythematosus
Structureless white (raised lesion)	Visible	Visible	Subsurface keratin or calcium deposits	Keratoacanthoma/SCC, well differentiated, pilomatrixoma if corresponding to subsurface keratin; calcinosis cutis if corresponding to calcium deposits
White rim (raised lesion)	Visible	Visible	Reactive epidermal hyperplasia	Pyogenic granuloma

but can also be found in lesions of cutaneous lupus erythematosus (10). White circles correspond to acanthosis of follicular epithelium with prominent hypergranulosis (6.8).

White dots or clods usually correspond to keratin filled cysts (milia). These are better seen with non-polarizing contact dermatoscopes (11). If multiple white dots or small round clods are present they usually point to a seborrheic keratosis (6.9) but are also seen in congenital nevi. Although multiple white dots and clods representing keratin filled cysts are a clue to seborrheic keratosis they are not unusual in basal cell carcinoma (6.10) and are also occasionally found in melanoma. The white clods of sebaceous gland hyperplasia are visible with polarized and with non-polarized der-

matoscopy (12, 13). Their white color is duller than polarizing-specific white clods or milia (6.11). Single white dots or clods may also represent pus in skin abscesses such as folliculitis (6.12) or furuncles, but also in myiasis (14).

Dots and clods that are only visible with polarized dermatoscopy (polarizing-specific white clods) do not correspond to milia. Polarizing-specific white clods have the same significance as polarizing specific white lines and correspond to dermal fibrosis and sclerosis. They nearly always appear together with polarizing specific white lines and are found in some basal cell carcinomas and melanomas (6.13, 6.14). Four white dots arranged in a square (four-dot clod) are a polarizing specific structure seen particularly in actinic keratoses, but also

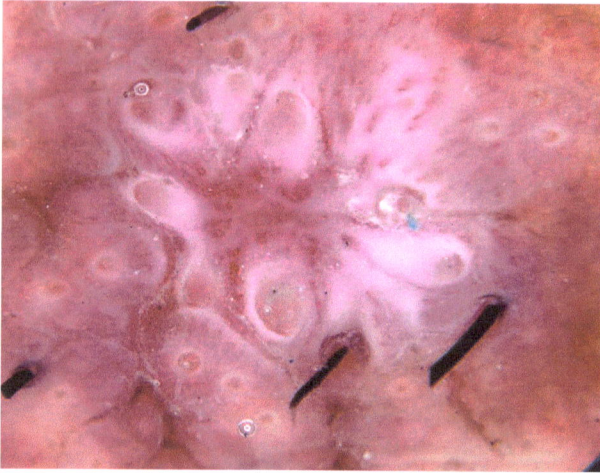

Figure 6.8: *White circles.*
White circles in two well differentiated squamous cell carcinomas.

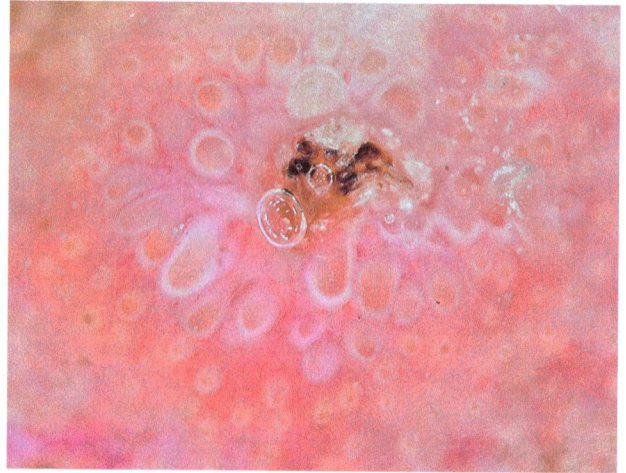

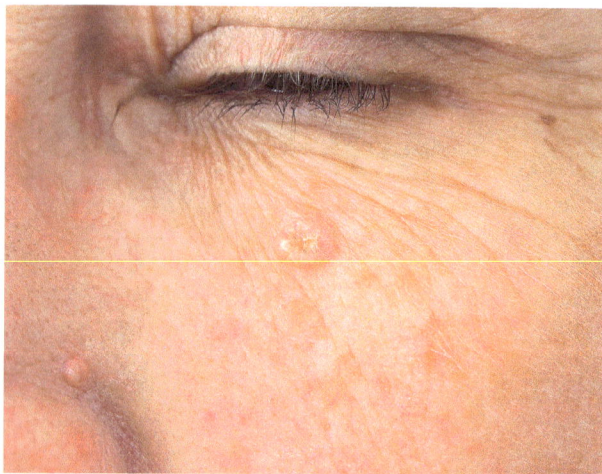

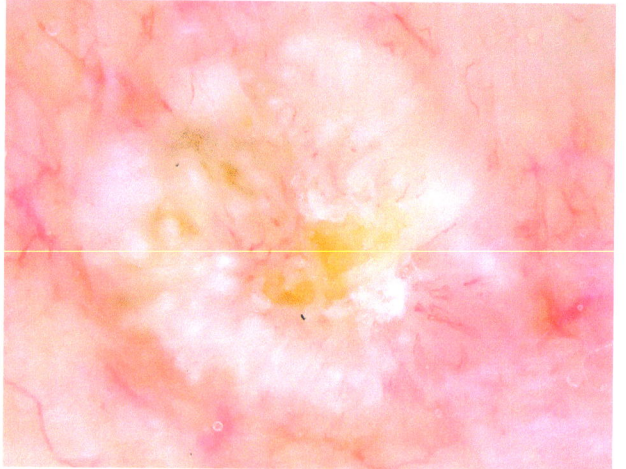

Figure 6.9: *White clods and dots in a seborrheic keratosis.*
*Although this lesion looks like a basal cell carcinoma clinically (**left**) it can be diagnosed as a seborrheic keratosis on dermatoscopy (**right**) based on white dots and clods (corresponding to milia), yellow clods, and the typical looped vessels.*

in other lesions, and even on severely sun-damaged skin without any discrete lesion (15). With non-polarized dermatoscopes, this structure may be seen less clearly as a single circle or clod.

A white structureless zone in a flat lesion usually corresponds to fibrosis or sclerosis. It can be found in flat melanomas and basal cell carcinomas but also in other flat lesions including inflammatory conditions such as lupus erythematosus and in flat scars. A white structureless zone in a raised lesion usually represents subsurface keratin as in well-differentiated squamous cell carcinomas/keratoacanthomas or in pilomatrixoma (6.15).

A peripheral white rim can be found in some pyogenic granulomas (16, 17). It corresponds to the reactive epidermal hyperplasia that surrounds the overgrowth of granulation tissue. For the sake of completeness it should be mentioned that necrotic tissue and calcinosis (6.16) may appear white on dermatoscopy.

Other clues

Scale, keratin, ulceration and white clues are not the only clues that help diagnose non-pigmented lesions. Most clues have already been mentioned in other chapters but the color yellow deserves special attention. Yellow color usually corresponds to keratin or a serum crust, which indicates ulceration. A yellow structureless zone can also be found when there is a dermal accumulation of macrophages that are replete with lipids (xanthoma cells). These xanthoma cells can

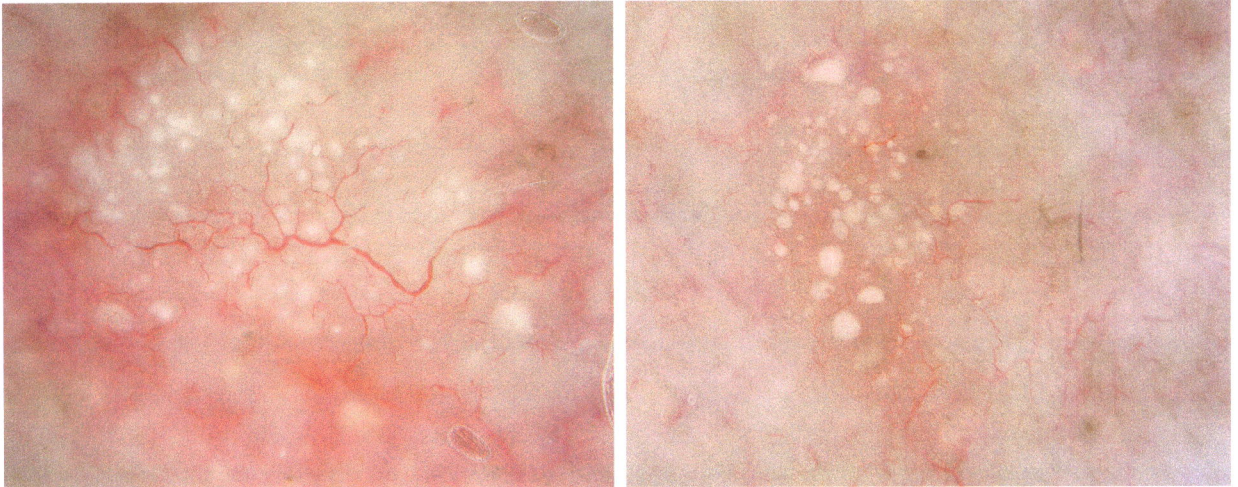

Figure 6.10: Two basal cell carcinomas with white dots and clods.
Although multiple white dots and clods are a clue to seborrheic keratosis they may be found in basal cell carcinomas.

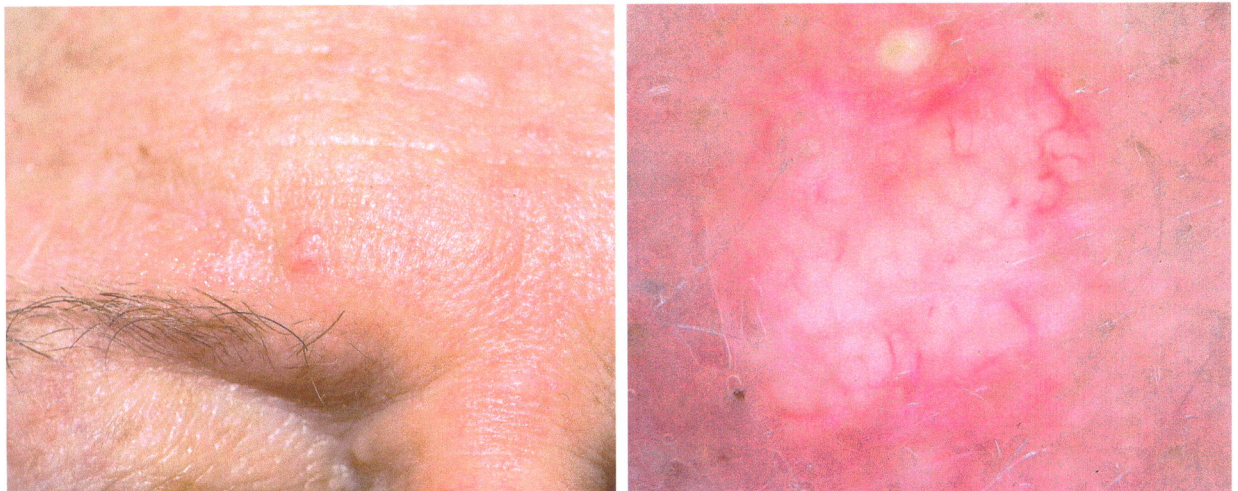

Figure 6.11: White clods of sebaceous gland hyperplasia.
In sebaceous hyperplasia, the white of the clods is duller than in milia or polarizing-specific white clods.

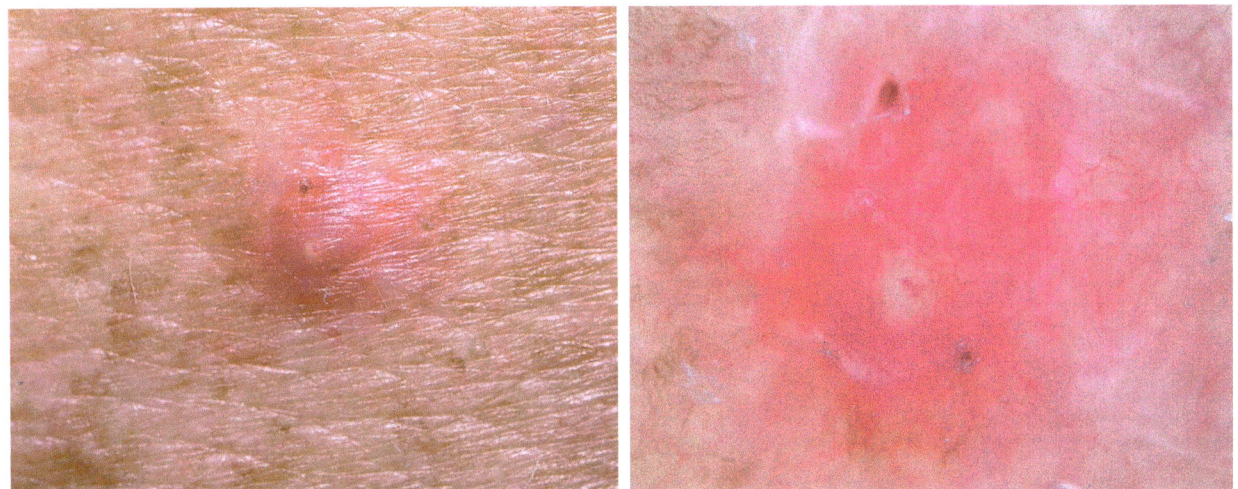

Figure 6.12: Folliculitis.
Pus in the center of folliculitis appears white.

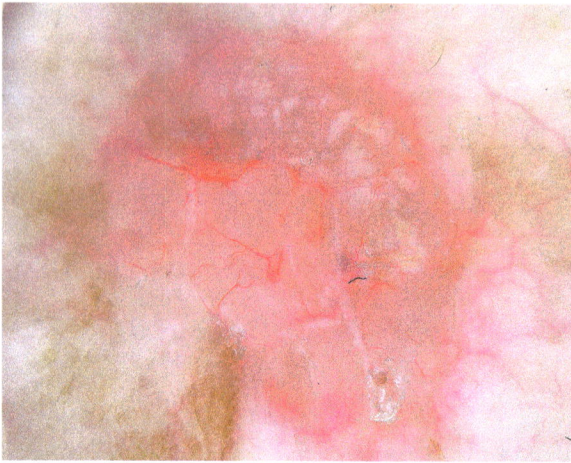

Figure 6.13: *Basal cell carcinoma with polarizing specific white lines and clods*

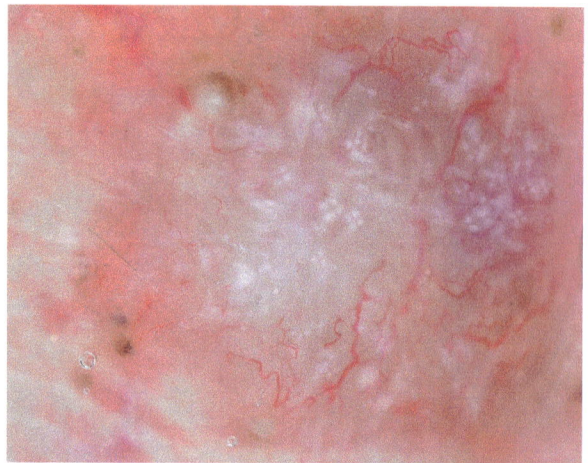

Figure 6.14: *Basal cell carcinoma with four-dot clod (for white dots arranged in a square)*

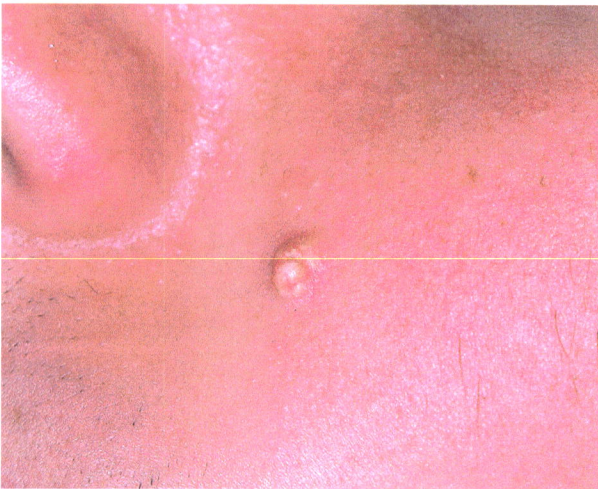

Figure 6.15: *White structureless zone in pilomatrixoma.*
Subsurface keratin in this pilomatrixoma appears as a white structureless zone on dermatoscopy (**right**).

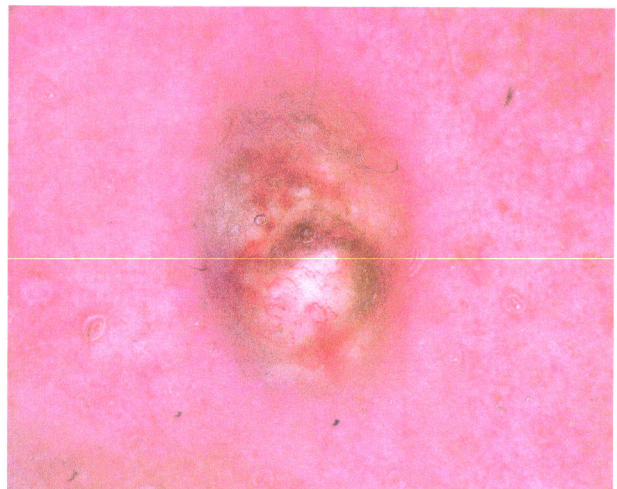

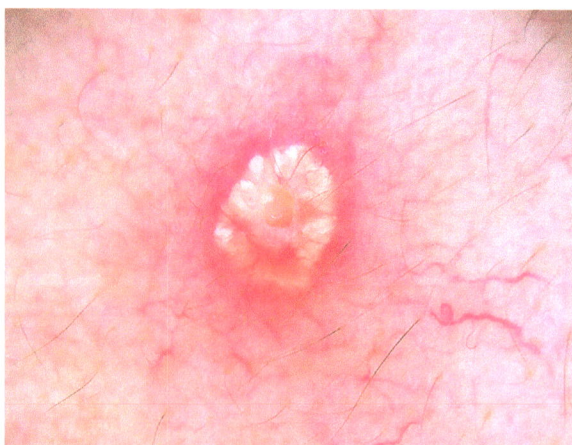

be found in any xanthomatous lesion, most notably in xanthelasma and in xanthogranuloma (18) *(6.17).* Yellow color can also be found in nevus sebaceous, in which the increased number of sebaceous glands is responsible for the yellow appearance on dermatoscopy *(6.18).* The yellow clods of initial cutaneous leishmaniasis most probably correspond to widened infundibula on the background of a granulomatous inflammation in the dermis whereas the yellow clods of lymphangioma correspond to dilated lymphatic vessels filled with lymphatic fluid (19).

Figure 6.16: *White structureless zone of calcinosis cutis*

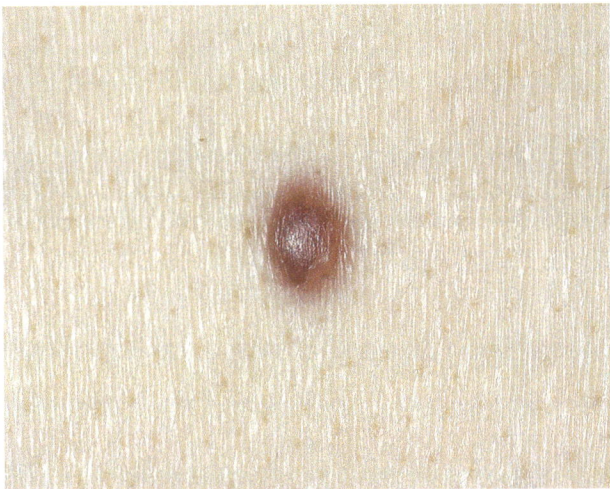

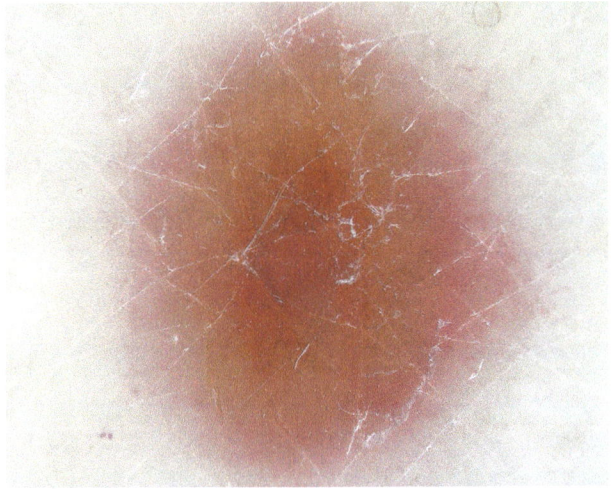

Figure 6.17: Yellow structureless zone of xanthogranuloma.
The structureless zone in the center of this xanthogranuloma in an adult is yellow and orange (dermatoscopy on the **right**).

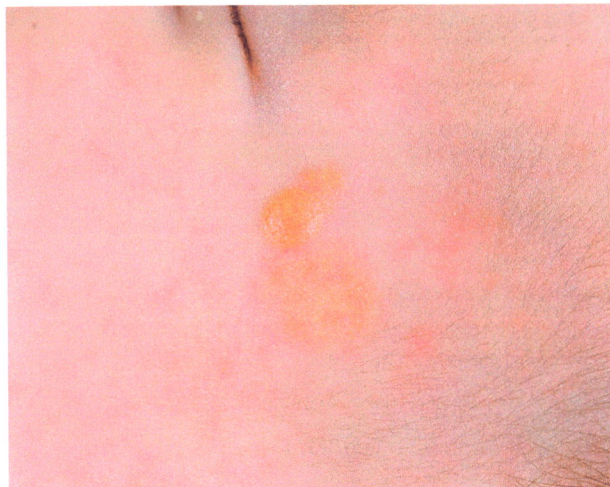

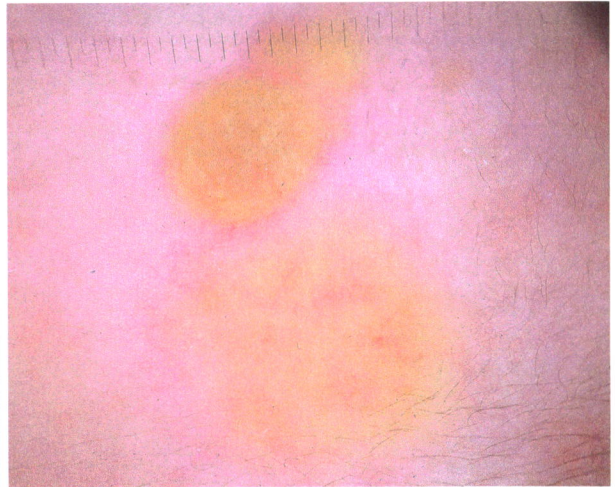

Figure 6.18: Yellow structureless zone of nevus sebaceous.
This nevus sebaceous in a newborn is structureless yellow on dermatoscopy **(right image)**.

6.2 Vascular patterns

In dermatoscopic assessment of pigmented lesions, blood vessel morphology is only ever accorded the status of being a clue to diagnosis, as patterns formed by vessels (20) are less specific and hence less important than pigment patterns and colors. The patterns formed by blood vessels are no more diagnostically specific in amelanotic lesions, but in the absence of melanin pigment, analysis of vessel patterns must assume greater importance.

The pattern of vessels is assessed using the principles detailed in chapter 3. Vessels may be seen as dots, clods or lines *(6.19)*. Lines may be straight, curved, looped, serpentine, helical or coiled. When one vessel type predominates, this is called a "monomorphous" pattern of vessels. When more than one type of vessel is seen, the pattern is called "polymorphous". In addition to the type of vessels, their arrangement – both how vessels are arranged relative to each other, and how vessels are distributed throughout the lesion – may also be of diagnostic significance *(6.20)*.

In the majority of cases, vessels appear to be distributed randomly, i.e. not arranged in any specific manner throughout the lesion. Vessels as dots or coils may be arranged in straight lines (linear arrangement) or in serpentine lines (serpiginous arrangement). When vessels as dots or coils are not uniformly distributed but

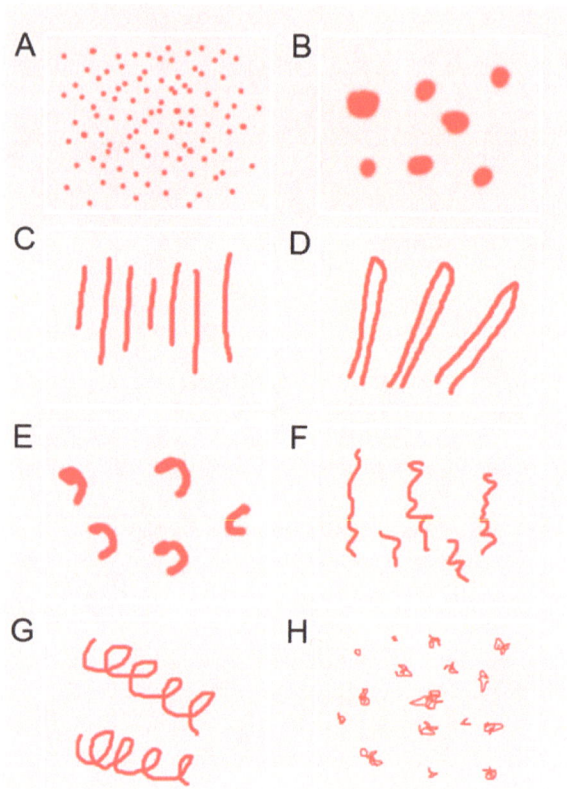

Figure 6.19: Type of vessels.
Vessels may be seen as dots (A), clods (B), or lines (C–H). Lines may be straight (C), looped (D), curved (E), serpentine (F), helical (G), or coiled (H).

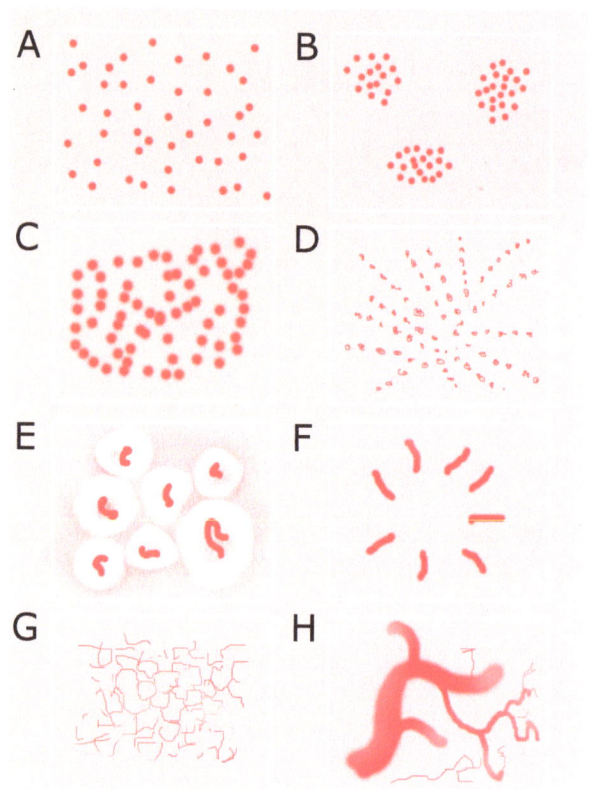

Figure 6.20: Arrangements of vessels.
Vessels may be randomly distributed (A), clustered (B), serpiginous (C) linear (D), centered (E), radial (F), reticular (G), or branched (H).

are denser at some sites than others, this arrangement is termed "clustered". Linear vessels of any type at the periphery that are oriented towards but do not cross the center are termed "radial". The arrangement of linear vessels (most commonly curved, sometimes serpentine or looped) in the center of skin colored or light brown clods is termed "centered". Straight linear vessels that intersect each other nearly at right angles have a "reticular" arrangement. Finally, serpentine vessels may be arranged such that multiple vessels originate from one common vessel; the derivative vessels typically originate from a thicker vessel. This arrangement is termed "branched".

Vessel morphology varies with lesion thickness. The capillary loops that rise from the superficial vascular plexus and extend towards the surface of the skin may appear as dots or curved or looped lines, depending on the angle from which they are viewed *(6.21)*. In flat lesions, most vessels are viewed end on and so appear as dots or short curved lines. As a lesion becomes thick-

er, there is a tendency for more vessels to be viewed obliquely and thus seen as loops. As malignant neoplasms become thicker, neovascularization becomes more common.

This variation means the same vessel morphology may have different diagnostic significance in nodules compared to flat lesions.

6.3 Differential diagnosis of non-pigmented lesions

General principles

As a general principle, even in a largely non-pigmented lesion, if there is any pigment at all that can be attributed to melanin (black, brown, blue or gray) one should first attempt to diagnose a lesion using a pigmented lesion algorithm *(6.22)*. Only if there truly is no pigment or if the pigmented features present are non-specific, should a non-pigmented algorithm be used. The meth-

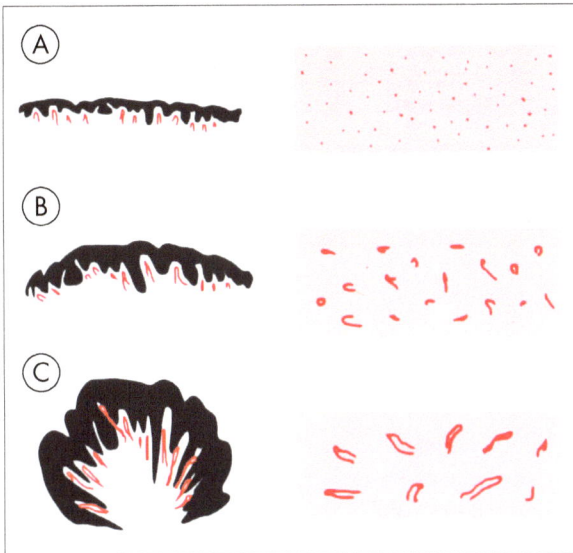

Figure 6.21: *Vessels in flat and raised lesions.*
The capillary loops that rise from the superficial vascular plexus and extend towards the surface of the skin may appear as dots or curved or looped lines, depending on the angle from which they are viewed.

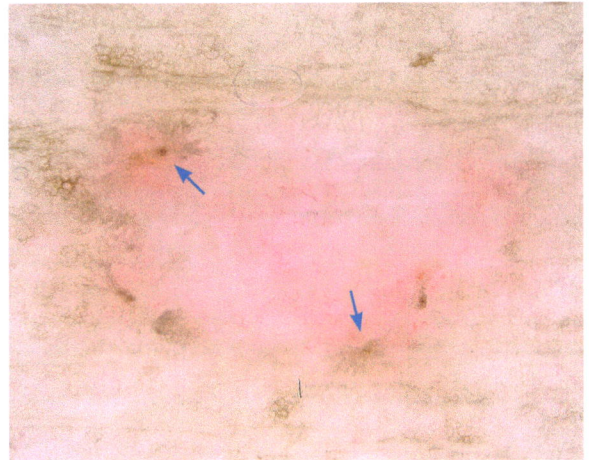

Figure 6.22: *Pigment first.*
Examine "non-pigmented" lesions carefully for any pigment before using a non-pigmented algorithm. On close inspection, two areas of converging radial lines are apparent, allowing a confident diagnosis of basal cell carcinoma.

od we present requires the integration of clinical and dermatoscopy features to reach an acceptable level of diagnostic accuracy.

As a matter of convenience, clinical features are usually assessed before dermatoscopy. These findings are then included in the diagnostic process as one proceeds with dermatoscopy.

The main features assessed clinically are whether the lesion is flat or raised; whether it is solitary or one of many; and the presence or absence of ulceration, scale, and keratin.

It is critical to differentiate between flat and raised non-pigmented lesions. When we speak of flat lesions we do not mean that the lesion must be so flat as to be impalpable. Rather, a lesion is termed flat when the horizontal diameter greatly exceeds height. Macules, flat papules and patches are flat whereas elevated papules and nodules are raised.

While it is true that neoplasms tend to be solitary and inflammatory conditions tend to be multiple, this is not always the case. In particular, actinic keratosis is often multiple. Most critically, a solitary non-pigmented neoplasm – most commonly Bowen's disease, but rarely even a non-pigmented melanoma – may be concealed amongst multiple patches of psoriasis.

As already mentioned, ulceration does not suggest a specific diagnosis but should (in the absence of trauma) prompt the consideration of malignancy.

Scale is an important hallmark of Bowen's disease and actinic keratosis but is obviously also found in inflammatory conditions. On the rare occasions scale is seen in superficial basal cell carcinoma or melanocytic lesions, it is usually a consequence of irritation such as rubbing or scratching. Occasionally nevi show a spongiotic reaction that leads to scaling (21). With severe chronic sun damage, the entire skin surface may be scaly, including that overlying lesions.

If keratin is present, the main differential diagnoses include well-differentiated squamous cell carcinomas/ keratoacanthomas, seborrheic keratoses and viral warts (22). Keratin can also be found in Unna or Miescher nevi (keratin plugs on the surface between papillomatous invaginations), in keratinizing adnexal proliferations such as pilomatrixoma (subsurface keratin) (23), in keratinizing cysts (subsurface keratin), and in angiokeratoma (surface keratin) (24). After clinical assessment one then proceeds to dermatoscopy.

Dermatoscopy of non-pigmented lesions

The first step in assessing non-pigmented lesions is to decide whether they are flat or raised. The vascular pattern is more diagnostically significant in flat lesions than in raised lesions. In raised lesions, other clues (ulceration, keratin, and white clues) take priority over vessel pattern analysis, just as pigmented structures take priority for pigmented lesions.

```
                                    Dots ──────── Melanocytic nevus
                                              ─── Inflammatory skin diseases (e.g. psoriasis)
                                                  (Bowen's disease)

                                    Clods ─────── Hemangioma
                                              ─── Vascular malformation
                                                  Hemorrhage

                                  Serpentine ──── Basal cell carcinoma

                 Monomorphous
                 vascular pattern   Coiled ────── Bowen's disease
                                                  (inflammatory skin diseases)

     Flat

                                  Vessels as ──── Exclude melanoma
                                  dots present

                 Polymorphous
                 vascular pattern  Vessels as ──── Basal cell carcinoma
                                  dots absent ──── Seborrheic keratosis
                                                   Bowen's disease
                                                   Something else
```

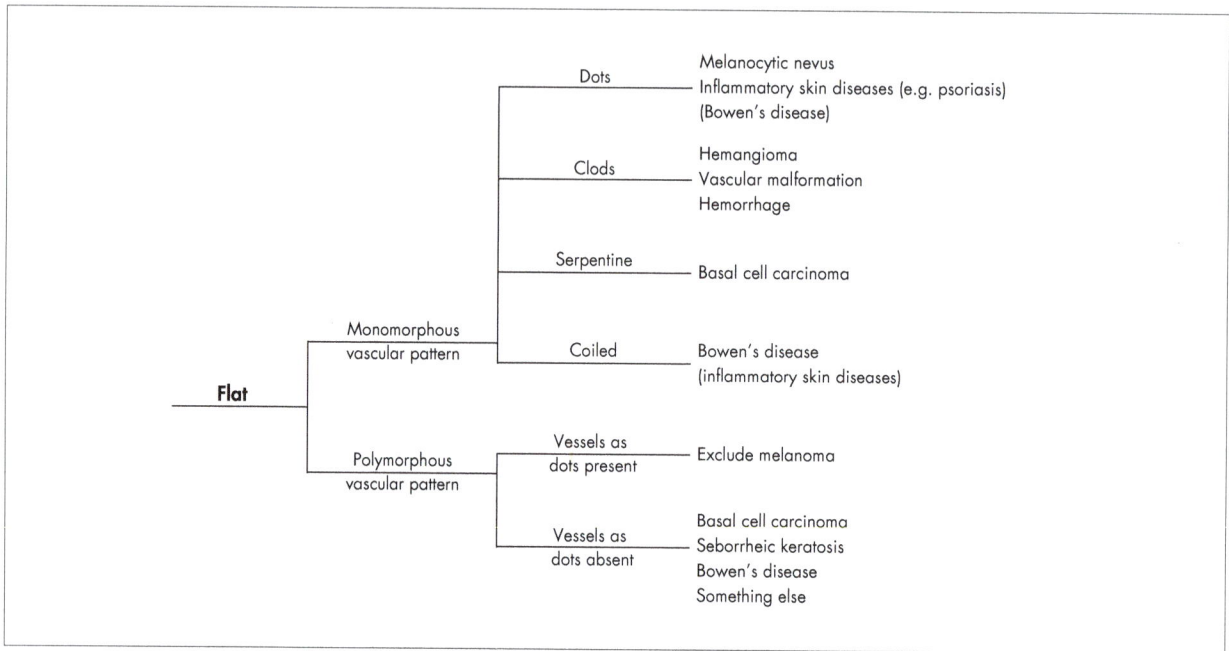

Figure 6.23: Algorithm for flat non-pigmented lesions with visible blood vessels

Flat non-pigmented lesions

Because nearly all pigmented lesions may also appear in a non-pigmented form, the differential diagnosis for flat non-pigmented lesions encompasses nearly the entire spectrum of melanocytic and non-melanocytic lesions discussed in chapter 2. In addition to this spectrum of neoplasms, various inflammatory skin diseases must also be considered. Melanocytic lesions that may appear as non-pigmented skin-colored to red macules or patches are Clark nevi, "superficial" or "superficial and deep" congenital nevi, Spitz nevi and, of course, melanoma. Keratinocytic cancers (actinic keratosis, Bowen's disease, superficial basal cell carcinoma) and many inflammatory skin diseases, for example psoriasis, nummular dermatitis, porokeratosis, lupus erythematosus and lichen planus occur mainly as flat pink lesions. We will discuss the dermatoscopic appearance of inflammatory lesions in greater detail in chapter 8. Rarely, even seborrheic keratosis and dermatofibroma may be flat and non-pigmented. The most common flat non-pigmented lesions and their appearance on dermatoscopy are shown in *table 6.2*.

If vessels are seen, there is a relatively simple algorithm for flat non-pigmented lesions, starting with the assessment of vascular patterns *(6.23)*. While it has proved useful in the hands of the authors, it lacks the specificity of algorithms to assess pigmented lesions. It should also be seen as evolving, rather than an algorithm carved in stone.

Next, one decides whether the vascular pattern is monomorphous or polymorphous.

When there is a monomorphous pattern of vessels, a distinction is made between vessels as dots, clods, and vessels as lines. In cases of vessels as dots, the differential diagnosis comprises Bowen's disease, inflammatory skin diseases such as psoriasis, and benign melanocytic lesions. There are exceptional cases of flat amelanotic melanomas on chronic sun-damaged skin that have a monomorphous pattern of dots, but a flat amelanotic melanocytic lesion with a monomorphous vascular pattern of dots is nearly always a nevus.

Scale (not always visible on dermatoscopy) is usually present in inflammatory lesions and Bowen's disease but not in melanocytic lesions. Further differentiation is then performed as far as possible on the basis of the clinical context and additional clues. The scale of psoriatic lesions is practically always white, whereas the scale of different types of dermatitis (for example nummular dermatitis or seborrheic dermatitis) is mixed with serum and appear yellow or orange (25). The scale of porokeratosis usually presents as a peripheral rim (26, 27) that should not be confused with delicate peripheral pigmentation of some flat basal cell carcinomas. The differentiation between psoriasis and Bowen's disease (intraepidermal carcinoma) can be challenging. The vessels of Bowen's disease are usually coils (28) and those of psoriasis usually dots (29) *(6.24)*. Sometimes, however, the coils of Bowen's disease are so small

Table 6.2: Flat non-pigmented (amelanotic) lesions

Diagnosis	Pattern of vessels	Clues
Actinic keratosis	Erythema around the openings of the infundibula	Face: In the center of the circular erythema there is a yellow or an orange clod; white circles; 4 white dots arranged in a square (polarized dermatoscopy); scale
Bowen's disease	Monomorphous, coiled or less often dot vessels, occasionally erythema (red or pink structureless area)	Coiled vessels arranged in clusters or in lines; scale
Basal cell carcinoma, superficial	Monomorphous or polymorphous, primarily serpentine vessels. Arrangement may be branched. Occasionally mainly erythema (red or pink structureless area).	Polarizing-specific (perpendicular) white lines; ulceration; adherent fiber sign may confirm ulceration
Telangiectasia macularis perstans (variant of cutaneous mastocytosis)	Thin reticular vessels	No scale
Seborrheic keratosis, flat	Monomorphous or polymorphous, vessels as lines (coiled, looped or serpentine)	White dots; white, yellow or orange clods
Angiomas and vascular malformations	Monomorphous, clods	None
Spider nevus (Nevus araneus)	Monomorphous, thick reticular vessels	Central red dot, sometimes pulsating
Dermatofibroma	vessels of many types can be seen but vessels as dots are most common	White structureless area or white lines in the center
Psoriasis	Monomorphous, dots	White scale
Pityriasis rosea	Monomorphous, dots	Peripheral scale
Spongiotic dermatitis (for example nummular dermatitis)	Monomorphous, dots	Yellow scale
Lupus erythematosus	Erythema, usually no discernable vessels	White circles, white structureless zones (advanced lesions with sclerosis)
Porokeratosis	Monomorphous, dots	Ring-shaped scale at the periphery (cornoid lamella)
Lichen planus	Monomorphous, dots	Thick white or skin colored lines (Wickham striae)
Clark nevus	Monomorphous, dots	No scale, flat (macule)
Superficial and deep congenital nevus	Monomorphous, dots, linear vessels (especially curved) in raised part	No scale, usually raised on the center
Spitz nevus	Monomorphous, dots	No scale, occasionally white or skin-colored lines, slightly raised
Melanoma	Polymorphous, dots and lines of all types	No scale, white lines, remnants of pigmentation dermatoscopically (especially brown structureless zones)

that the vessels appear as dots and in long standing, elevated lesions of psoriasis the vessels may appear as coils. In psoriasis the vessels tend to be randomly distributed over the lesions whereas in Bowen's disease they tend to be arranged in clusters or lines. In contrast to Bowen's disease (often dull white or yellow scales) the scales of psoriasis tend to be shiny white.

As discussed in Chapter 3, a monomorphous pattern of red clods (vessels as clods) indicates a hemangioma or a vascular malformation.

As well as Bowen's disease, coiled vessels may be seen in psoriasis, lichen simplex chronicus, and other inflammatory diseases. Serpentine vessels are seen in superficial basal cell carcinoma (6.25), but this diagnosis is more reliable when other specific clues to basal cell carcinoma are present.

The reticular pattern of vessels is not included in the algorithm because it is too unspecific (it occurs, for instance, on chronic sun-damaged skin). Thin reticular vessels are found in lesions of a specific type of mastocytosis,

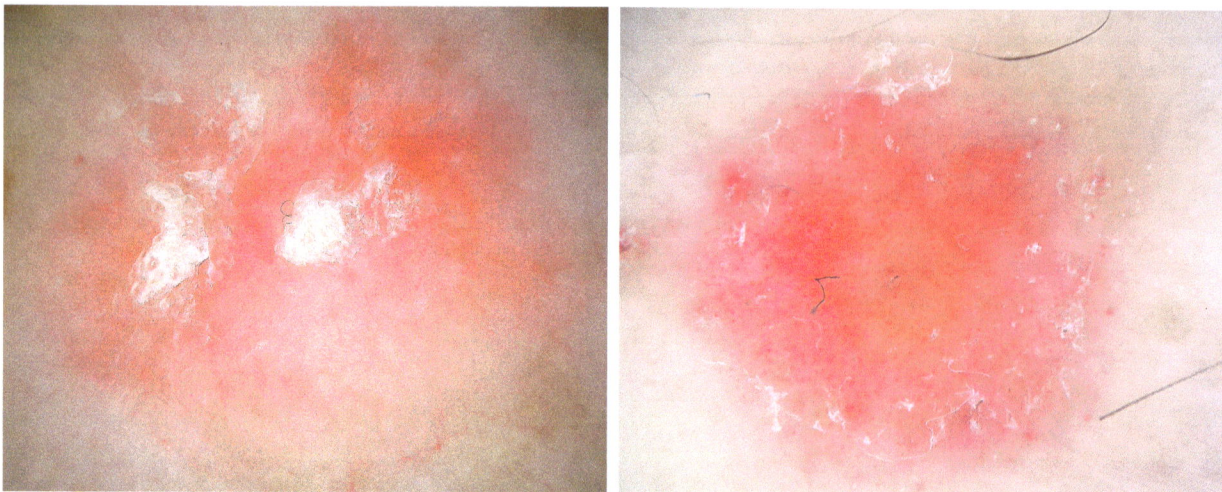

Figure 6.24: *Dermatoscopy of psoriasis and Bowen's disease.*
Psoriasis on the left is typified by vessels as dots that are randomly distributed and shiny white scales. Bowen's disease on the right is characterized by coiled vessels (here the coils are very small and imitate vessels as dots).

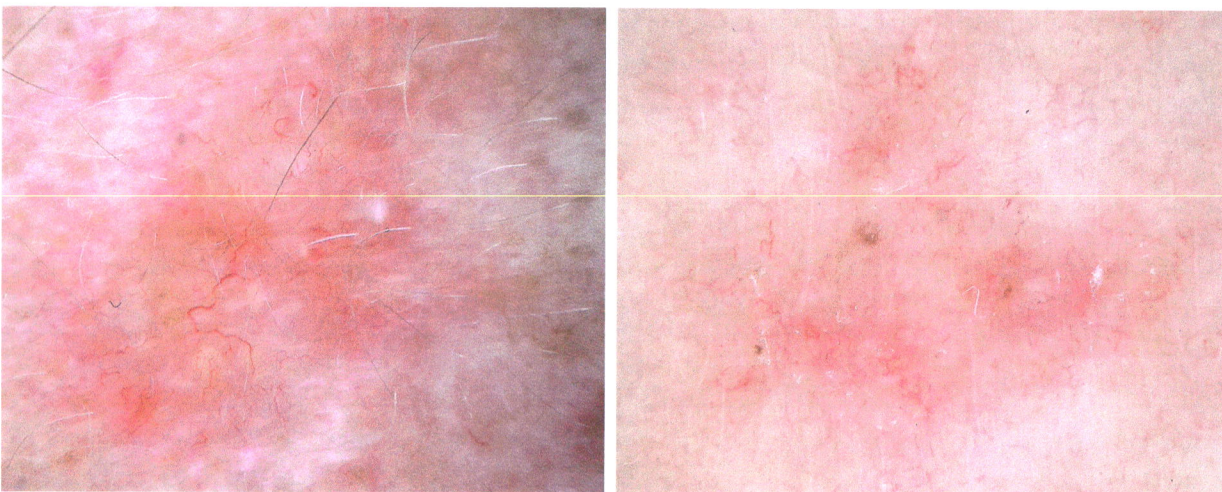

Figure 6.25: *Dermatoscopy of flat basal cell carcinomas.*
Flat basal cell carcinomas are typified be the presence of serpentine vessels. **On the left:** *Dermatoscopy of a flat basal cell carcinoma of the face.* **On the right:** *Dermatoscopy of a flat basal cell carcinoma of the trunk.*

telangiectasia macularis eruptiva perstans (30–32). Thick reticular vessels are found in "spider nevus" (nevus araneus). A central dot vessel (the supplying arteriole) is commonly seen, sometimes with visible pulsations. Dermatofibromas are occasionally non-pigmented (4). If they are flat they usually show a vascular pattern of dots or coils, and may also show a typical central white structureless area or central polarizing-specific white lines.

When the vascular pattern is polymorphous, one should proceed in a stepwise manner, as in cases of pigmented lesions with more than one pattern. The investigator first determines whether vessels as dots are present. As in all vascular patterns, a few vessels as dots are not significant; to constitute a pattern they must cover a significant part of the lesion. In *6.26* and *6.27* we show flat non-pigmented lesions with *(6.26)* and without *(6.27)* vessels as dots. If the vascular pattern is polymorphous and includes vessels as dots *(figure 6.26,* middle and bottom row) a melanoma cannot be excluded with certainty and the lesion should be submitted for histopathology. If it is difficult to decide

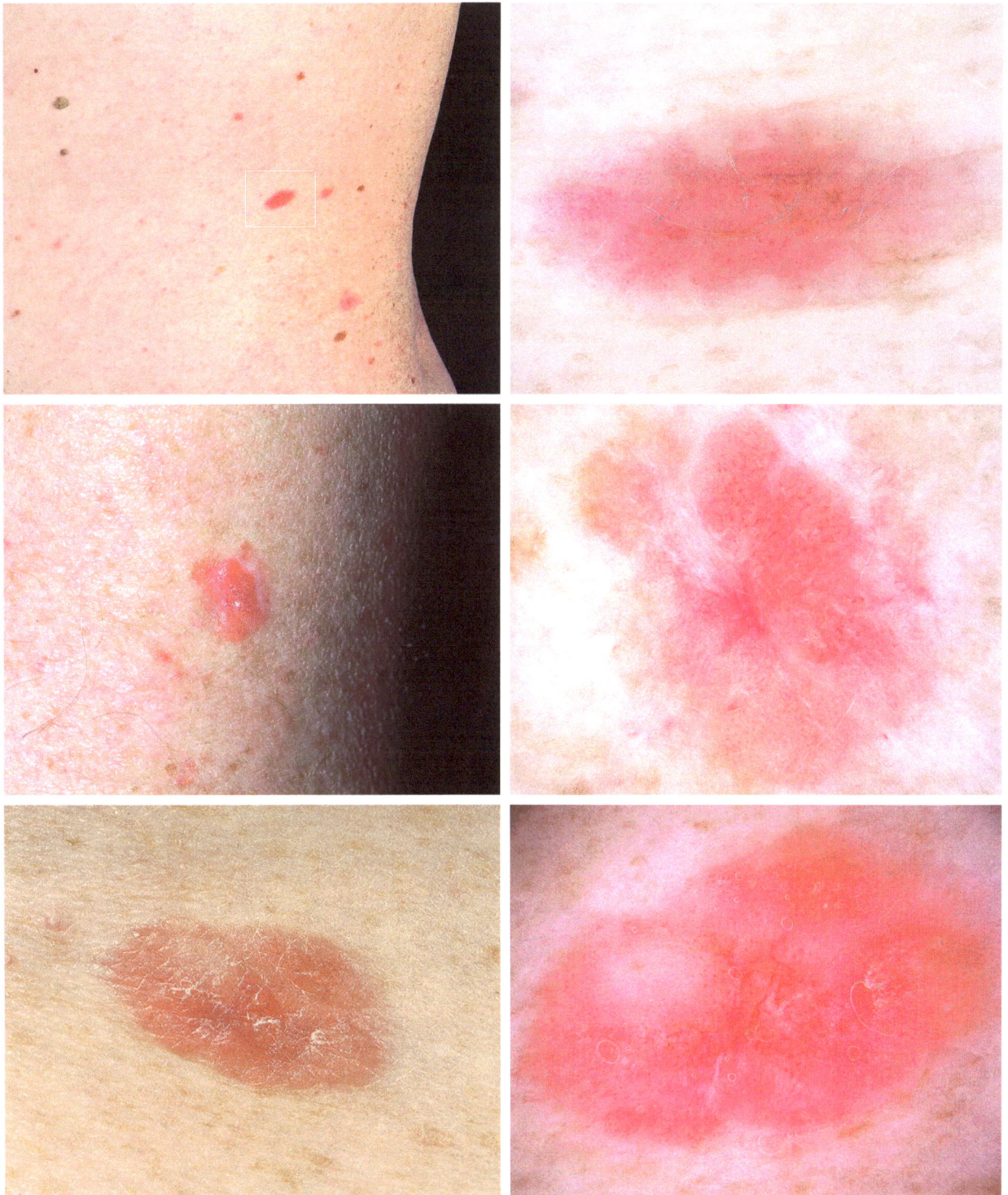

Figure 6.26: Flat non-pigmented lesions with vessels as dots.
Clinical view **left,** dermatoscopy **right. Top:** Monomorphous pattern of vessels (only vessels as dots) in a Clark nevus. **Middle:** Polymorphous pattern of vessels (vessels as dots and serpentine linear vessels) in a melanoma (< 1 mm). **Bottom:** Polymorphous pattern of vessels (vessels as dots and serpentine linear vessels) in a melanoma (< 1 mm).

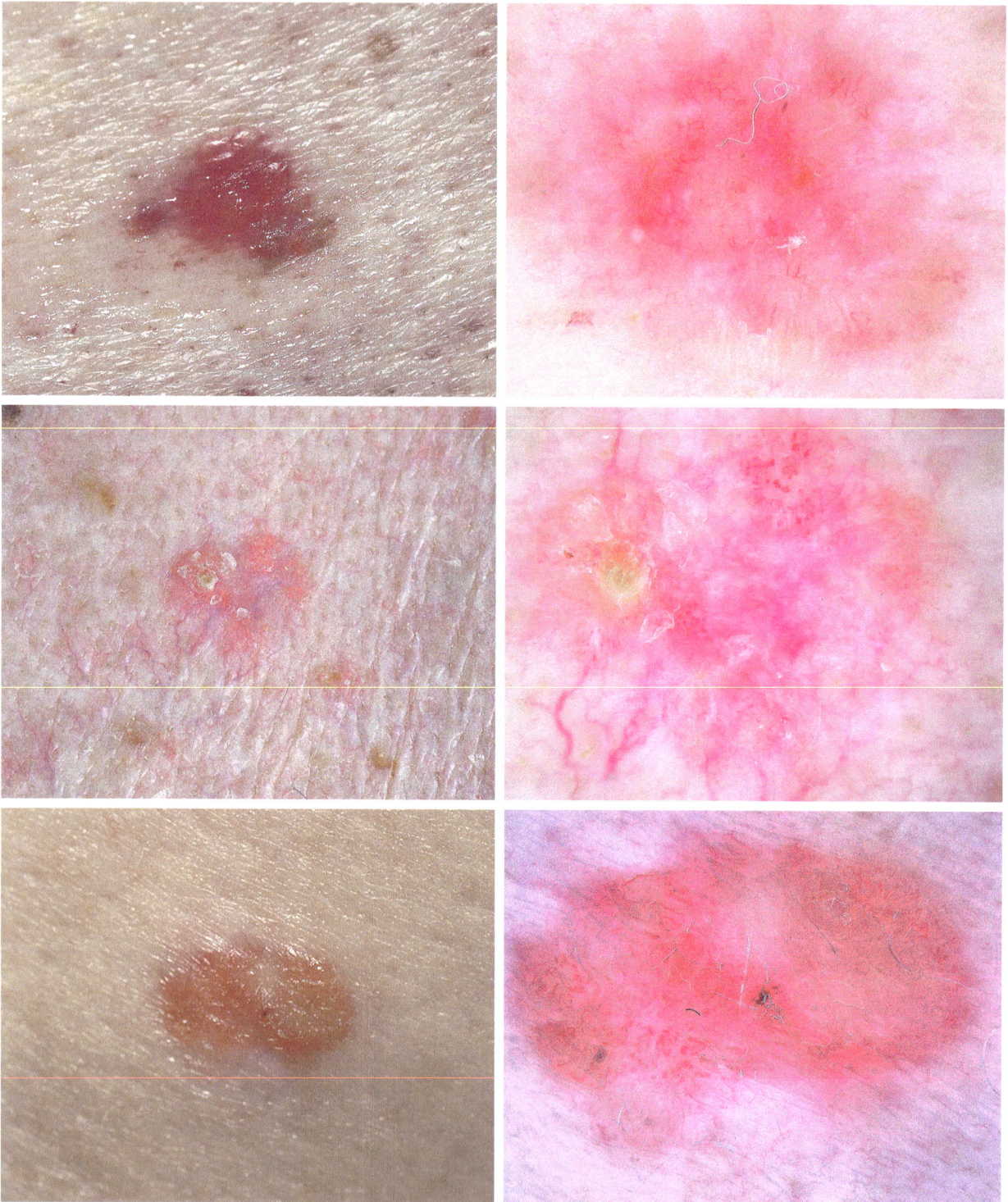

Figure 6.27: *Flat non-pigmented lesions without vessels as dots.*
*Clinical view **left**, dermatoscopy **right**. **Top:** Monomorphous pattern of vessels (only serpentine vessels) in a basal cell carcinoma on the trunk (note: ulceration and adherent fiber sign). **Middle:** Monomorphous pattern (coiled vessels) in Bowen's disease (note the presence of scale). **Bottom:** Polymorphous pattern of vessels (serpentine and coiled vessels) in a basal cell carcinoma on the trunk.*

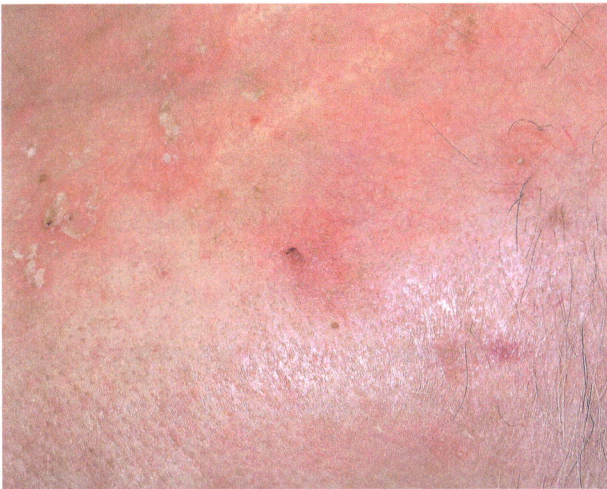

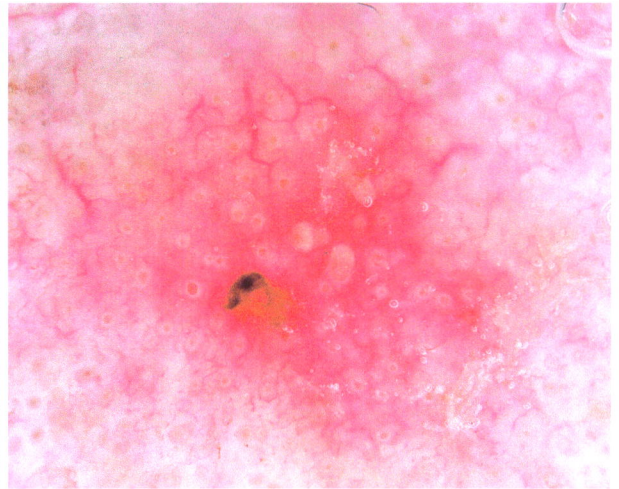

Figure 6.28: Actinic keratosis.
Facial actinic keratoses typically show erythema without vessels and sometimes show white circles around follicular openings. The serpentine vessels seen peripherally are those of chronic sun-damaged skin and are not part of the lesion (image courtesy of Iris Zalaudek).

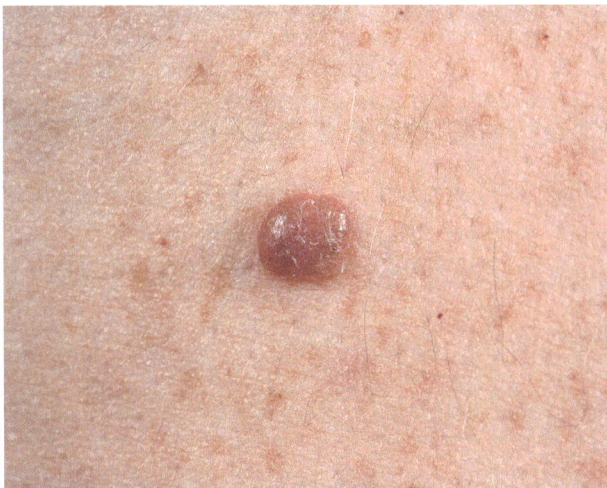

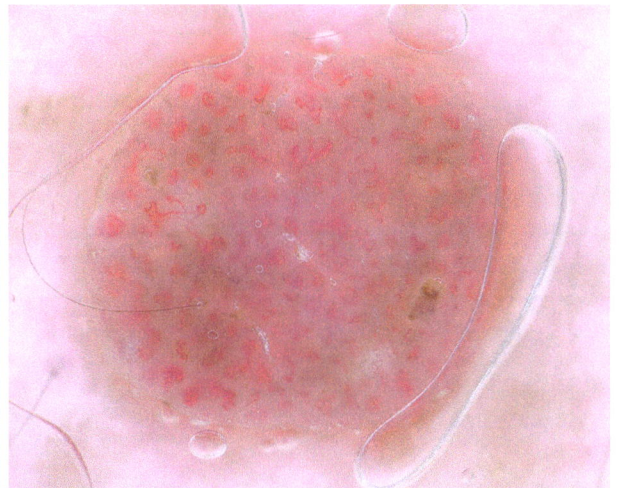

Figure 6.29: Non-pigmented seborrheic keratosis.
A non-pigmented seborrheic keratosis presenting as a nodule with looped, serpentine and coiled vessels. A few white dots and yellow clods are the only clues that point to seborrheic keratosis. A seborrheic keratosis cannot be diagnosed with certainty and it is better to remove the lesion by shave biopsy for histopathologic evaluation.

whether the pattern is one of dots or small coils, it is prudent to assume they are dots and thus keep melanoma in the differential diagnosis.

When there are no vessels as dots but polymorphous linear vessels (including coiled, serpentine, and looped vessels) the investigator should consider superficial basal cell carcinoma, Bowen's disease or seborrheic keratosis. In cases of superficial basal cell carcinoma the predominant structures are thin serpentine vessels (33), whereas Bowen's disease is marked by coiled vessels (28). Ulceration is more common in flat basal

cell carcinomas, scale is more common in Bowen's disease. Seborrheic keratosis may have all types of vessels as lines, including looped vessels (34). However, in most cases there will be one or more of white dots and white, yellow or orange clods.

When no vessels are visible or when a diffuse erythema is seen in a flat lesion, dermatoscopy is of no significant benefit unless other clues are present. Actinic keratoses *(6.28)* often have an erythematous background without discernable vessels. Facial actinic keratosis may have white circles (8), but white circles should also lead to a consideration of invasive squamous cell carcinoma (9). Erythema and white circles are also found in lupus erythematosus (10). When sclerosis becomes prominent, lesions of lupus erythematosus show white structureless zones, especially in the center. The polarizing specific "four dot clod" can be found in actinic keratosis and in lupus erythematosus (15).

Nodular non-pigmented lesions

The assessment of non-pigmented nodular lesions is one of the biggest challenges in dermatoscopy. The differential diagnosis to be taken into account is vast. Benign nodular non-pigmented non-melanocytic lesions include seborrheic keratoses *(6.29),* dermatofibromas (4), warts (22) (including molluscum contagiosum, *6.30 middle),* infectious nodules (for example Leishmaniasis (19)), all forms of prurigo (35) (for example picker's nodule), angioma (including pyogenic granuloma, *6.3),* sebaceous gland hyperplasia (12, 13) *(6.11),* clear cell acanthoma (36) *(6.31),* common benign neoplasms such as pilomatrixoma (23) *(6.15)* and rare ones such as eccrine poroma (37, 38) *(6.32)* or trichoepithelioma (39) *(6.33),* and all kind of cysts including epidermal cysts or mucoid (myxoid) finger cysts (40) *(6.34).* Non-melanocytic malignancies include poorly (41) *(6.30 top, 6.35 bottom left)* and well differentiated squamous cell carcinomas (9) (including keratoacanthoma, *6.35, top left),* basal cell carcinoma (33) *(6.36),* rare cutaneous malignancies like Merkel cell carcinoma (42) *(6.37),* and cutaneous metastases of any malignancy. In melanocytic lesions the differential diagnoses are limited to Unna or Miescher nevus *(6.38),* Spitz nevus and melanoma *(6.35 bottom right, 6.39).*

The principal nodular non-pigmented lesions and their dermatoscopic appearances are listed in *table 6.3.* Based on the descriptions of individual lesions it becomes clear that the morphology of vessels assists little in diagnosis. Unlike flat lesions, the distinction between monomorphous and polymorphous patterns of vessels has no diagnostic significance for nodules. With the exception of some specific arrangements discussed below, vascular patterns have poor specificity for nodular non-pigmented lesions. Therefore, ulceration, keratin and white clues are given priority over vessel pattern analysis when assessing nodules.

As stated previously, in the absence of a clear and convincing history of trauma, any solitary ulcerated non-pigmented nodule should be submitted for histopathology. In most ulcerated non-pigmented nodules it will not be possible to come to a specific diagnosis by dermatoscopy. Nodular basal cell carcinomas are the commonest nodular malignancy and they are frequently ulcerated, but any other malignant neoplasm like Merkel cell carcinoma and melanoma can also be ulcerated. Benign conditions that may present as ulcerated nodules include pyogenic granulomas, nodular prurigo (picker's nodule) and some infectious diseases (e.g. leishmaniasis).

If surface keratin is present in an amelanotic nodule, the principal diagnoses are well-differentiated squamous cell carcinoma/keratoacanthoma, warts, and seborrheic keratosis. The presence of keratin helps to distinguish well-differentiated squamous cell carcinomas or keratoacanthomas from other raised non-pigmented neoplastic lesions such as basal cell carcinomas, Merkel cell carcinomas and amelanotic melanomas. Unna or

Table 6.3: Raised non-pigmented lesions

Diagnosis	Pattern of vessels	Dermatoscopic clues and clues beyond dermatoscopy
Basal cell carcinoma	Serpentine, branched vessels	Dermatoscopic clues: Ulceration, white lines, structureless white
Keratoacanthoma	Radially arranged vessels as lines that may be straight, curved, serpentine, looped or branched	Dermatoscopic clues: Central keratin plug (stronger clue when branched serpentine vessels are adjacent to keratin plug), surface keratin, white structureless areas and white circles
Squamous cell carcinoma (well differentiated)	All types of vessels as lines, including coiled ones, occasionally also branched vessels	Dermatoscopic clues: Surface keratin, white structureless areas and white circles
Squamous cell carcinoma (poorly differentiated)	All types of vessels as lines, including coiled ones, occasionally also branched vessels, vessels cover more than 50 % of the lesion	Dermatoscopic clues: absence of surface keratin, white structureless areas and white circles

Diagnosis	Pattern of vessels	Dermatoscopic clues and clues beyond dermatoscopy
Clear cell acanthoma	Coiled or dot vessels in serpiginous arrangement	None
Eccrine poroma	Coiled, serpentine and branched vessels, polymorphous vessels	Dermatoscopic clues: The linear vessels are thin Other clues: Anatomic site (most commonly occurs on palms and soles)
Hemangiomas and vascular malformations (including pyogenic granuloma)	Vessels as clods	Dermatoscopic clues: Discrete vessels as lines or dots usually absent, Pyogenic granuloma: Thick white or skin colored intersecting lines, white or brown margin Other clues to pyogenic granuloma: Recent history of trauma
Prurigo (picker's nodule)	Radial vessels (if centrally ulcerated), serpiginous arrangement of vessels occasionally	Clinical context, distribution of lesions, history, number of lesions
Viral warts	Verruca plana: Monomorphous vessels as dots Verruca vulgaris: Skin-colored to white clods, each with a central dot vessel Verruca plantaris/palmaris: Yellow structureless zone with red to black dots and lines (hemorrhage)	Clinical context, distribution of lesions, history, number of lesions
Leishmaniasis	Polymorphous vascular pattern	Dermatoscopic clues: Yellow clods, ulceration Other clues: Clinical context, history, recent travel in endemic area
Metastasis	Polymorphous with linear vessels, branched vessels	Clinical context, history, number of lesions
Molluscum contagiosum	Radial vessels	Dermatoscopic clues: Central white or skin-colored or orange clod
Merkel cell carcinoma	Branched vessels and other vessels as lines	None
Sebaceous gland hyperplasia	Radial vessels, usually curved or serpentine	Dermatoscopic clues: Central white or yellow clods. Vessels do not cross center.
Dermatofibroma	Vessels as dots	Dermatoscopic clues: Polarizing-specific white lines or reticular white lines or white structureless area in the center Other clues: Firm to the touch, "dimple sign"
Calcinosis cutis	Serpentine Vessels	Dermatoscopic clues: Structureless white zone Other clues: Firm to the touch (even firmer than dermatofibroma)
Pilomatrixoma	Serpentine Vessels	Dermatoscopic clues: Structureless white zone, dermal hemorrhage (blue structureless zone) Other clues: Firm to the touch (even firmer than dermatofibroma)
Unna or Miescher nevus	Thick curved vessels in the center of skin-colored clods, occasionally no vessels visible	Dermatoscopic clues: Skin-colored polygonal clods, seborrheic keratosis-like findings like white dots, yellow or orange clods Other clues: Clinical context (usually multiple similar lesions)
Spitz nevus	Vessels as dots	Dermatoscopic clue: White or skin-colored lines Other clues: Classic non-pigmented Spitz nevi most commonly occur on the face
Melanoma or metastasis of melanoma	Vessels of all types arranged randomly	Dermatoscopic clue: White lines. Helical vessels or vessels as pink or red clods Other clues: in the case of melanoma metastasis: clinical context, history, and number of lesions

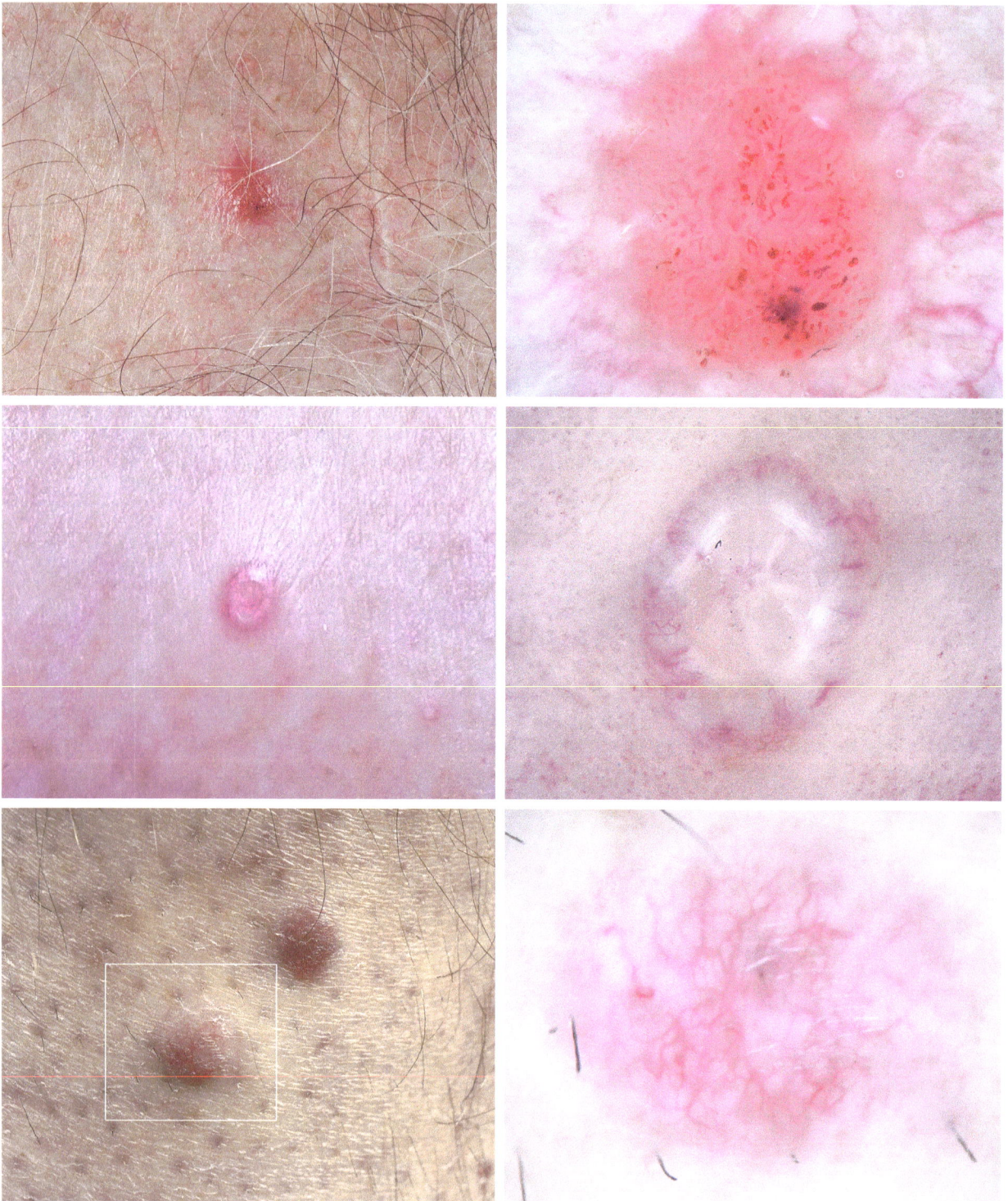

Figure 6.30: *Nodular non-pigmented lesions.*
Dermatoscopy **right column. Top:** *Polymorphous vessels arranged randomly (looped vessels, coiled vessels, clods) in a squamous cell carcinoma.* **Middle:** *Serpentine and loop vessels arranged radially in a molluscum contagiosum.* **Bottom:** *Serpentine branched vessels in a melanoma metastasis.*

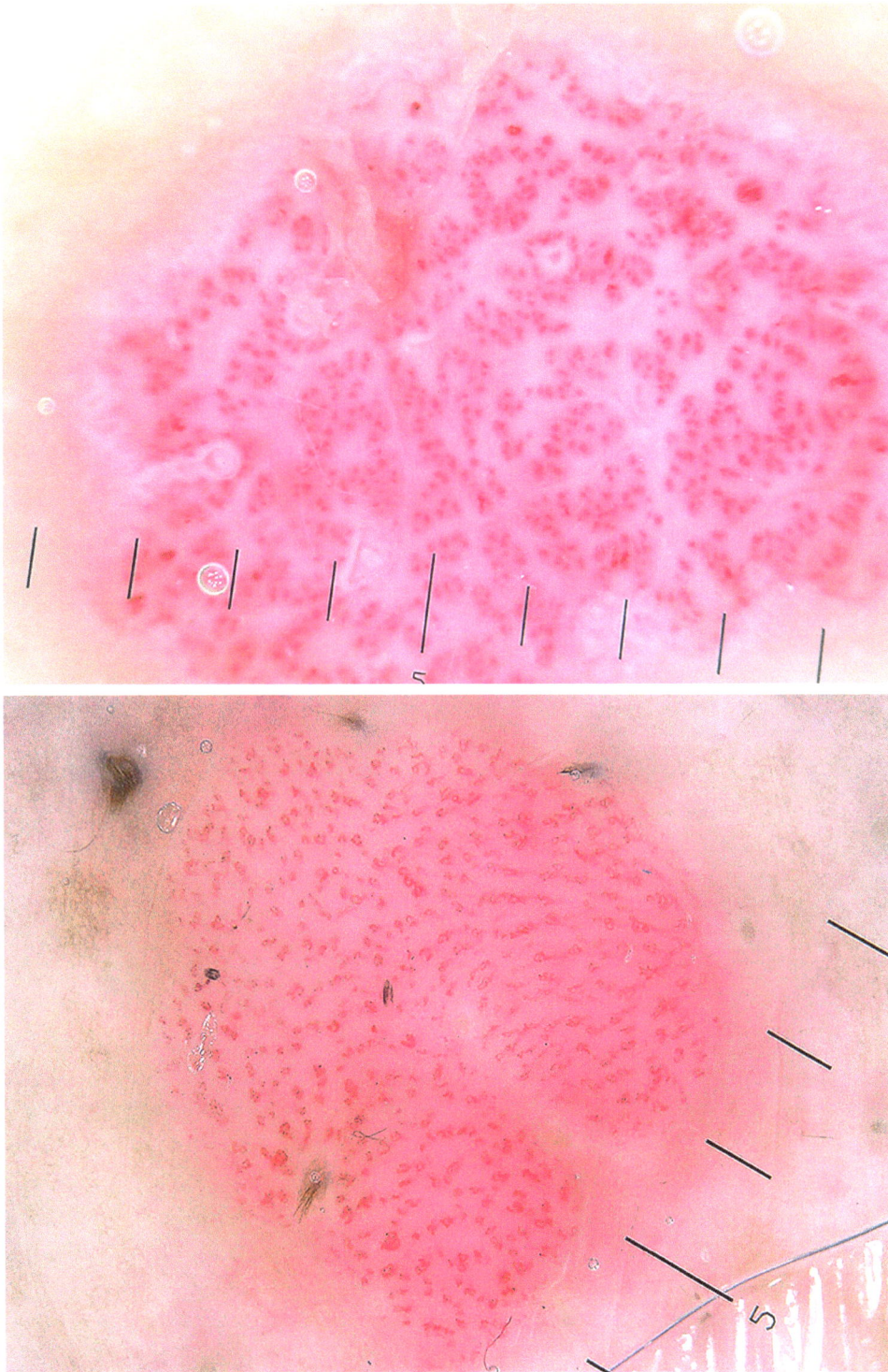

Figure 6.31: Clear cell acanthoma.
Two clear cell acanthomas with the dermatoscopy showing the characteristic serpiginous arrangement of small coiled vessels.

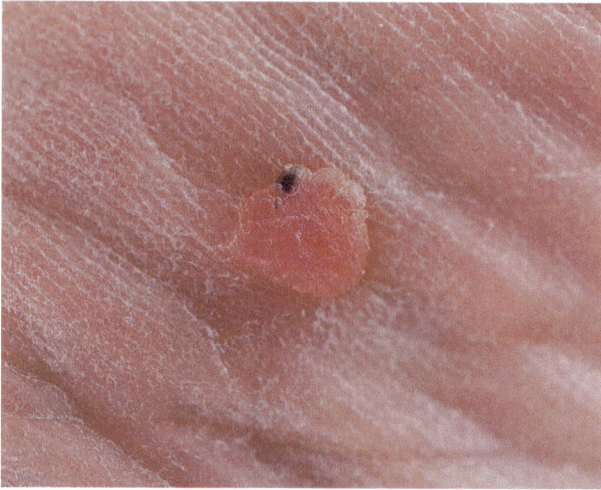

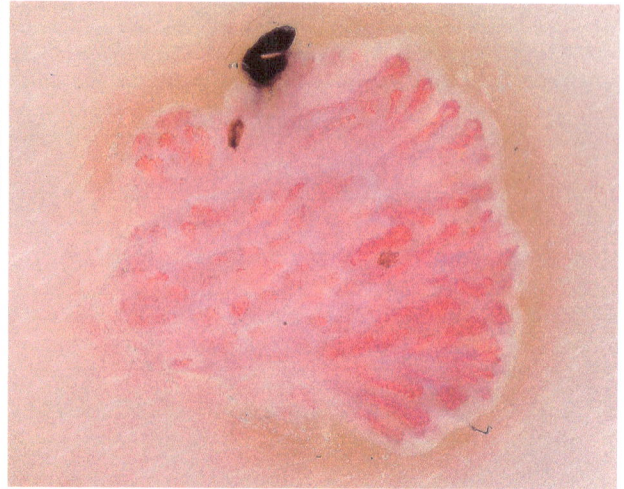

Figure 6.32: Eccrine poroma.
Eccrine poroma typically, but not exclusively, occurs on acral sites like the one depicted here. On dermatoscopy **(right)** one can see the looped and serpentine vessels with coiled ends.

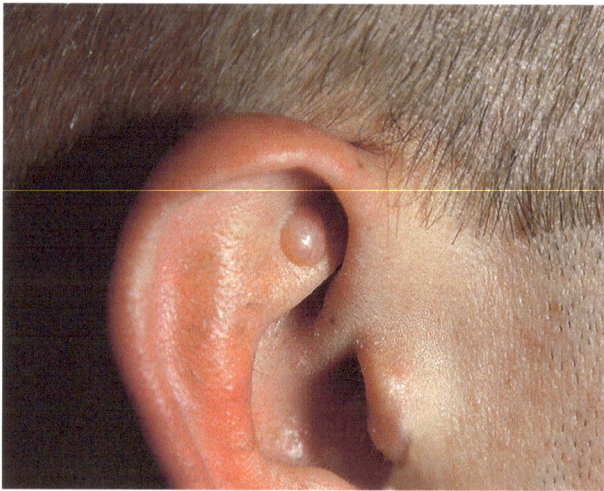

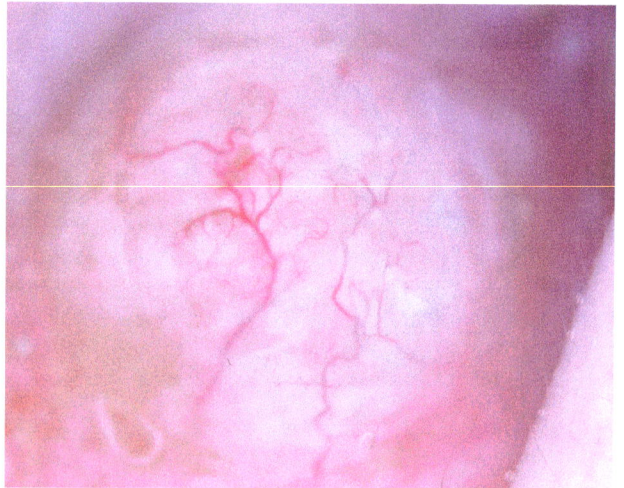

Figure 6.33: Trichoepithelioma.
Serpentine branched vessels are not specific for basal cell carcinoma. Trichoepithelioma is a benign neoplasm with follicular differentiation that shows serpentine branched vessels indistinguishable from those in basal cell carcinoma.

Miescher nevus or papillomatous parts of congenital nevi may show surface keratin in the epidermal invaginations. Pilomatrixoma is typified by subsurface keratin, which is characterized by a white structureless zone dermatoscopically. The subsurface keratin of epidermal cysts is hardly ever visible by dermatoscopy. Keratin may also be present in viral warts and angiokeratoma. A single central plug of keratin usually indicates a keratoacanthoma, but it is not possible to reliably distinguish between well-differentiated squamous cell carcinoma and keratoacanthoma dermatoscopically.

Blood spots in keratin are a good clue to the diagnosis of well-differentiated squamous cell carcinomas and keratoacanthomas (6.6).
While keratin is a good clue to well differentiated squamous cell carcinomas, poorly differentiated squamous cell carcinomas usually do not produce keratin.
Occasionally dermatoscopy does not permit a clear distinction between a central keratin plug and a central ulcer, particularly when a keratin plug contains bloods spots. This is an important distinction because radially arranged vessels may be found around an

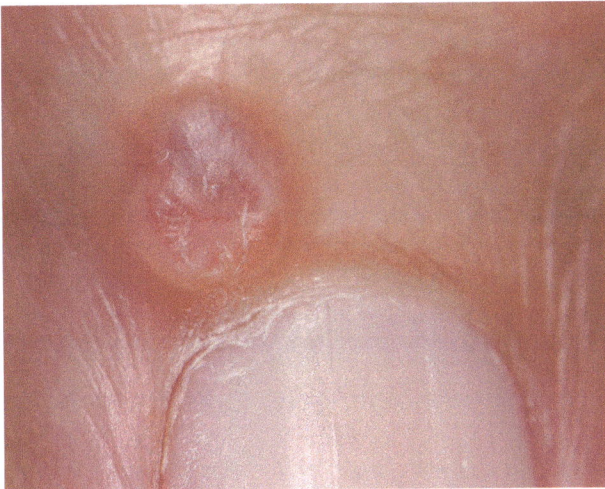

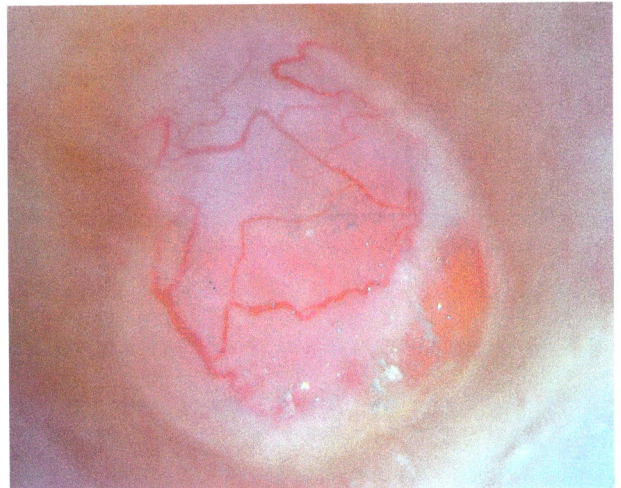

Figure 6.34: *Digital mucoid (myxoid) cyst.*
*Mucoid finger cysts may also show serpentine branched vessels on dermatoscopy **(right)**. Any tumor underneath the superficial vascular plexus including cysts can present with serpentine branched vessels.*

ulcer, regardless of the lesion's etiology. For example, ulcerated basal cell carcinomas may show radial vessels *(6.35 top, right)*.
Polarizing specific white lines and white clods can be found in malignant neoplasms (e.g. basal cell carcinoma, melanoma) and in some benign conditions (e.g. dermatofibroma, Spitz nevus, pyogenic granuloma). Reticular white lines may be present in melanoma or Spitz nevi and in some dermatofibromas. As a general rule, non-pigmented nodules with white lines should be biopsied or excised unless an unequivocal benign diagnosis can be made based on clues beyond dermatoscopy.
White circles in a nodular lesion point to keratoacanthoma/well-differentiated squamous cell carcinoma. Rarely, other lesions may show white circles, for example some basal cell carcinomas.
If ulceration, keratin and white clues are absent the specific diagnosis of nodular lesions becomes even more challenging.
In some cases, a specific vascular arrangement will help to narrow down the differential diagnosis. Three arrangements have high specificity for benign conditions, allowing these lesions to be excluded from further assessment.
The serpiginous arrangement of coiled vessels is so specific for clear cell acanthoma that no other diagnosis needs to be considered.
Linear vessels seen in the center of polygonal skin-colored clods is termed a centered arrangement. These vessels may be polymorphous. When this includes thick curved vessels, this is indicative of an Unna nevus or a

Miescher nevus. Centered vessels may also be found in seborrheic keratoses. The clods only pattern is specific for hemangioma. It is crucial that no vessels as lines are present as this can be a clue to malignancy.
The differential diagnoses of the other specific vessel arrangements include both benign and malignant tumors. Radially arranged vessels are found in sebaceous gland hyperplasia (additional clue: several white or yellow clods in central location), in molluscum contagiosum (additional clue: singular skin-colored or orange clod in central location) and in keratoacanthoma (additional clue: a keratin plug in central location, which may be white, yellow or orange). The radially arranged vessels in keratoacanthoma may be looped, linear, curved or branched-serpentine. The specificity of branched serpentine vessels for basal cell carcinoma is frequently overestimated. Of course basal cell carcinoma is the most common diagnosis in cases of non-pigmented nodular lesions with branched vessels, but in principle any invasive tumor in the dermis lying below the superficial vascular plexus may have this pattern of vessels. This is true for cysts, benign adnexal tumors (e.g. trichoblastoma or poroma), keratoacanthoma/ well differentiated squamous cell carcinoma and other types of neoplasms. It is true for the rare Merkel cell carcinoma, and cutaneous metastases regardless of the origin of the primary malignancy. In the absence of a confident specific benign diagnosis, non-pigmented nodules with branched serpentine vessels should be submitted for histopathology.
Eccrine poroma is characterized by a combination of coiled, serpentine and branched vessels. The peculiar

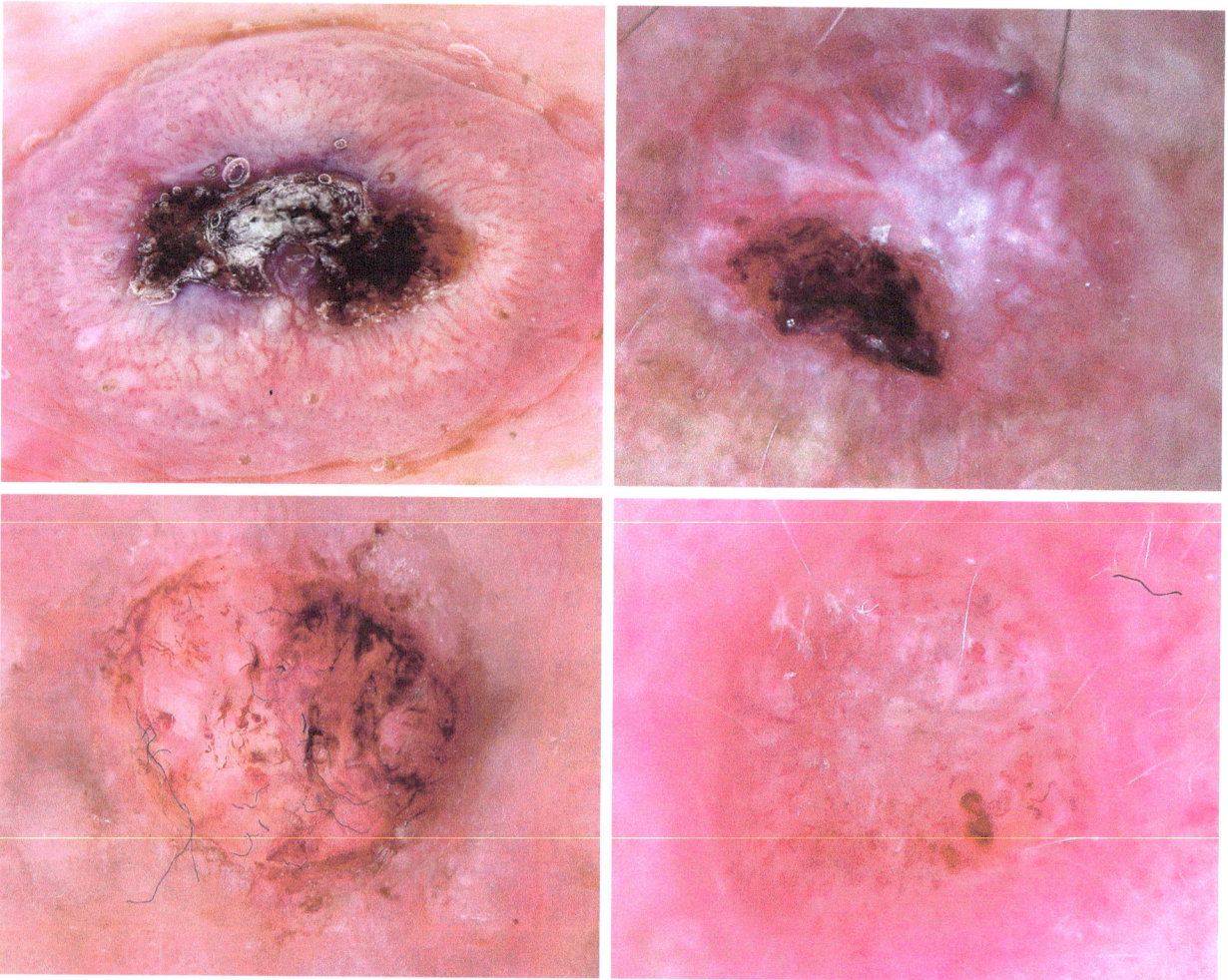

Figure 6.35: Nodular amelanotic lesions.
Top left: Keratoacanthoma with central keratin plug (with blood spots) and radial vessels. **Top right:** Basal cell carcinoma with radial vessels and serpentine branched vessels. The radial vessels in this basal cell carcinoma are unusual and due to ulceration. **Bottom left:** Polymorphous vessels without a specific arrangement in a poorly differentiated squamous cell carcinoma (note ulceration and adherent fibers). **Bottom right:** Polymorphous vessels without a specific arrangement in a melanoma (invasion thickness: > 1 mm). Note the presence of helical vessels.

combination of coiled and serpentine vessels evoked the metaphor of "cherry blossom" vessels *(figure 6.32),* which is of course dispensable.

When a melanoma occurs as a non-pigmented nodule, the vessels are usually polymorphous and randomly arranged *(6.35 bottom right, 6.39 bottom, 6.40 bottom).* According to Menzies (43), vessels in amelanotic nodular melanoma are often arranged in the center of the lesion. Helical vessels are not common, but when seen are quite specific for melanoma, usually primary but sometimes metastatic *(6.35 bottom right).* Pink or red clods, and white lines also should be viewed with caution when seen in conjunction with vessels as dots or lines.

Summary

In summary, the investigator is confronted with the limits of dermatoscopy when trying to assess non-pigmented lesions. Nevertheless, in some cases dermatoscopy may yield clues that point in the right direction – clues that may remain hidden to observation by the naked eye. Because diagnostic uncertainty is greater for non-pigmented lesions than in pigmented ones, histopathology will be required more often to establish an accurate diagnosis. Importantly, the investigator must recognize this greater uncertainty, and avoid making decisions that exceed the limitations of the method.

We can, however, apply some simple general rules, which can be summarized into a very rudimentary

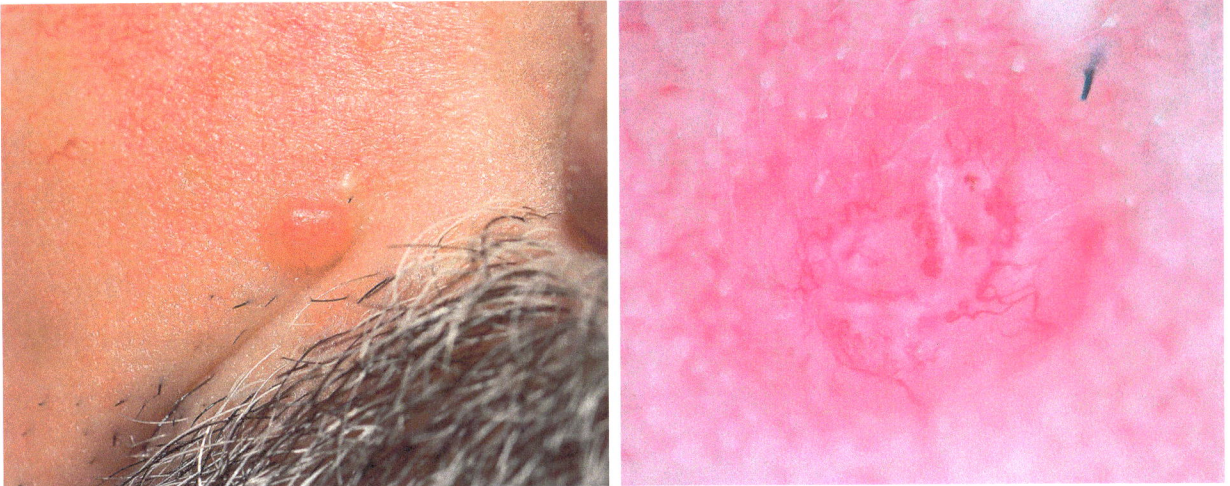

Figure 6.36: *Basal cell carcinoma.*
Serpentine branched vessels in a basal cell carcinoma.

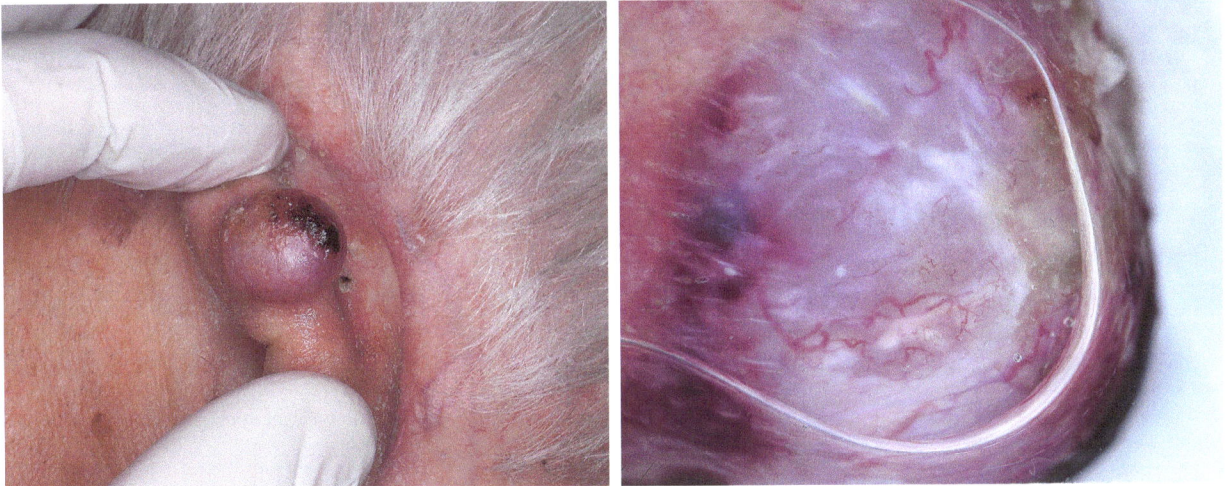

Figure 6.37: *Merkel cell carcinoma.*
A Merkel cell carcinoma presenting as non-pigmented ulcerated nodule with serpentine branched vessels on dermatoscopy **(right).** *Images courtesy of Jean-Yves Gourhant.*

short algorithm (44). Any non-pigmented lesion that is ulcerated or has white clues (white lines in any lesion and in raised lesions, keratin, white circles or white structureless areas) should be biopsied or excised to rule out malignancy. If ulceration and white clues are absent one should try to make a specific diagnosis based on other clues (e.g. keratin, scale, yellow color, white dots etc.) and vascular patterns. If a specific benign diagnosis cannot be made with confidence the lesion should be biopsied or excised to rule out malignancy. Some examples to demonstrate the usefulness of this rule are given in figures 6.40 to 6.42.

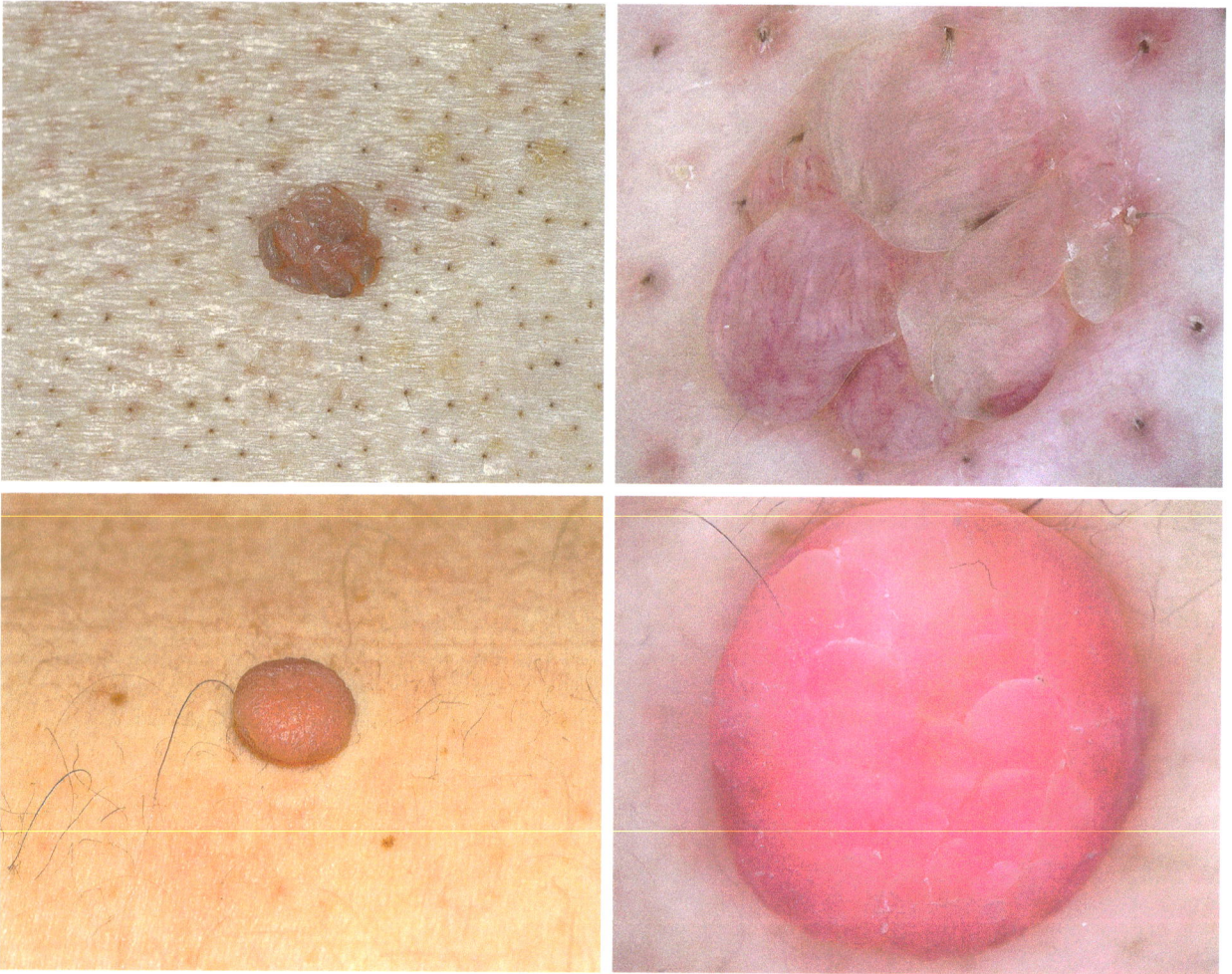

Figure 6.38: Unna nevi ("dermal nevi").
*Unna nevi often are amelanotic nodules. On dermatoscopy **(top and bottom right)** one can see skin colored clods. The top case shows the typical specific arrangement of linear vessels in the center of the clods.*

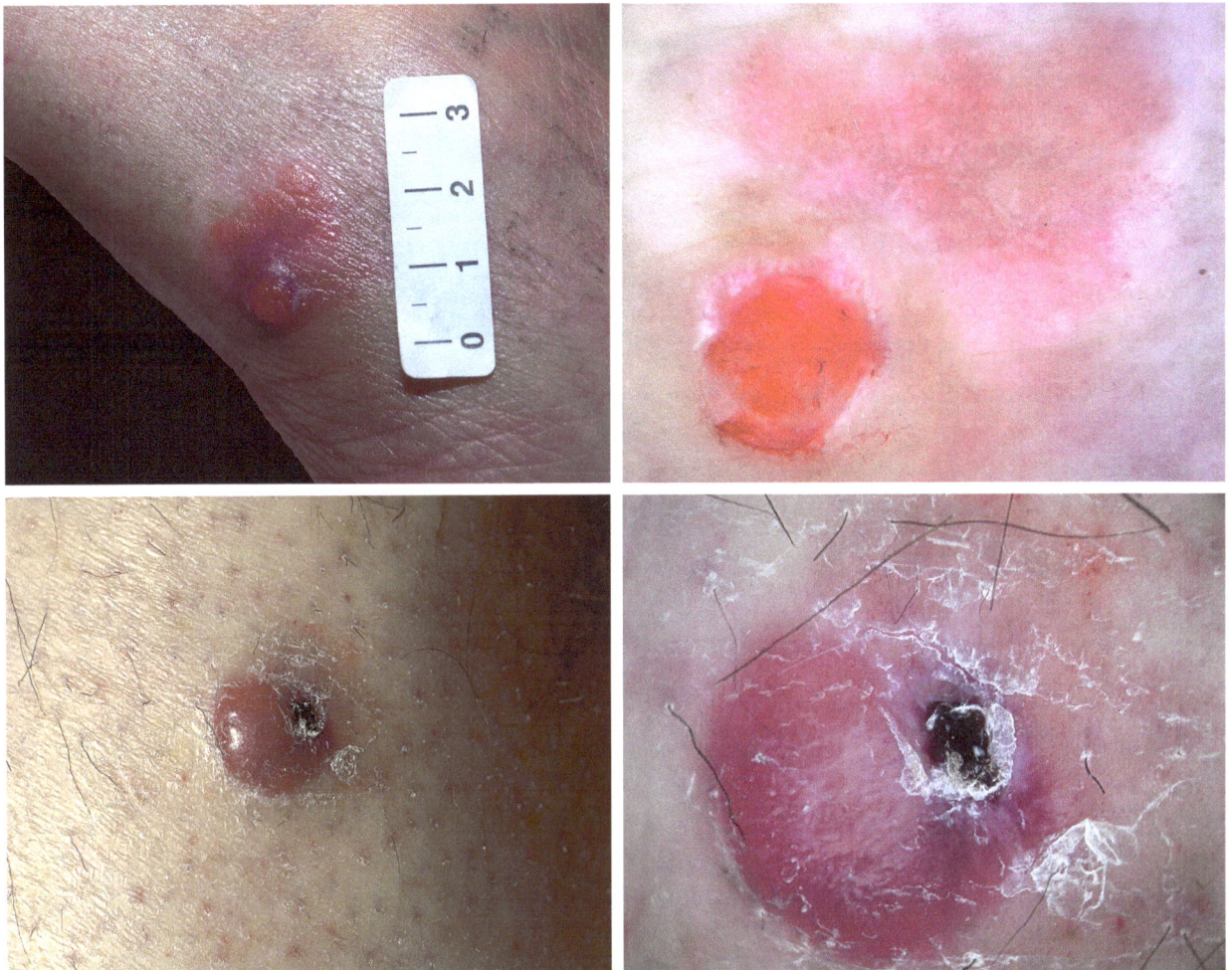

Figure 6.39: *Amelanotic melanomas.*
Top: *This melanoma (> 1 mm) consists of a nodular and a flat portion. The nodular portion is marked by polymorphous vessels arranged randomly. The flat portion shows vessels as dots, which confirms the diagnosis of melanoma.* **Bottom:** *A nodular lesion that primarily shows vessels as dots on dermatoscopy, but also other types of vessels which do not follow any special arrangement. The hemorrhagic crust due to ulceration (seen as a single black clod) is a clue to malignancy in the absence of trauma. A further clue to melanoma is the presence of white lines. Diagnosis: Melanoma (> 1 mm).*

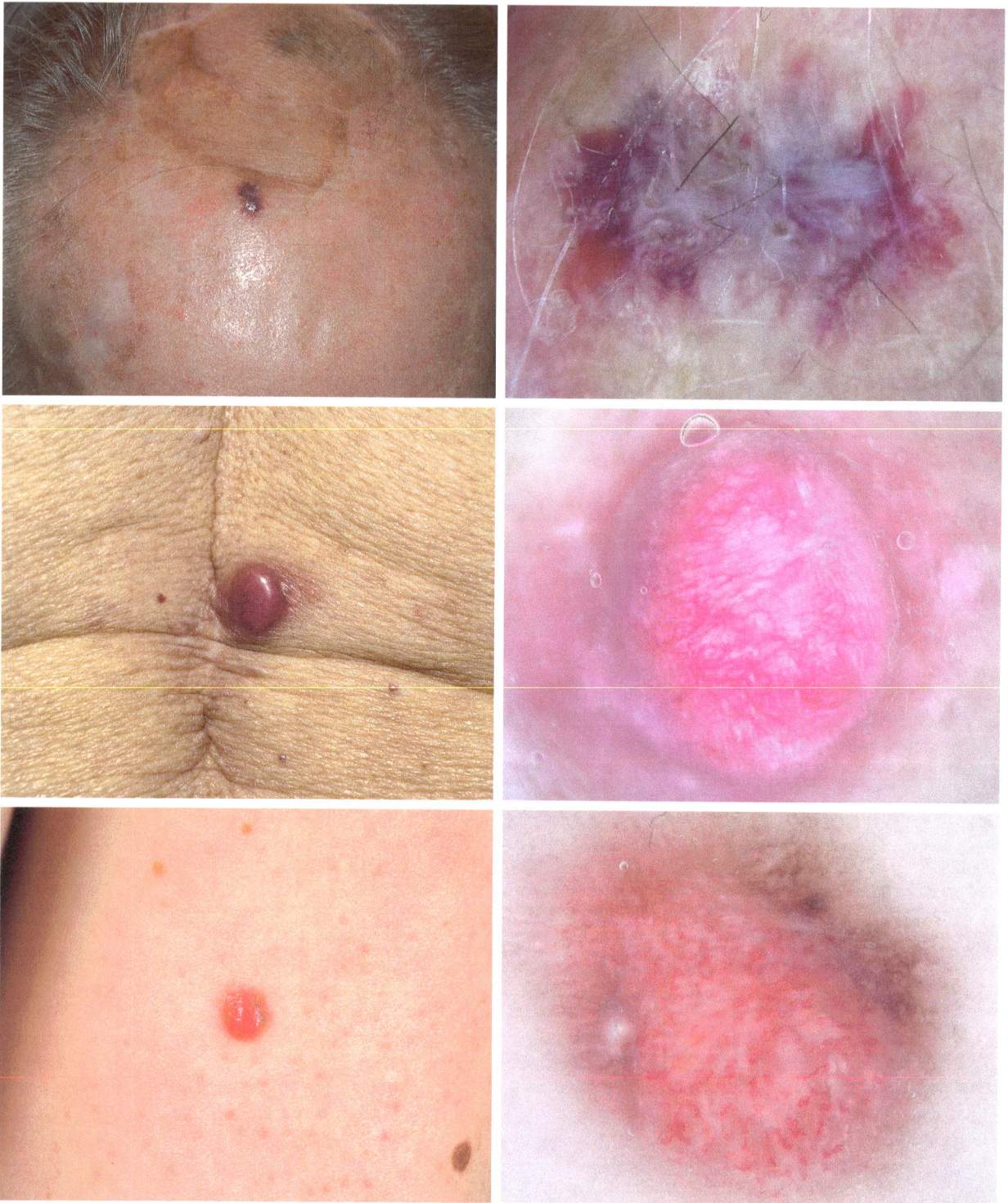

Figure 6.40: *Examples to demonstrate a simple algorithm for non-pigmented lesions.*
Top: *A flat lesion with white lines on dermatoscopy requires histology to rule out malignancy. On dermatoscopy there is only an erythematous background. Vessels are not visible. Diagnosis: Atypical fibroxanthoma.* **Middle:** *A nodule with white lines on dermatoscopy requires histology to rule out malignancy. The serpentine branched vessels are not specific for basal cell carcinoma. Any tumor underneath the superficial vascular plexus including cysts can present with serpentine branched vessels – in this case a malignant peripheral nerve sheath tumor.* **Bottom:** *A nodule without specific clues except remnants of brown pigmentation in the periphery. A confident benign diagnosis is not possible. The vessels are polymorphic including coils and loops. The diagnosis is melanoma (> 1 mm thickness).*

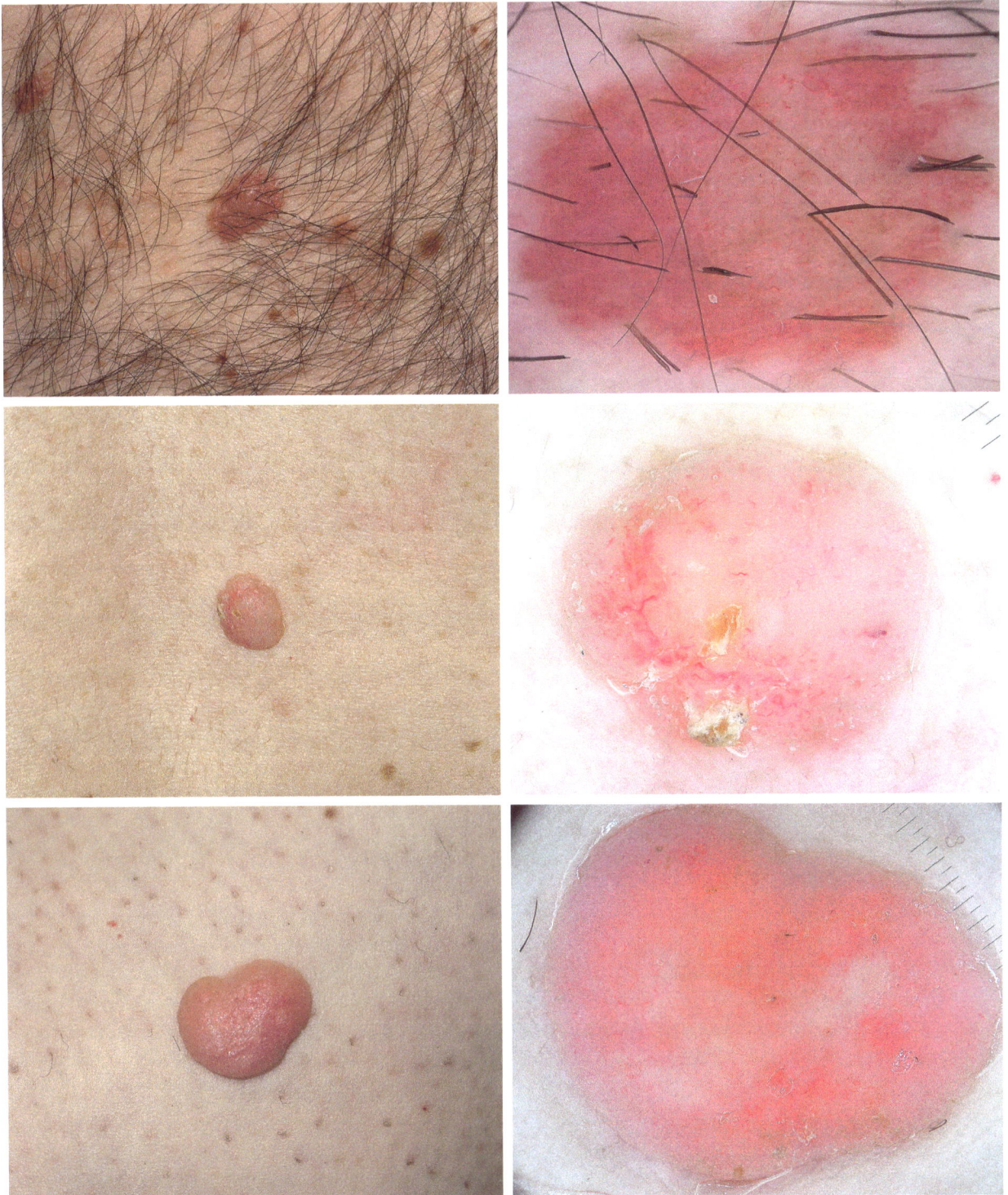

Figure 6.41: *Examples to demonstrate a simple algorithm for non-pigmented lesions.*
Top: *A flat lesion with a raised center without any specific clues and short linear vessels in the raised center. Skin colored clods in the center are barely visible. It depends on how confident one can diagnose a congenital nevus here to decide if this lesion should be excised or not. The physician who took care of this patient was confident enough to leave this lesion.* ***Middle:*** *A non-pigmented nodule that is ulcerated on dermatoscopy should be excised or biopsied to rule out malignancy. Histopathologic diagnosis: Fibroepithelioma of Pinkus (a variant of basal cell carcinoma).* ***Bottom:*** *A non-pigmented nodule without specific clues. Because a confident benign diagnosis is not possible it is advisable to remove the lesion to rule out malignancy. Histopathologic diagnosis: Fibroepithelioma of Pinkus (a variant of basal cell carcinoma). Image courtesy of G. Argenziano and I. Zalaudek.*

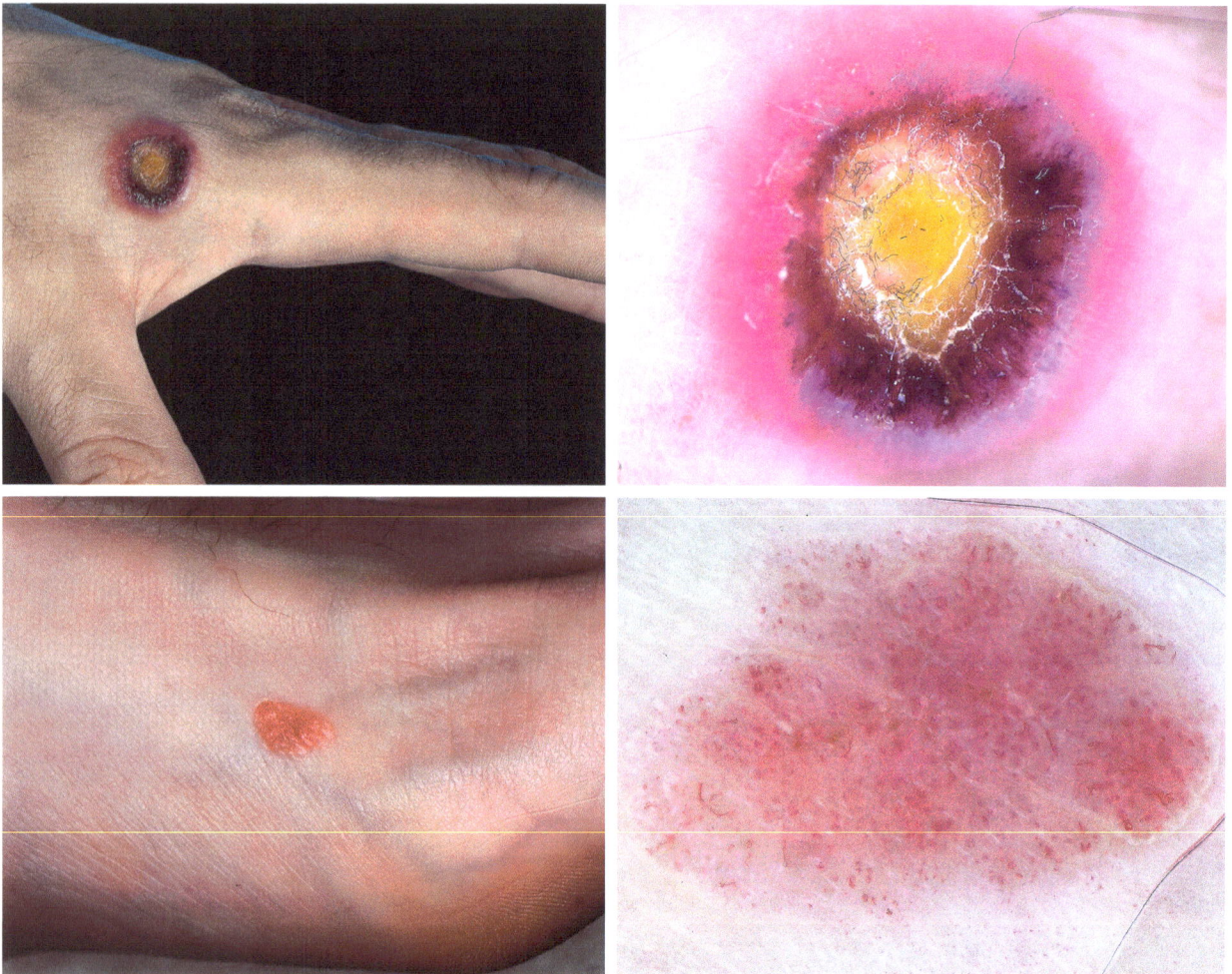

Figure 6.42: Examples to demonstrate a simple algorithm for non-pigmented lesions.
Top: *An ulcerated nodule with a yellow serum crust on dermatoscopy should be excised or biopsied to rule out malignancy. Histopathologic diagnosis: Large cell anaplastic T-cell lymphoma.* **Bottom:** *A non-pigmented nodule with coiled and looped vessels but no specific clues. Because a confident benign diagnosis is not possible it is advisable to remove the lesions to rule out malignancy. Histopathologic diagnosis: Eccrine poroma. Images courtesy of G. Argenziano, I. Zalaudek, J-Y. Gourhant and P. Zaballos.*

References

1   Agero AL, Taliercio S, Dusza SW, Salaro C, Chu P, Marghoob AA. Conventional and polarized dermoscopy features of dermatofibroma. Arch Dermatol. 2006; 142: 1431–1437.

2   Arpaia N, Cassano N, Vena GA. Dermoscopic patterns of dermatofibroma. Dermatol Surg. 2005; 31: 1336–1339.

3   Puig S, Romero D, Zaballos P, Malvehy J. Dermoscopy of dermatofibroma. Arch Dermatol. 2005; 141: 122.

4   Zaballos P, Puig S, Llambrich A, Malvehy J. Dermoscopy of dermatofibromas: a prospective morphological study of 412 cases. Arch Dermatol. 2008; 144: 75–83.

5   Zaballos P, Puig S, Malvehy J. Dermoscopy of atypical dermatofibroma: central white network. Arch Dermatol. 2006; 142: 126.

6   Balagula Y, Braun RP, Rabinovitz HS, et al. The significance of crystalline/chrysalis structures in the diagnosis of melanocytic and nonmelanocytic lesions. J Am Acad Dermatol. 2012; 67: 194 e191–198.

7   Lozzi GP, Piccolo D, Micantonio T, Altamura D, Peris K. Early melanomas dermoscopically characterized by reticular depigmentation. Arch Dermatol. 2007; 143: 808–809.

8   Zalaudek I, Giacomel J, Argenziano G, et al. Dermoscopy of facial nonpigmented actinic keratosis. Br J Dermatol. 2006; 155: 951–956.

9   Rosendahl C, Cameron A, Argenziano G, Zalaudek I, Tschandl P, Kittler H. Dermoscopy of squamous cell carcinoma and keratoacanthoma. Arch Dermatol. 2012; 148: 1386–1392.

10   Lallas A, Apalla Z, Lefaki I, et al. Dermoscopy of discoid lupus erythematosus. Br J Dermatol. 2013; 168: 284–288.

11   Benvenuto-Andrade C, Dusza SW, Agero AL, et al. Differences between polarized light dermoscopy and immersion contact dermoscopy for the evaluation of skin lesions. Arch Dermatol. 2007; 143: 329–338.

12   Bryden AM, Dawe RS, Fleming C. Dermatoscopic features of benign sebaceous proliferation. Clin Exp Dermatol. 2004; 29: 676–677.

13   Zaballos P, Ara M, Puig S, Malvehy J. Dermoscopy of sebaceous hyperplasia. Arch Dermatol. 2005; 141: 808.

14   Bakos RM, Bakos L. Dermoscopic diagnosis of furuncular myiasis. Arch Dermatol. 2007; 143: 123–124.

15   Liebman TN, Scope A, Rabinovitz H, Braun RP, Marghoob AA. Rosettes may be observed in a range of conditions. Arch Dermatol. 2011; 147: 1468.

16   Zaballos P, Carulla M, Ozdemir F, et al. Dermoscopy of pyogenic granuloma: a morphological study. Br J Dermatol. 2010; 163: 1229–1237.

17   Zaballos P, Llambrich A, Cuellar F, Puig S, Malvehy J. Dermoscopic findings in pyogenic granuloma. Br J Dermatol. 2006; 154: 1108–1111.

18   Song M, Kim SH, Jung DS, Ko HC, Kwon KS, Kim MB. Structural correlations between dermoscopic and histopathological features of juvenile xanthogranuloma. J Eur Acad Dermatol Venereol. 2011; 25: 259–263.

19   Llambrich A, Zaballos P, Terrasa F, Torne I, Puig S, Malvehy J. Dermoscopy of cutaneous leishmaniasis. Br J Dermatol. 2009; 160: 756–761.

20   Argenziano G, Zalaudek I, Corona R, et al. Vascular structures in skin tumors: a dermoscopy study. Arch Dermatol. 2004; 140: 1485–1489.

21   Meyerson LB. A peculiar papulosquamous eruption involving pigmented nevi. Arch Dermatol. 1971; 103: 510–512.

22   Tschandl P, Rosendahl C, Kittler H. Cutaneous human papillomavirus infection: manifestations and diagnosis. Curr Probl Dermatol. 2014; 45: 92–97.

23   Zaballos P, Llambrich A, Puig S, Malvehy J. Dermoscopic findings of pilomatricomas. Dermatology. 2008; 217: 225–230.

24   Zaballos P, Daufi C, Puig S, et al. Dermoscopy of solitary angiokeratomas: a morphological study. Arch Dermatol. 2007; 143: 318–325.

25   Lallas A, Argenziano G, Apalla Z, et al. Dermoscopic patterns of common facial inflammatory skin diseases. J Eur Acad Dermatol Venereol. 2014; 28: 609–614.

26   Delfino M, Argenziano G, Nino M. Dermoscopy for the diagnosis of porokeratosis. J Eur Acad Dermatol Venereol. 2004; 18: 194–195.

27   Pizzichetta MA, Canzonieri V, Massone C, Soyer HP. Clinical and dermoscopic features of porokeratosis of Mibelli. Arch Dermatol. 2009; 145: 91–92.

28   Zalaudek I, Argenziano G, Leinweber B, et al. Dermoscopy of Bowen's disease. Br J Dermatol. 2004; 150: 1112–1116.

29   Pan Y, Chamberlain AJ, Bailey M, Chong AH, Haskett M, Kelly JW. Dermatoscopy aids in the diagnosis of the solitary red scaly patch or plaque-features distinguishing superficial basal cell carcinoma, intraepidermal carcinoma, and psoriasis. J Am Acad Dermatol. 2008; 59: 268–274.

30   Akay BN, Kittler H, Sanli H, Harmankaya K, Anadolu R. Dermatoscopic findings of cutaneous mastocytosis. Dermatology. 2009; 218: 226–230.

31   Arpaia N, Cassano N, Vena GA. Lessons on dermoscopy: pigment network in nonmelanocytic lesions. Dermatol Surg. 2004; 30: 929–930.

32 Vano-Galvan S, Alvarez-Twose I, De las Heras E, et al. Dermoscopic features of skin lesions in patients with mastocytosis. Arch Dermatol. 2011; 147: 932–940.

33 Carroll DM, Billingsley EM, Helm KF. Diagnosing basal cell carcinoma by dermatoscopy. J Cutan Med Surg. 1998; 3: 62–67.

34 Zalaudek I, Kreusch J, Giacomel J, Ferrara G, Catricala C, Argenziano G. How to diagnose nonpigmented skin tumors: a review of vascular structures seen with dermoscopy: part II. Nonmelanocytic skin tumors. J Am Acad Dermatol. 2010; 63: 377–386; quiz 387–378.

35 Errichetti E, Piccirillo A, Stinco G. Dermoscopy of prurigo nodularis. J Dermatol. 2015; 42: 632–634.

36 Akin FY, Ertam I, Ceylan C, Kazandi A, Ozdemir F. Clear cell acanthoma: new observations on dermatoscopy. Indian J Dermatol Venereol Leprol. 2008; 74: 285–287.

37 Ferrari A, Buccini P, Silipo V, et al. Eccrine poroma: a clinical-dermoscopic study of seven cases. Acta Derm Venereol. 2009; 89: 160–164.

38 Nicolino R, Zalaudek I, Ferrara G, et al. Dermoscopy of eccrine poroma. Dermatology. 2007; 215: 160–163.

39 Ardigo M, Zieff J, Scope A, et al. Dermoscopic and reflectance confocal microscope findings of trichoepithelioma. Dermatology. 2007; 215: 354–358.

40 Salerni G, Gonzalez R, Alonso C. Dermatoscopic pattern of digital mucous cyst: report of three cases. Dermatol Pract Concept. 2014; 4: 65–67.

41 Lallas A, Pyne J, Kyrgidis A, et al. The clinical and dermoscopic features of invasive cutaneous squamous cell carcinoma depend on the histopathological grade of differentiation. Br J Dermatol. 2015; 172: 1308–1315.

42 Jalilian C, Chamberlain AJ, Haskett M, et al. Clinical and dermoscopic characteristics of Merkel cell carcinoma. Br J Dermatol. 2013; 169: 294–297.

43 Menzies SW, Kreusch J, Byth K, et al. Dermoscopic evaluation of amelanotic and hypomelanotic melanoma. Arch Dermatol. 2008; 144: 1120–1127.

44 Rosendahl C, Cameron A, Tschandl P, Bulinska A, Zalaudek I, Kittler H. Prediction without Pigment: a decision algorithm for non-pigmented skin malignancy. Dermatol Pract Concept. 2014; 31: 59–66.

7 Clues and Clichés

As we have seen in previous chapters, clues are important hints that help to solve the differential diagnosis produced by analysis of pattern and color. They usually point towards a diagnosis, but very few clues are specific for a particular diagnosis in all contexts. Studies which state that a particular clue has a given sensitivity and specificity should be interpreted with caution as there is always a selection bias (usually admitted) in the choice of included lesions, the series may not be large, and all too often the clue is only evaluated in a limited context, most commonly of distinguishing nevus from melanoma. Clues must always be interpreted in context, otherwise a good clue may become a cliché. This chapter will look at a selection of clues that deserve special attention, and at some common clichés.

7.1 Clues

Adherent fiber
Adherent fiber is a dermatoscopic clue to ulceration. Ulceration may of course be caused by trauma to normal skin or benign lesions, but malignant neoplasms and especially basal cell carcinomas may ulcerate after trivial irritation. The serum or blood that leaks onto the skin has adhesive properties which persist when it dries out and this may trap fibers of clothing fabric, other exogenous debris or the patient's own dislodged hair. Adherent fiber may be found on basal cell carcinomas even when ulceration was not observed prior to dermatoscopy. As ulceration is often an important clue to malignancy, so is the presence of dermatoscopically observed adherent fiber *(7.1)*.

Branched fine lines in flat acral lesions
Brown or gray branched fine lines sprinkled with dots in a flat acral lesion is a very distinctive pattern. When uniformly distributed over the whole lesion *(7.2)*, it is pathognomonic for tinea nigra (1). As tinea nigra commonly occurs on the feet where surgery is technically difficult, the diagnosis is best confirmed by a successful trial of treatment with topical antifungal cream. This leads to resolution of the lesion within 3 weeks and avoids a biopsy to exclude melanoma.

Branched serpentine vessels adjacent to keratin
The presence of branched serpentine vessels adjacent to keratin is a strong clue to keratoacanthoma *(7.3)*. Commonly keratoacanthomas are symmetrical lesions with a central keratin plug and vessels (linear, looped, serpentine, coiled or polymorphous) arranged in a radial pattern and with this morphology they are easily identified (2). The clue of branched serpentine vessels adjacent to keratin is particularly useful when the presentation is not typical, but it is also often present in the more typical cases. There is an ongoing controversy among different schools of dermatopathologists whether keratoacanthomas are benign lesions or highly differentiated variants of squamous cell carcinoma (3). However, even the proponents of the concept that a keratoacanthoma is a benign neoplasm agree that lesions that appear as keratoacanthomas clinically or dermatoscopically should be excised to rule out squamous cell carcinoma.

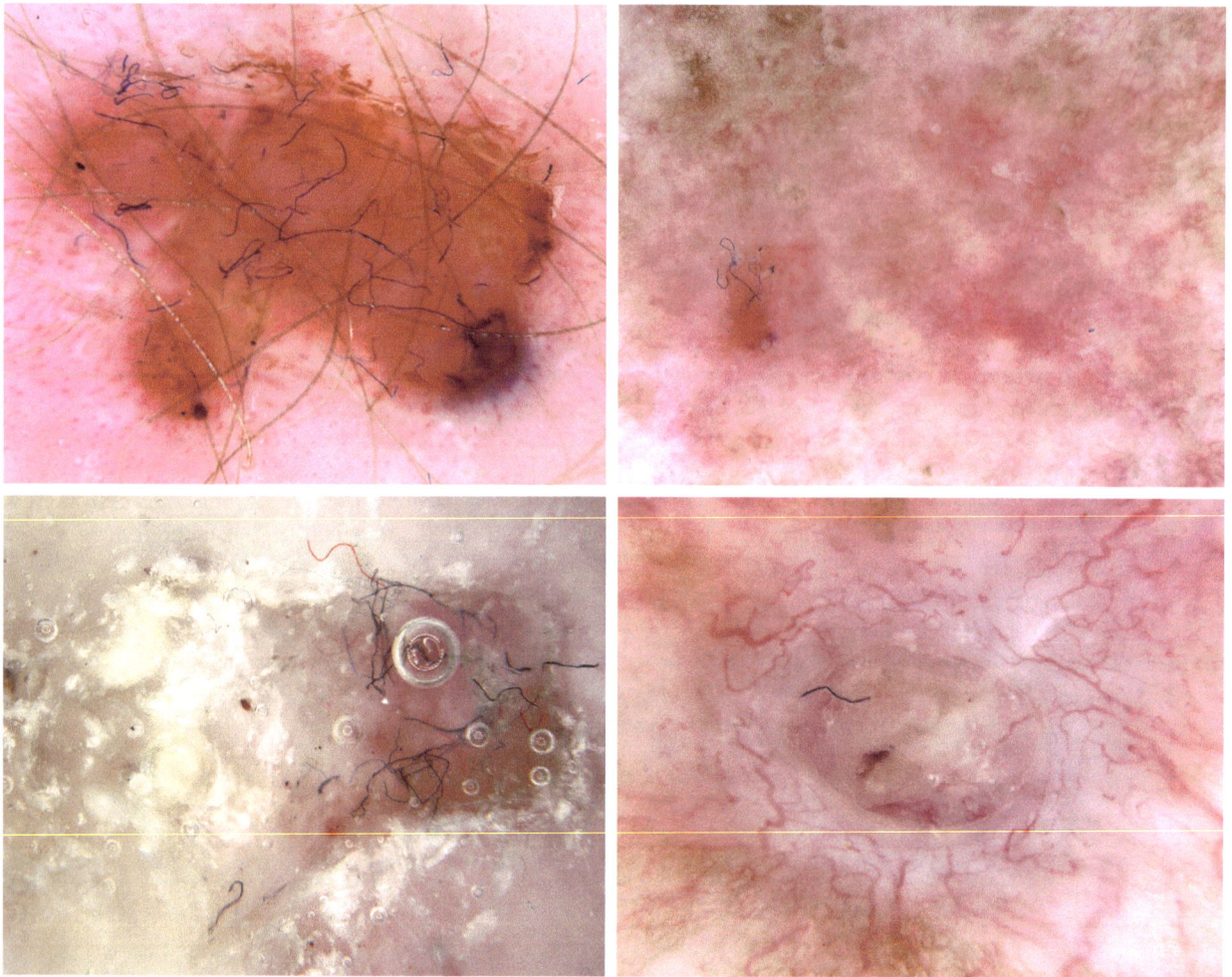

Figure 7.1: Adherent fiber as a clue to ulceration.
Top left: Adherent fabric fiber can easily be distinguished from intact hair on this ulcerated basal cell carcinoma. **Top right:** Adherent fiber lies over a focal ulcer on the surface of this basal cell carcinoma. **Bottom left:** Fabric fiber reveals the presence of ulceration which was not evident clinically on the surface of this squamous cell carcinoma. **Bottom right:** Focal ulceration on a nodular portion of a basal cell carcinoma is identified by a single adherent fabric fiber. The ulceration was not evident clinically and may have been missed dermatoscopically except for the adherent fiber.

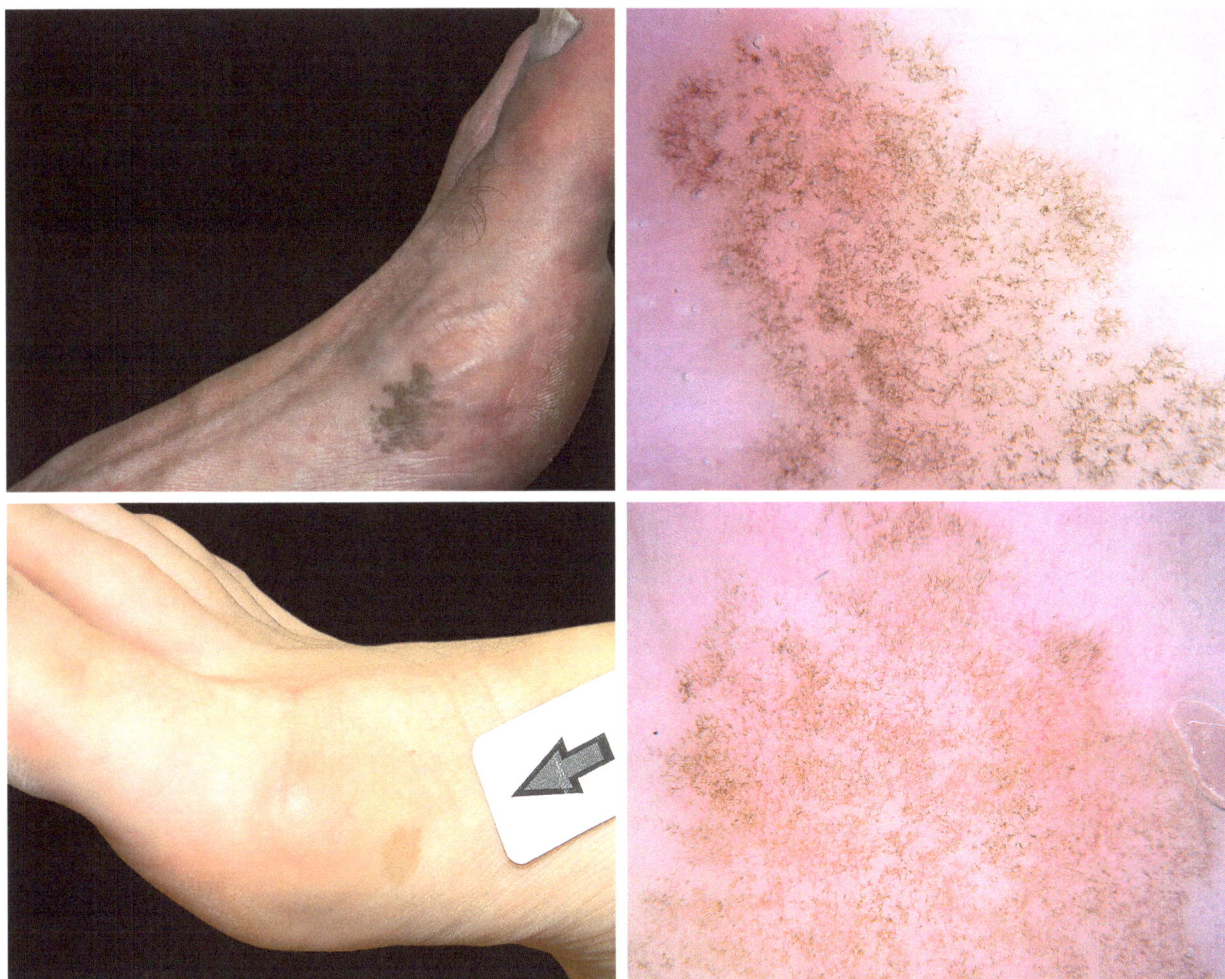

Figure 7.2: *Dermatoscopy of tinea nigra.*
Dermatoscopy on the right. These 2 cases of tinea nigra were confirmed histopathologically when biopsied to exclude melanoma.

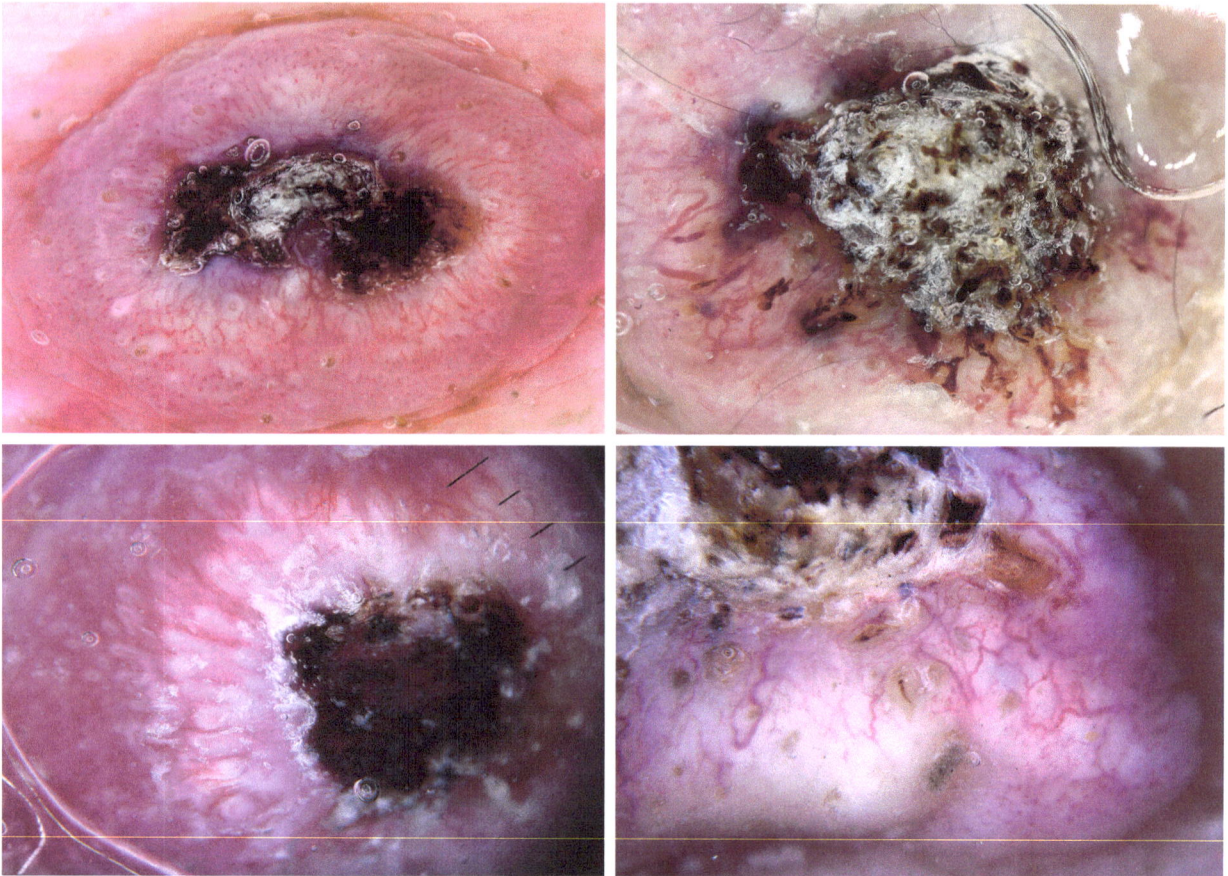

Figure 7.3: Branched serpentine vessels adjacent to keratin as a clue to keratoacanthoma.
Each of these keratoacanthomas has the typical morphology of a central keratin plug with vessels surrounding it in a radial pattern. **Top left:** *Keratoacanthoma with polymorphous vessels (coiled and looped) including a focus of serpentine branched vessels just inferior to the central part of the keratin plug. The arrangement of vessels is radial.* **Top right and bottom left and right:** *Keratoacanthomas with serpentine branched vessels adjacent to keratin.*

Circles, ovals, and distorted circles

A pattern of circles on non-facial skin, not correlating to infundibulae and in conjunction with ovals and distorted circles is a strong clue to a seborrheic keratosis *(7.4)*. The circles, ovals and distorted circles are produced by elongation and broadening of rete ridges due to acanthosis of the epidermis *(7.5)*. Pigmentation of these structures is due to hyperpigmentation of basal keratinocytes.

Double reticular lines

Occasionally it is apparent on higher magnification that the individual "lines" forming a reticular pattern are actually double lines enclosing a hypopigmented space. The double line corresponds to pigmented basal keratinocytes. The hypopigmented space between the pair of lines indicates that the rete ridges are not filled with pigment. If this pattern is found throughout a lesion it usually indicates a benign lesion. It usually indicates a junctional Clark nevus *(7.6)*. If, on the other hand, the rete ridges are broadened and filled with pigment (filled with neoplastic melanocytes) the hypopigmented space becomes pigmented and instead of double lines one sees thick reticular lines, which is a clue to melanoma. Occasionally one finds thick reticular lines in a seborrheic keratosis. In this case the rete ridges are not filled with neoplastic melanocytes but with pigmented keratinocytes.

Four dots in a square (four-dot clod)

These structures were first described by Marghoob and Cowell (4) who called them "rosettes" (see also chapter 4). They are only seen with a polarizing dermatoscope *(7.7)*, and are composed of 4 white dots arranged in a square or as a rhomboid. With a non-polarizing dermatoscope, this structure is seen as a simple white

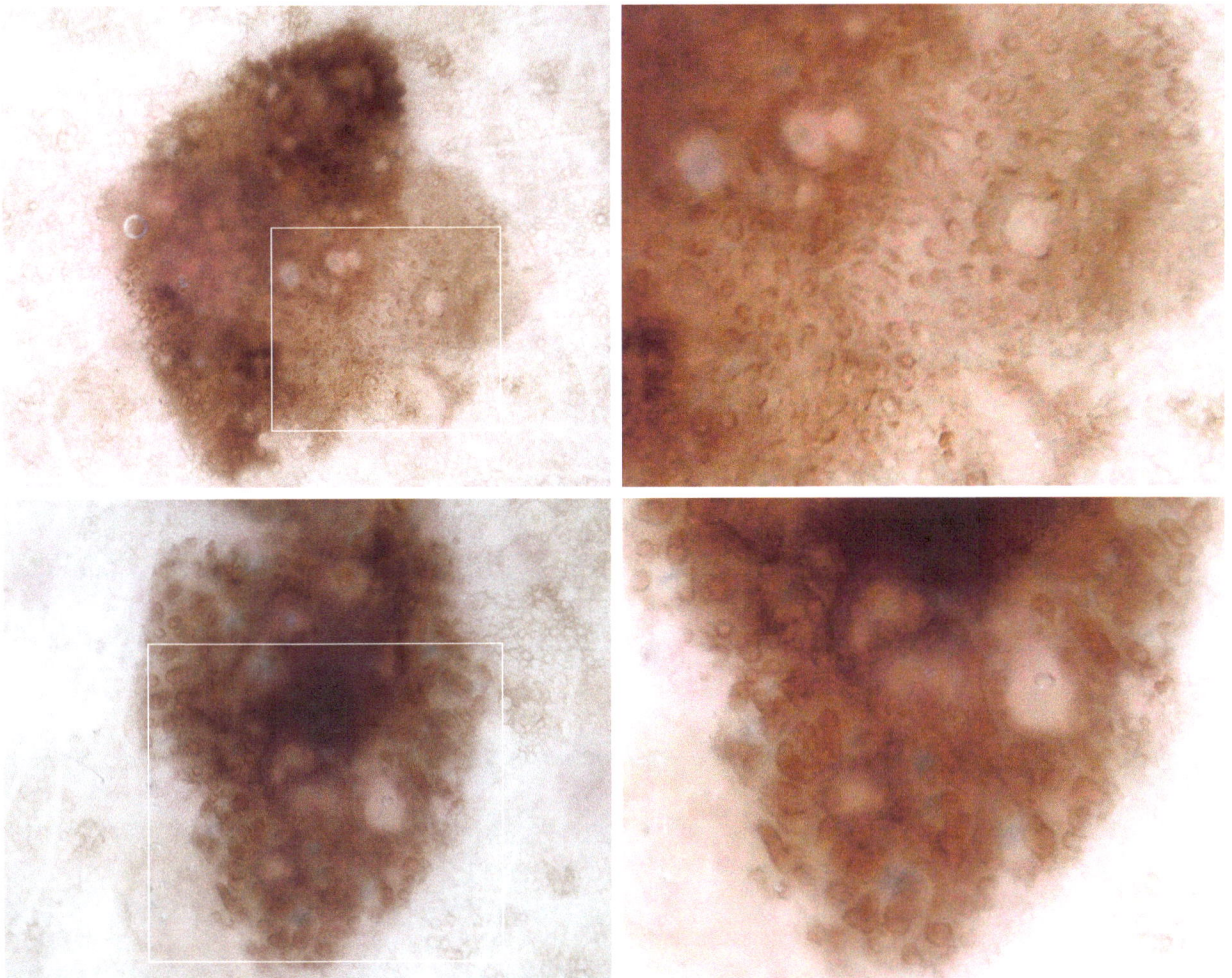

Figure 7.4: Circles, ovals and distorted circles as a clue to seborrheic keratosis.
Circles, ovals, and distorted circles in two seborrheic keratoses. In the **bottom** lesion one can see the transformation of circles to parallel curved lines.

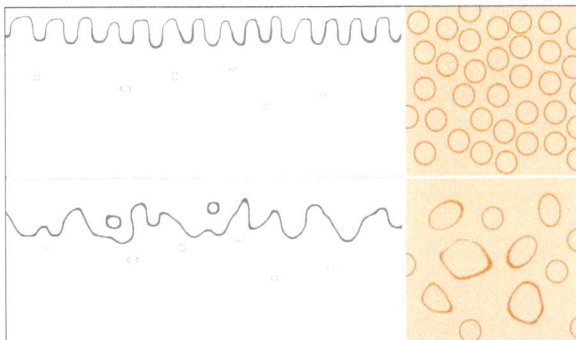

Figure 7.5: Dermatoscopic-pathologic correlation of circles and distorted circles on non-facial skin.
If the rete ridges are thin and regular and the basal keratinocytes are hyperpigmented one sees reticular lines (like for example in solar lentigo and Clark nevi) and if the rete ridges are broadened by regular acanthosis (like in dermatofibroma) one sees small regular circles **(top).** If the rete ridges are broadened because of irregular acanthosis and the basal keratinocytes are hyperpigmented (like in some seborrheic keratoses) one sees distorted circles on dermatoscopy **(bottom).**

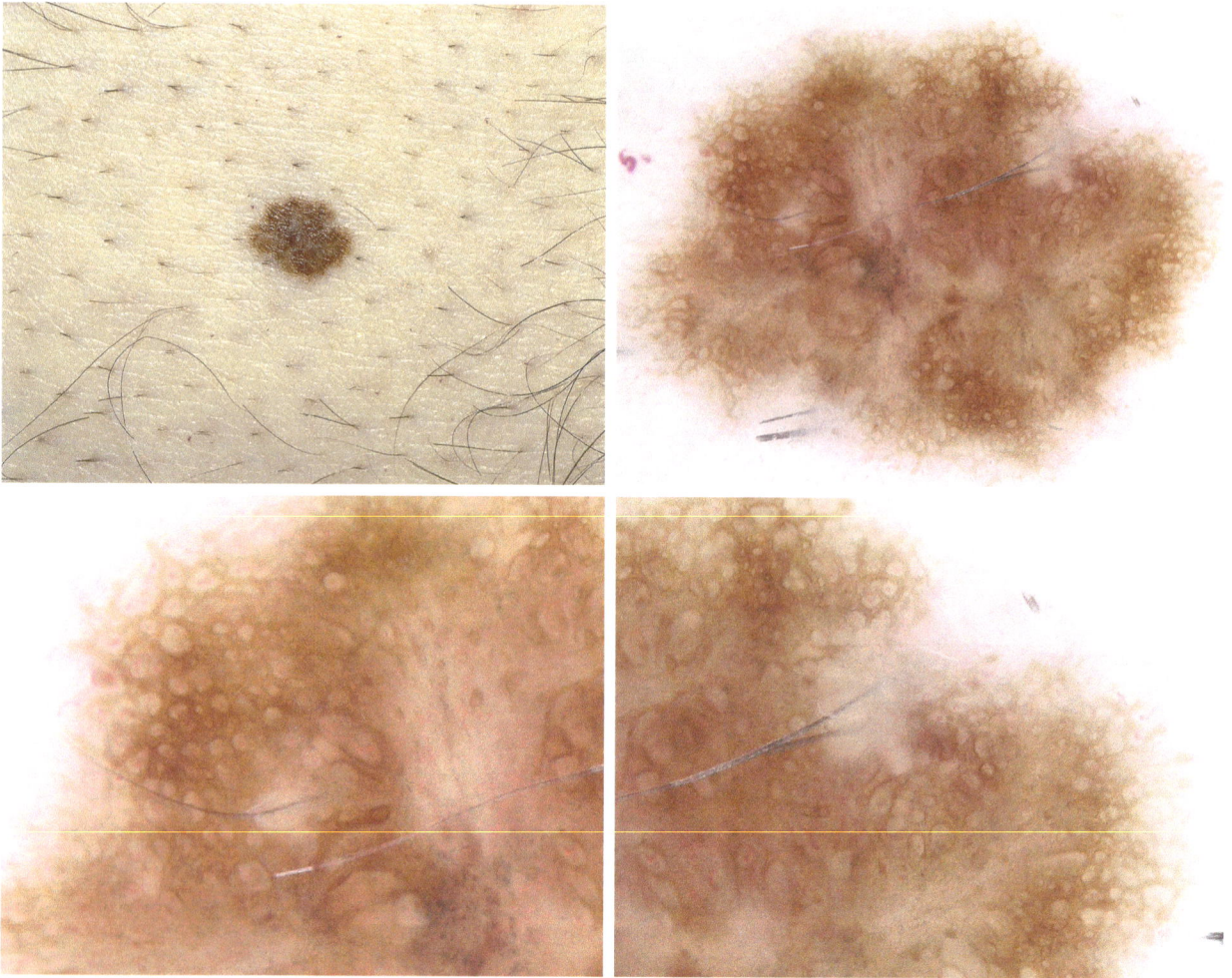

Figure 7.6: *Double reticular lines as a clue to Clark nevus.*
Clinical (**top left**) *and dermatoscopic* (**top right**) *view of a Clark nevus. At high magnification* (**bottom row**) *double reticular lines throughout the lesion are obvious. The double lines have a small hypopigmented space between them.*

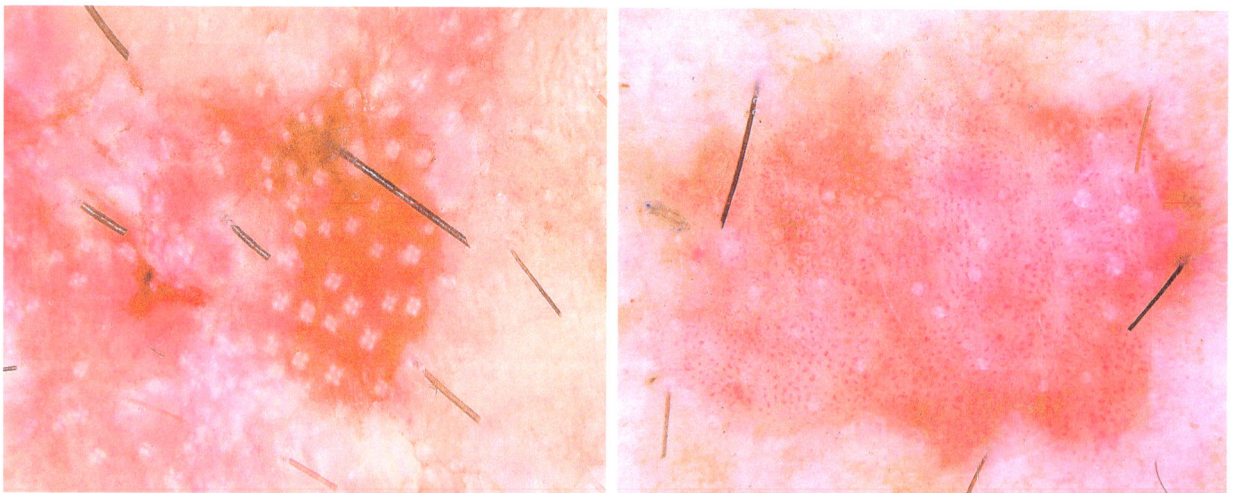

Figure 7.7: *Four dots in a square (four-dot clod) as clue to actinic keratosis or superficial squamous cell carcinoma.*
Left: *With polarized light the 4-dots are seen very clearly on the pigmented portion of this actinic keratosis.* **Right:** *Four dots in a square as a clue to superficial squamous cell carcinoma (Bowen's disease) in this case in collision with a solar lentigo which accounted for the reticular lines.*

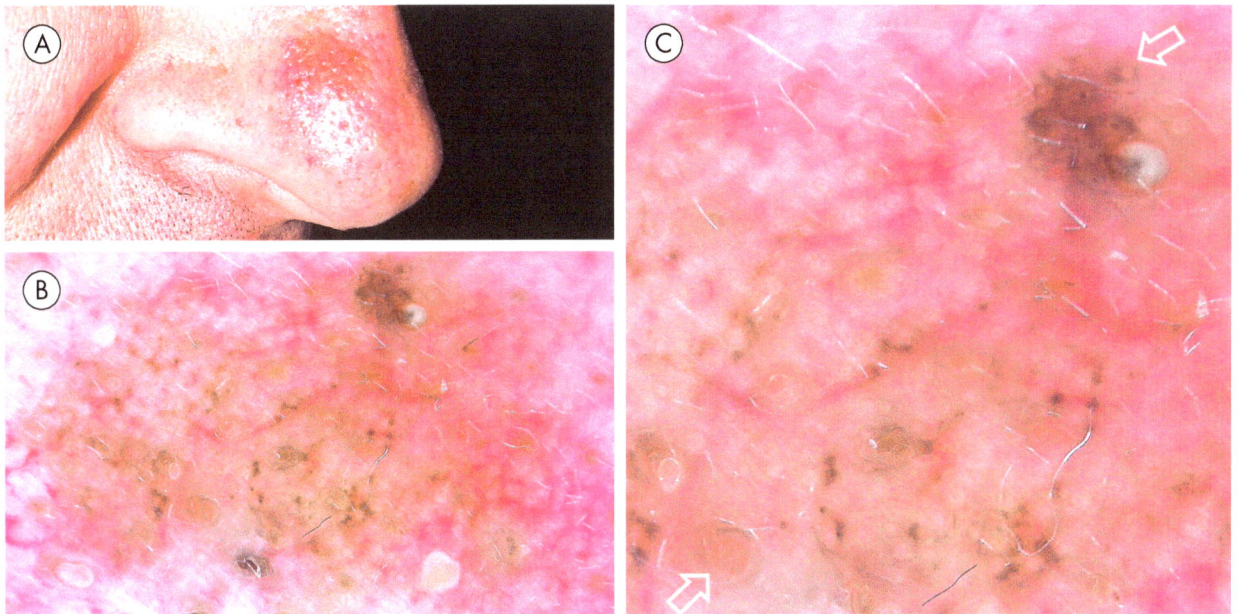

Figure 7.8: Thin gray circles as a clue to melanoma in situ.
Clinically this pigmented macule on the nose looks insignificant **(A).** Dermatoscopically **(B, C)** there are only thin gray circles on a brown structureless background. This is not the pattern of lichen-planus-like keratosis or pigmented actinic keratosis. Excision biopsy revealed it to be an in-situ melanoma.

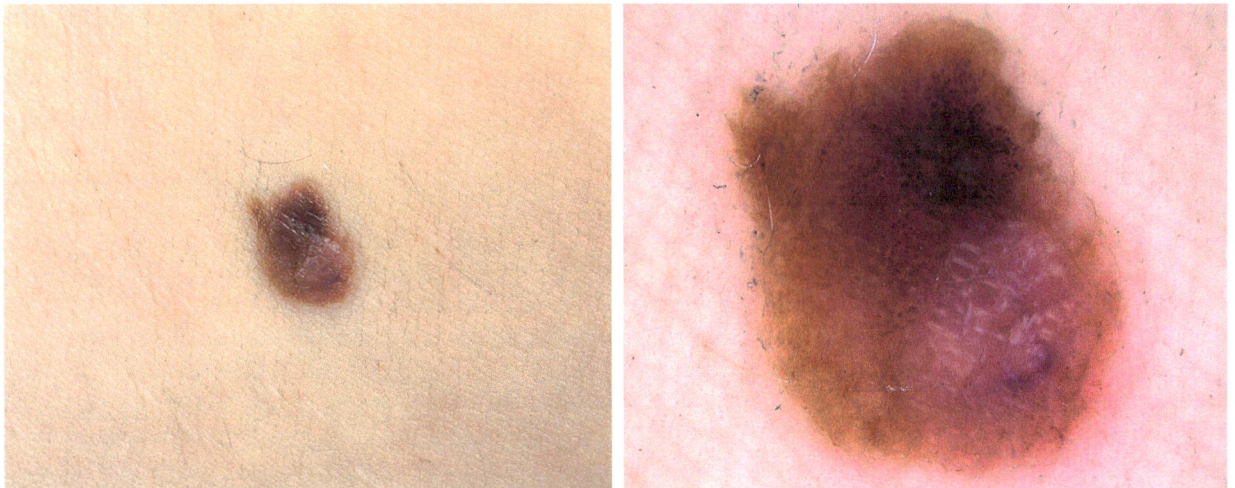

Figure 7.9: White lines.
Short white lines in an invasive melanoma arising in a pre-existing nevus (dermatoscopy on the **right).**

clod. In the appropriate context it is a clue to actinic keratosis or superficial squamous cell carcinoma but it is not as specific as initially thought. It can even be found on normal skin.

Gray circles versus gray dots on the face

We consider that any dermatoscopic gray in head or neck lesions should be regarded as a clue to melanoma (5), with a differential diagnosis of lichen planus-like keratosis and pigmented actinic keratosis. When the gray is seen as thin gray circles, this is a far stronger clue to melanoma than gray dots, even when the dots are arranged as circles *(7.8).*

White lines

White lines may be short or long, thin or thick. They may be arranged in a reticular pattern or perpendicular to each other but without crossing each other. Reticular

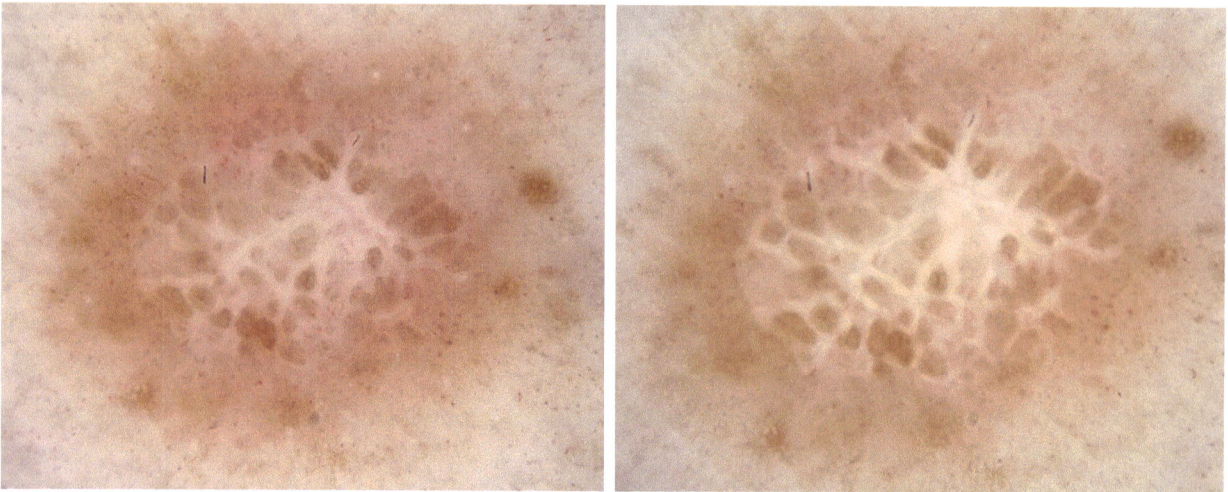

Figure 7.10: Reticular white lines in a dermatofibroma.
*Reticular white lines are seen in this dermatofibroma with both non-polarized **(left)** and polarized **(right)** dermatoscopy. They are brighter with polarized dermatoscopy.*

white lines have also been termed "reticular depigmentation" (6) or "negative pigment network" (7) but for reasons of clarity we use only the objective language of pattern analysis.

Most white lines correspond to fibrosis or sclerosis in the dermis, some to hypergranulosis (for example the white lines seen in lichen planus), and some to a combination of both (8). Superficial fibrosis (i.e. fibrosis in the papillary dermis) and hypergranulosis are seen as white lines regardless of whether the dermatoscope uses polarized or non-polarized light. In other situations, white lines are only seen when dermatoscopes with a polarizing light source are used (9). Polarizing specific white lines are seen as two groups of parallel lines, with the groups at right angles to each other (perpendicular white lines), and correspond to fibrosis in deeper parts of the dermis.

In the short "Chaos and Clues" algorithm presented in chapter 5, any white lines seen either with polarizing or non-polarizing dermatoscopy are a clue to malignancy if they are whiter than normal skin. In pattern analysis, the interpretation of white lines depends on the context. White lines are not highly specific, being seen commonly in melanomas (7) and Spitz nevi (10, 11) *(7.9),* and basal cell carcinomas and dermatofibromas (12) *(7.10).* White lines are seen occasionally in a wide variety of other lesions. White reticular lines rule out a basal cell carcinoma with a similar high degree of certainty as pigmented reticular lines *(7.11).*

Angulated lines (polygons)

Angulated lines (polygons) were first described as a clue to flat melanomas on non-facial, chronic sun-damaged skin by Keir (13) *(7.12).* These melanomas often mimic solar lentigo and may lack other, more conventional, melanoma clues. As defined by Keir, angulated lines (polygons) form multi-sided geometrical shapes which may be completely or incompletely enclosed. In a recent study by Jaimes and Keir (14) angulated lines were found in 44% of flat melanomas on non-facial, chronic sun-damaged skin. Facial angulated lines have been termed rhomboids (15) or zig-zag pattern (16) by others. Like angulated lines on non-facial skin, they are a clue to melanoma. Angulated lines on facial skin can also be found in pigmented solar keratosis (5).

White circles

White circles are a clue to actinic keratosis and squamous cell carcinoma (including keratoacanthomas) (2) especially on, but not limited to the face *(7.13).* In flat pigmented lesions on the face which have evenly distributed gray dots (differential diagnosis: melanoma in situ, lichen planus-like keratosis, and pigmented actinic keratosis) the presence of white circles helps to make the diagnosis of pigmented actinic keratosis (5) *(7.14).*

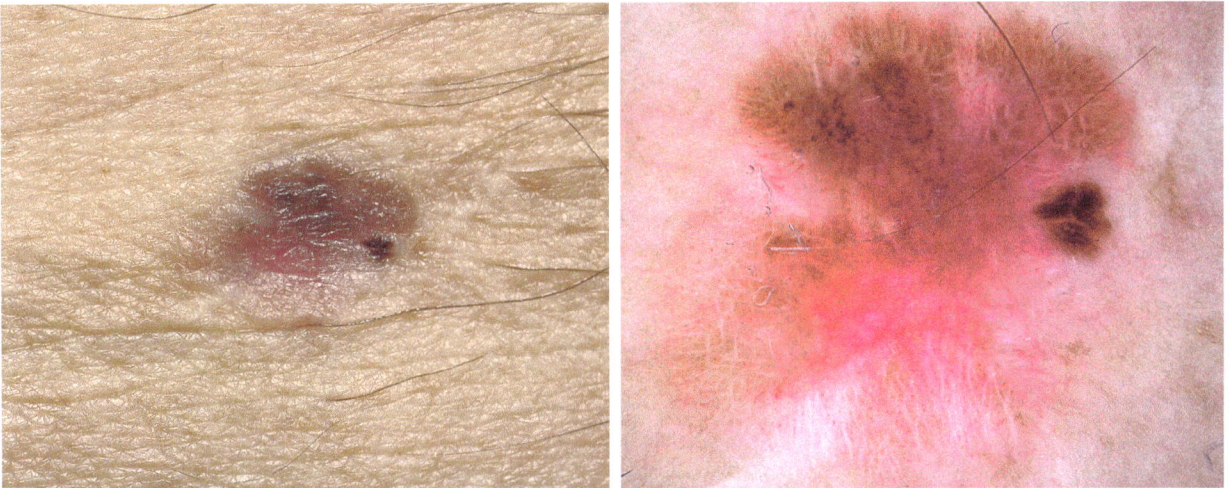

Figure 7.11: *White reticular lines as clue to differentiate melanoma from pigmented basal cell carcinoma.*
*The clinical image on the **left** may be interpreted as pigmented basal cell carcinoma or as melanoma. On dermatoscopy the lesion is chaotic with both polarizing specific and reticular white lines (6 o'clock). Reticular white lines rule out basal cell carcinoma. The diagnosis is melanoma (invasive, < 1 mm).*

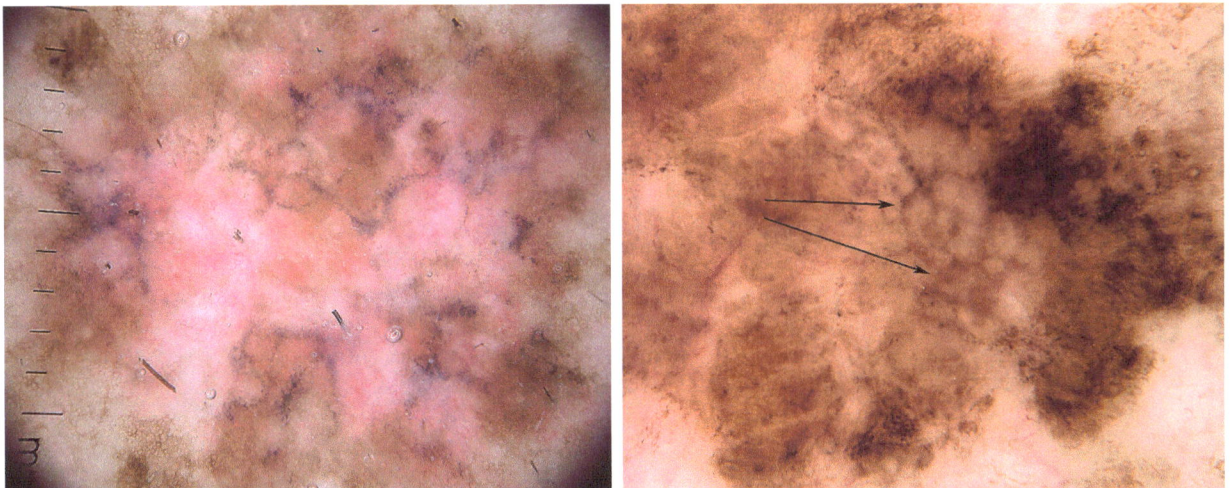

Figure 7.12: *Polygons in flat melanomas on non-facial skin.*
Left: *This invasive melanoma is asymmetric with clues to malignancy including gray dots and eccentric structureless areas. The gray dots are arranged in lines making incompletely closed polygonal shapes.* **Right:** *This in-situ melanoma has some features suggestive of solar lentigo (curved lines, circles, scalloped border). Arrows point to some lines forming completely enclosed polygonal shapes.*

7.2 Common Clichés

"Pigment network" is a melanocytic criterion
Reticular lines (pigment network) are created by melanin located on the rete ridges. Because this pigment can be in keratinocytes as well as melanocytes, no conclusion can be drawn about melanocytic status from this criterion alone (17) *(7.15)*. While it is true that most lesions with reticular lines due to melanin pigment are melanocytic, there are frequent exceptions (see also chapter 2 for examples of non-melanocytic lesions with reticular lines). Reticular lines also occur in seborrheic keratoses, solar lentigines and dermatofibromas. Only the pathologist can see melanocytes and the pathologist must be the arbiter of melanocytic status.

Curved lines ("fingerprint like structures") identify a lesion as a solar lentigo/flat seborrheic keratosis
This is the most dangerous of all invalid interpretations of dermatoscopic clues because it exempts the lesion

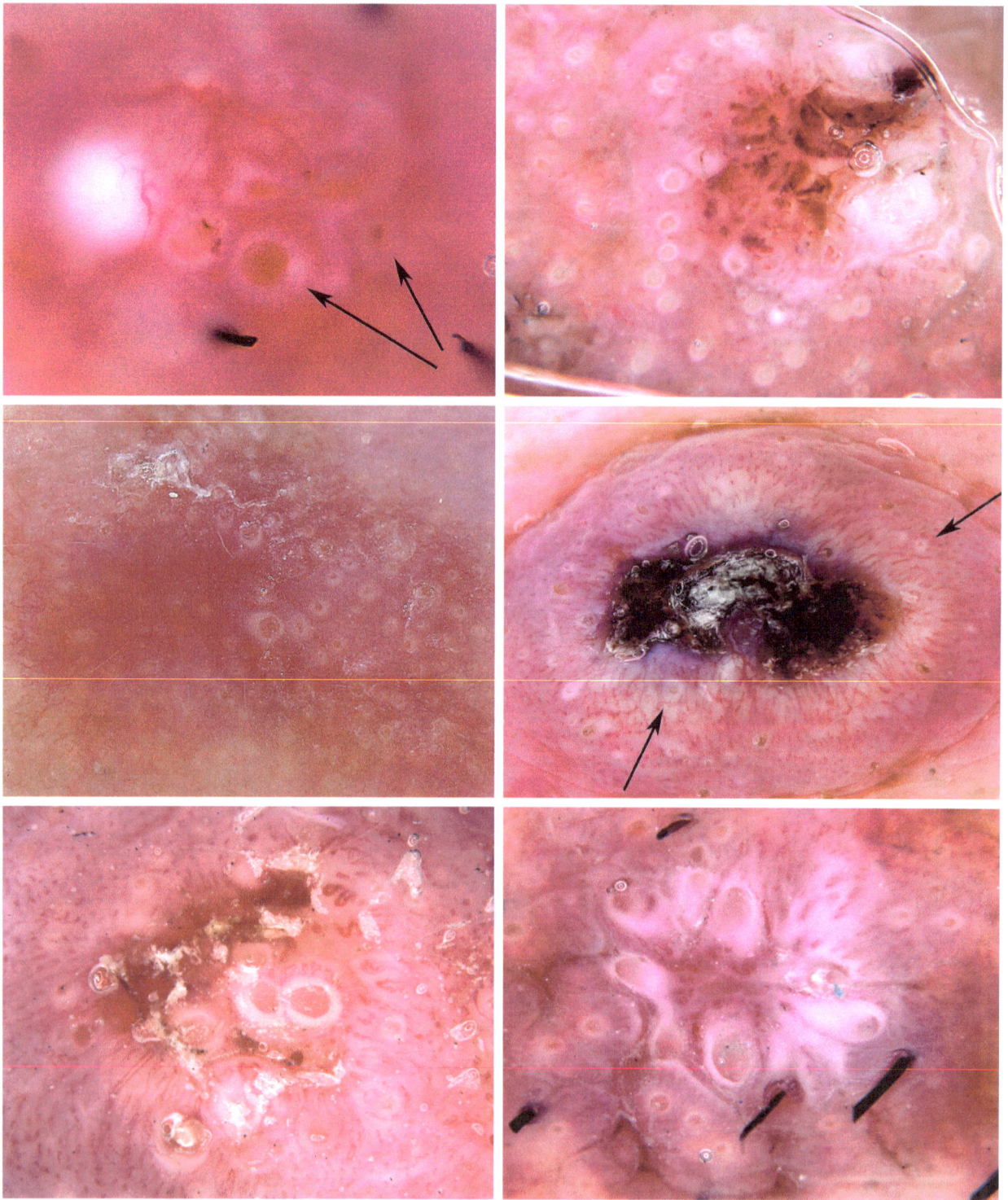

Figure 7.13: White circles as a clue to squamous cell carcinoma.

An unequivocal pattern of white circles is present in each of these lesions. **Top left:** Squamous cell carcinoma on the face (arrows point to white circles). The white circles contrast with vascular erythema surrounding them. **Top right:** White circles form a pattern in a squamous cell carcinoma on the ear. **Middle left:** Squamous cell carcinoma arising in an actinic keratosis on the nose. The white circles contrast with vascular erythema surrounding them. Yellow clods occupy the center in each of these white circles. **Middle right:** White circles in a kerato-acanthoma. **Bottom left:** Squamous cell carcinoma on the ear. **Bottom right:** Squamous cell carcinoma on the neck.

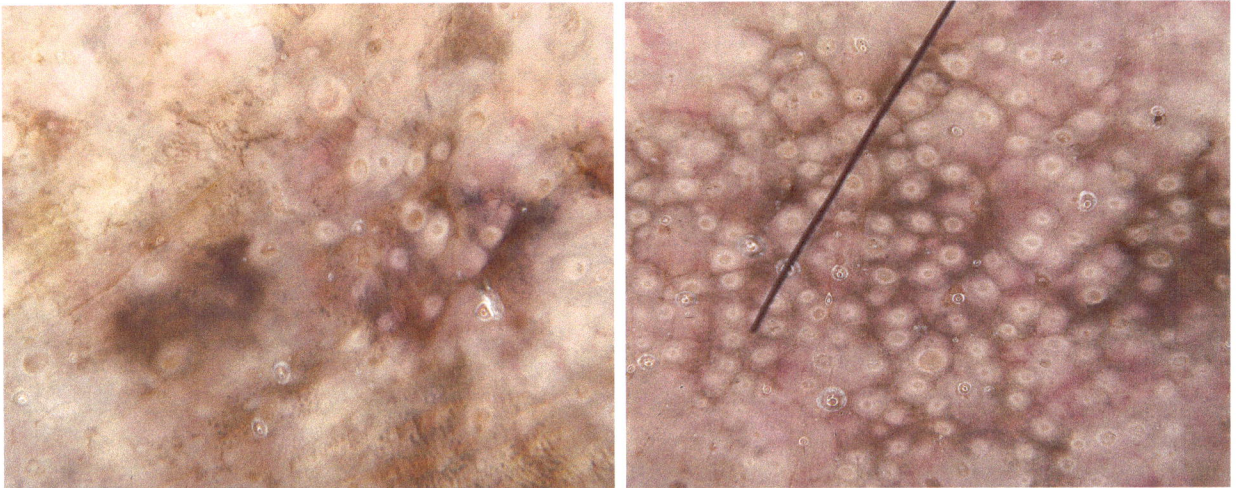

Figure 7.14: *Dermatoscopy of two pigmented actinic keratoses on the forehead.*
Left and right: *Dermatoscopy of pigmented actinic keratosis on the forehead. Note that the pigment occupies the space between the white circles. The differential diagnosis includes melanoma in situ, lichen planus-like keratosis, and pigmented actinic keratosis. The clue of white circles identifies these lesions as pigmented actinic keratosis.*

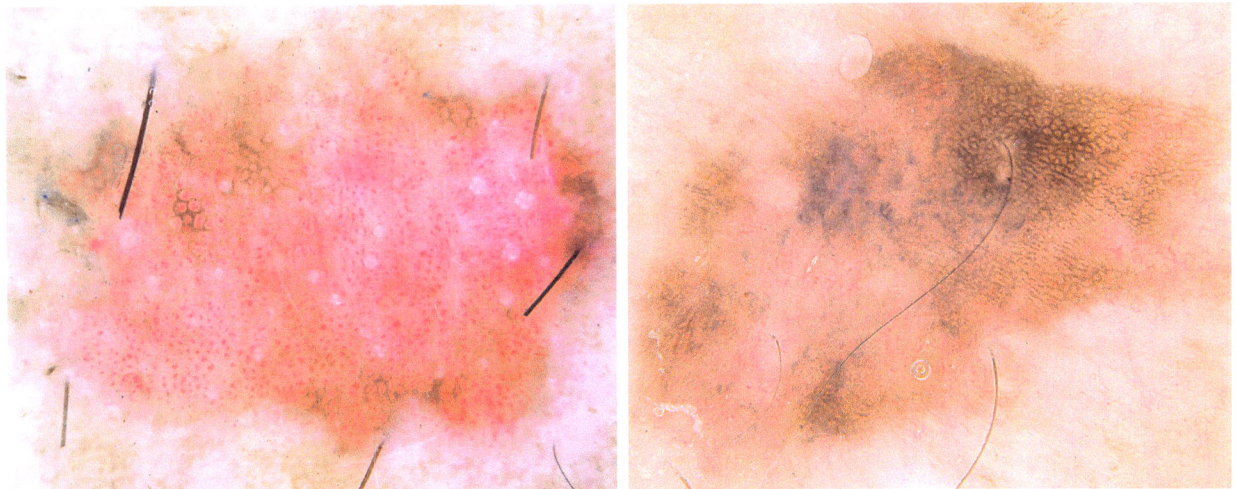

Figure 7.15: *Reticular lines in non-melanocytic lesions.*
Left: *This lesion has areas of reticular lines. It was Bowen's disease colliding with a solar lentigo and the solar lentigo produced the reticular lines. There was no melanocytic proliferation in any part of this lesion.* **Right:** *This lesion was excised (correctly) to exclude melanoma. It was reported as pigmented Bowen's disease. The reticular lines were due to collision with a seborrheic keratosis. Both are non-melanocytic!*

from further assessment to exclude melanoma. While in most cases this clue does correctly identify solar lentigines or flat seborrheic keratoses, this pattern may also be seen in melanoma. The example shown in *figure 7.16* very emphatically illustrates the danger of interpreting patterns and clues without taking into account the whole context.

White dots and clods ("milia") indicate a seborrheic keratosis

White dots and clods (milia) are produced by small intraepidermal accumulations of keratin. Although white dots and clods are most commonly found in seborrheic keratosis, they also occur in malignancies such as basal cell carcinoma and melanoma *(7.17)*. Seborrheic keratosis should never be diagnosed on the basis of white dots and clods alone.

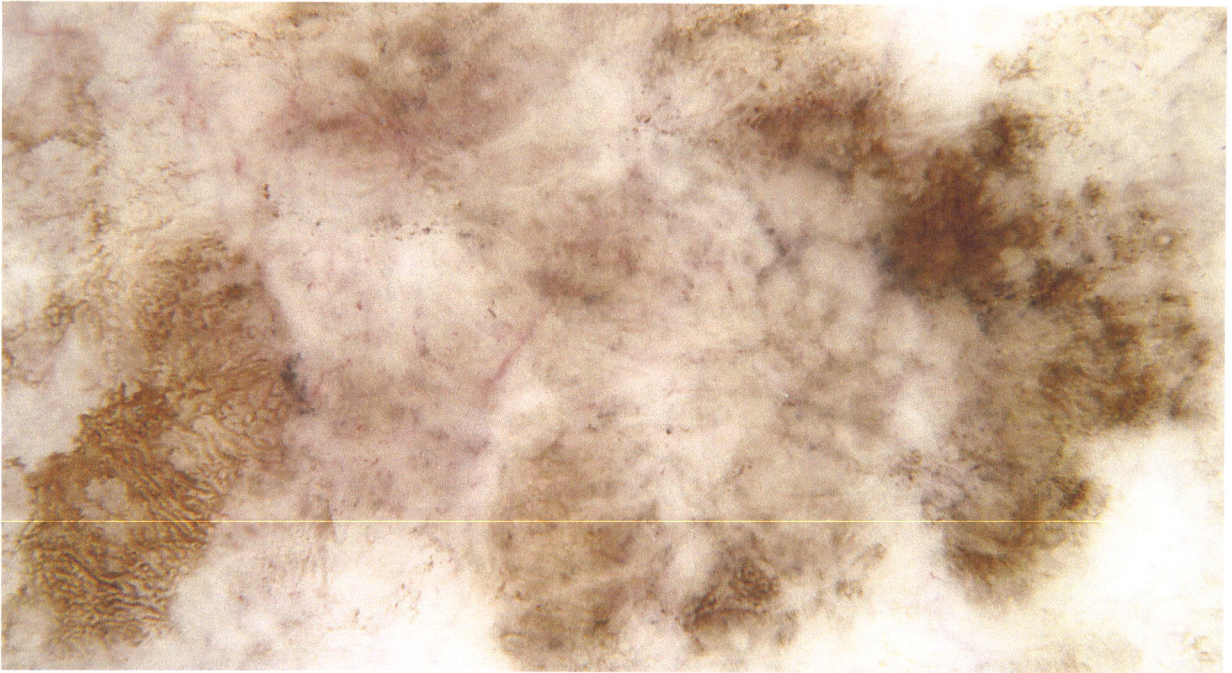

Figure 7.16: Curved lines ("fingerprint like structures") as a misleading clue to solar lentigo/flat seborrheic keratosis.
This is a lesion with curved lines ("light-brown fingerprint like structures" in the metaphoric language) that could be easily discarded as a solar lentigo/flat seborrheic keratosis. However, it is asymmetric with a clue to malignancy by virtue of gray dots. Furthermore, it lacks a well-demarcated, scalloped border. This is melanoma in situ.

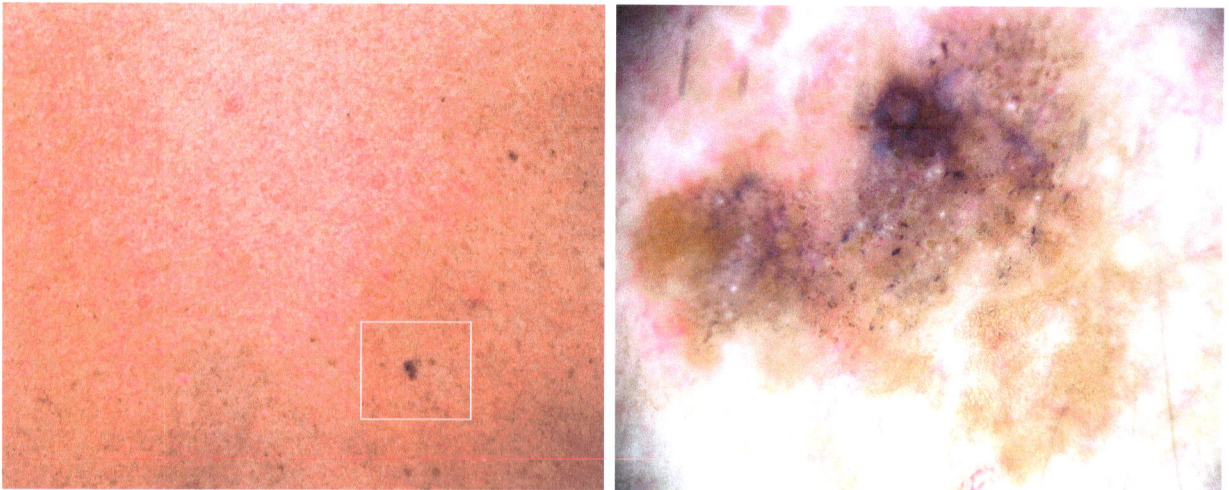

Figure 7.17: White dots ("milia") can occur in any type of lesion, not only seborrheic keratosis.
Melanoma with multiple white dots and clods ("milia"). This lesion could easily be mistaken for a seborrheic keratosis if it is not assessed in context. Clinically (left) this is a solitary lesion, whereas seborrheic keratoses usually are seen in large numbers. This anomaly should arouse suspicion and lead to careful assessment. Dermatoscopically (right) there are no yellow or orange clods, the border is poorly demarcated, and the vessels are neither looped nor centered in hypopigmented clods. Therefore there is little support for a proposed diagnosis of seborrheic keratosis, even if white dots are the standout feature of this lesion. The presence of gray dots always raises the possibility of melanoma, and this was confirmed on histopathology (invasive < 1 mm).

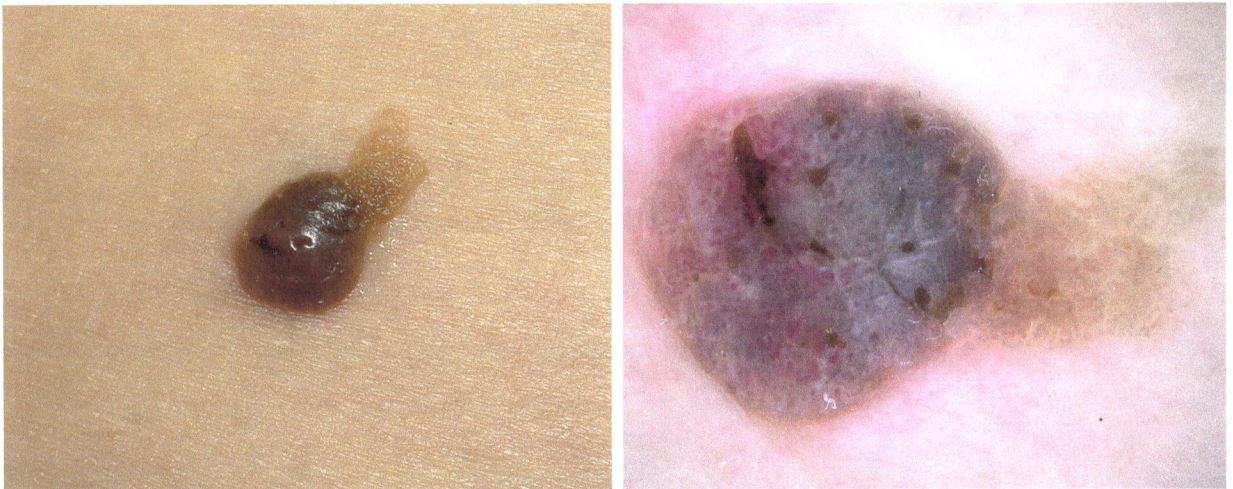

Figure 7.18: Blue structureless area ("blue veil") in a seborrheic keratosis.
*Clinical view on the **left,** dermatoscopic view on the **right.** Like many seborrheic keratosis this lesion is chaotic. An unequivocal blue structureless area ("blue veil") is present on the dermatoscopic image, a finding not uncommon in acanthotic seborrheic keratosis.*

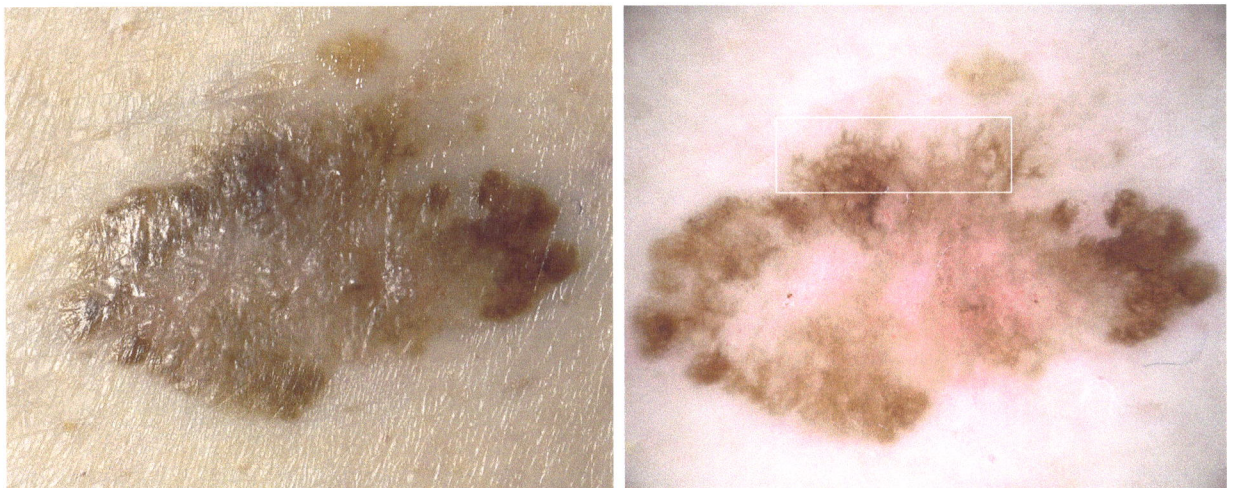

Figure 7.19: Pseudopods in a seborrheic keratosis.
*Clinical view on the **left,** dermatoscopic view on the **right.** This seborrheic keratosis is chaotic, has reticular lines, and a few pseudopods at the periphery in the area indicated by the white rectangle. Whilst reticular lines are in synchrony with the diagnosis of a seborrheic keratosis, pseudopods are an unexpected finding. The scalloped and sharply demarcated border is a clue to seborrheic keratosis. White dots ("milia") are not visible in this image taken with polarized dermatoscopy.*

Blue structureless area ("blue veil") indicates melanoma

A blue structureless area is a good clue to differentiate a melanoma from a nevus. It is not a good clue to differentiate a melanoma from a seborrheic keratosis because acanthotic seborrheic keratoses frequently show a blue structureless area *(7.18).* Other clues are needed in this context.

Segmental pseudopods or segmental radial lines indicate a melanoma

Although pseudopods are admittedly a very strong clue to melanoma they can be found in other lesions too. *Figure 7.19* shows a seborrheic keratosis with pseudopods. Segmental radial lines can be found in basal cell carcinoma, pigmented Bowen's disease, recurrent nevi, Reed nevi, and rarely also in Clark nevi.

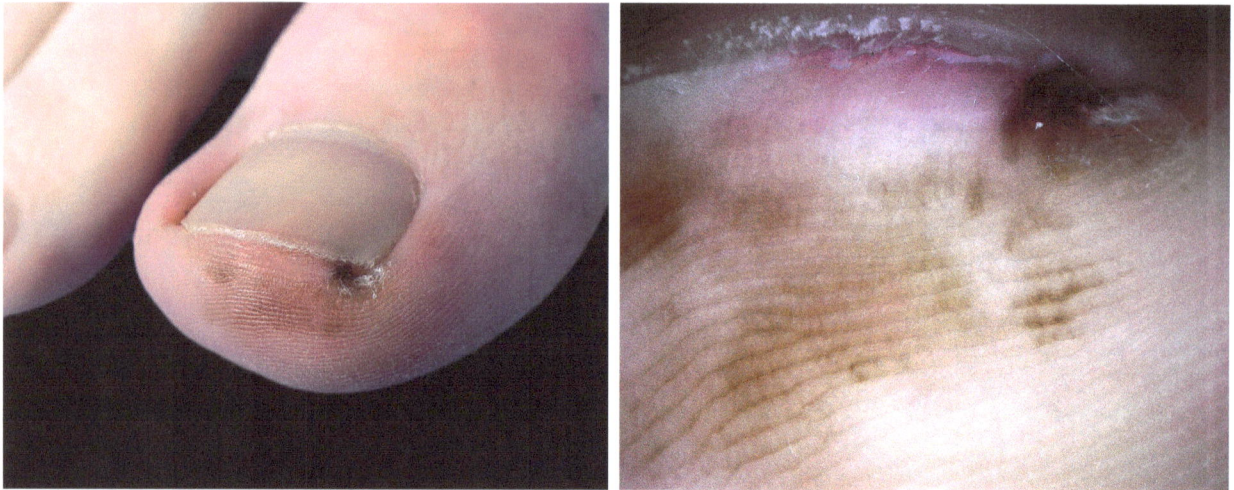

Figure 7.20: *Parallel furrow pattern in an acral melanoma.*
The absence of a parallel ridge pattern and the presence of a parallel furrow pattern in acral lesions does not exclude acral melanoma.
This is melanoma because it is chaotic and there are clues to malignancy (eccentric structureless zone). The presence of a parallel furrows
pattern does not make this a benign lesion!

A parallel furrows pattern indicates a benign acral lesion

The absence of a parallel ridge pattern and the presence of a parallel furrow pattern in acral lesions does not exclude acral melanoma (18) *(7.20)*. The general principles of pattern analysis also apply to acral lesions. If there is chaos and a clue to melanoma then the lesion is suspicious for melanoma regardless of whether parallel lines are situated in the furrows or on the ridges.

Serpentine branched vessels indicate a basal cell carcinoma

While it is true that most basal cell carcinomas, especially when they are nodular, have serpentine branched vessels ("arborizing vessels"), it is not true that this arrangement of vessels is highly specific for basal cell carcinomas. Any tumor underneath the superficial vascular plexus may show serpentine branched vessels in dermatoscopy including other neoplasms (19), cysts (20), deposits, and inflammatory lesions (21) *(7.21)*.

Malignant neoplasms are chaotic

Although most pigmented cutaneous malignant neoplasms are chaotic by dermatoscopy there are important exceptions: Small melanomas, nodular melanomas, and flat facial and acral melanomas are often symmetrical *(7.22)*. Whilst in large and flat lesions chaos takes precedence over clues, clues are more important than chaos in small (5 mm and less) and nodular lesions. Very rarely chaos may be absent even in large and flat melanomas *(7.23)*. In these cases, information beyond dermatoscopy like the clinical context ("ugly duckling") or the history given by the patient ("changing lesion") may draw the attention of the examiner to the lesion.

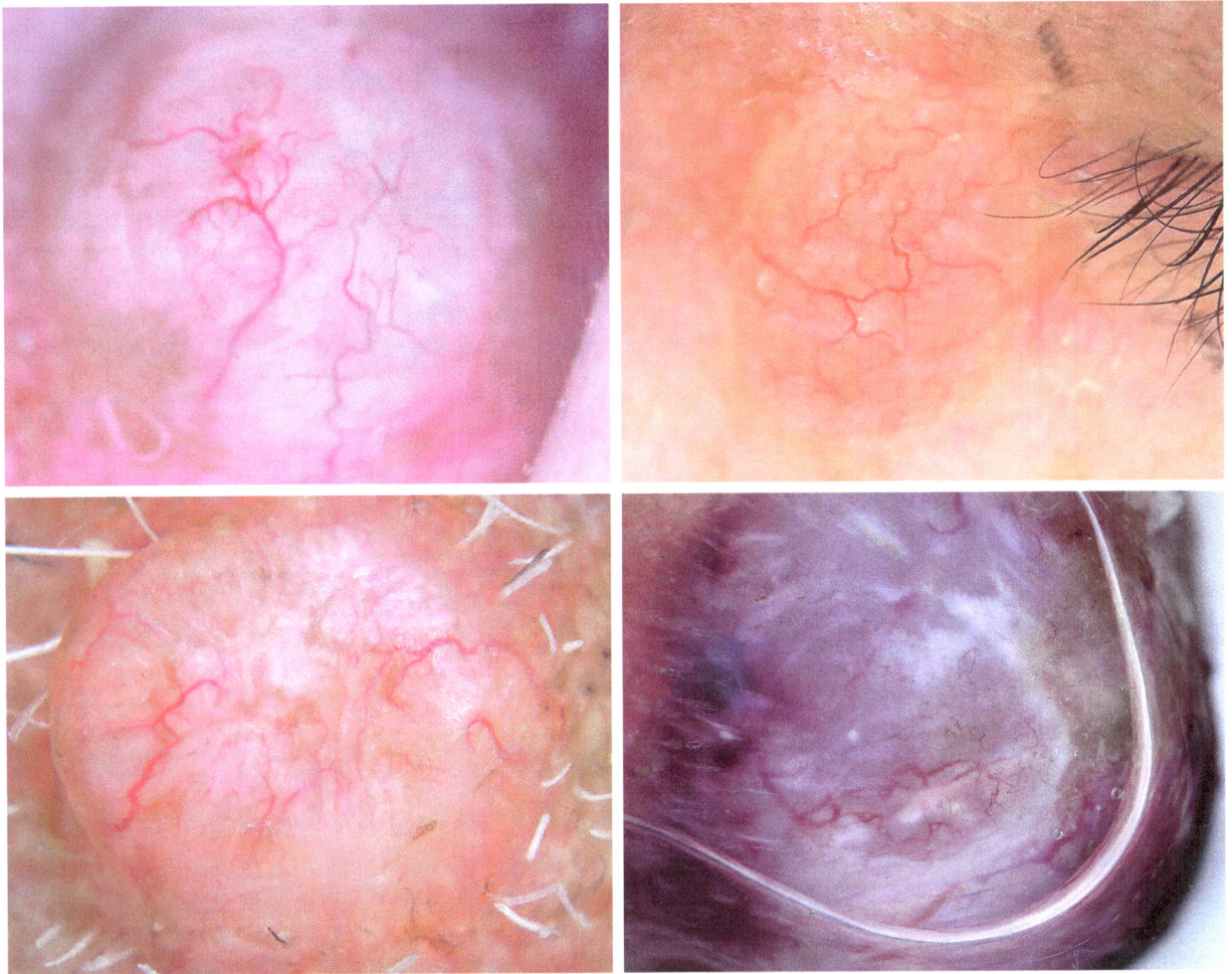

Figure 7.21: *Benign and malignant neoplasms and cysts with serpentine branched vessels on dermatoscopy. Serpentine branched vessels can be found in any tumor that is situated underneath the superficial vascular plexus, not only in basal cell carcinomas. Four examples are trichoepithelioma* (**top left**), *eccrine hidrocystoma* (**top right**), *pilar sheath acanthoma* (**bottom left**), *Merkel cell carcinoma* (**bottom right**). *Images courtesy of Nisa Akay, Jean-Yves Gourhant, Iris Zalaudek and Giuseppe Argenziano).*

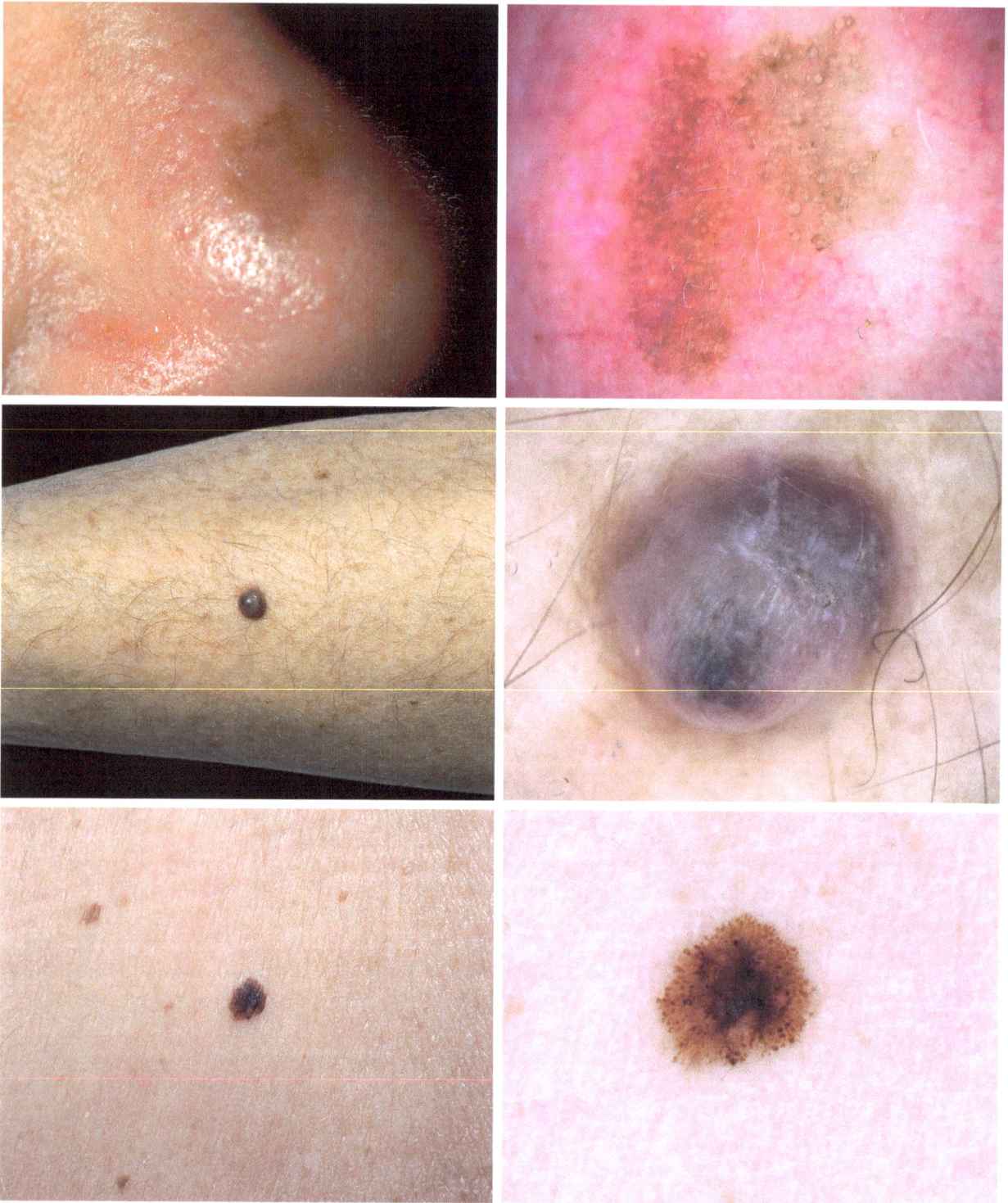

Figure 7.22: *Flat facial melanomas, nodular melanomas, and small melanomas may be symmetrical, not chaotic. Clinical view on the **left**, dermatoscopic view on the **right**. **Top row:** Flat facial melanomas (usually in situ) may be symmetrical. The discrete gray circles (not dots arranged as circles) on dermatoscopy allow the diagnosis of melanoma in situ with confidence. **Middle row:** Melanomas that grow quickly may present as nodules and often lack chaos. The diagnosis of melanoma can be suspected because of white lines and a blue structureless area. In nodular lesions, clues are more important than chaos. **Bottom row:** Small melanoma (5 mm in diameter) that is not chaotic on dermatoscopy but has gray and blue clods in the center. In small lesions clues are more important than chaos.*

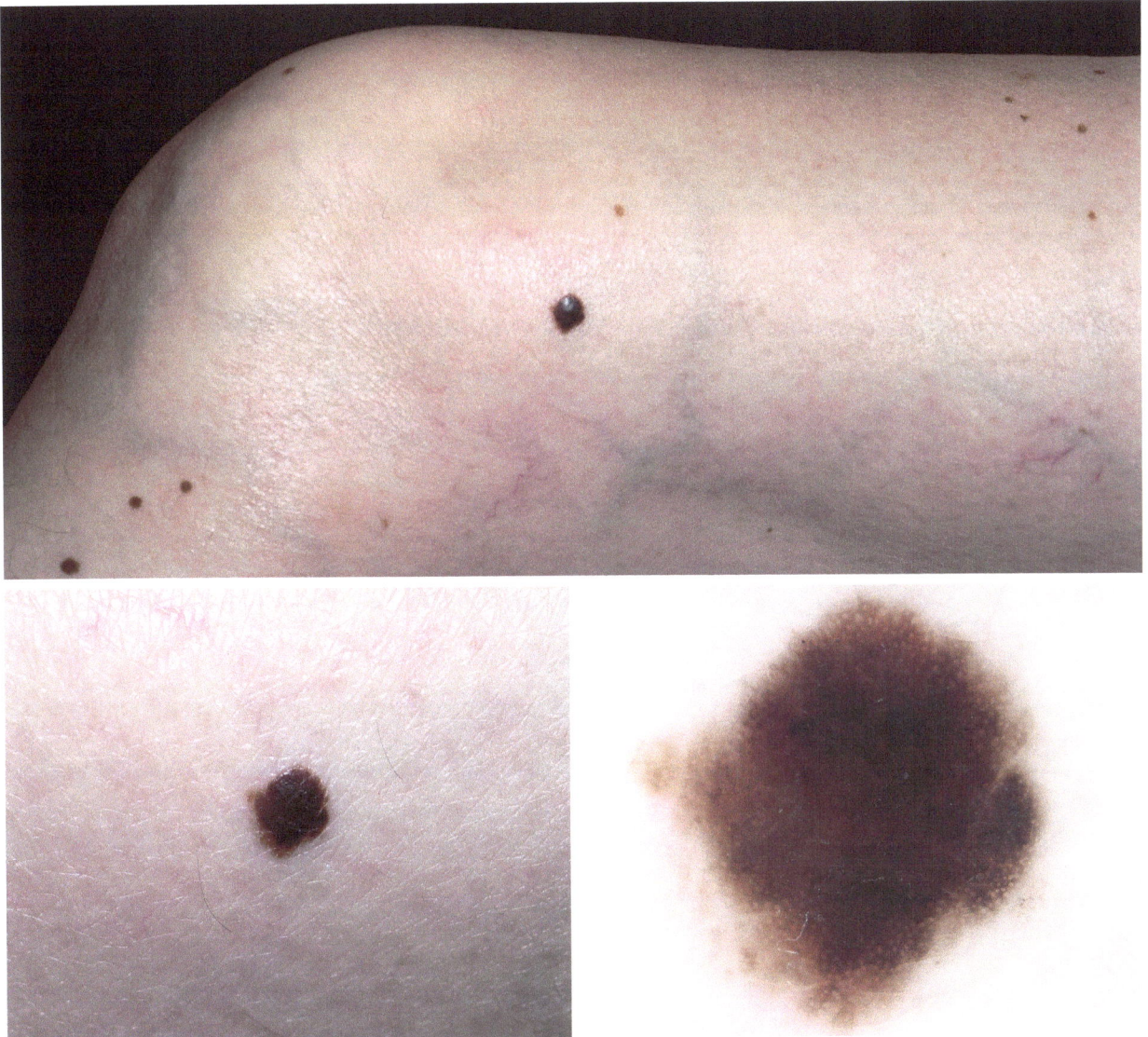

Figure 7.23: *The clinical context helps to diagnose melanomas that are not chaotic.*
On the clinical overview **(top)** *this pigmented lesion is different than the other pigmented lesions in this area ("ugly duckling"). The clinical close-up image* **(bottom left)** *reveals a symmetrical brown plaque. On dermatoscopy there is no chaos* **(bottom right).** *There are, however, thick reticular lines as clues to melanoma.*

References

1   Piliouras P, Allison S, Rosendahl C, Buettner PG, Weedon D. Dermoscopy improves diagnosis of tinea nigra: a study of 50 cases. Australas J Dermatol. 2011; 52(3): 191–194.

2   Rosendahl C, Cameron A, Argenziano G, Zalaudek I, Tschandl P, Kittler H. Dermoscopy of squamous cell carcinoma and keratoacanthoma. Arch Dermatol. 2012; 148(12): 1386–1392.

3   Selmer J, Skov T, Spelman L, Weedon D. SCCs and KAs are biologically distinct and can be diagnosed by light microscopy. Histopathology. 2016; 69(4): 535–41.

4   Marghoob AA, Cowell L, Kopf AW, Scope A. Observation of chrysalis structures with polarized dermoscopy. Arch Dermatol. 2009; 145(5): 618.

5   Tschandl P, Rosendahl C, Kittler H. Dermatoscopy of flat pigmented facial lesions. J Eur Acad Dermatol Venereol. 2015; 29(1): 120–127.

6   Lozzi GP, Piccolo D, Micantonio T, Altamura D, Peris K. Early melanomas dermoscopically characterized by reticular depigmentation. Arch Dermatol. 2007; 143(6): 808–809.

7   Pizzichetta MA, Talamini R, Marghoob AA, et al. Negative pigment network: an additional dermoscopic feature for the diagnosis of melanoma. J Am Acad Dermatol. 2013; 68(4): 552–559.

8   Pizzichetta MA, Canzonieri V, Soyer PH, Rubegni P, Talamini R, Massone C. Negative pigment network and shiny white streaks: a dermoscopic-pathological correlation study. Am J Dermatopathol. 2014; 36(5): 433–438.

9   Braun RP, Scope A, Marghoob AA. The "blink sign" in dermoscopy. Arch Dermatol. 2011; 147(4): 520.

10 Botella-Estrada R, Requena C, Traves V, Nagore E, Guillen C. Chrysalis and negative pigment network in Spitz nevi. Am J Dermatopathol. 2012; 34(2): 188–191.

11 Moscarella E, Lallas A, Kyrgidis A, et al. Clinical and dermoscopic features of atypical Spitz tumors: A multicenter, retrospective, case-control study. J Am Acad Dermatol. 2015; 73(5): 777–784.

12 Balagula Y, Braun RP, Rabinovitz HS, et al. The significance of crystalline/chrysalis structures in the diagnosis of melanocytic and nonmelanocytic lesions. J Am Acad Dermatol. 2012; 67(2): 194 e191–198.

13 Keir J. Dermatoscopic features of cutaneous non-facial non-acral lentiginous growth pattern melanomas. Dermatol Pract Concept. 2014; 4(1): 77–82.

14 Jaimes N, Marghoob AA, Rabinovitz H, et al. Clinical and dermoscopic characteristics of melanomas on nonfacial chronically sun-damaged skin. J Am Acad Dermatol. 2015; 72(6): 1027–1035.

15 Lallas A, Tschandl P, Kyrgidis A, et al. Dermoscopic clues to differentiate facial lentigo maligna from pigmented actinic keratosis. Br J Dermatol. 2016; 174(5): 1079–1085.

16 Slutsky JB, Marghoob AA. The zig-zag pattern of lentigo maligna. Arch Dermatol. 2010; 146(12): 1444.

17 Tschandl P, Rosendahl C, Kittler H. Accuracy of the first step of the dermatoscopic 2-step algorithm for pigmented skin lesions. Dermatol Pract Concept. 2012; 2(3): 203a208.

18 Lallas A, Kyrgidis A, Koga H, et al. The BRAAFF checklist: a new dermoscopic algorithm for diagnosing acral melanoma. Br J Dermatol. 2015; 173(4): 1041–1049.

19 Tschandl P. Dermatoscopic pattern of a spiradenoma. Dermatol Pract Concept. 2012; 2(4): 204a209.

20 Salerni G, Gonzalez R, Alonso C. Dermatoscopic pattern of digital mucous cyst: report of three cases. Dermatol Pract Concept. 2014; 4(4): 65–67.

21 Rudnicka L, Olszewska M, Rakowska A, Slowinska M. Trichoscopy update 2011. J Dermatol Case Rep. 2011; 5(4): 82–88.

8 Special situations

8.1 Nails

Pigmentations of the nail plate are frequently – probably too frequently – biopsied in order to exclude a melanoma of the nail matrix. However, the decision to biopsy nail pigmentation should not be made lightly – biopsies of the nail matrix are not only painful, they also may cause irreversible abnormalities of nail growth. By keeping a few basic principles in mind, the number of biopsies can be reduced without increasing the risk of missing a melanoma.

In principle, melanomas may occur anywhere in the nail unit, but in practice almost all originate in the nail matrix. Nail matrix pigmented neoplasms create longitudinal pigmentation of the nail plate, known as longitudinal melanonychia. Melanomas that do not arise in the nail matrix but in the nail bed do not produce longitudinal melanonychia. Initially the nail changes produced by nail bed melanoma may be mistaken for "nail dystrophy" or "onychomycosis" and thus remain unrecognized. Fortunately these are exceedingly rare neoplasms.

The following applies exclusively to melanomas that arise from the nail matrix.

Anatomy of the nail

In order to understand nail pigmentation, one must understand the anatomy of the nail organ. The nail plate is a convex 0.5-mm-thick plate composed of keratin. It is the final product of keratinocytes in the nail matrix. The nail plate lies on the nail bed. Its lateral margins are surrounded by the lateral nail fold while its proximal end is spanned by the proximal nail fold. These margins are also known as the nail wall or the paronychium. The narrow cornified portion of proximal nail fold which glides on 1 to 2 mm of the nail plate is known as the cuticle. The nail matrix itself lies below the lunula, the white arc at the proximal end of the nail plate (8.1).

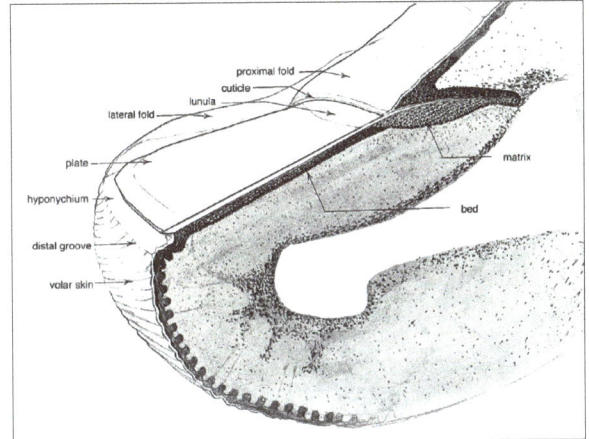

Figure 8.1: Anatomy of the nail plate.
(Adapted from Ackerman and Boer, Histologic diagnosis of inflammatory skin diseases. An algorithmic method based on pattern analysis, 3rd edition).

Dermatoscopy of nail pigmentation

Dermatoscopy of the nail plate requires a high viscosity ("stiff") contact fluid like ultrasound gel. Thinner fluids like paraffin oil and alcohol do not stay in place due to the highly irregular contour of the nail organ. A contact fluid also improves visualization when performing dermatoscopy with polarized light (1–4).

The most commonly seen pattern on dermatoscopy is a parallel pattern of lines (8.2). In longitudinal melanonychia, these parallel lines extend continuously from the lunula to the free end of the nail plate. Longitudinal melanonychia usually occupies just a part, and less frequently the entire width, of the nail plate. It is attributable to the increased production of melanin in the nail matrix, which may or may not be caused by a proliferation of melanocytes.

Gray pigmentation of lines is usually attributable to an increase of melanin, but it is not associated with proliferation of melanocytes in the nail matrix. The most common causes of gray parallel lines are lentigines (melanotic macules) of the nail matrix, ethnic hyperpigmentation, drug induced hyperpigmentation, hyperpigmentation during pregnancy, and traumatic or inflammatory hyperpigmentation (4). Traumatic hyperpigmentation occurs on finger nails mainly due to manipulation of the nail

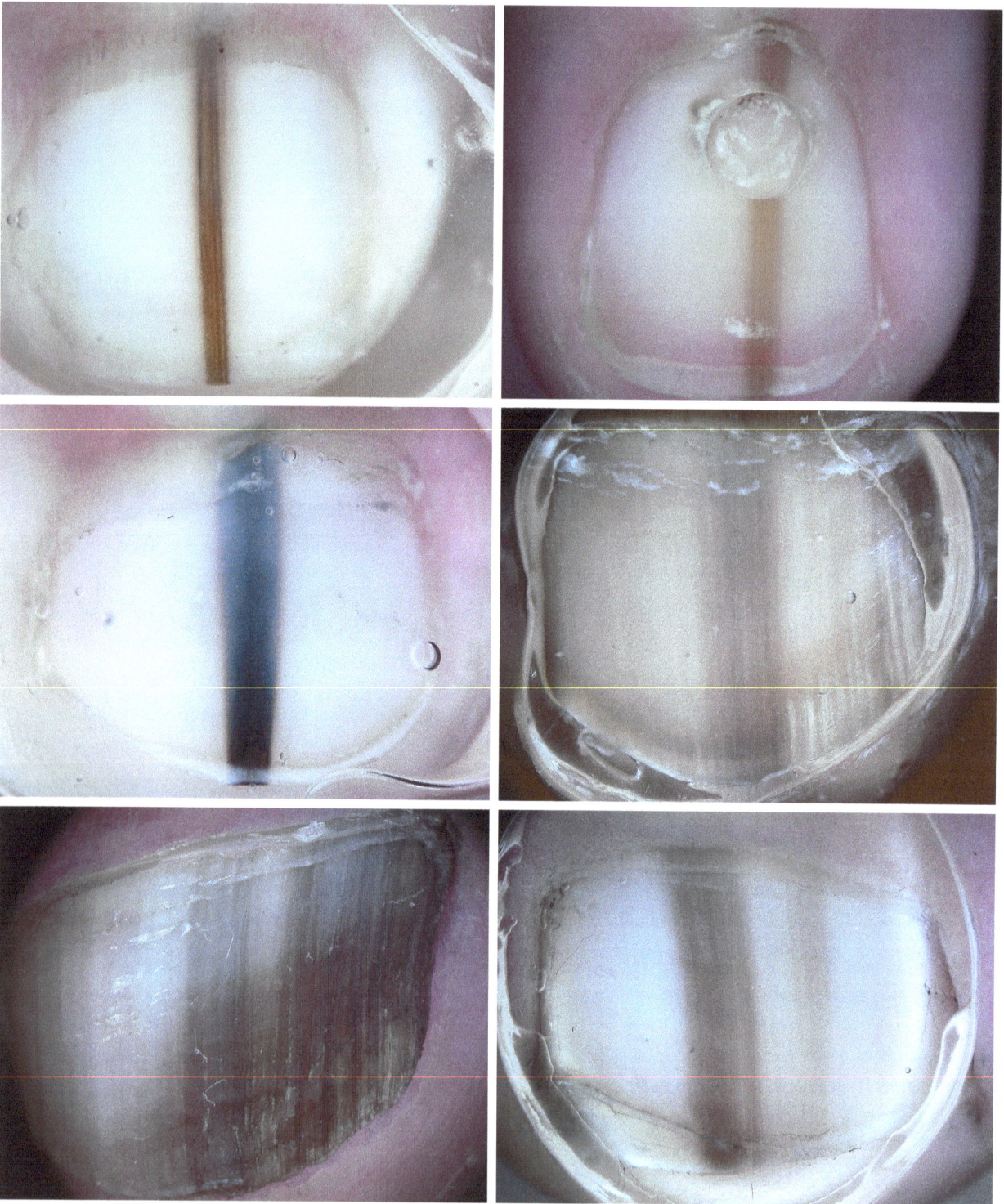

Figure 8.2: *Parallel lines in the nail plate.*
Top row, left: *Regularly arranged brown parallel lines in a nevus of the nail matrix.* **Top row, right:** *Light-brown parallel lines arranged regularly (the lines are equally spaced) in a nevus of the nail matrix. Note that the wrong site was selected for the biopsy: it is too far distal. Melanocytic lesions originate in the nail matrix, further proximally below the lunula.* **Middle row, left:** *A congenital nevus of the nail matrix in a 5-year-old child. The fact that the lesion is broader in its proximal portion than in its distal portion is a sign of rapid growth.* **Middle row, right:** *Gray parallel lines due to manipulation ("onychotillomania") in a finger nail.* **Bottom row, left:** *Brown and gray parallel lines due to chronic friction trauma of the nail of the big toe. A biopsy of the nail matrix is needed to exclude melanoma.* **Bottom row, right:** *In situ melanoma of the nail matrix with light-brown lines arranged unevenly (the distance between the lines varies).*

organ (so-called onychotillomania, *8.2 middle, right)*, whereas on the toe nails it primarily occurs due to friction. Friction induced pigmentation of the toe can sometimes show a mix of brown and gray lines and then it is difficult to differentiate this condition from melanocytic lesions *(8.2, bottom left)*. The brown lines caused by trauma are created by a mixture of hemorrhage and post-inflammatory hyperpigmentation. In some of these cases a biopsy is unavoidable.

Gray parallel lines are seen in many inflammatory conditions; for instance, onychomycosis (dermatophytes and even Candida *albicans* may produce melanin), lichen planus and (more rarely) psoriasis. Rare causes of gray parallel lines are the Laugier-Hunziker syndrome, Addison's disease or HIV disease (1). Drugs (e.g. tetracycline, AZT, amiodarone) and radiotherapy may also cause gray pigmentation of the nail plate. In all of these conditions, more than one nail is nearly always involved.

Brown or black parallel lines are usually caused by proliferation of melanocytes in the nail matrix. This indicates the presence of a nevus or a melanoma. In cases of nevus, the lines are (approximately) the same color and width, equally spaced, and arranged in a strictly parallel manner *(8.2, top)*. In cases of melanoma, however, they are "chaotic", which means that they vary in color and width, the distance between the lines varies *(8.2 bottom right, 8.3)*, and the lines are no longer all parallel (4).

The so-called Hutchinson's sign is defined as a macroscopically visible pigmentation of the proximal or lateral nail fold while the micro-Hutchinson sign refers to pigmentation of the cuticle *(8.4)*. These are both

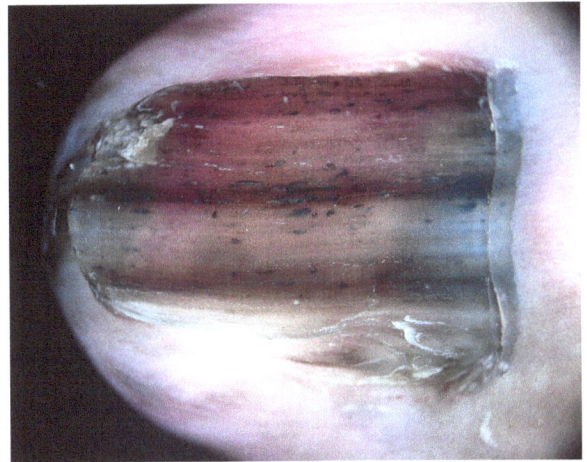

Figure 8.3: Melanoma of the nail plate.
This melanoma of the nail plate is more advanced than those shown in figure 8.2 bottom right and in figure 8.4. Apart from pigmentation of the nail plate one can see delicate pigmentation of periungual skin (Hutchinson's sign). The parallel lines of the nail plate vary in color and thickness. Note that there are blood spots, which show that a single criterion can be misleading if the context is ignored. This is a pattern of a melanoma and the unusual finding of blood spots should not alter your diagnosis.

clues to melanoma. The Hutchinson sign and the micro-Hutchinson sign must not be confused with the pseudo-Hutchinson sign *(8.5)*. The pseudo-Hutchinson sign occurs when pigmentation of the nail plate is visible through the cuticle. The pseudo-Hutchinson sign is not a clue to melanoma.

Melanoma in the nail matrix usually is found on the big toe, thumb or index finger; other digits are rarely affected. As a rule, melanomas of the nail matrix do

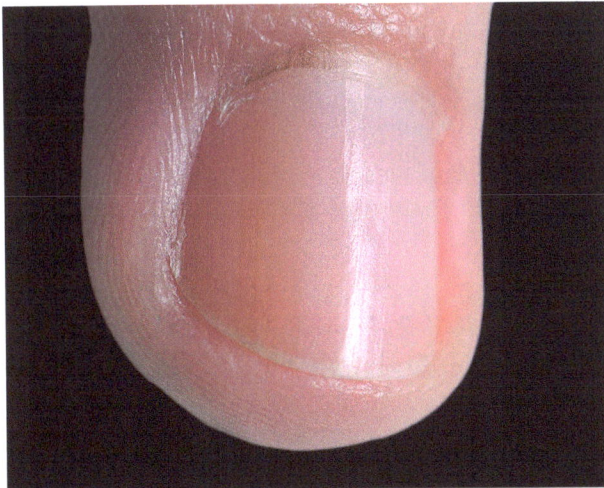

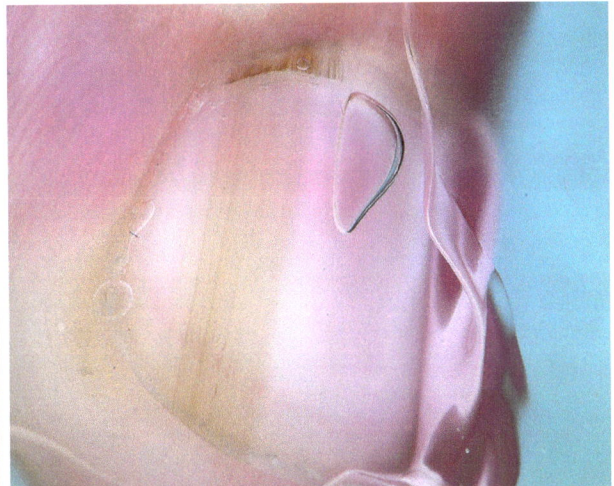

Figure 8.4: Melanoma in situ with micro-Hutchinson sign.
While clinically (**left**) *pigmentation is subtle, dermatoscopy on the* **right** *clearly shows pigmentation of the cuticle (micro-Hutchinson sign), a clue to melanoma.*

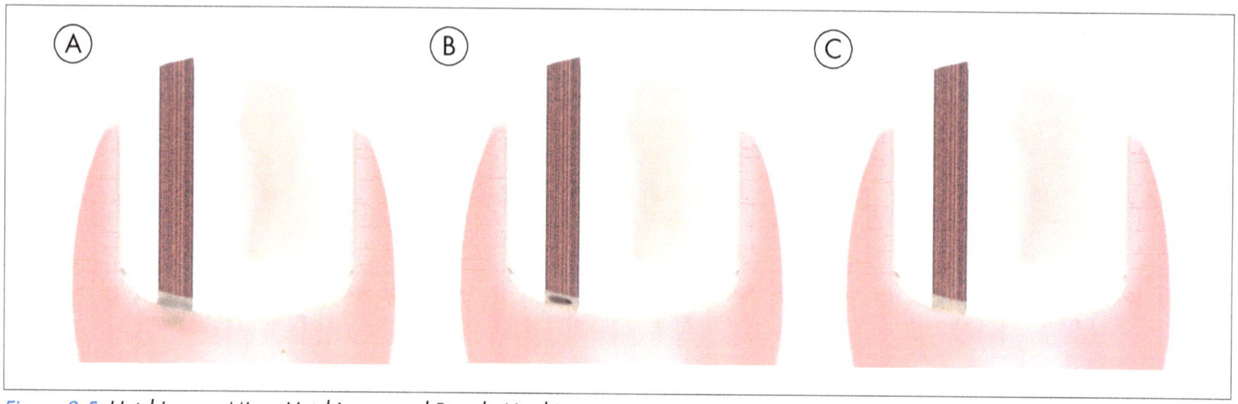

Figure 8.5: Hutchinson-, Micro-Hutchinson, and Pseudo-Hutchinson sign.
Hutchinson sign **(A)** is pigmentation of the proximal (or lateral) nail fold. Pigmentation of the cuticle is termed Micro-Hutchinson sign **(B)**. Pigmentation of the nail plate visible through the cuticle is termed Pseudo-Hutchinson sign. The cuticle bears no pigment **(C)**. Only A and B are clues to melanoma.

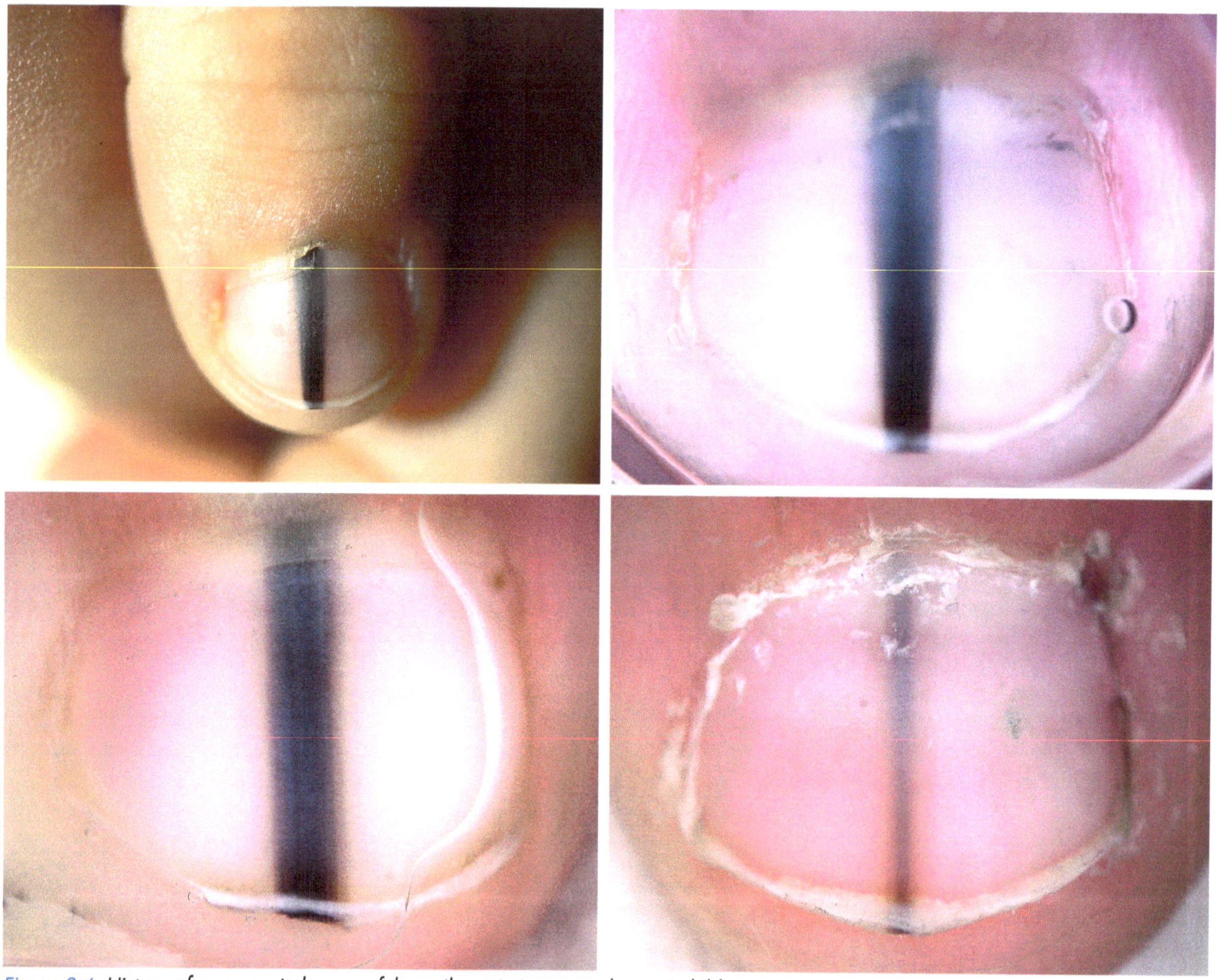

Figure 8.6: History of a congenital nevus of the nail matrix in a prepubescent child.
The clinical image is **top left**, the other images show a chronologic sequence of dermatoscopic images. At the first visit **(top right)** the pigmentation is broader in the proximal nail plate than in the distal nail plate, which indicates that the lesion is still growing. One year later **(bottom left)** the pigmentation in the proximal and distal nail plate have the same width, which indicates that the lesion stopped growing. Three years later the nevus is much smaller.

not occur in children (5). The exceptional reports of melanoma of the nail matrix in prepubescent children are most probably congenital nevi that have been misdiagnosed as melanomas. Congenital nevi of the nail matrix (which may not be visible at birth) commonly show clues to melanoma including signs of growth. In growing lesions the pigmentation is broader in the proximal part of the nail plate and smaller in the distal part *(8.6).* While this feature would be regarded as a clue to malignancy in adults one should not be too concerned if it occurs in children. Usually this sign of growth will disappear if the lesion is monitored for some months.

Therefore, even if clues to malignancy are present, biopsy of the nail matrix in prepubertal children should be performed very rarely, and only after careful consideration.

Apart from parallel lines, nail pigmentation may also be seen as dots, clods or a structureless pattern. These patterns occur in isolation or in combination with parallel lines. In most cases dots, clods and structureless areas are a sign of bleeding and therefore not caused by melanin but by hemoglobin *(8.7).* The distinction between hemorrhage and pigmentation of the nail due to melanin is usually made quite easily. Hemorrhage tends to be red or purple and the pigmentation appears structureless. Pigmentation of the nail plate caused by melanin is usually brown or occasionally black, and usually seen as longitudinal melanonychia, i.e. parallel lines extending the whole length of the nail plate. Parallel lines may also be found in hemorrhage, but not only will they be a different color, the lines do not extend continuously from the proximal to the free distal end of the nail plate. Growth of the nail plate causes pigmentation to advance distally. Pigmentation from hemorrhage advances very slowly; in toe nails it may be as little as 1 mm per month. Over time, a growing, non-pigmented healthy piece of nail will be found between the pigmentation and the proximal nail fold. The pigmentation produced by hemorrhage normally resolves spontaneously, regardless of the pattern seen. Renewed bleeding may occur in case of repetitive trauma and prevent complete outgrowth of the pigmentation. This is especially true for toe nails; at this site the trauma tends to remain unnoticed.

Because neoplasms may bleed, signs of hemorrhage do not entirely rule out a malignancy of the nail unit *(8.3).* For this reason it is advisable to perform a follow-up examination after three months in patients with subungual hemorrhage who are unable to recall an explicit incident of trauma.

Fungal infections may be accompanied by a structureless brown discoloration of the nail; in very rare cases there may also be parallel lines *(8.8).* This brown pigmentation is due to the fact that fungi may produce melanin. Usually there are additional clues to fungal infections such as thickening of the nail, subungual hyperkeratoses and whitish discoloration of the nail, which usually extends from proximal to distal. Sometimes fungal microscopy or culture may be the only way to establish the diagnosis. There are also pigment-forming bacteria like for example *Pseudomonas aeruginosa (8.9),* which is characterized by green discoloration of the nail plate (chloronychia).

Rarely, melanomas of the nail organ do not produce longitudinal melanonychia. Melanomas of the nail bed and nail fold may produce other patterns of pigmentation, and amelanotic melanomas are of course non-pigmented. Dermatoscopy features of these rare situations have not yet been described, and diagnosis must be based on clinical features.

Biopsies of the nail matrix
Longitudinal melanonychia originates in the nail matrix, which means any biopsy must be performed not from the nail bed, but from the matrix, at the proximal end of the pigmentation. Dermatoscopy of the free end of the nail helps to identify the zone of the matrix that is responsible for the pigmentation of the nail plate (6). When the pigmentation is mainly in the deeper layers of the nail plate, the biopsy should be performed in the distal part of the nail matrix. Pigmentation in the more superficial layers of the nail plate requires a biopsy from the proximal part of the matrix. These biopsies from the proximal nail matrix are associated with a higher risk of disrupted nail growth.

In narrow lesions (less than 3 mm in diameter) biopsy can be performed by punch excision. In these cases it will be adequate to insert the punch through the nail plate into the nail matrix after folding back the proximal portion of the nail fold. For slightly larger lesions (3 to 6 mm) located in the center of the nail, biopsy can be by transverse excision or shave of the nail matrix, ideally including the entire lesion (1).

For this purpose the nail plate is fenestrated and the nail matrix exposed.

In lesions larger than 6 mm diameter, usually one is only able to perform a partial biopsy – in most cases a punch biopsy – to confirm the diagnosis. Partial biopsies have a major disadvantage, as they make the already demanding histological investigation even more difficult. False negative histopathology reports due to inadequate partial biopsies are not rare.

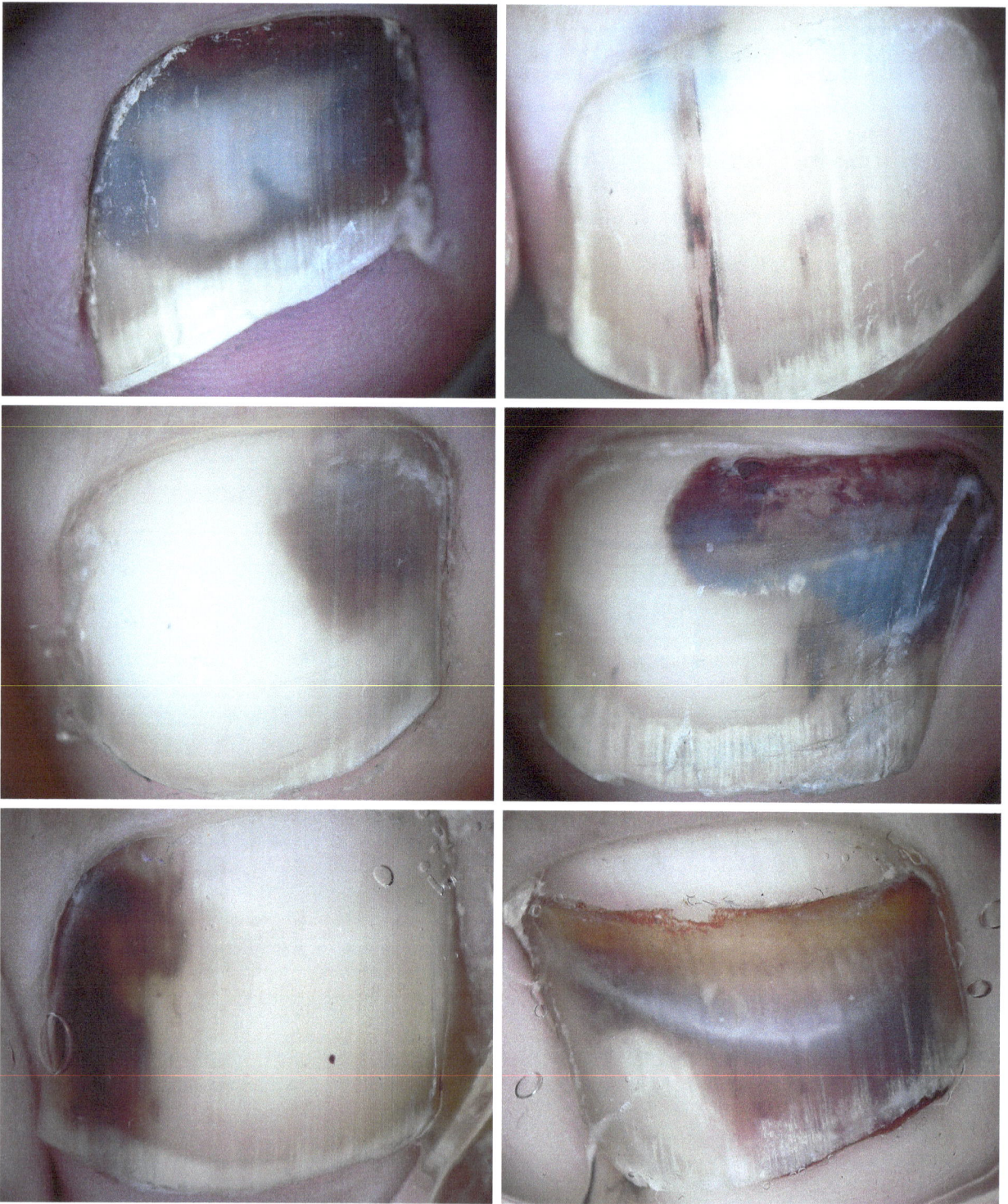

Figure 8.7: Subungual bleeding.
Manifestations of subungual bleeding. The red or red-brown color, the structureless pattern or clods, and pigmentation that does not extend continuously from proximal to distal are characteristic features of this condition.

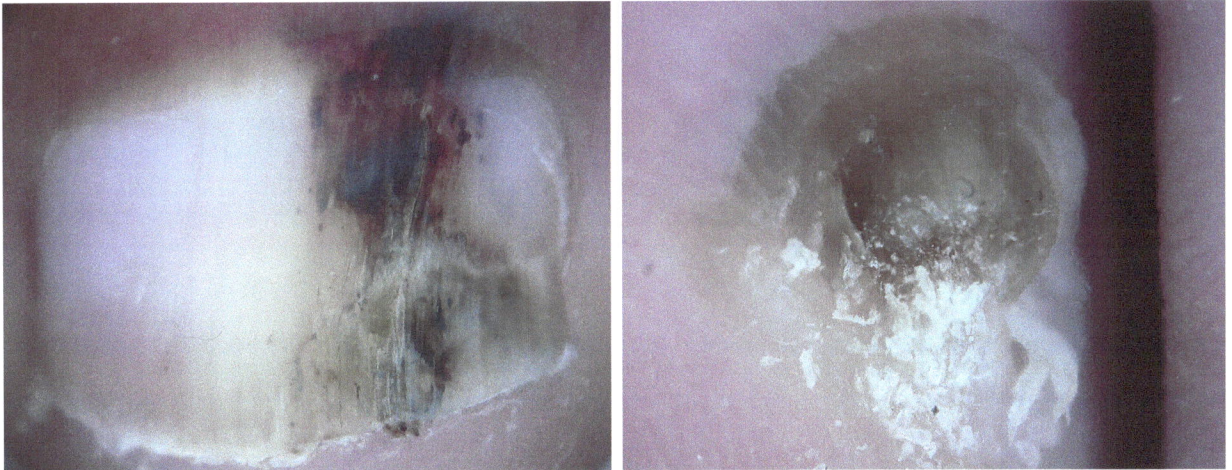

Figure 8.8: *Fungal infection of the nail plate.*
Left: *Fungal infection with hemorrhage.* **Right:** *Fungal infection of the small toenail with gray discoloration of the hyperkeratotic nail plate.*

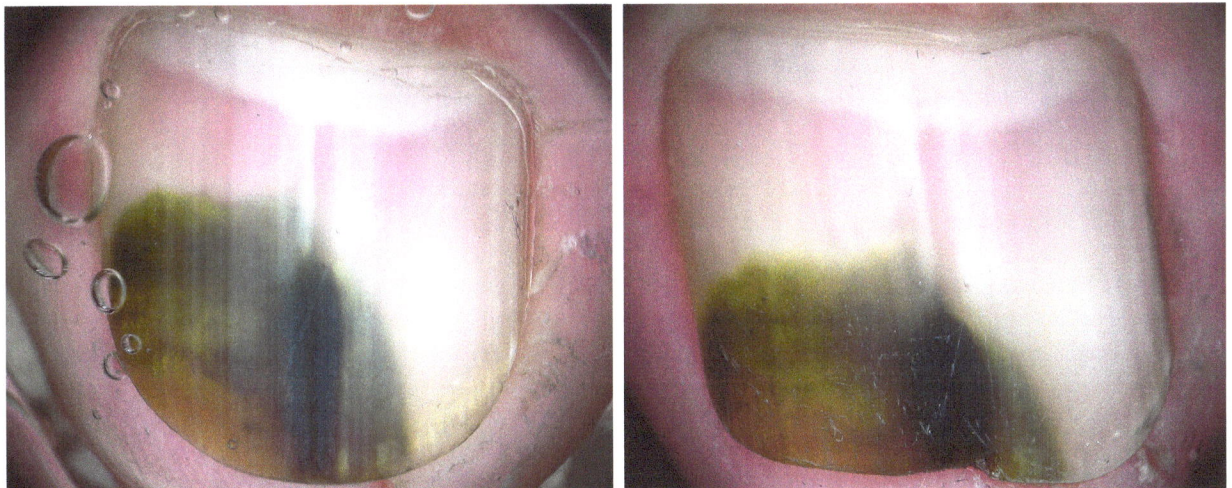

Figure 8.9: *Infection of the nail plate by Pseudomonas aeruginosa.*
*Green discoloration of the proximal nail due to infection with Pseudomonas aeruginosa before **(left)** and shortly after **(right)** treatment with oral quinolone.*

When the longitudinal melanonychia is to one side and not in the center of the nail, a longitudinal nail biopsy is performed. The entire lateral nail matrix and nail bed is removed, and lateral nail fold sutured to the nail plate (1). The pathology laboratory should be instructed to section the specimen longitudinally rather than transversely.

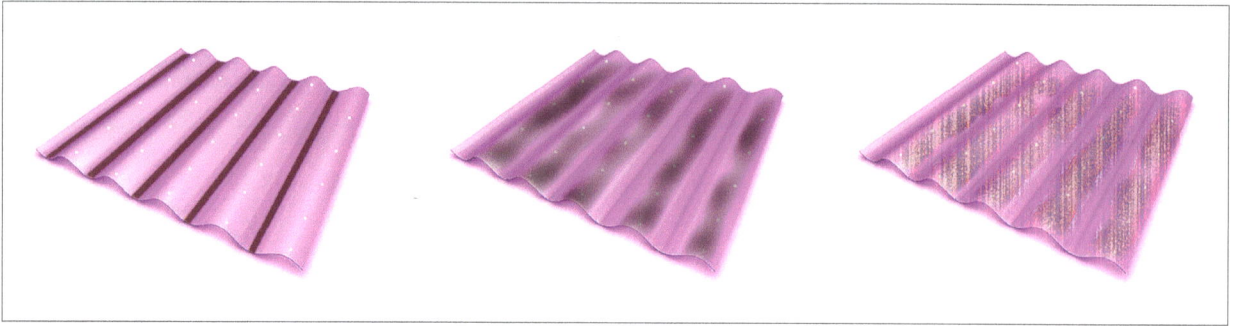

Figure 8.10: *Various arrangements of parallel lines on acral skin.*
Parallel lines in furrows **(left)**, *on ridges* **(middle)** *or crossing ridges* **(right)**. *We are grateful to Masaru Tanaka for teaching us the correct arrangement of parallel lines crossing the ridges.*

8.2 Acral lesions

The diagnosis of acral lesions by dermatoscopy is based on the same principles as those at other locations, but the common patterns seen do vary by site. While circles predominate on the face and reticular lines on the trunk and the proximal extremities, the predominant pattern of acral melanocytic lesions is parallel lines *(8.10)*.

Clinicians and dermatopathologists rarely agree on nomenclature, but both call a benign acral melanocytic proliferation an "acral nevus" without further differentiation. In fact, while some nevi preferentially occur at specific anatomical locations (Clark nevi are found nearly exclusively on the trunk and the proximal extremities, but very rarely on the face or acral skin), nearly all types of nevi may occur on acral skin *(8.11, 8.12, 8.13)*. Whenever possible, a specific diagnosis such as Spitz, Reed, "superficial" or "superficial and deep" congenital nevus should be used instead of the term "acral nevus". There is only one type of nevus which has no counterpart at other locations, the "classical acral nevus" *(8.11)*. Clinically it is seen as a uniformly light-brown macule, at dermatopathology one finds small melanocyte nests mainly at the dermo-epidermal junction.

Although parallel lines are the most common pattern of acral melanocytic proliferations, other patterns may also be seen. Dots, clods and the structureless pattern are seen quite frequently, circles and reticular lines less often, radial lines and pseudopods rarely. Parallel lines may be seen in the furrows, on the ridges, or crossing both furrows and ridges. One pattern may merge into another, most commonly the furrow pattern merging with the crossing pattern. The crossing pattern preferentially occurs at sites of greatest pressure, i.e. the heels and the lateral part of the sole (7, 8). While the furrow pattern is the most common

pattern in acral nevi of all types *(8.11, 8.13)*; several types of furrow pattern exist (7, 9). Usually there is just one pigmented line in every furrow; but sometimes there are two. These single or double lines may be composed of dots, rather than being continuous. In another variant, the parallel lines in the furrows are connected by crosswise lines *(8.11, middle row, 8.13 middle row)*. The furrow pattern may be combined with dots or clods, more rarely even circles. In lesions with more than one pattern, the same principles apply as for other sites of the body, i.e. pattern and color plus clues lead to the diagnosis.

Beginners may find it difficult to distinguish between ridges and furrows (10). However, with some practice the distinction can be made quite easily because ridges are wider than furrows, and the eccrine ducts (visible as hypopigmented dots) open out onto the ridges. In heavily pigmented acral lesions it may be difficult to identify the pattern because pigmentation is found both on ridges and in furrows. In these cases, the pattern can usually be identified as ridge or furrow at the lesions' periphery, where pigmentation is lighter.

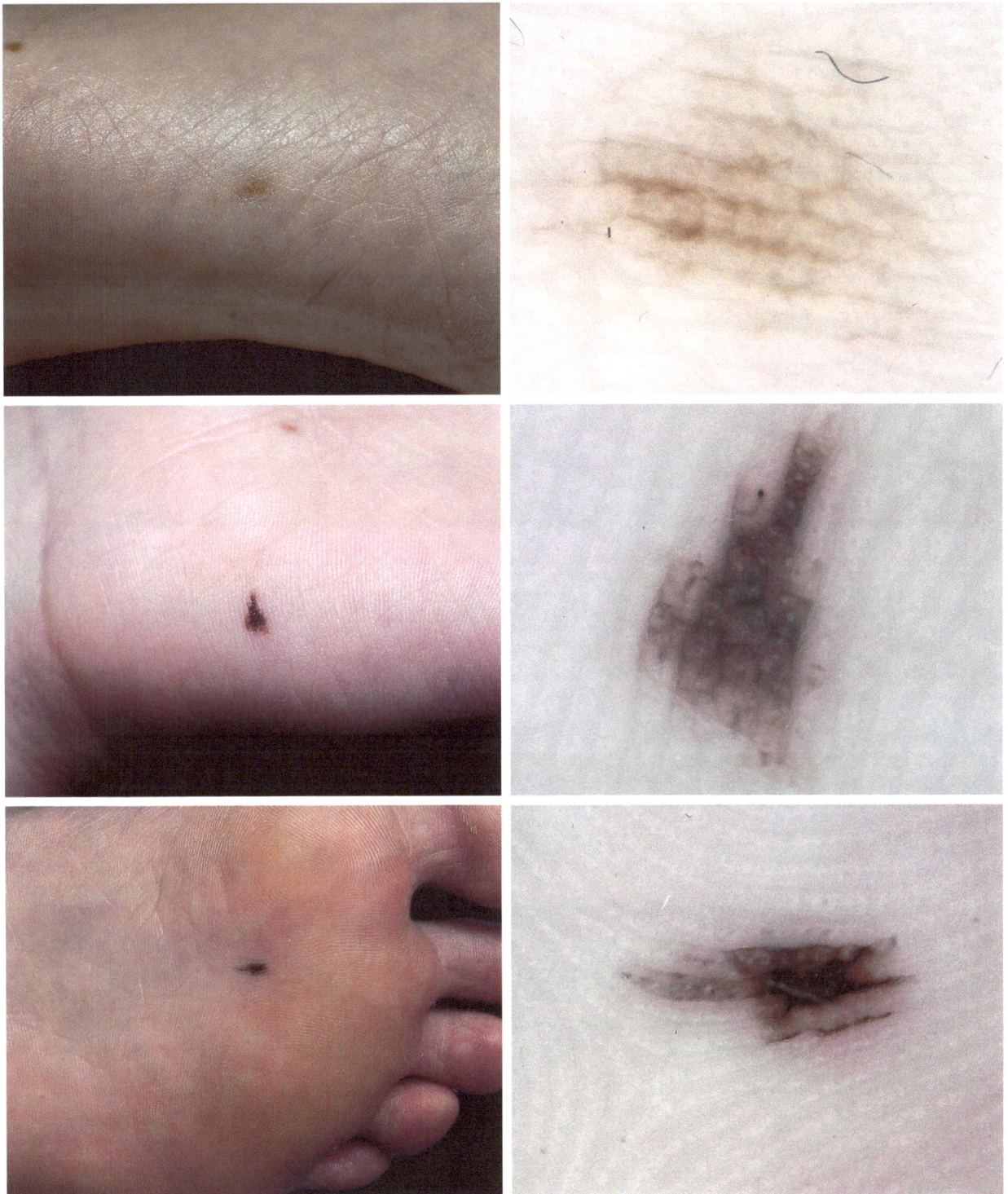

Figure 8.11: *Acral nevi.*
Clinical **left column,** dermatoscopy **right column.** *Parallel lines in the furrows are the typical pattern of classical acral nevi.* **Top:** *Classical acral nevus with parallel lines in the furrows.* **Middle:** *This acral nevus shows a variant of the parallel furrow pattern. The parallel lines in the furrows are connected by crosswise lines, giving an impression of reticular lines.* **Bottom:** *This classical acral nevus shows two patterns: structureless centrally and parallel lines in the furrows peripherally. Note that although there is some pigment on the ridges, the lines are in a furrow pattern.*

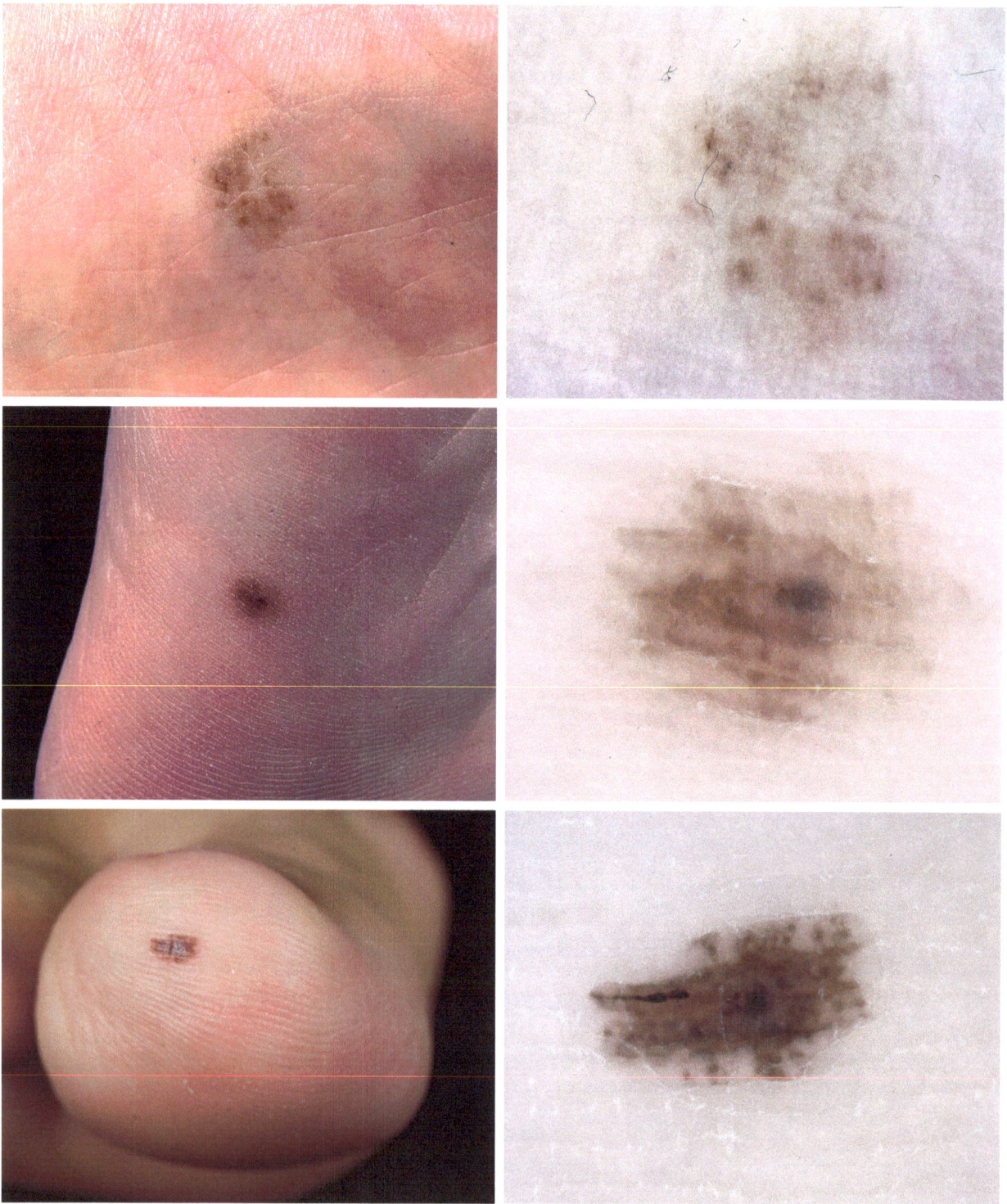

Figure 8.12: *Acral nevi.*
*Nevi on acral skin may show any pattern, not just parallel lines. The general diagnostic method of dermatoscopy (pattern + color + clues = diagnosis) applies, regardless of location. **Top:** One pattern, reticular lines, light-brown and variegate, no clues to melanoma. Histopathological diagnosis: "Superficial" congenital nevus. **Middle:** One pattern, brown clods, no clues to melanoma. Histopathological diagnosis: "Superficial and deep" congenital nevus. **Bottom:** More than one pattern, clods and structureless, but no unequivocal clues to melanoma. Histopathological diagnosis: "Superficial" congenital nevus.*

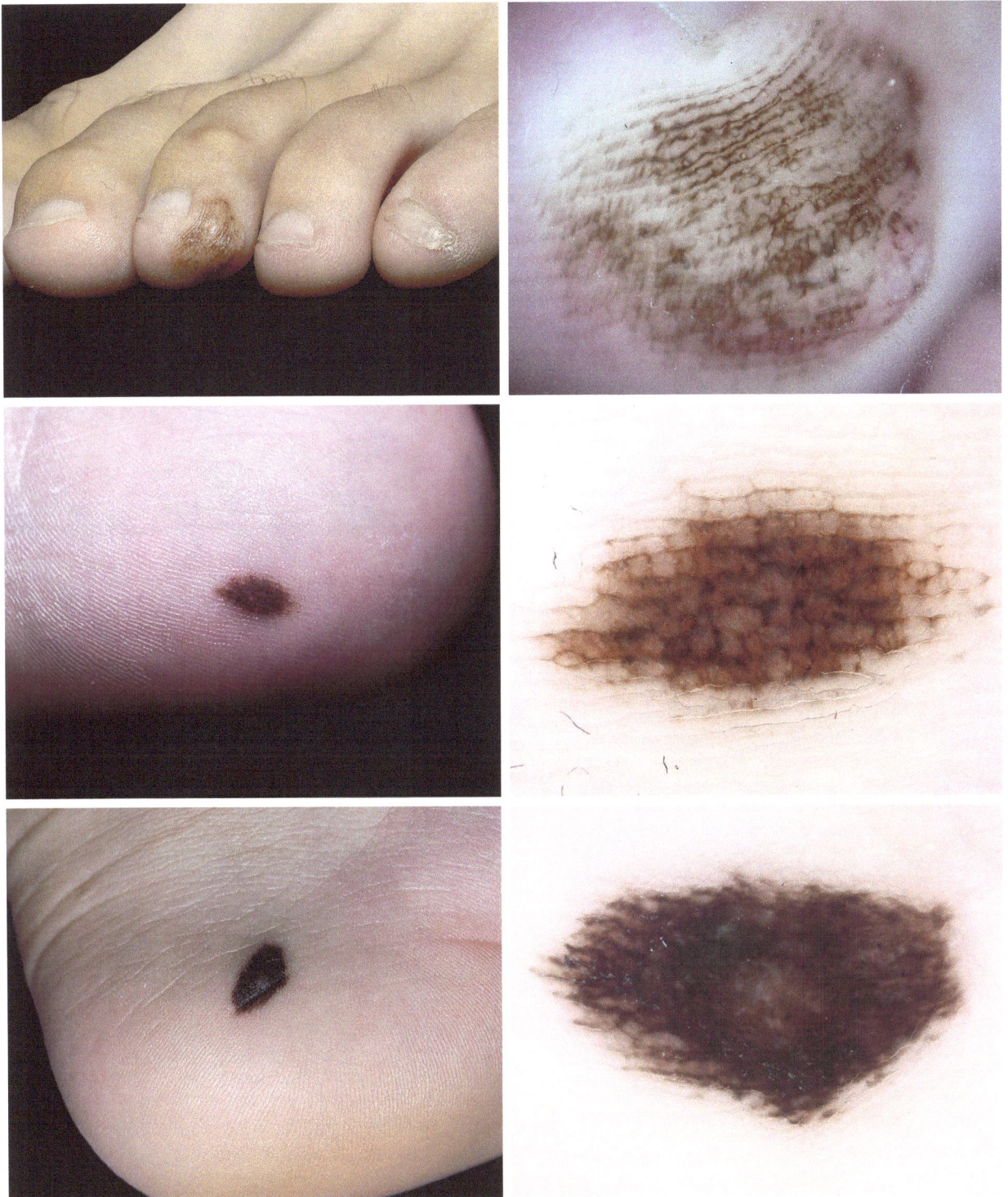

Figure 8.13: *Complex patterns of acral nevi.*
The general diagnostic method of dermatoscopy (pattern + color + clues = diagnosis) applies, regardless of location. **Top:** *More than one pattern, parallel lines in the furrows and circles, no clues to melanoma. Histopathological diagnosis: "Superficial and deep" congenital nevus.* **Middle:** *More than one pattern, parallel lines in the furrows (with intersecting connecting lines) and circles. A few gray clods as a clue to melanoma make it advisable to perform a diagnostic excision. Histopathological diagnosis: "Superficial and deep" congenital nevus.* **Bottom:** *More than one pattern, parallel lines in the furrows at the periphery, and structureless in the center. There are a few gray clods as a clue to melanoma, but symmetry usually overrules any single clue. Histopathological diagnosis: "Superficial and deep" congenital nevus.*

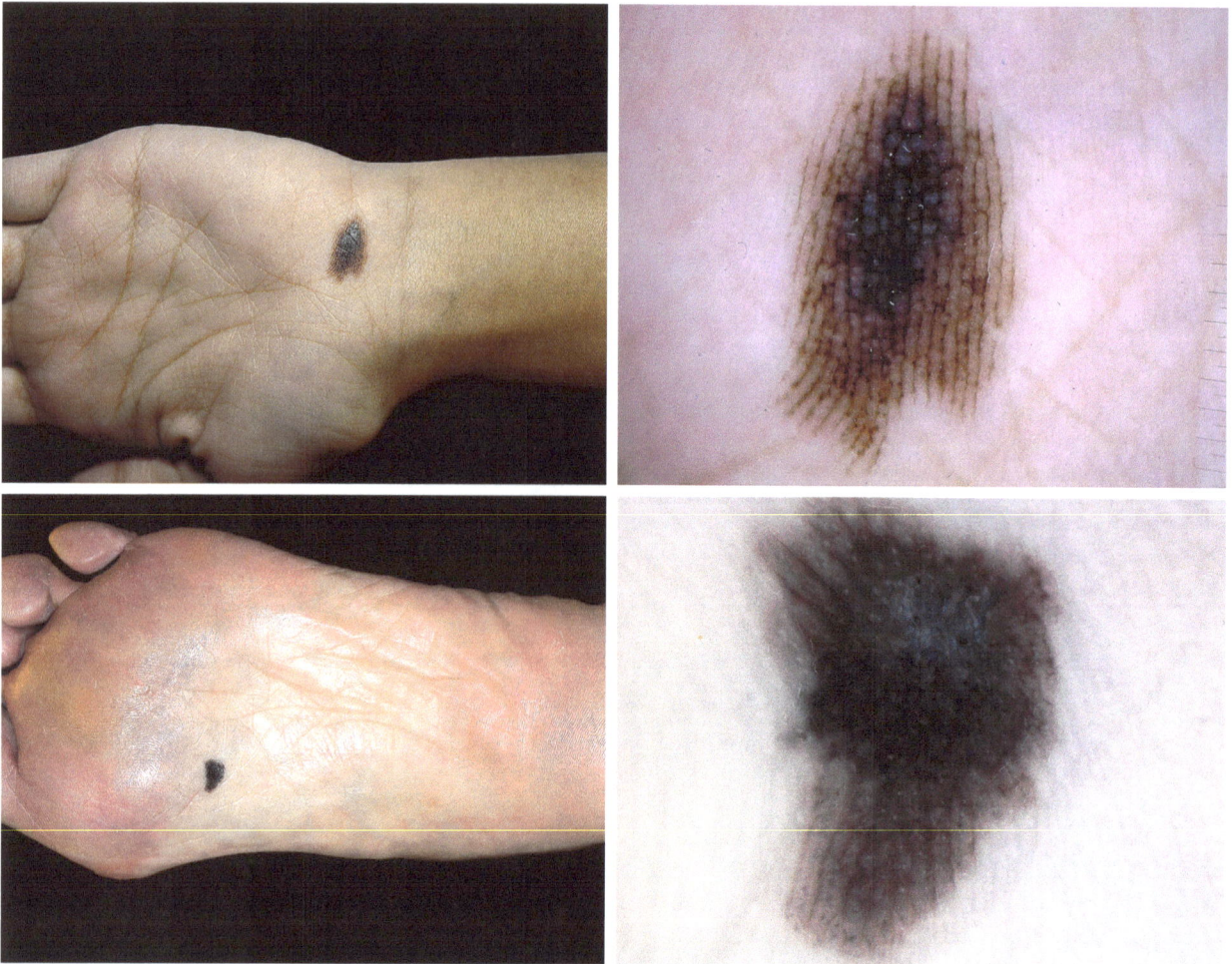

Figure 8.14: Congenital nevus versus melanoma on acral skin.
*The general principles of pattern analysis also apply to acral lesions. The congenital nevus of the palm shown in the **top row** is symmetric and lacks chaos on dermatoscopy **(top right).** Note the parallel furrow pattern at the periphery. The invasive acral melanoma on the sole **(bottom row)** is chaotic and has several melanoma clues (gray structures, black dots and clods at the periphery) on dermatoscopy **(bottom right).** Note that the parallel lines of this melanoma are situated in the furrows mainly and not on the ridges. The absence of a parallel ridge pattern does not exclude the diagnosis of melanoma in a chaotic lesion!*

The general principles to distinguish nevi from melanomas at other sites also apply to acral lesions *(8.14).* Analogous to in situ melanomas on the face or the trunk, which may only demonstrate circles or reticular lines, acral in situ melanomas may show only one pattern, namely parallel lines on the ridges (11, 12). This pattern is the most important melanoma-specific clue on acral skin, and is so specific that even in the absence of chaos one should consider biopsy of acral lesions with parallel lines on the ridges *(8.15, top row).* Of course any other melanoma-specific clue may also be seen in acral melanomas *(8.15, middle and bottom row).* Invasive acral melanomas usually are chaotic (more than one pattern and more than one color arranged asymmetrically) with at least one additional clue to melanoma. In general, as acral melanomas become thicker, they more closely resemble melanomas found at non-acral sites. Importantly, when clues to melanoma are seen in large lesions with more than one pattern, parallel lines in the furrows do not rule out an acral melanoma *(8.14 bottom, 8.16).*

In addition to melanocytic proliferations, hemorrhage may create pigmented lesions on acral skin. When blood flows out of the dermis it usually reaches the epidermis along the outside of the eccrine duct openings. A small bleed will be limited to the ridges (the

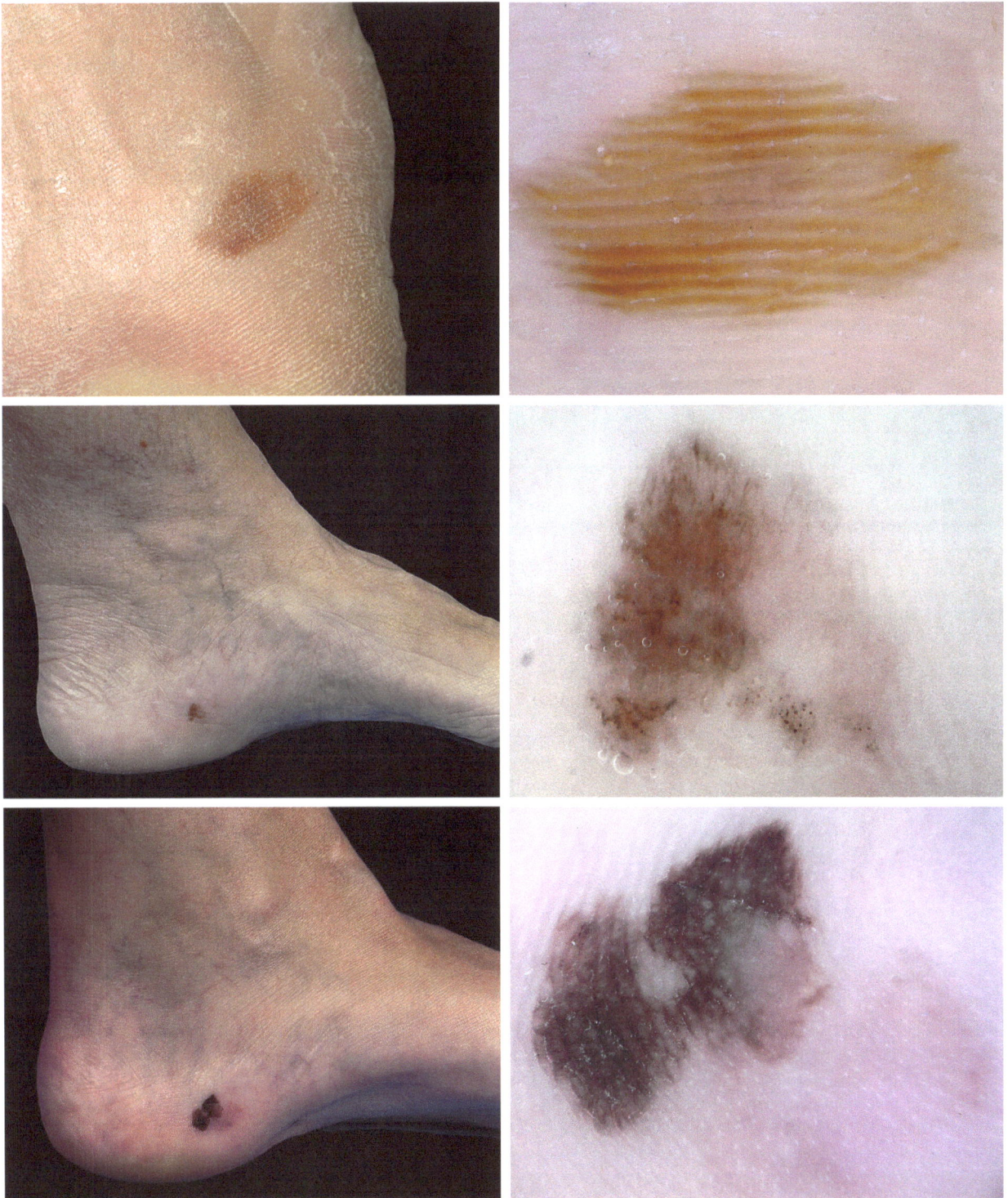

Figure 8.15: Acral melanoma.

Top: *Parallel lines on the ridges are the most important clue to in situ melanomas on acral skin. Histopathological diagnosis: Melanoma in situ.* **Middle:** *More than one pattern, structureless and dots, arranged asymmetrically, more than one color, black and gray dots and a structureless area in eccentric location as clue to melanoma, lead to the diagnosis of melanoma. Histopathological diagnosis: Melanoma (< 1 mm).* **Bottom:** *More than one pattern, parallel lines and structureless, arranged asymmetrically, more than one color, peripheral black dots and an eccentric structureless area as clues to melanoma, lead to the diagnosis of melanoma. Histopathological diagnosis: Melanoma (< 1 mm) in a pre-existing nevus.*

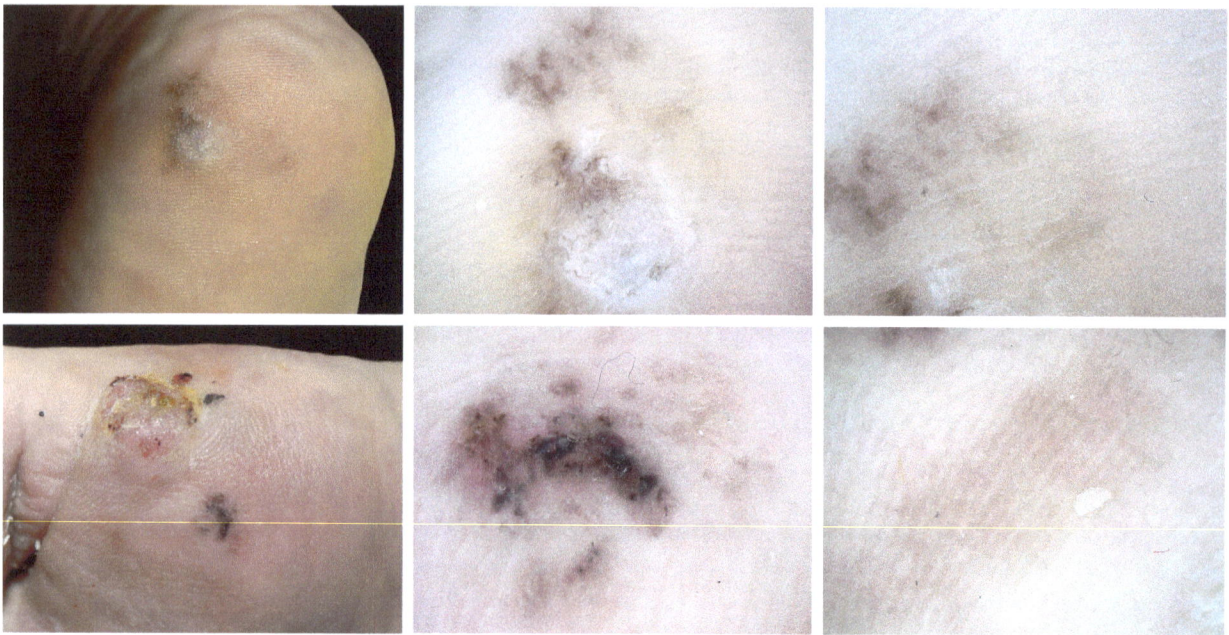

Figure 8.16: Large acral melanomas.
Top: *An acral melanoma with a structureless pattern and variegate pigmentation. Dermatoscopy* **top middle and right:** *structureless pattern with chaotic arrangement of colors. Histopathological diagnosis: Melanoma (< 1 mm).* **Bottom:** *More than one pattern, clods and parallel lines, arranged asymmetrically, and gray clods as a clue to melanoma. Histopathological diagnosis: Melanoma (< 1 mm). Note that the parallel lines are mostly in the furrows and not on the ridges, but the clue of gray clods remains a clue to melanoma, regardless of both parallel furrow pattern and lesion site.*

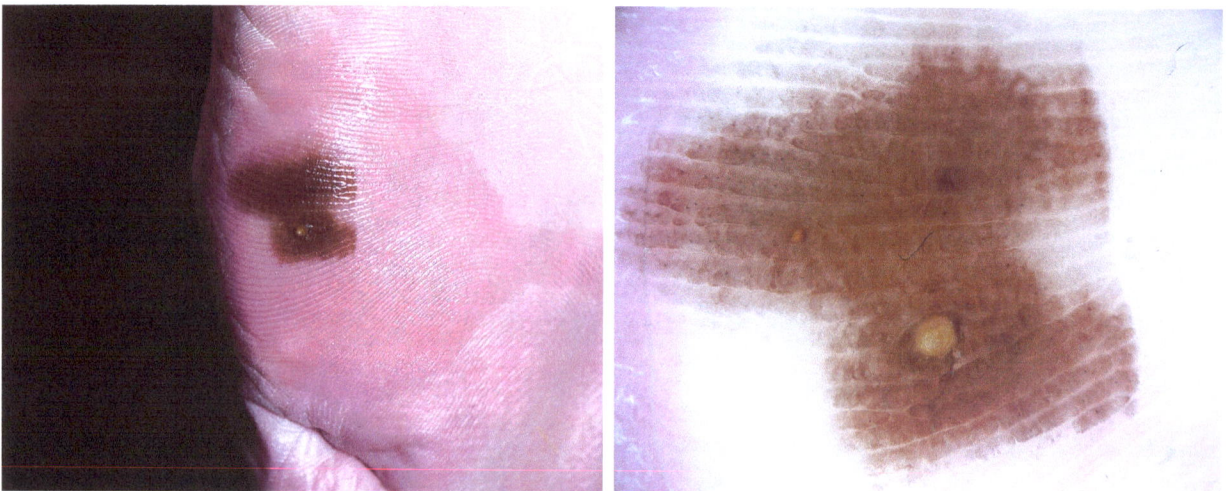

Figure 8.17: Exogenous pigmentation.
Parallel lines on the ridges may also occur in exogenous pigmentation. Here a plantar wart was treated by applying a silver nitrate cautery pen.

eccrine ducts open out onto the ridges) and so creates a parallel ridge pattern. A larger hemorrhage overflows from the ridges and creates a structureless pattern. Red clods at the lesion's periphery ("satellite clods") are characteristic of hemorrhage, but are not always seen (13). Whether the pattern is lines, clods or structureless, hemorrhages are nearly always red or black and can therefore be easily differentiated from (brown) melanocytic proliferations on the basis of their color. However, rarely hemorrhage may be brown – which makes it more difficult to distinguish from melanocytic lesions. The sharp demarcation from

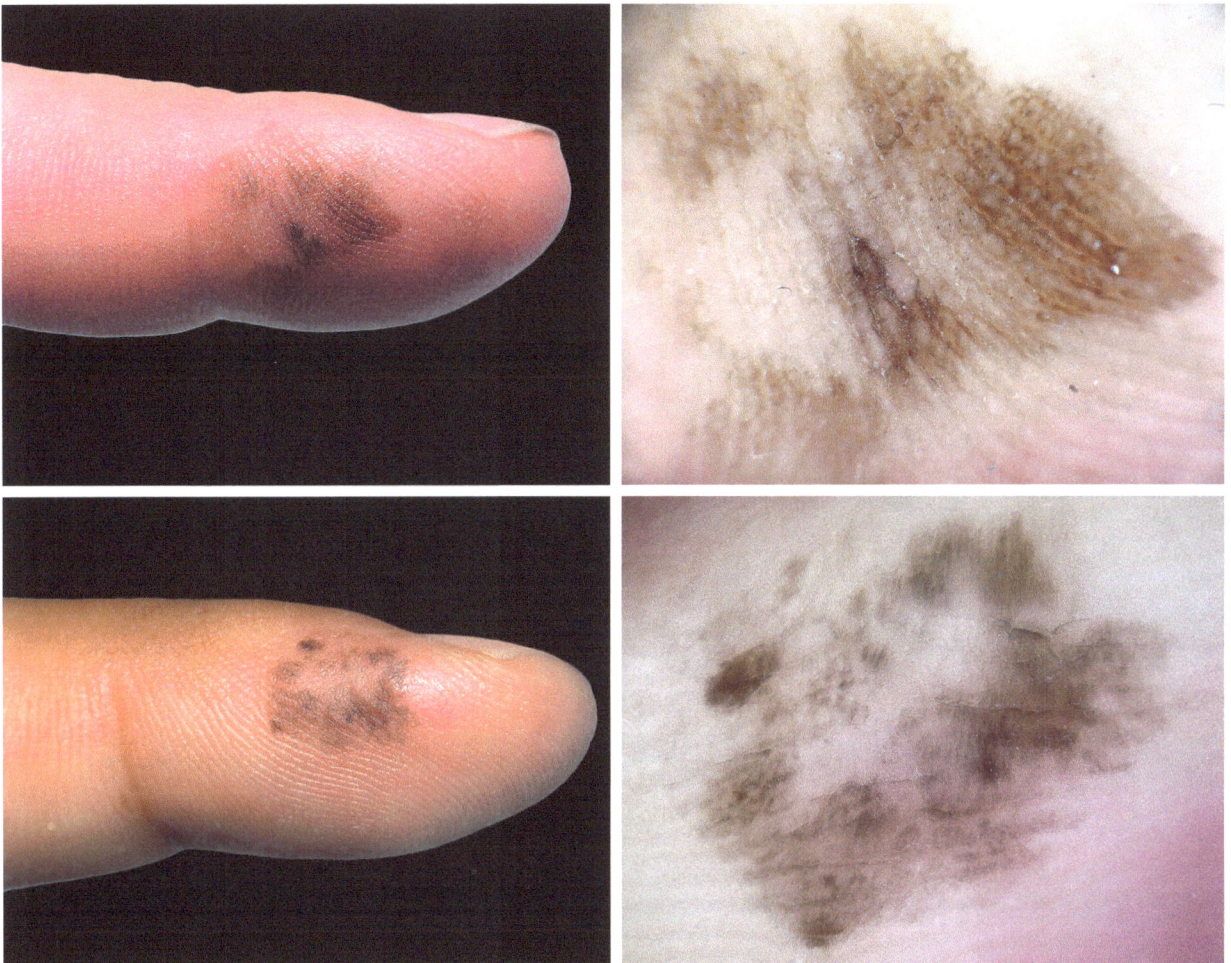

Figure 8.18: *Acral melanoma versus periungual pigmented Bowen's disease (intraepidermal carcinoma).*
Top: *Acral melanoma in situ on an index finger with the parallel ridge pattern (between 12 and 3 o'clock) on dermatoscopy* **(top right).**
Bottom: *Periungual pigmented Bowen's disease (intraepidermal carcinoma) with the structureless pattern on dermatoscopy* **(bottom right).**

the surrounding skin and the typical satellite clods of a hemorrhage usually point to the correct diagnosis. If doubt still remains, one may try to carefully shave off the blood with a scalpel. With bleeding that is mainly confined to the stratum corneum this will be easy. With melanocytic lesions, of course, it will be impossible (13).

In addition to acral hemorrhage, exogenous pigmentation may also have a parallel ridge pattern. These lesions may also be difficult to distinguish from melanocytic proliferations on the basis of their morphology alone, as in the case shown in *figure 8.17.* The correct diagnosis of exogenous pigmentation can usually be established by taking a careful history.

A rare differential diagnosis of acral melanoma is acral (usually periungual) pigmented Bowen's disease (intraepidermal carcinoma), which is usually induced by human papilloma virus infection. The most common pattern of periungual pigmented Bowen's disease is (as at other sites) structureless brown. Less commonly, dots arranged in lines are also visible. The parallel ridge pattern is usually absent in Bowen's disease. The typical vascular pattern of Bowen's disease is also usually absent. Despite some distinguishing features, it can be very challenging to differentiate periungual pigmented Bowen's disease from acral melanoma *(8.18)*.

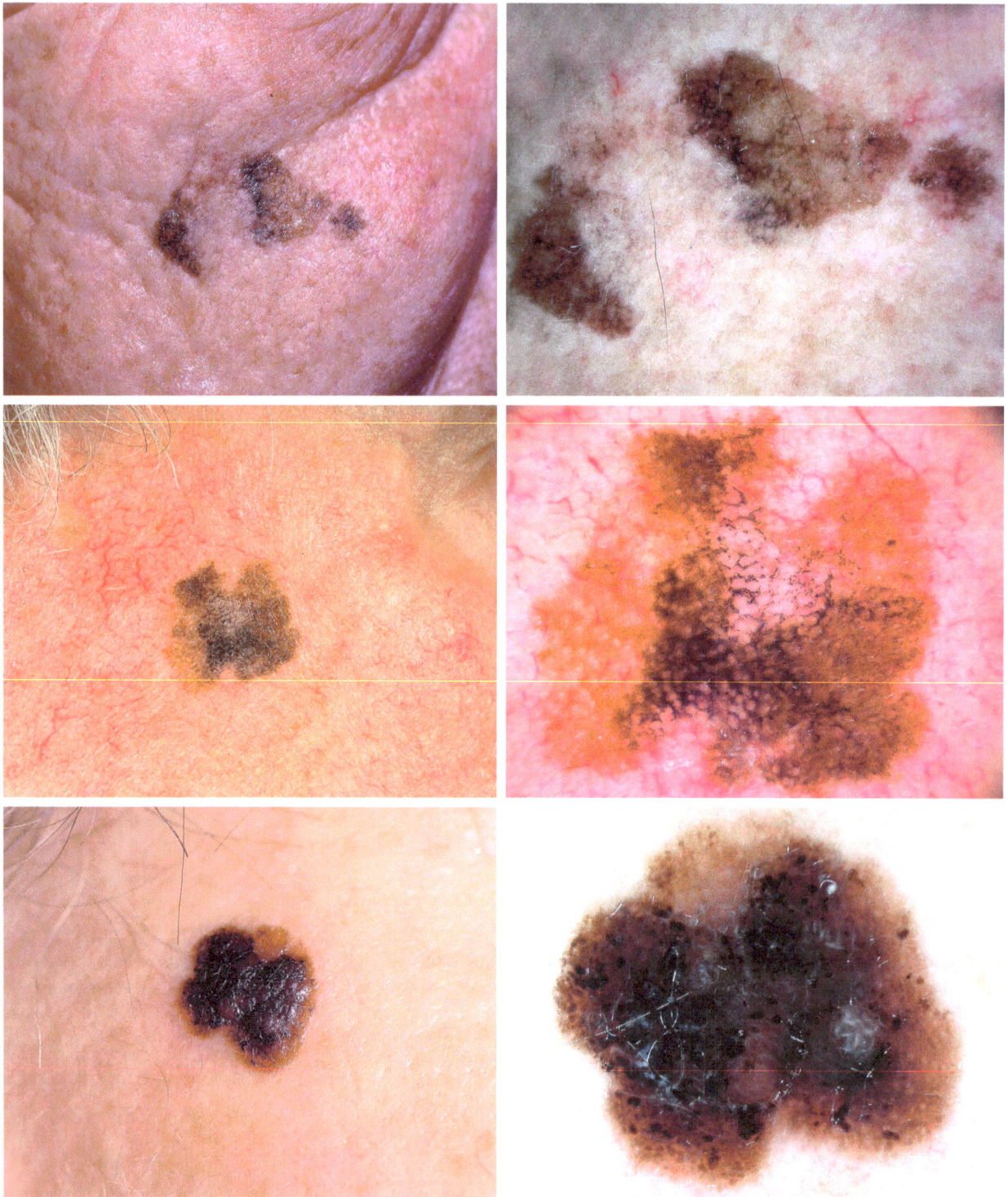

Figure 8.19: *Most invasive facial melanomas are chaotic and have clues to malignancy.*
Top: *Invasive facial melanoma with regression. Dermatoscopy* **(right)** *shows chaos and gray structures.* **Middle:** *Invasive facial melanoma. Dermatoscopy shows chaos and grey structures and angulated lines (polygons).* **Bottom:** *Invasive facial melanoma: Dermatoscopy shows chaos and a pattern of clods with black clods at the periphery.*

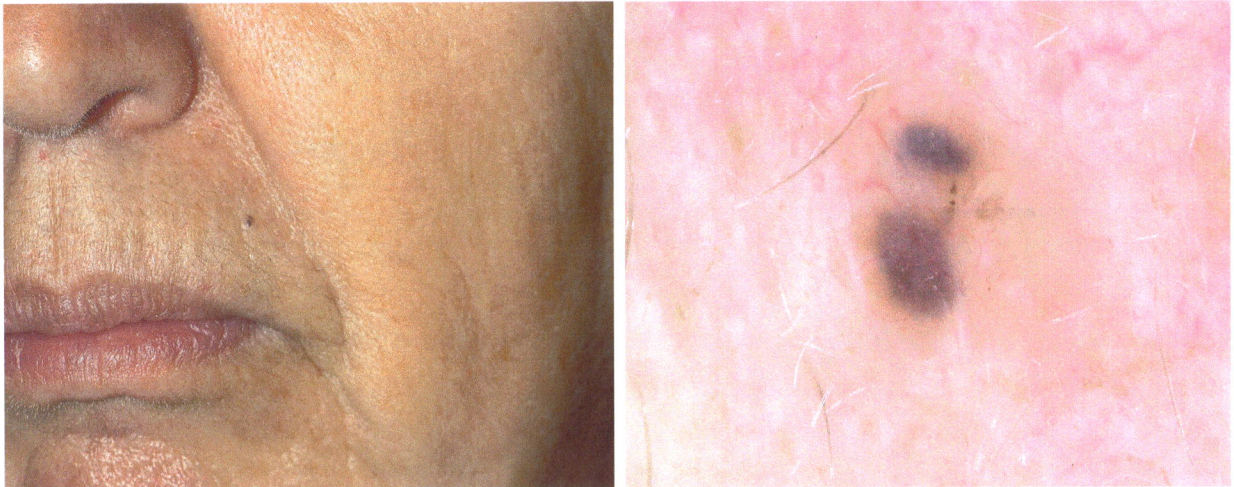

Figure 8.20: An embryonic basal cell carcinoma.
An embryonic basal cell carcinoma measuring 2 mm in diameter that can be diagnosed with confidence based on the dermatoscopic findings of gray clods and serpentine vessels.

8.3 The face

Dermatoscopic diagnosis of pigmented lesions on the face follows the same principles as those used to diagnose lesions at other locations. For many lesions, the face is not a "special situation" at all. Advanced neoplasms of all types show the same features on the face as elsewhere. Advanced melanomas on facial skin are usually chaotic and have the same clues to malignancy seen at other locations *(8.19)*. The diagnosis of facial basal cell carcinomas is not different than at any other anatomic site, even when they are in an embryonic stage *(8.20)*. Other lesions that commonly occur on the face *(8.21)* are Miescher nevi (a type of largely dermal, probably congenital nevus), blue nevi, and Spitz nevi (typically the non-pigmented type) in younger persons, and of course seborrheic keratosis *(8.22)* in elderly persons (14). On the face one may also find proliferations with differentiation of sebaceous glands (e.g. sebaceous gland hyperplasia) or benign neoplasms with follicular differentiation (e.g. trichoepithelioma), and of course inflammatory conditions like rosacea or lupus erythematosus but these lesions are usually not pigmented. The dermatoscopy of inflammatory diseases is discussed in more detail later in this chapter.

Facial location assumes critical importance in the differential diagnosis of flat pigmented neoplasms; flat nevi, early melanoma, solar lentigo especially when in regression (lichen planus-like keratosis), and pigmented actinic keratosis/Bowen's disease. The remainder of this section is devoted to the challenging task of differentiating these lesions.

Although any pattern may be seen, the predominant dermatoscopic patterns for flat facial lesions are circles, dots, structureless, angulated lines, curved lines, and reticular lines *(8.23)*. The anatomy of the facial skin explains the relatively high frequency of circles and the structureless pattern in flat facial lesions (15). Hair follicles are both more frequent and more prominent on the face than at other sites.

Furthermore, in the course of one's life the rete ridges tend to flatten. If the rete ridges are flattened, hyperpigmentation of basal keratinocytes is seen not as reticular lines, but as a structureless brown area interrupted by round non-pigmented follicular openings *(8.23C)*. We do not recommend the term "pseudo-network" as it is important to recognize this pattern as structureless.

Many solar lentigines have a structureless pattern and are usually only brown. In some solar lentigines, however, the rete ridges may be elongated which results in a pattern of reticular or curved lines. Common patterns of solar lentigines are shown in *figure 8.24*. Contrary to common belief, a reticular pattern on chronic sun-damaged facial skin is therefore a clue for a non-melanocytic and not for a melanocytic lesion. A pattern of circles in flat pigmented facial lesions requires careful assessment, especially if the circles are gray. A pattern of thin gray circles is the most specific clue to early facial melanoma, but only when the pigmentation is confluent, and not grey dots arranged as circles *(8.25, 8.26)*. As a facial melanoma in situ progresses, circles may thicken and in some areas coalesce to create a structureless zone, *(8.27)* but

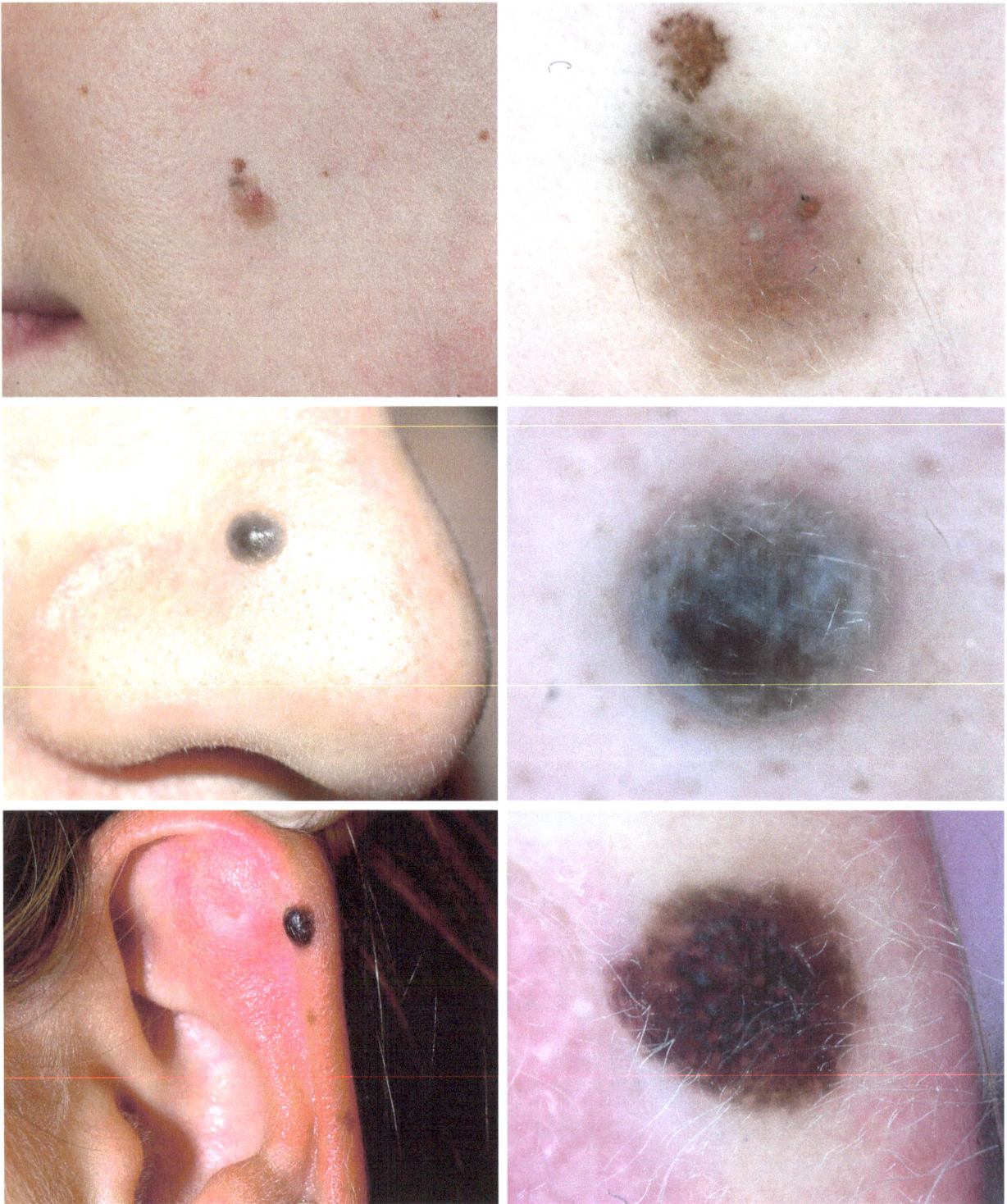

Figure 8.21: *Nevi on the face.*
In addition to Miescher nevi, other nevi – primarily congenital ones – may occur on the face. The general diagnostic method of derma-toscopy (pattern + color + clues = diagnosis) applies regardless of the location on the face. **Top:** *A brown and blue structureless lesion in which the colors are arranged asymmetrically must be excised in order to exclude a melanoma. Histopathological diagnosis: Combined congenital nevus.* **Middle:** *One pattern, structureless, one color, blue – these are clues to a blue nevus.* **Bottom:** *One pattern, clods, more than one color, brown and gray, with the colors arranged symmetrically, are most likely indicative of a nevus. Histopathological diagnosis: "Superficial and deep" congenital nevus.*

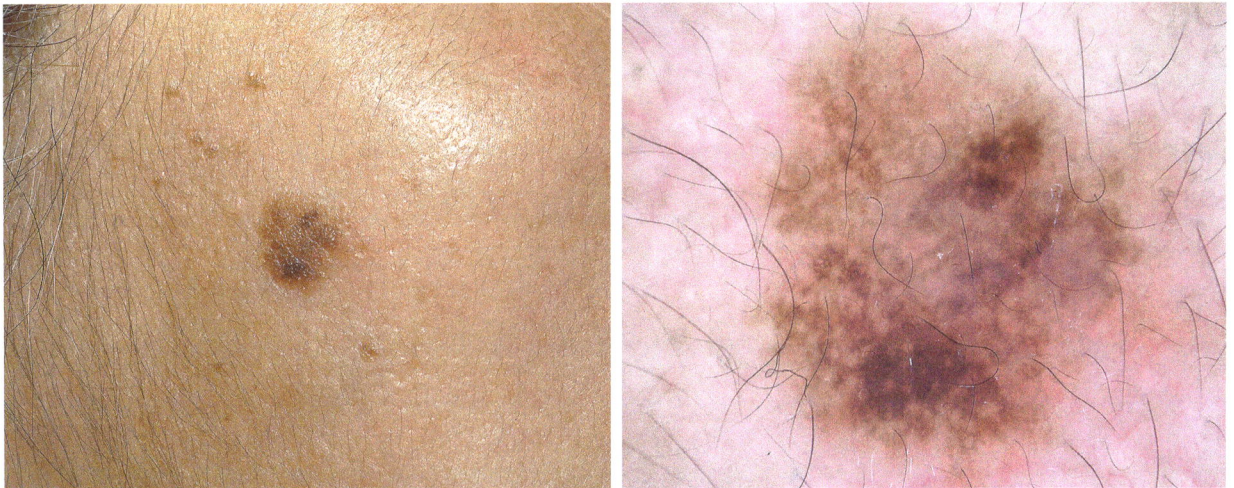

Figure 8.22: *Facial seborrheic keratosis.*
A flat seborrheic keratosis that shows a reticular pattern on dermatoscopy (**right**). *The color is only brown. Note that other clues to seborrheic keratosis are missing. There are no white dots or clods and the border is not sharply demarcated.*

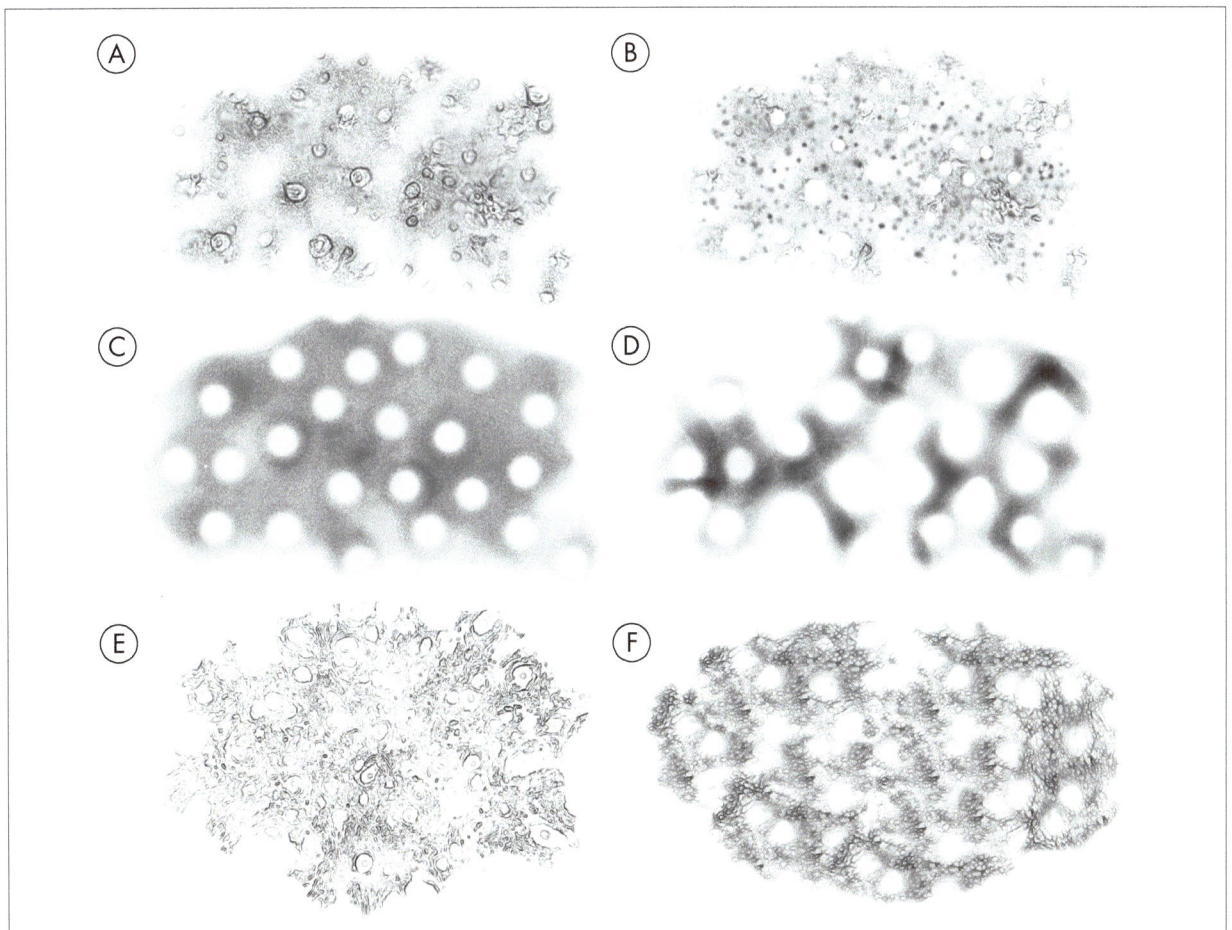

Figure 8.23: *Schematic presentations of patterns of flat facial pigmented lesions.*
A: *Circles.* **B:** *Dots.* **C:** *Structureless. This pattern has been termed "pseudo-pigment network", a term which is discouraged because it is misleading – the pattern is structureless, not "network".* **D:** *Angulated lines (polygons).* **E:** *Curved lines.* **F:** *Reticular lines.*

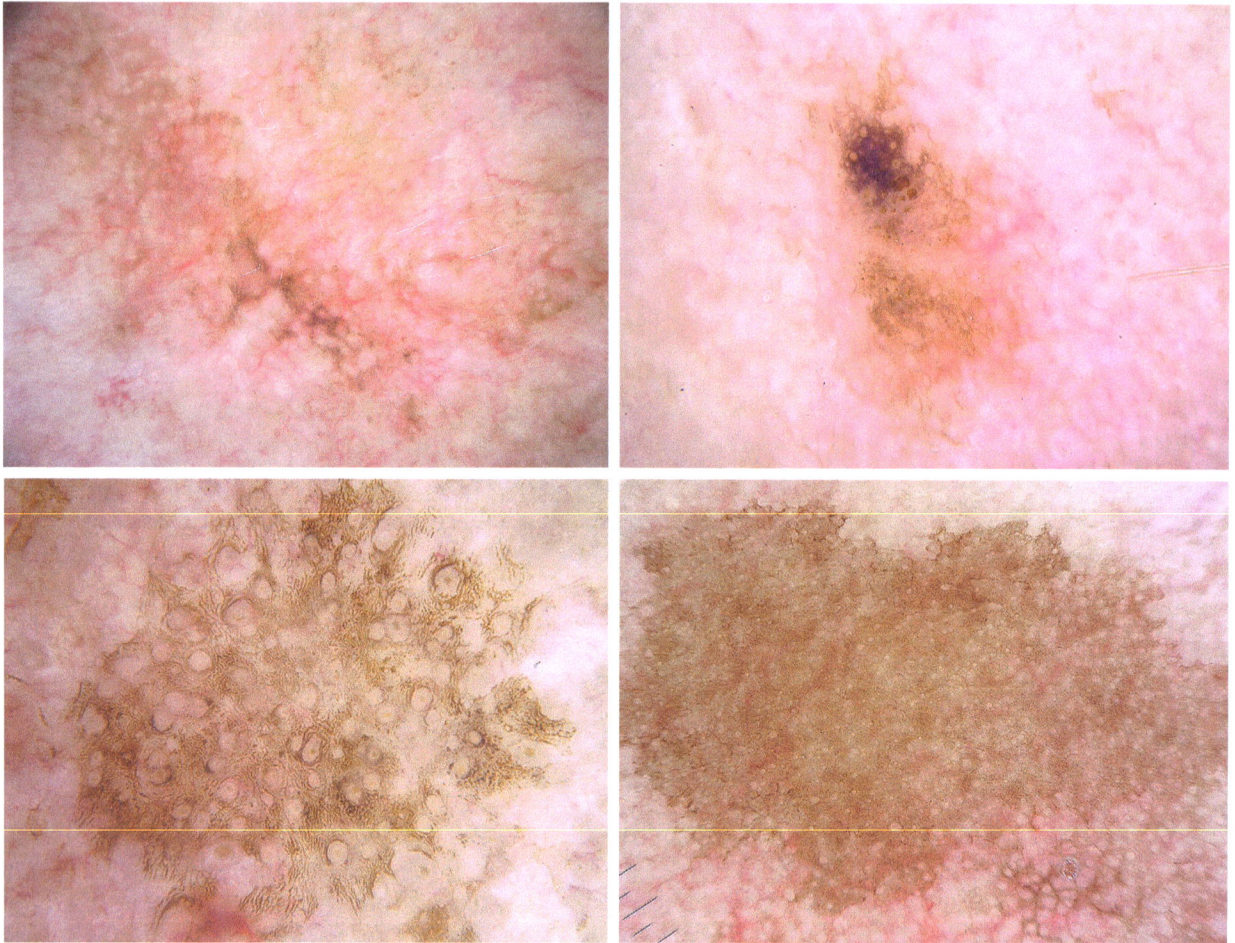

Figure 8.24: Common patterns of facial solar lentigines on dermatoscopy.
Top left: Solar lentigo with a reticular pattern. There are also some brown circles. Note that some of the brown circles are incomplete ("asymmetric follicular openings"), which is not a specific clue in this context. There is no gray. **Top right:** A solar lentigo with a reticular pattern. There are also some brown dots and small clods, which indicate a transition to a flat seborrheic keratosis. **Bottom left:** Solar lentigo with curved lines. Note that the color is only brown and the sharply demarcated scalloped border, which is also a clue to solar lentigo. **Bottom right:** Solar lentigo with structureless pattern. The color is only brown. The sharply demarcated scalloped border is another clue to solar lentigo.

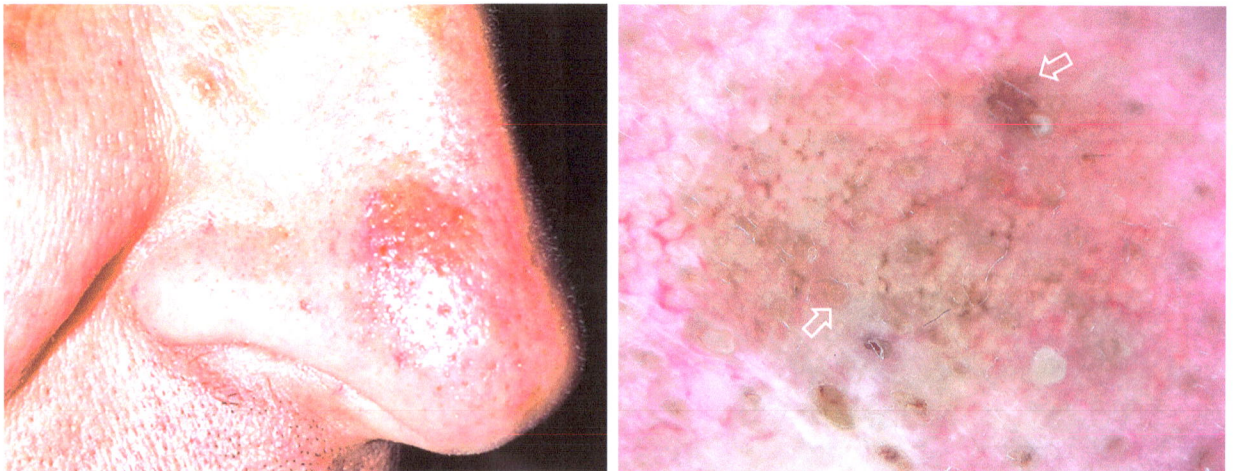

Figure 8.25: Subtle gray circles in a melanoma in situ.
Clinically **(left)** this is an inconspicuous brown macule. On dermatoscopy **(right)** one finds discrete gray circles (arrows). The histological diagnosis is in situ melanoma.

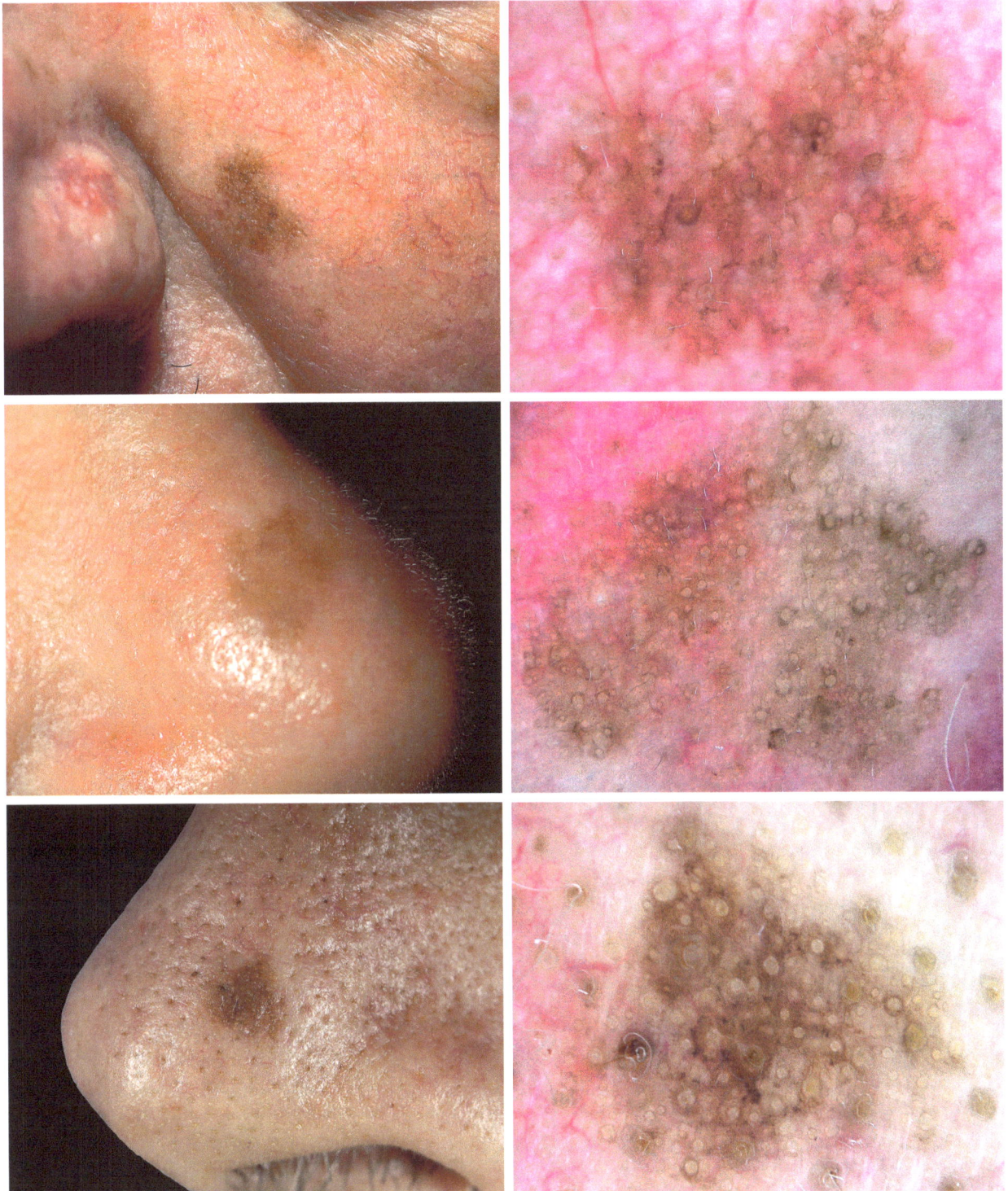

Figure 8.26: *Three facial melanomas in situ with circles as the main pattern.*
Dermatoscopy on the right. **Top, middle:** *In situ melanomas with gray and brown circles.* **Bottom:** *An in situ melanoma with brown circles only.*

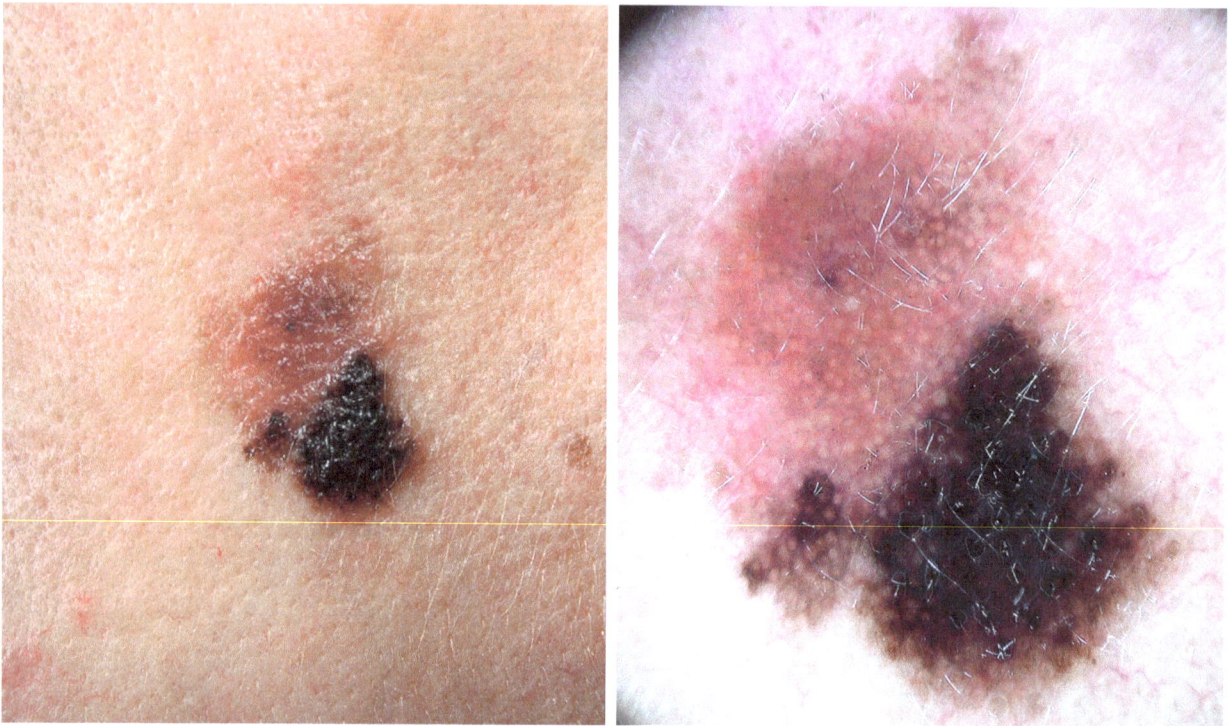

Figure 8.27: A facial melanoma with more than one pattern.
*Dermatoscopy on the **right**. Melanoma with circles (upper part) and angulated lines (left lower part). The more advanced right lower part shows a structureless pattern.*

the pattern of circles usually remains visible in other parts. Sometimes the circles in melanoma in situ are brown and not gray *(8.26 bottom)* and then it can be very difficult to differentiate melanoma in situ from solar lentigo. In solar lentigo, however, other clues are usually present such as reticular and curved lines and a sharply demarcated, scalloped border. Although some say incomplete circles ("asymmetric follicular openings") are a clue to melanoma in situ, we consider this feature of limited value because incomplete circles are commonly found in solar lentigines and in pigmented actinic keratoses (i.e. the clue has poor specificity). A circle in a circle (concentric circles) is a quite specific clue to facial melanoma in situ, but it is rarely present (i.e. the clue has poor sensitivity) *(8.28)*. Furthermore, this clue is usually found in larger lesions with other (less subtle) clues which make the diagnosis of melanoma obvious. In a study by Tschandl et al (16) the clue of "circle in a circle" was found in only 4.2 % of facial flat melanomas.

Similar to flat melanomas on chronic sun damaged non-facial skin, the pattern of angulated lines is also common in facial melanoma in situ *(8.29, 8.30)*. (16) However, on the face, angulated lines are not

highly specific for melanoma; they are also found in pigmented actinic keratoses and lichen planus-like keratosis. Facial angulated lines probably correspond to what has been previously described as rhomboids by Stolz et al. (15)

Although gray pigmentation may appear in benign facial lesions (as in lichen planus-like keratosis) it is an important clue to malignancy in flat lesions *(8.31)*. In a study by Tschandl et al (16) the sensitivity of gray pigmentation for melanoma in situ was 96 % and the specificity was 31 %.

Because of the rather poor specificity, the decision to biopsy a lesion should not be based on the clue of gray pigmentation alone. Other clues including the presence or absence of benign clues (for example clues to solar lentigo) should be also considered. However, if gray circles are present, especially if the circles are thin, the diagnosis of melanoma in situ (lentigo maligna) should be favored over the other diagnoses.

Pigmented actinic keratoses are common on facial skin and can mimic melanoma in situ *(8.32)*. Clues to pigmented actinic keratosis are scale, background erythema, white circles, and, although less specific,

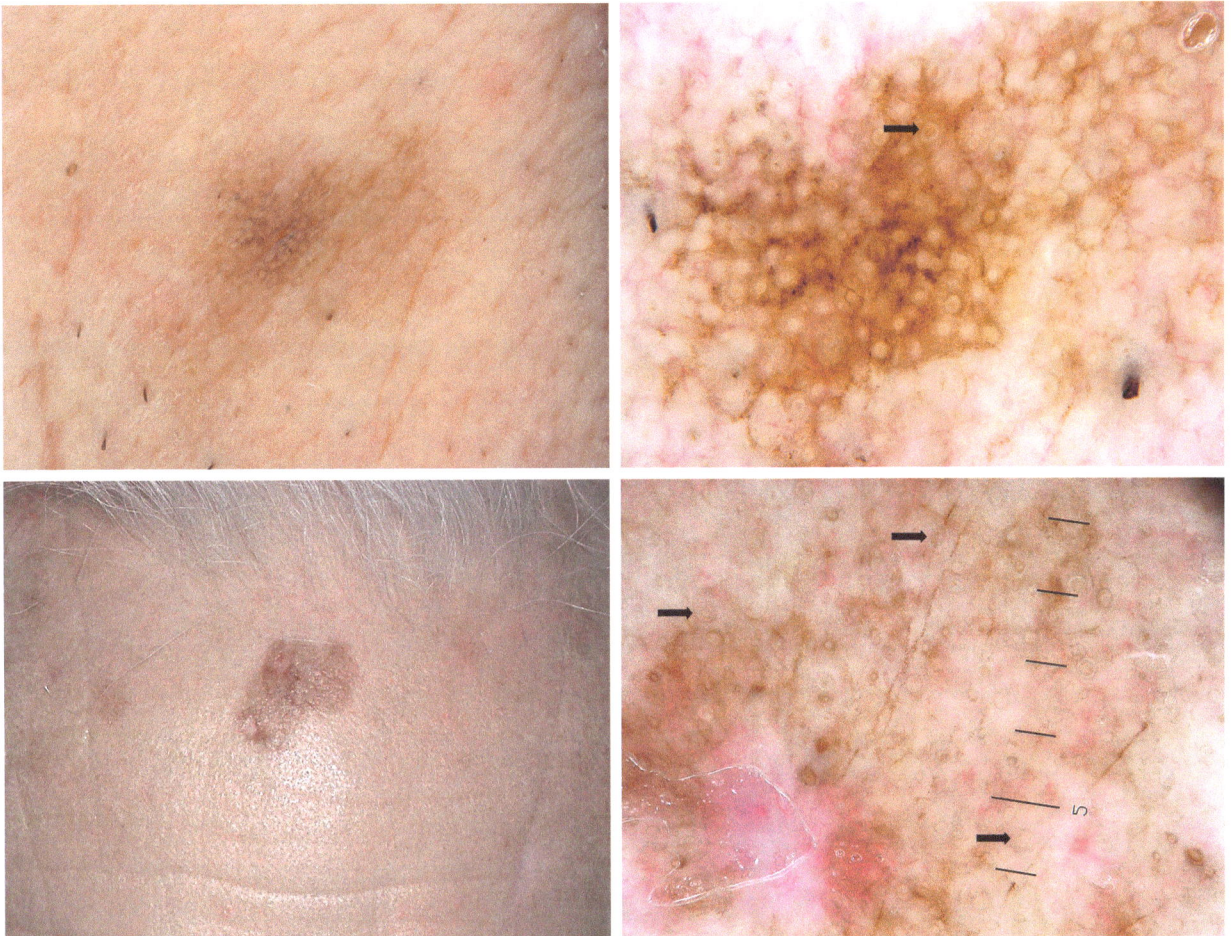

Figure 8.28: *Two facial melanomas with the clue of "circle within a circle".*
Dermatoscopy on the **right.** *Melanoma with concentric circles (circle within a circle) on dermatoscopy (black arrows).*

four dots in a square. Pigmented actinic keratosis may show many patterns including circles, structureless, dots and even reticular and curved lines. Reticular and curved lines in a pigmented actinic keratosis usually indicate a collision with solar lentigo. Lichen planus-like keratosis may also mimic facial melanoma in situ. Lichen planus-like keratosis is a solar lentigo in the stage of regression *(8.33).* As a consequence of inflammation, melanophages accumulate in the papillary dermis and appear as grey dots under the dermatoscope. Hence these lesions are frequently biopsied. The gray dots in lichen-planus like keratosis are usually distributed between the follicular openings *(8.33 bottom)* and not arranged in circles around follicular openings.

Other parts of the lesion may show remnants of a solar lentigo. Angulated lines may occur in lichen planus like-keratosis but only rarely and usually only in the part of the lesion in which regression occurs *(8.33 top).*

While Clark nevi may mimic melanoma in situ, they are very rare on facial skin. Clinicians should be very reluctant to accept a histopathologic diagnosis of Clark nevus (often referred to as "dysplastic" nevus) on facial skin, especially if the diagnosis is based on a partial biopsy. Dermatopathologists may err too.

Collisions are very common on the face. Melanoma in situ, solar lentigo and actinic keratosis are all common lesions on chronic sun damaged skin, meaning collisions will occur by chance.

Histopathologically, solar lentigines are commonly found adjacent to facial melanomas in situ, but this does not prove a causal relationship between solar lentigo and melanoma in situ, as has been proposed in the concept of "unstable lentigo". Solar lentigines are also found in conjunction with actinic keratoses,

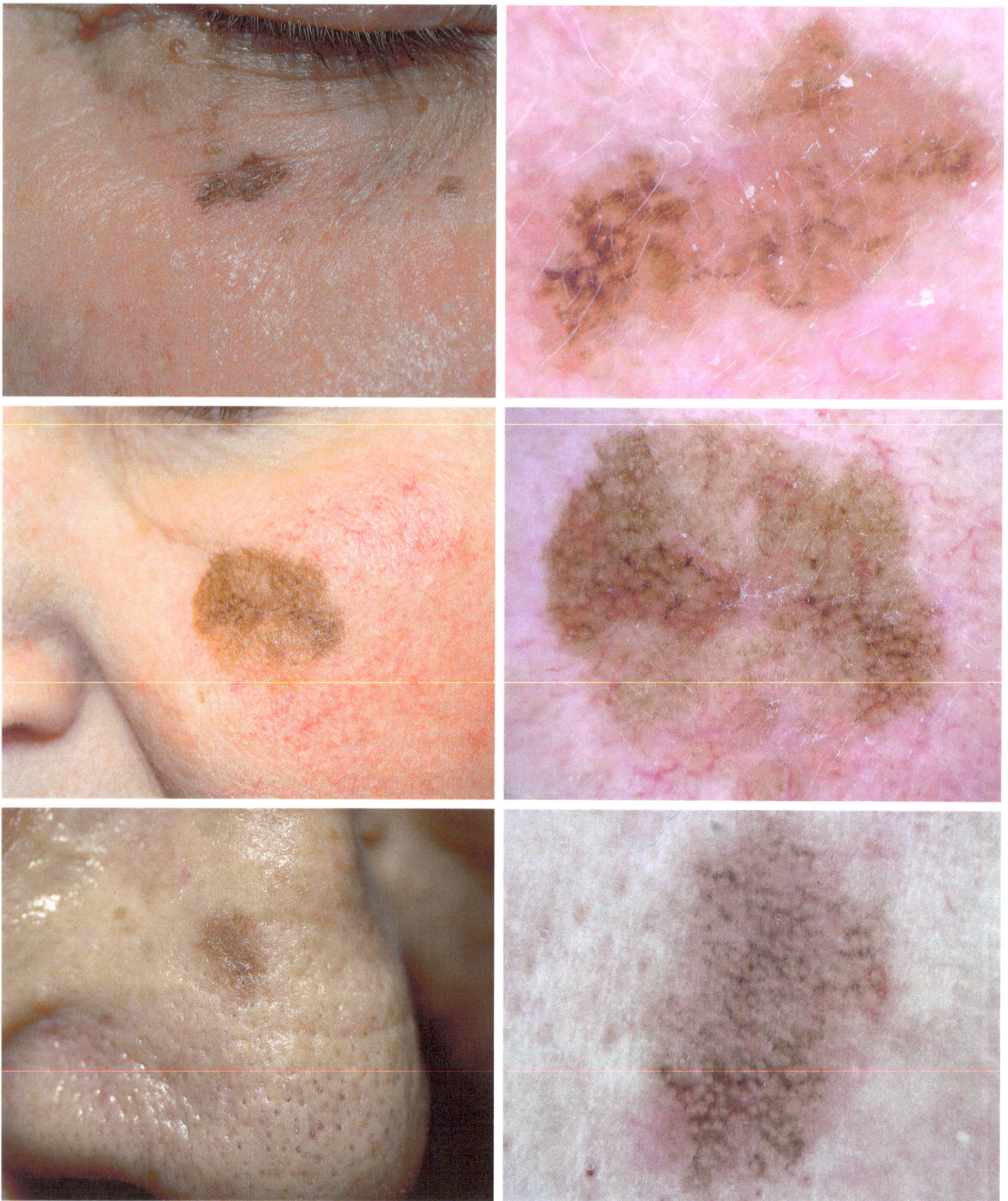

Figure 8.29: *Facial melanomas (in situ) with angulated lines.*
Dermatoscopy on the **right. Top:** *Melanoma in situ with angulated lines. Note that there is only very subtle gray color.* **Middle:** *Melanoma in situ with angulated lines, some of which are gray.* **Bottom:** *Melanoma in situ with gray dots and angulated lines.*

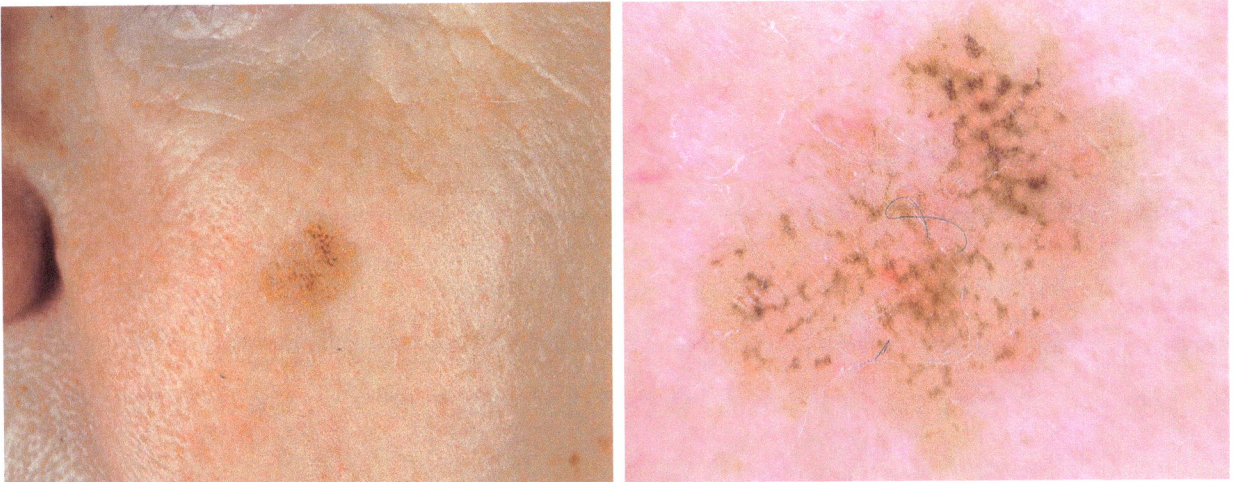

Figure 8.30: *Melanoma in situ with angulated lines as the only clue.*
Melanoma in situ with angulated lines as the main pattern. The color is brown. Note that there are no clues that point to solar lentigo (such as a sharply demarcated scalloped border). In more difficult lesions, the absence of benign clues may raise suspicion that one is dealing with a melanoma in situ.

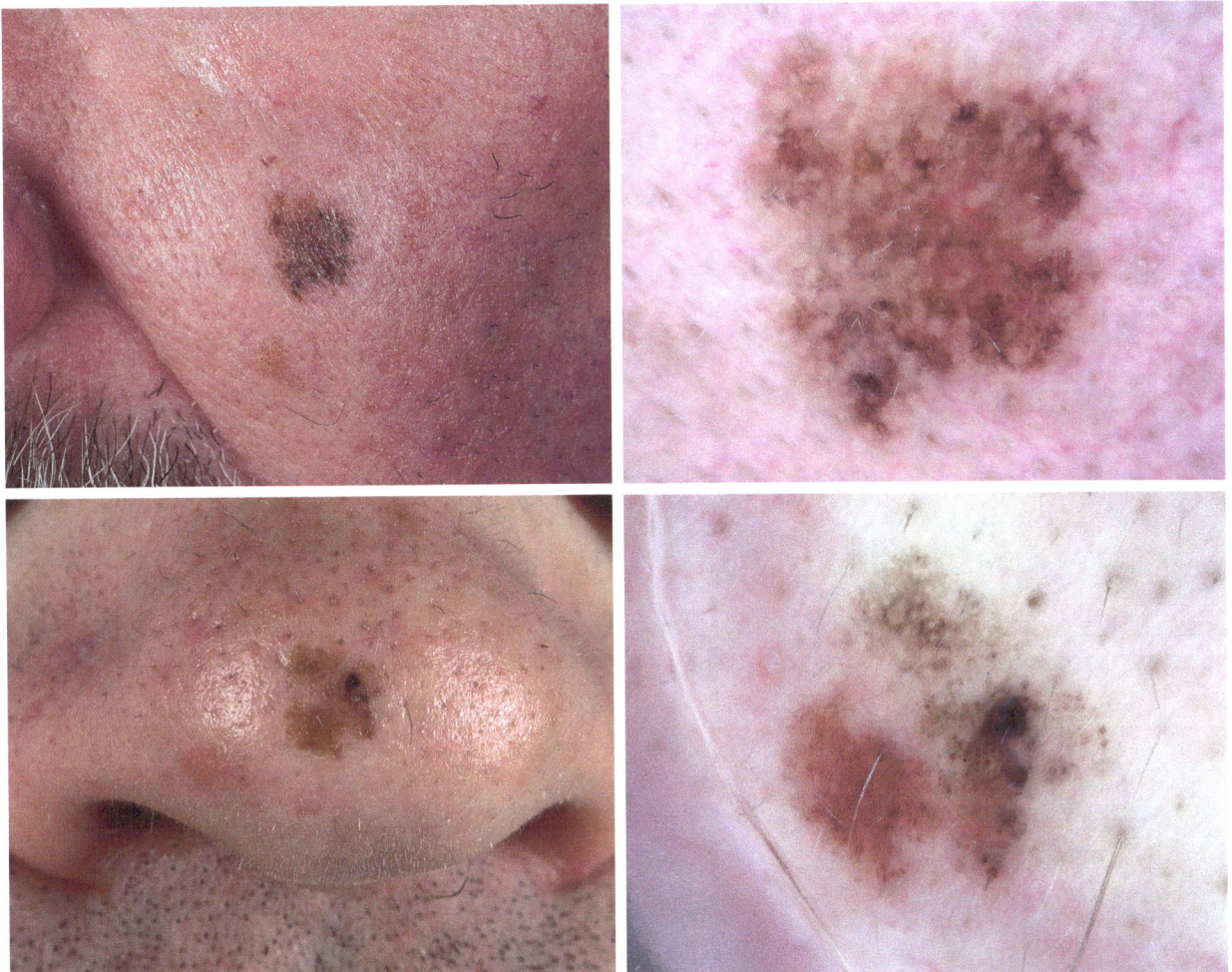

Figure 8.31: *Gray structures as a clue to facial melanoma.*
*Clinical **left column**, dermatoscopy **right column.** The general diagnostic method of dermatoscopy (pattern + color + clues = diagnosis) applies regardless of the location on the face. **Top:** One pattern, reticular, more than one color, variegate, gray lines and circles as clues to melanoma, lead to the diagnosis of an in situ melanoma. **Bottom:** More than one pattern, clods and structureless, arranged asymmetrically, gray clods and dots as a clue to melanoma, lead to the diagnosis of melanoma. Note that in both cases, there are no clues to a benign lesion.*

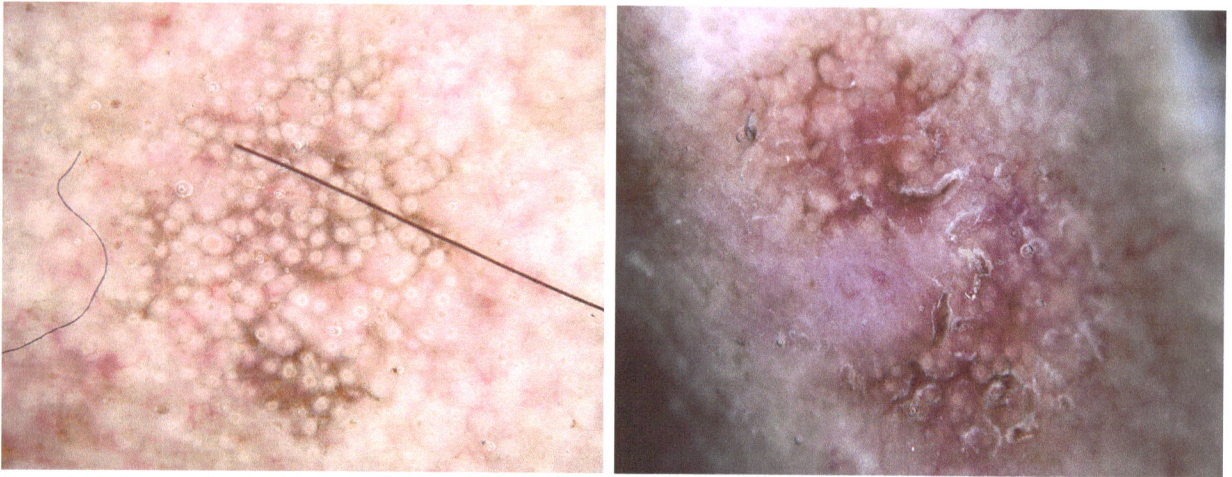

Figure 8.32: *Pigmented actinic keratosis.*
Two pigmented actinic keratoses with a pattern of angulated lines. Additional clues to pigmented actinic keratosis are white circles (left), and white circles, scale and background erythema (right).

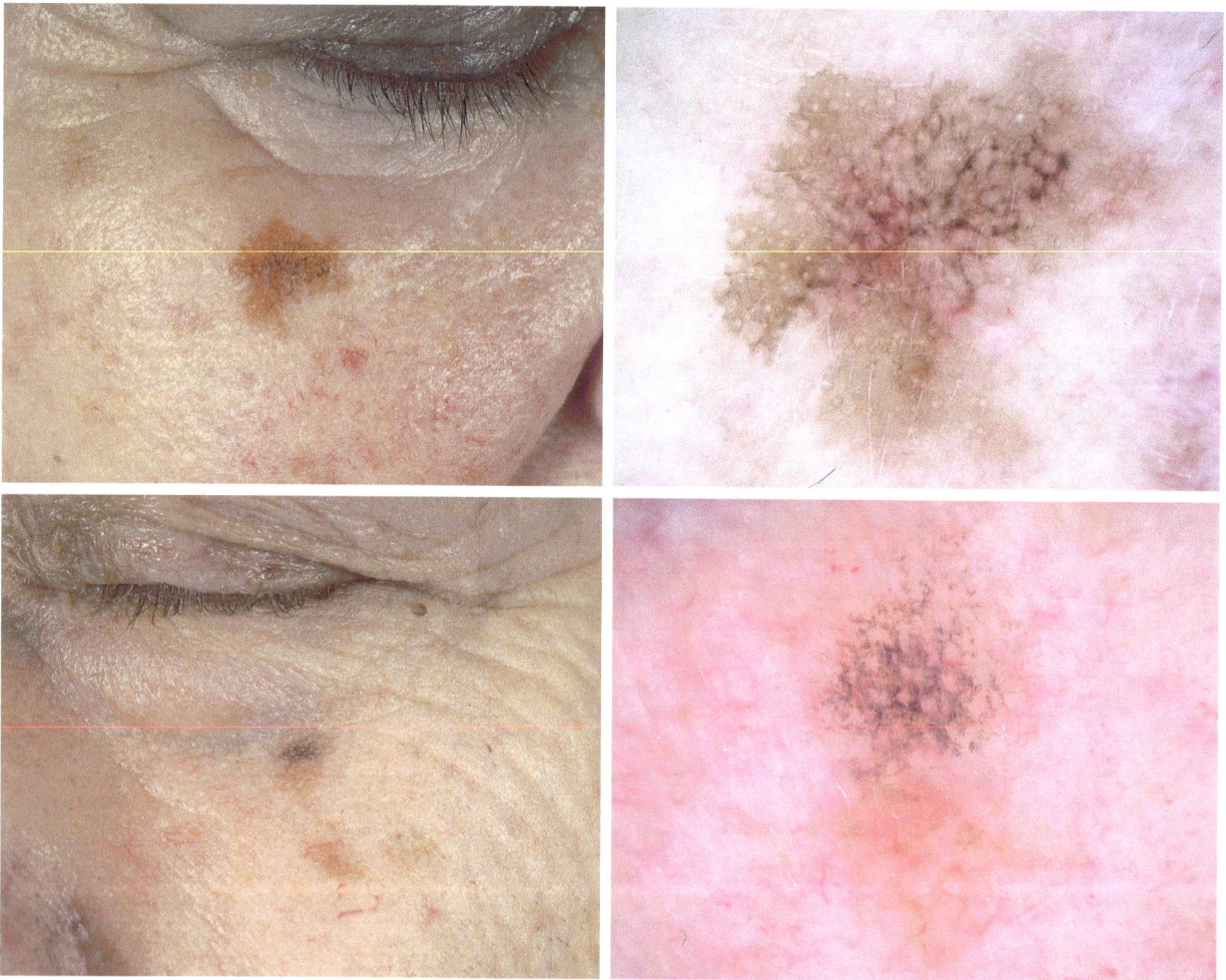

Figure 8.33: *Solar lentigines with regression (Lichen-planus like keratosis).*
Clinical **left column**, dermatoscopy **right column. Top:** *Solar lentigo in regression (lichen planus-like keratosis) with a structureless brown pattern and a few brown circles at the periphery. In the center one can see gray structures which are best described as angulated lines. A typical feature of solar lentigo is the sharply demarcated scalloped margin. However, a biopsy is required to rule out an in situ melanoma.*
Bottom: *Solar lentigo in regression (lichen planus-like keratosis) with a few gray dots and lines in the upper part of the lesion. Note that the grey dots are distributed between the follicular openings and not around the follicular openings. A biopsy or examination with reflectance confocal microscopy is required to exclude an in situ melanoma.*

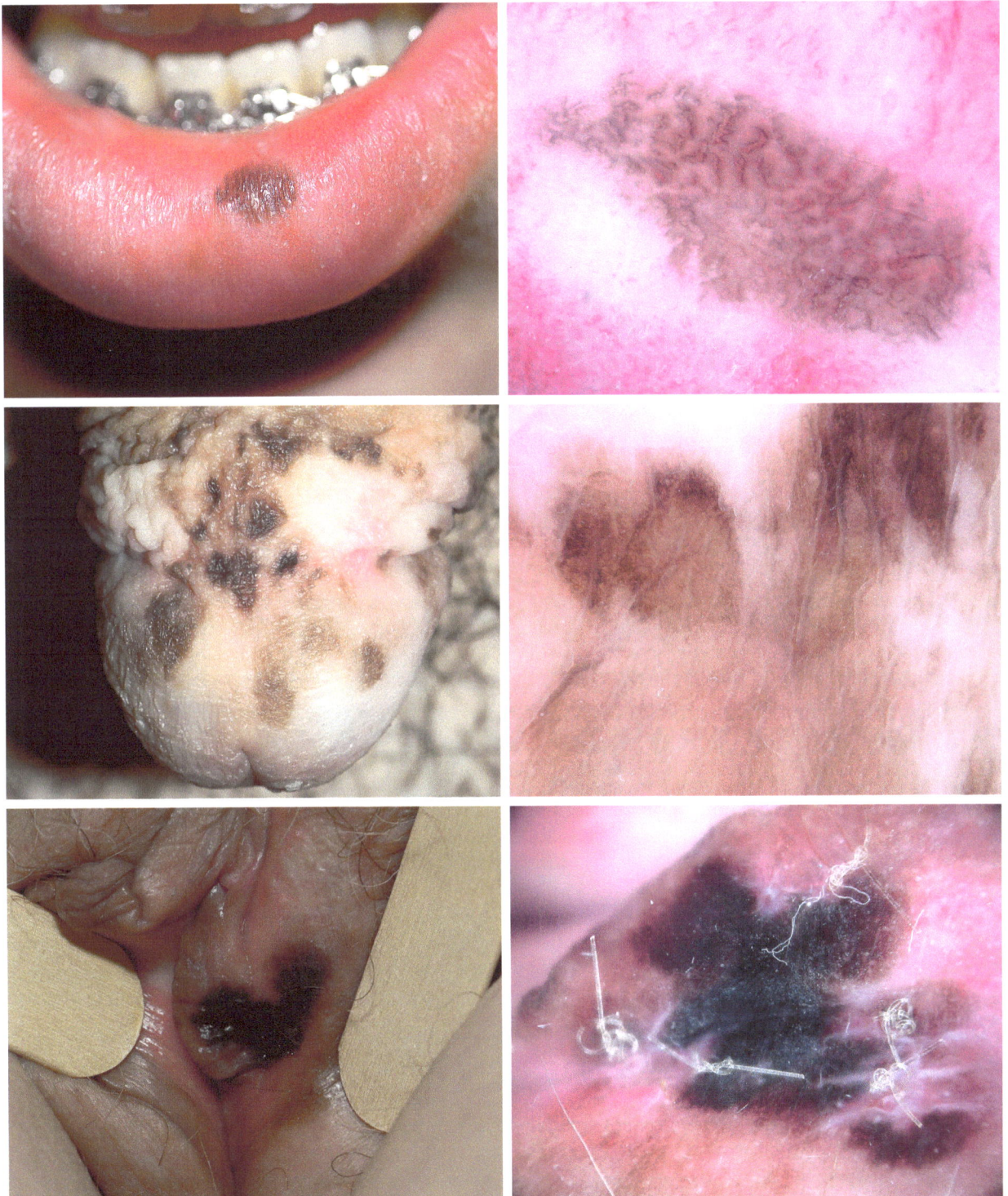

Figure 8.34: Dermatoscopy of mucosal lesions.
Clinical **left column,** dermatoscopy **right column. Top:** Typical labial lentigo. On dermatoscopy one finds curved lines and circles which is a common pattern on mucosal sites. **Middle:** Penile lentiginosis with multiple light brown and dark brown macules. On dermatoscopy one finds brown circles and a brown structureless area but no gray, blue, black or white areas. **Bottom:** Vulvar melanoma that is already clinically obvious. On dermatoscopy one finds a large black and blue structureless area located eccentrically which is a clue to melanoma.

especially in pigmented actinic keratosis, without being precursor lesions.

Even with dermatoscopy it is sometimes difficult or even impossible to distinguish between facial melanoma in situ, lichen-planus like keratosis and pigmented actinic keratosis. If dermatoscopy does not allow a specific diagnosis with confidence, biopsy is required. In the specific context of flat facial pigmented lesions with equivocal dermatoscopy findings, consideration may be given to using reflectance confocal microscopy as an adjunctive diagnostic procedure to increase specificity (reduce the number of biopsies required). (17, 18)

8.4 Mucosal lesions

Lentigines (melanotic macules) are the most common pigmented lesions on the lip, the oral mucosa, and the genital area. Lentigines are typically light-brown or dark-brown spots *(8.34 top row).* On the lip they often occur as single lesions, usually on the lower lip. "Mucosal lentiginosis" refers to the presence of multiple lesions. Genital lentiginosis is much more diverse in terms of morphology than labial or oral lentiginosis *(8.34 middle row).*

As a reliable distinction between this entity and a mucosal melanoma cannot be made on the basis of clinical investigation alone, these lesions are frequently biopsied. The most common dermatoscopic patterns of mucosal pigmented lesions are structureless, curved lines, and circles, but any pattern may be seen. Color may be more important than structure in diagnosing mucosal lesions. A recent study suggests any blue, gray or white area should raise the suspicion for a malignant neoplasm especially when combined with structureless areas (19).

Mucosal melanomas are usually diagnosed late when the clinical diagnosis is already obvious *(8.34 bottom row).* Dermatoscopy is of limited additional value at this stage, but may be useful in less advanced cases (20, 21).

8.5 Recurrent melanocytic lesions

Nevi and melanomas often recur after incomplete removal. Recurrent nevi may mimic melanoma dermatoscopically and pathologically, creating a diagnostic challenge for both the clinician and the dermatopathologist. When submitting recurrent pigmented lesions, the clinician must alert the pathologist to the previous surgical procedure and (when available) provide the original histopathologic diagnosis.

Not every incompletely removed nevus becomes a clinically apparent recurrent nevus. Risk factors for

clinical recurrence seem to be young age and location on the trunk. Usually nevi recur after a superficial shave biopsy of a small congenital nevus or a dermal nevus (Miescher nevus or Unna nevus), with the shave removing only the epidermal and superficial dermal parts but not the deeper dermal parts of the nevus. If these residual melanocytes repopulate the epidermis, this produces visible pigmentation inside the scar.

Recurrent nevi may have any pattern but the most common patterns are radial lines and pseudopods *(8.35, top and middle).* When radial lines and/or pseudopods are found over the entire circumference, a recurrent nevus mimics a Reed nevus. More worryingly, radial lines and/or pseudopods may be seen only in some segments of the periphery, creating a recurrent nevus which mimics melanoma dermatoscopically.

There are clues to help distinguish recurrent nevus from melanoma. Most important is the relationship of the pigmentation to the scar of the original procedure. In recurrent nevi the pigmentation is nearly always confined to the scar. If a melanoma recurs the pigmentation is also present outside the scar *(8.35 bottom).* While a recurrent nevus with a pattern of radial lines and/or pseudopods may mimic a melanoma, these patterns are usually not seen in an actual recurrent melanoma. In contrast to recurrent nevi, which are more common on the trunk, recurrent melanomas more frequently occur on the face and on acral skin, simply because melanomas are more often removed incompletely at these sites. Not only is obtaining surgical margins more difficult, facial and acral melanomas commonly have a lentiginous growth pattern (single melanocytes in the epidermis predominate over nests), making it more difficult for both clinician and pathologist to distinguish the margins of the melanoma.

Fortunately, a lentiginous growth pattern is correlated with slow growth rate, so if these melanomas recur, they recur slowly. This explains the apparent paradox that nevi usually recur faster than melanomas. In a study by Blum et al (22) the median time to treatment of recurrence was 8 months for nevi and 25 months for melanoma.

8.6 Difficult lesions

What is difficult? The answer to this question depends on the investigator. Beginners find a lot of things difficult which experts find easy, but that is not the focus of this chapter. There are, however, some types of lesions that challenge even a well-trained investigator *(8.36).* These lesions may be equally consistent with several differential diagnoses, because they demonstrate insuf-

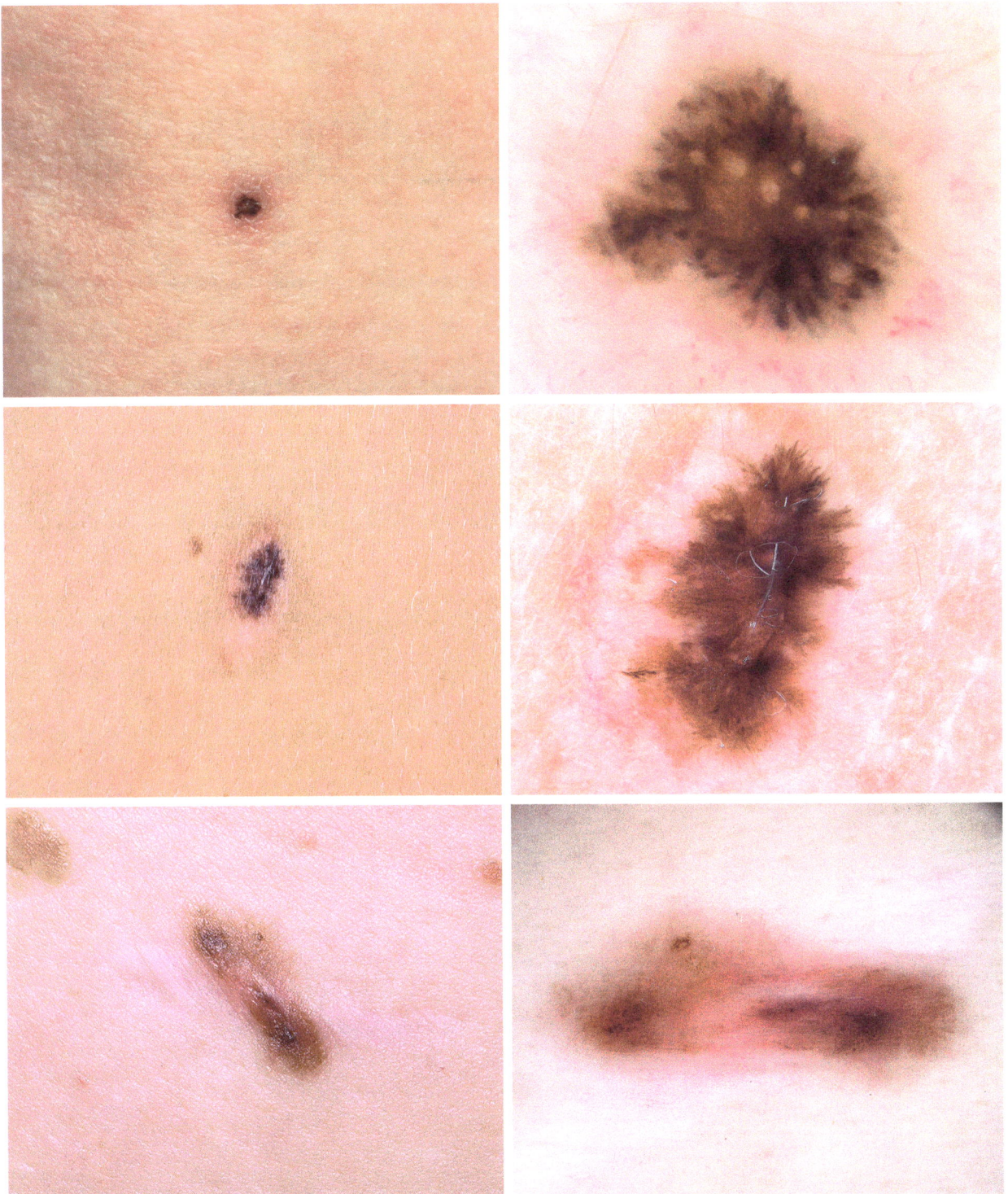

Figure 8.35: *Recurrent nevi and recurrent melanoma.*
Clinical **left column,** dermatoscopy **right column. Top:** *Recurrent nevus with pseudopods on dermatoscopy. The pigmentation stays within the scar.* **Middle:** *Recurrent nevus with radial lines on dermatoscopy. The pigmentation stays within the scar.* **Bottom:** *Recurrent melanoma with clods and a structureless pattern. The pigmentation crosses the scar.*

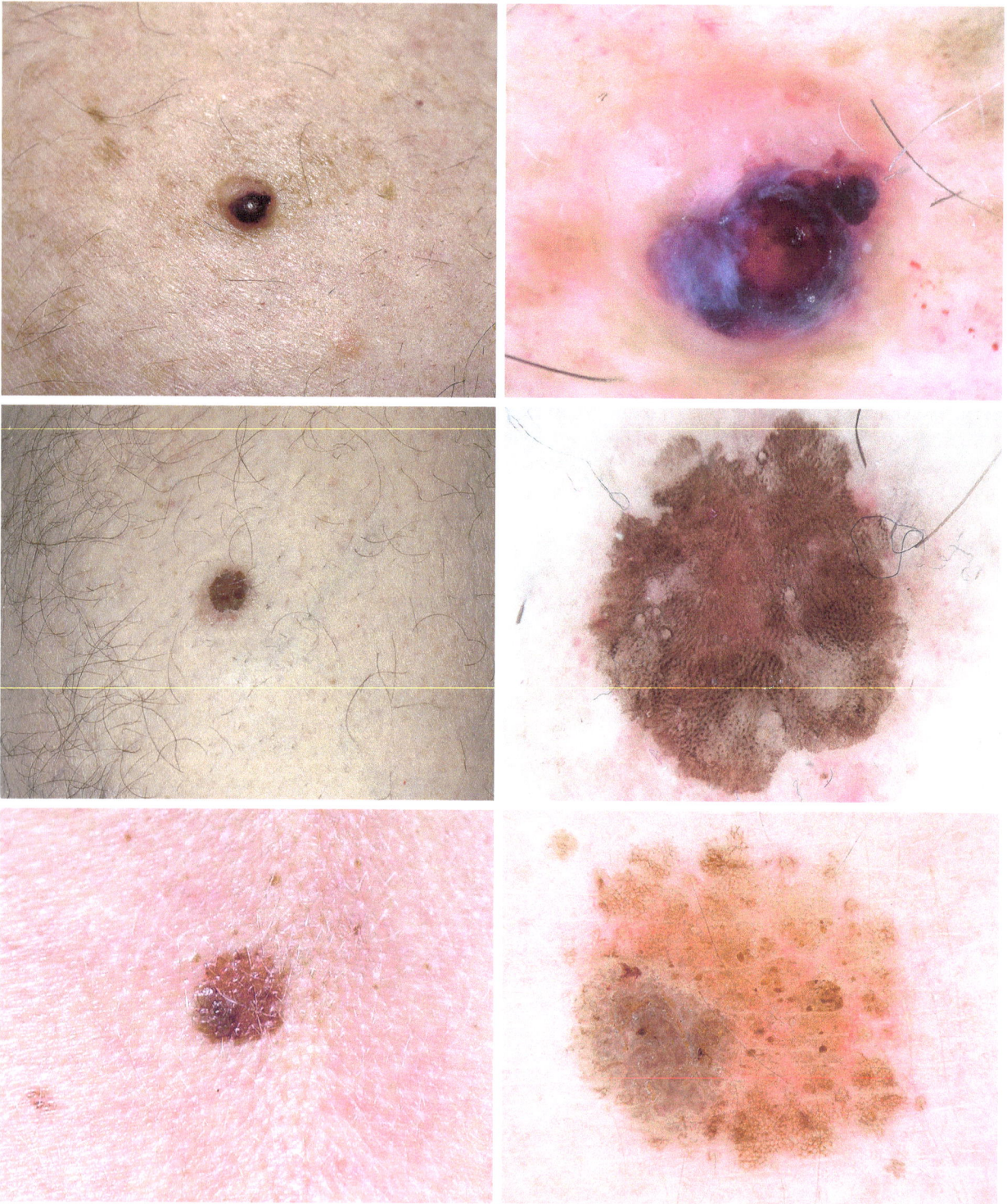

Figure 8.36: Examples of "difficult" lesions.
Clinical **left column,** dermatoscopy **right column. Top row:** Structureless is the least specific pattern. The list of differential diagnoses is long. In this example there are red or purple and skin-colored structureless areas. The list of differential diagnoses includes a basal cell carcinoma, melanoma, or a metastasis. In principle, however, every malignant neoplasm must be considered. The serpentine vessels (which most commonly indicate basal cell carcinoma) are misleading. Histopathological diagnosis: Melanoma (> 1 mm). **Middle row:** Curved lines, circles, dots, and a sharply demarcated margin, are strongly indicative of solar lentigo. These are all misleading clues as this lesion is actually an intracorneal hemorrhage in unusual location. **Bottom row:** Collision lesion with thick curved lines between 6 o'clock and 9 o'clock (seborrheic keratosis) and reticular lines (Clark nevus).

ficient or contradictory clues. In the extreme case there are lesions with misleading clues, which are difficult to reconcile with the diagnosis even retrospectively, i.e. after the histopathology is known.

Too many differential diagnoses

Some patterns give rise to a long list of differential diagnoses that cannot be clearly and reliably distinguished from each other, even with the presence of additional clues. For example, when one follows the algorithm for the structureless pattern, one is confronted with a large number of potential diagnoses. A large number of differential diagnoses are also generated when the investigator is unable to make a confident decision at a certain point in the algorithm. For instance, when the investigator cannot decide whether two patterns are arranged symmetrically or asymmetrically, all diagnoses at the ends of both symmetric and asymmetric branches of the algorithm must be considered. This is a major reason why beginners perform more excisions – they distrust their observations more frequently than experts do, and the list of the potential diagnoses is therefore longer. The difficulty of too many differential diagnoses is unpleasant but rarely causes any serious error because diagnostic uncertainty usually results in a histopathological investigation.

No specific clues

Non-pigmented lesions are considered difficult because usually the pattern of vessels is the only clue to diagnosis (23). Without pigment, a lesion lacks not only color but also structure (= pattern). The specificity of the patterns of vessels is very poor compared to that of pigmented structures, meaning there is greater diagnostic uncertainty for non-pigmented lesions (24). The consequence is a more frequent need for histopathology.

Contradictory clues

We call the clues seen in a lesion "contradictory" when some of the clues favor one particular diagnosis, but other clues favor another diagnosis. For instance, a lesion which has some clues such as blue clods, radial lines and serpentine vessels indicating a basal cell carcinoma, but other clues like reticular lines which render this diagnosis unlikely, one is confronted with a conflict of clues. Handling such apparent contradictions is made easier when the potential causes of contradictory clues are kept in mind.

The commonest cause of contradictory clues is misinterpretation on the part of the investigator. Once this possibility has been ruled out, the investigator should consider the presence of a collision lesion (25–28).

In theory, any type of collision may occur. However, some collisions occur more frequently than others. For instance, solar lentigines are very common on chronic UV-damaged skin, meaning that these solar lentigines are seen to collide with all manner of other lesions simply by chance. In our previous example, one would observe the clues of basal cell carcinoma as well as those of solar lentigo (reticular lines!); the different parts can usually be quite easily distinguished from each other. Whether one is confronted with a simple coincidence or a causal link, i.e. one lesion (usually a malignant one) arising from another lesion – is usually mere speculation. The presence of a coincidence is especially likely when the two lesions are fundamentally different. For instance, it would be difficult to explain how a melanocytic lesion (a melanoma) could arise from an epithelial lesion (a solar lentigo).

Collisions with solar lentigines are common, regardless of whether the second lesion is a basal cell carcinoma, a melanoma, or a superficial squamous cell carcinoma. These combinations should not be a reason to construe a causal association. Collisions between seborrheic keratoses and superficial squamous cell carcinomas of the Bowen's type and collisions of dermatofibromas and basal cell carcinomas are less common, but do occur. Of course one should also interpret melanomas that arise in a pre-existing nevus as collision lesions. Last but not least, it should be mentioned that pathologists tend to mention in their reports only those diagnoses that they consider relevant. For instance, when there is a collision between a basal cell carcinoma and a solar lentigo, the latter is not always mentioned. In these cases the dermatoscopist's findings may remain inexplicable.

Misleading clues

Clues that suggest an incorrect diagnosis are misleading. They commonly give rise to serious errors. Dermatoscopy is not a perfect method, even in the hands of an experienced investigator. Sometimes the histological diagnosis does not concur at all with the dermatoscopic appearance.

Nevertheless, one's confidence in the method should not be shaken by such instances. On the contrary, when dermatoscopic findings cannot be made to concur with the histopathological diagnosis, one should speak to one's pathologist and not to one's psychiatrist! Never forget that even pathology reports may be incorrect. Errors are very rare in specimen handling and report transcription, but they do occur. More commonly, a different diagnosis is reached after the pathologist reviews the specimen or seeks a second opinion from a colleague.

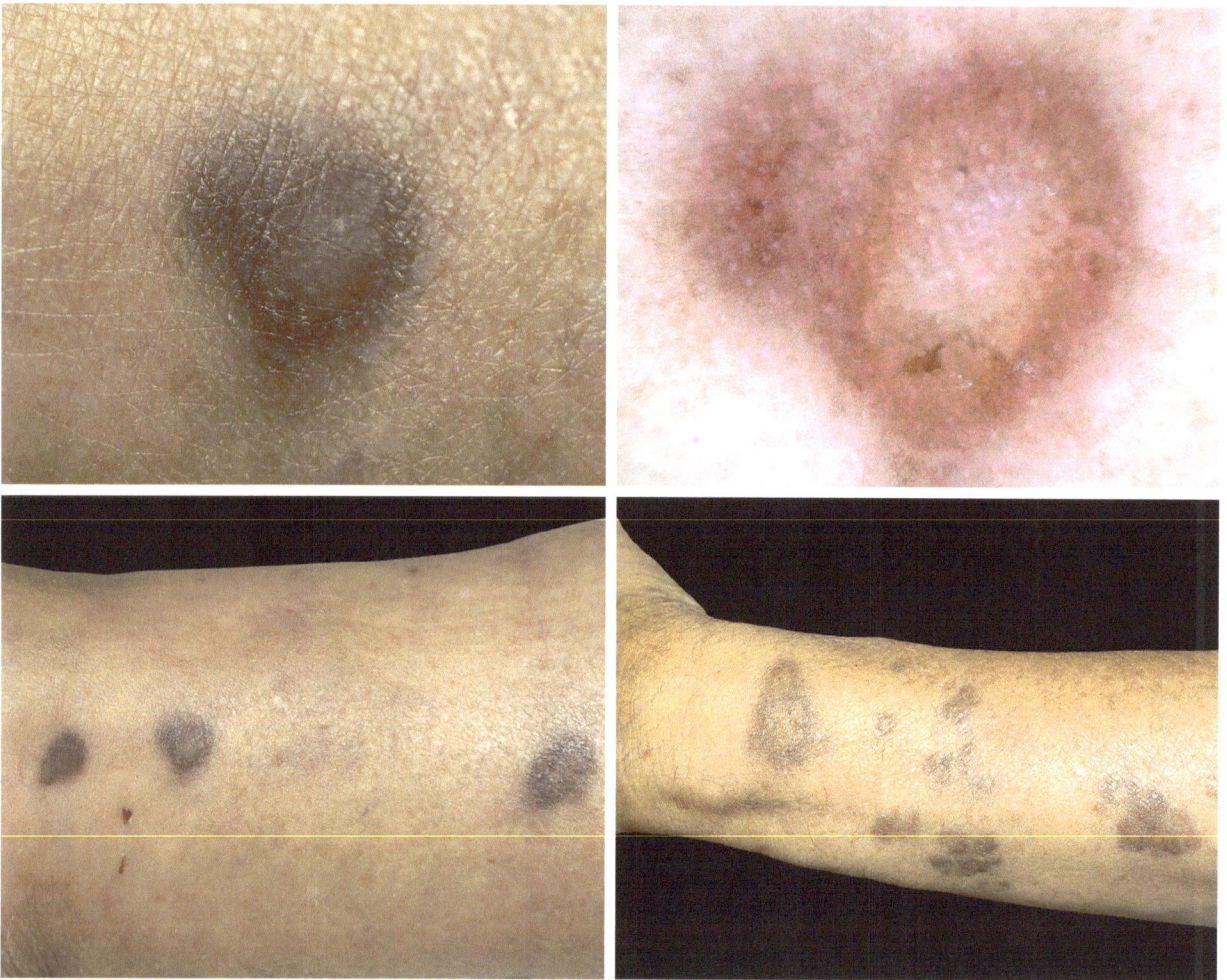

Figure 8.37: *The dermatoscopic interpretation depends on the clinical context.*
Top row: *Clinical close-up* **(left)** *and dermatoscopic image* **(right)** *are best interpreted as dermatofibroma.* **Bottom row:** *The clinical context is the clue to the correct diagnosis of Kaposi sarcoma.*

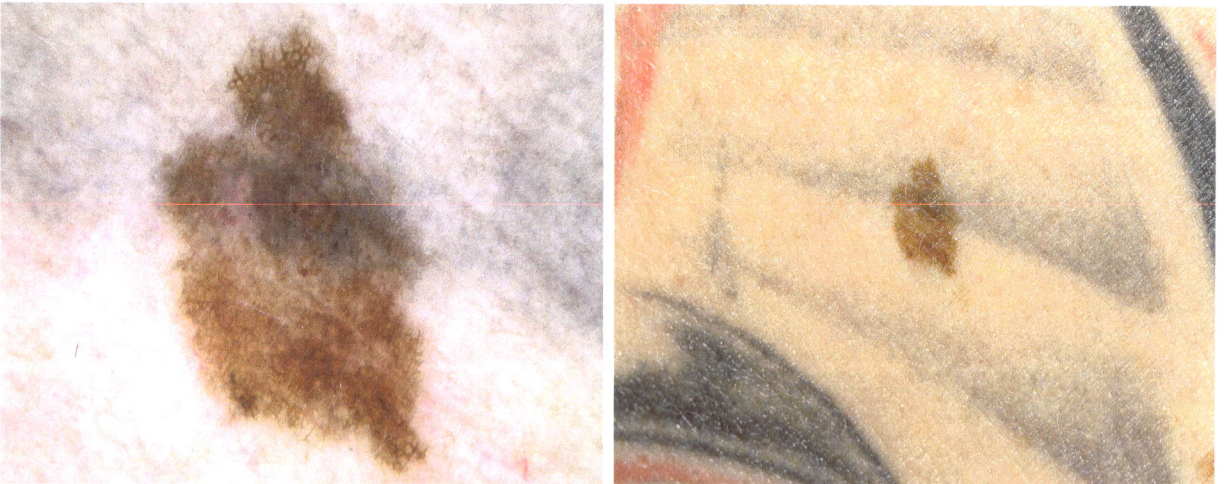

Figure 8.38: *The dermatoscopic interpretation depends on the clinical context.*
Left: *Dermatoscopic view of a reticular lesion with gray structures that may be interpreted as a clue to melanoma.* **Right:** *The clinical context reveals that the gray structures belong to a tattoo.*

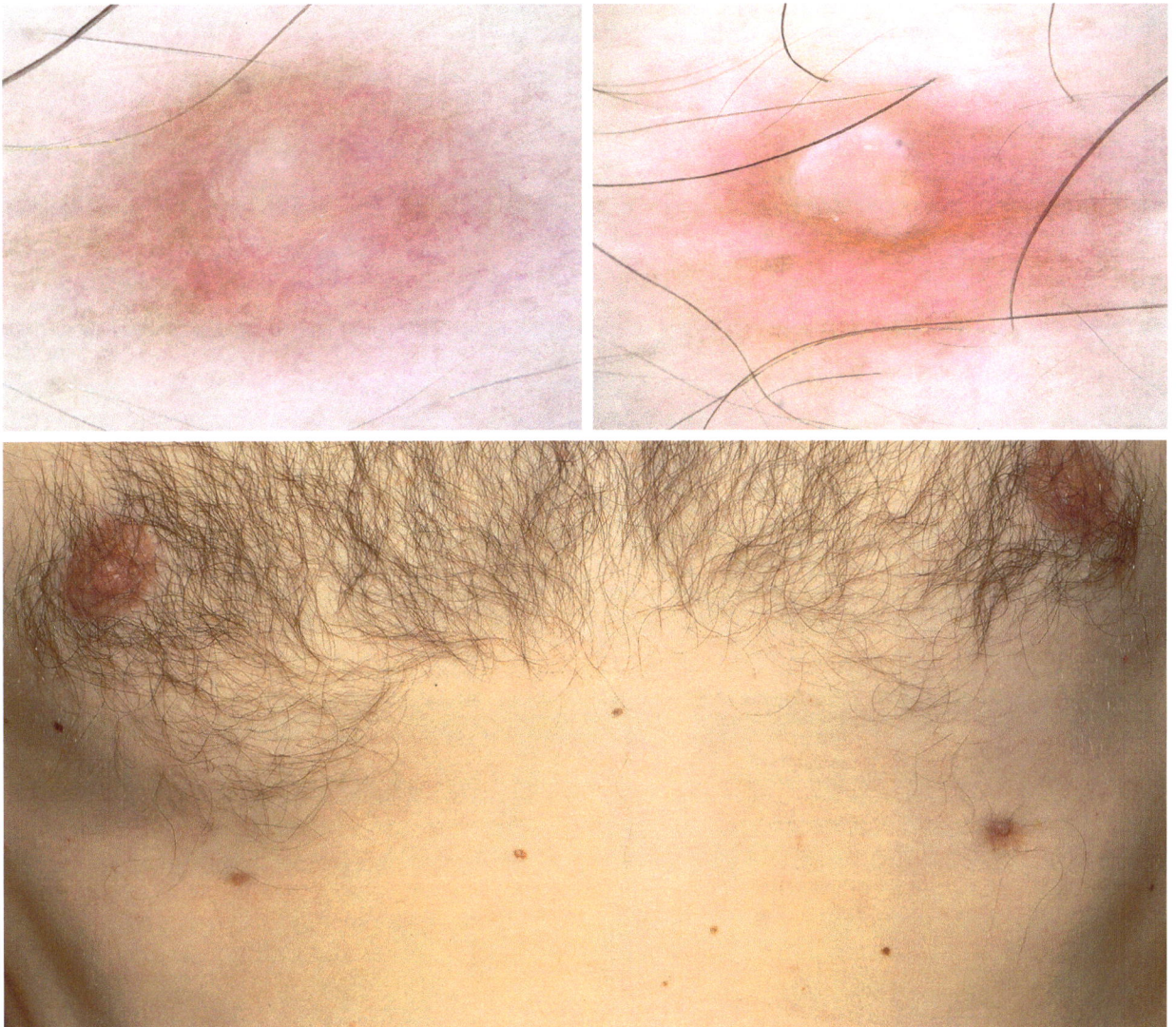

Figure 8.39: *The dermatoscopic interpretation depends on the clinical context.*
Top row: *Dermatoscopic images of two pigmented lesions from the same patient. The best diagnosis for both lesions is either congenital nevus or dermatofibroma.* **Bottom:** *The clinical context reveals that both lesions are localized along the milk line, therefore the diagnosis is accessory nipples.*

Table 8.1: Dermatoscopy of common inflammatory and infectious skin diseases	
Diagnosis	Dermatoscopic clues
Psoriasis	Monomorphous vessels as dots or coils, white scales
Spongiotic dermatitis (e.g. contact dermatitis, nummular dermatitis, seborrheic dermatitis)	Monomorphous vessels as dots, yellow scales
Pityriasis rosea	Monomorphous vessels as dots, peripheral scales
Porokeratosis	Brown or gray raised circle as border and/or scale within this circle, vessels as dots
Lichen planus	Red to brown structureless zone intersected by thick white branched lines (Wickham striae)
Lupus erythematosus	Erythema, yellow clods (follicular keratin plugs), white circles (perifollicular), white structureless zone
Sarcoidosis, sarcoidal rosacea	Yellow structureless zone, serpentine vessels
Grover's disease	Yellow serum crust in the center
Molluscum contagiosum	White to yellow clods or structureless zone in the center, curved vessels at the periphery which do not cross the center
Verruca plana	Monomorphous vessels as dots
Verruca vulgaris	Skin-colored to white clods, each with centered vessels, vessels can be dots or lines (if wart is more elevated)
Verruca plantaris/palmaris	Yellow structureless zone with red to black dots and lines (hemorrhage)
Verruca genitalis	White reticular lines
Tinea nigra	Very thin brown branched lines
Trichomycosis palmellina	Yellow, red or black structureless zone around the (axillary) hair
Scabies	Thick curved/serpentine line (burrow), mite as a triangle at the end of the thick line: black dots in the burrow
Pediculosis	Identification of the parasite and the nits (clods): full (brown oval) and empty (transparent with a flat end)
Tungiasis	Round red to black structureless zone with a central black clod/dot, Brown edge around the structureless zone

Avoidance of error

One could fill a whole book with good suggestions for avoiding errors in dermatoscopy. However, these few points are most important:

1. Assess lesions in an unbiased way, i.e. without giving preference to a pre-conceived diagnosis. Avoid making instant ("blink") diagnoses.
2. Describe the lesion as objectively as possible
3. Use an objective method – ideally pattern analysis – to interpret the clues.
4. Trust the method and not your feelings.
5. Justify your diagnosis with logical arguments based on the features as you have described them.
6. Evaluate the lesion in the clinical context (8.37–8.39)

If you follow this advice you will soon become an expert in dermatoscopy if you are not one already.

8.7 Inflammatory skin diseases

Dermatoscopy is not limited to the examination of pigmented and non-pigmented neoplasias. It may also be helpful in the diagnosis of infectious and non-infectious inflammatory skin diseases (table 8.1). Dermatoscopy is extremely useful in diagnosing some parasitic diseases. A new term has been coined for this purpose: Entomodermatoscopy. This is a neologism derived from entomology (the study of insects) and dermatoscopy (29). In all inflammatory diseases, whether they are caused by living organisms or not, dermatoscopy is at best an auxiliary investigation to complement the clinical evaluation. The diagnosis is nearly always established by clinical examination. In inflammatory diseases one usually finds multiple lesions (e.g. psoriasis or scabies); only rarely one finds single lesions (e.g. larva migrans).

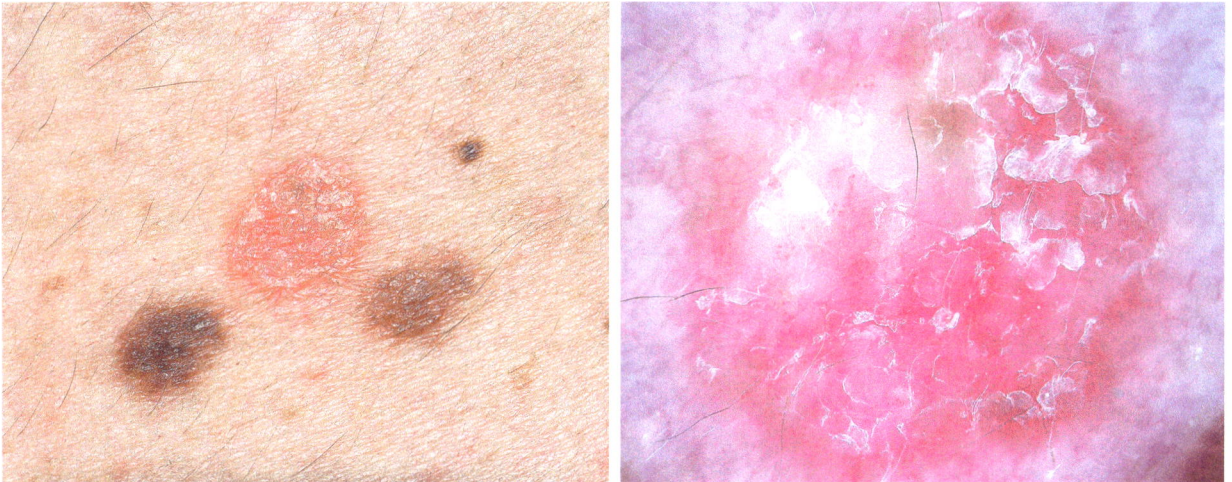

Figure 8.40: *Dermatoscopy of psoriasis.*
Clinical appearance **left,** *dermatoscopy* **right.** *The dermatoscopy of psoriasis is characterized by white scale, and vessels as dots or small coils, randomly distributed.*

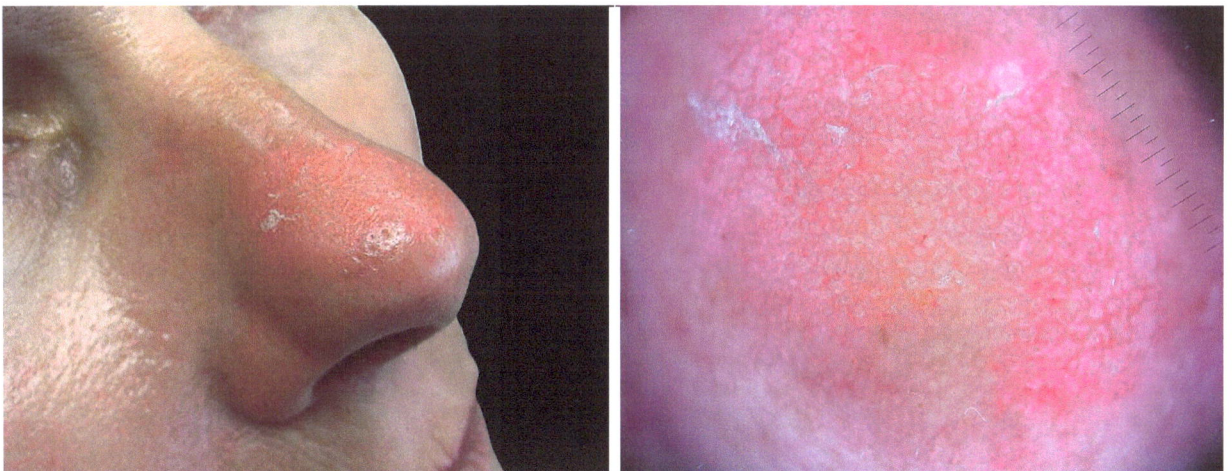

Figure 8.41: *Cutaneous lupus erythematosus.*
Clinical appearance **left,** *dermatoscopy* **right.** *Note the characteristic follicular keratin plugs seen as small white and yellow clods, the background erythema, and scale. Images courtesy Ian McColl.*

Non-infectious inflammatory diseases

The dermatoscopic appearance of psoriasis has already been discussed in detail in chapter 6. Psoriasis is marked by a monomorphous pattern of vessels as either dots or small coiled vessels. A further clue is white scale (30). These features mean it is often necessary to differentiate psoriasis from Bowen's disease. In Bowen's disease, vessels are usually coiled. The distribution of vessels is usually random in psoriasis, whereas in Bowen's disease they tend to be arranged in clusters (31). These characteristics, however, are relatively non-specific and may not permit differentiation from Bowen's disease based on dermatoscopy alone.

Scale in psoriasis is usually white *(8.40)*. The scale of spongiotic dermatitis (e.g. nummular dermatitis, seborrheic dermatitis, contact dermatitis) is more frequently yellow because the stratum corneum contains serum. The scale of pityriasis rosea is found peripherally. In lesions of chronic cutaneous lupus erythematosus one finds, in addition to erythema, small, white, yellow or orange clods on dermatoscopy. These correspond to the follicular keratin plugs seen on histology *(8.41)*. In addition, scale may occur. In older lesions of lupus erythematosus one finds white circles around follicular openings and, as a consequence of sclerosis, white structureless zones *(8.42)*.

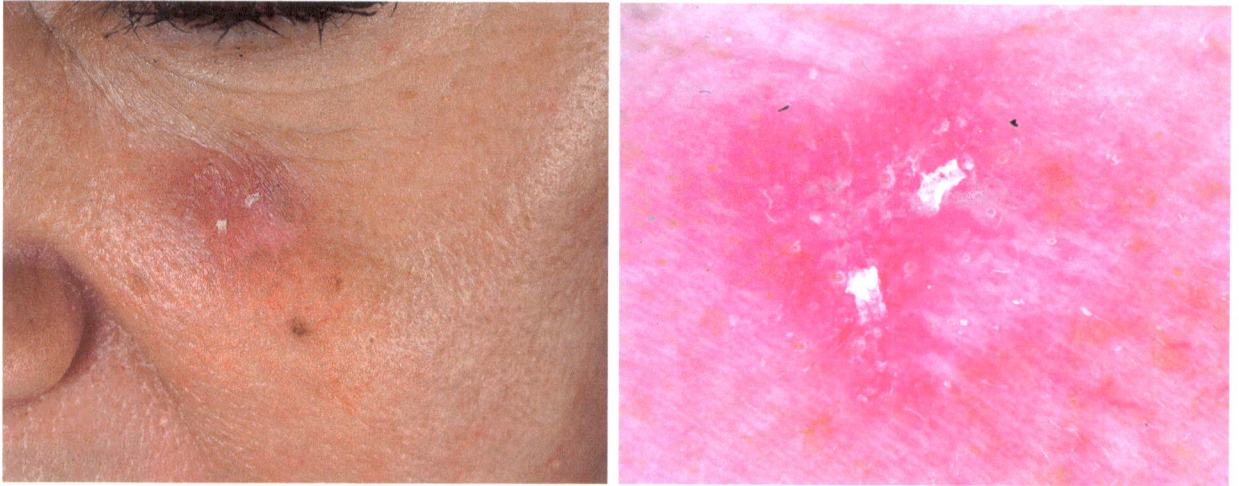

Figure 8.42: Cutaneous lupus erythematosus.
Clinical appearance **left,** dermatoscopy **right.** This is an older lesion of cutaneous lupus erythematosus with more sclerosis. Note the background erythema, white circles, the white structureless zone, and scale.

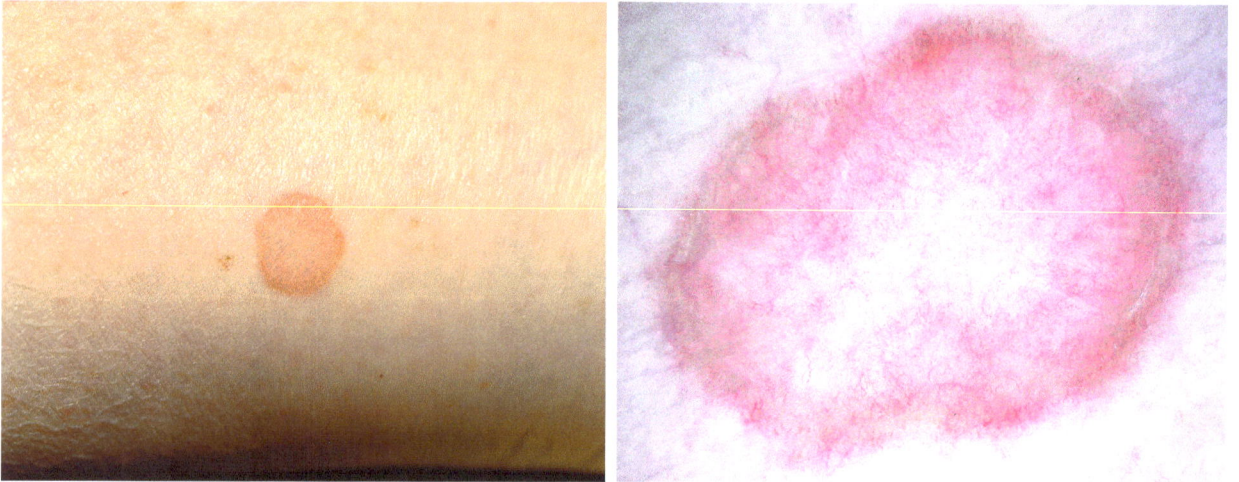

Figure 8.43: Dermatoscopy of porokeratosis.
Clinical appearance **left,** dermatoscopy **right.** The dermatoscopy shows a subtle yellow circle or rim at the border of the lesion. The vascular pattern in the center, which is composed of vessels as dots and linear vessels, is not specific.

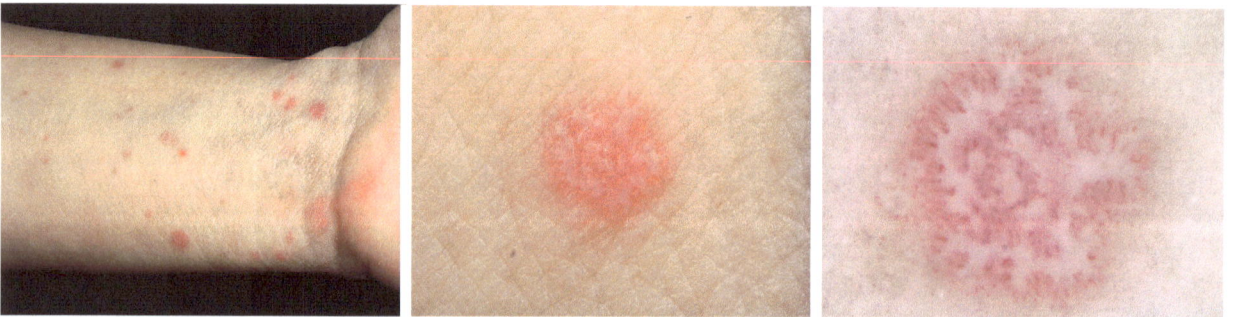

Figure 8.44: Lichen planus.
Overview **(left)**, detail **(middle)** and dermatoscopic appearance **(right)**. On dermatoscopy the Wickham striae appear as thick white lines. The findings are so specific that a biopsy is not needed to confirm the diagnosis.

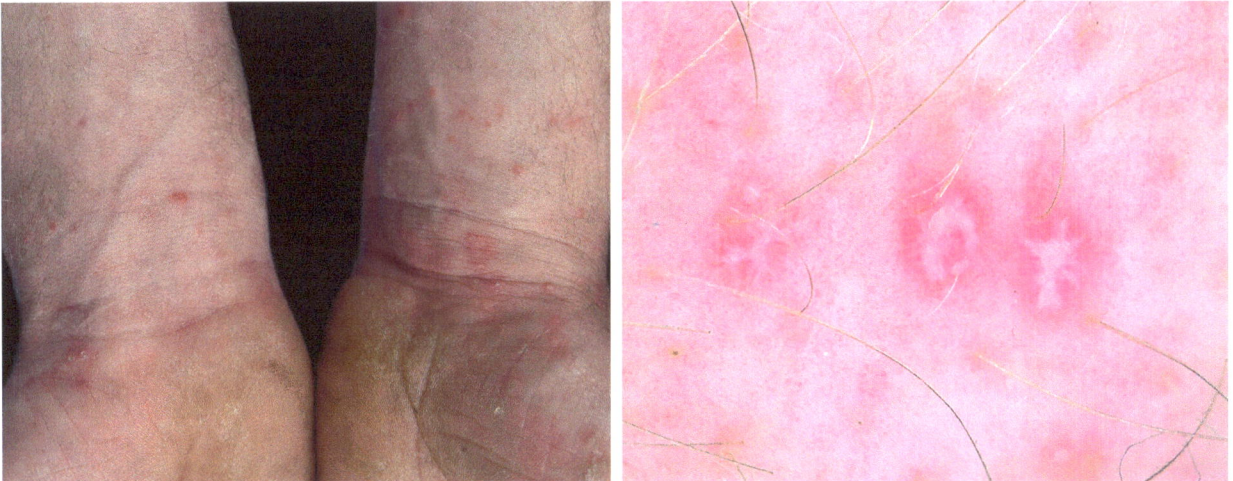

Figure 8.45: Lichen planus.
Clinical appearance **left,** *dermatoscopy* **right.** *The specific dermatoscopy of lichen planus is already present in very small lesions.*

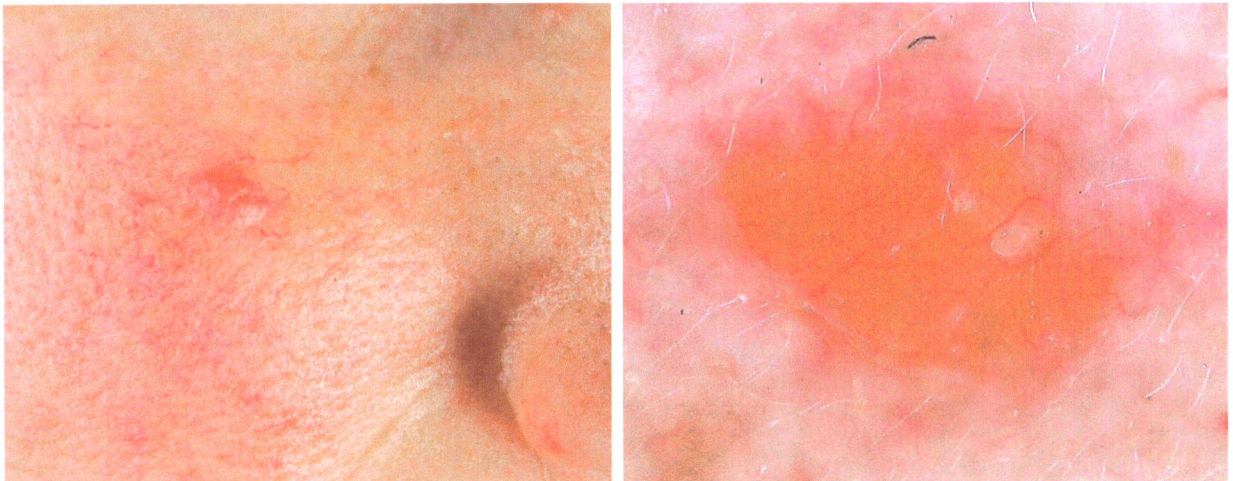

Figure 8.46: Sarcoidosis and sarcoidal rosacea.
Clinical appearance **left,** *dermatoscopy* **right.** *In this case of sarcoidal rosacea one finds the typical structureless yellow zone and serpentine branched vessels.*

Porokeratosis, a disorder of keratinization with various phenotypes, is typified by the so-called cornoid lamella – a column of parakeratotic cells in the stratum corneum, visible only on histopathology. On dermatoscopy this appears as a white or yellow hyperkeratotic circle defining the border of the lesion *(8.43).* Centrally there may be a monomorphous pattern of vessels as dots, or a brown and white structureless area as a sign of atrophy (32).

In lichen planus one finds structureless red to brown areas intersected by thick white branched lines or white clods *(8.44).* The white branched lines correspond to the so-called Wickham striae (30, 33). The dermatoscopic features of lichen planus are quite specific and can be seen even in very small lesions *(8.45).* In sarcoidosis (including the sarcoidal variant of rosacea) one finds a yellow or orange structureless zone and serpentine vessels *(8.46).* Cutaneous amyloidosis is characterized by a red structureless zones on dermatoscopy *(8.47).* Vessels are typically absent. Transient acantholytic dyskeratosis, also known as Grover's disease, is characterized by a central yellow clod that is often star-shaped, and most likely corresponds to the superficial erosions topped with a serum crust that are typical for this itchy disease *(8.48).*

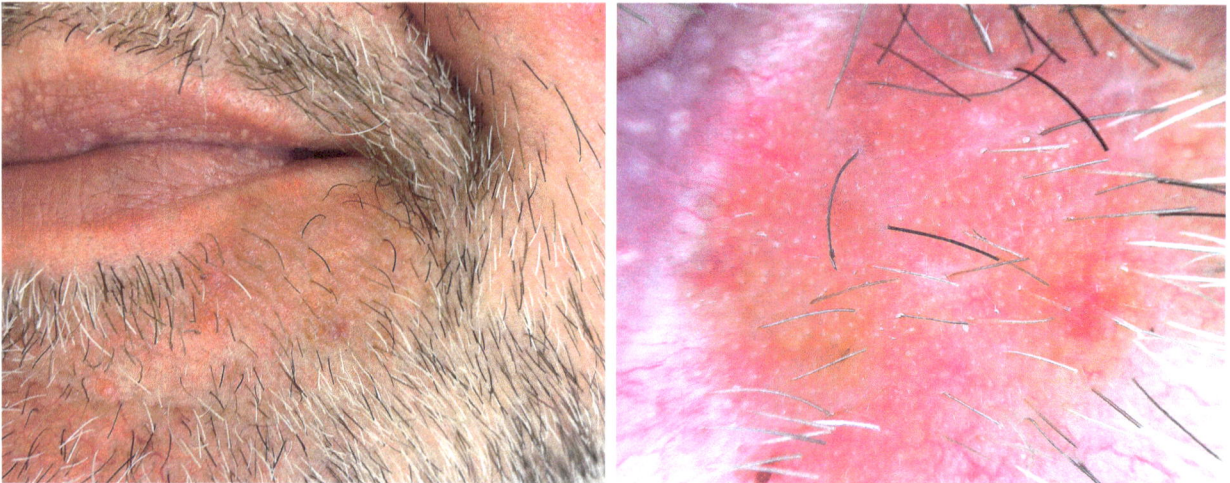

Figure 8.47: Cutaneous amyloidosis.
*Clinical appearance **left**, dermatoscopy **right.** The dermatoscopic findings are not very specific. One finds a red and yellow structureless zone without any vessels.*

Figure 8.48: Grover's disease.
Dermatoscopy of Grover's disease. The yellow star-shaped clod in the center most probably corresponds to an erosion covered by a serum crust induced by scratching. Image courtesy of Iris Zalaudek.

Infections and Infestations

Viruses

Of the large number of skin lesions that may be caused by viruses we will confine ourselves here to a small selection of those lesions whose diagnosis is facilitated by dermatoscopy. Molluscum contagiosum is caused by a poxvirus. These lesions are manifested as skin-colored papules that reveal, on dermatoscopy, white or yellow clods and/or a structureless area in the center *(8.49, top)*. At the periphery of the lesion one finds radially arranged vessels that do not cross the center of the lesion (29, 34, 35). Various human papillomaviruses (HPV) are the cause of viral warts (verrucae). Viral warts have many different clinical appearances, but are almost never pigmented. Verrucae planae (plane warts) have vessels as dots on a light-brown or yellow structureless background. Verrucae vulgares or common verrucae *(8.49, bottom)* have skin-colored or pink clods with vessels in the center (centered vessels). When a viral wart occurs at the sole of the foot or the palm it is known as a plantar or palmar verruca. These merely have a yellow structureless zone that corresponds to the hyperkeratosis with red or black dots and short lines, corresponding to hemorrhage and vessels, and can be differentiated from a callus or a clavus (36).

Fungi

Tinea nigra is a rare disease in Europe, North America and southern Australia, but more common in tropical

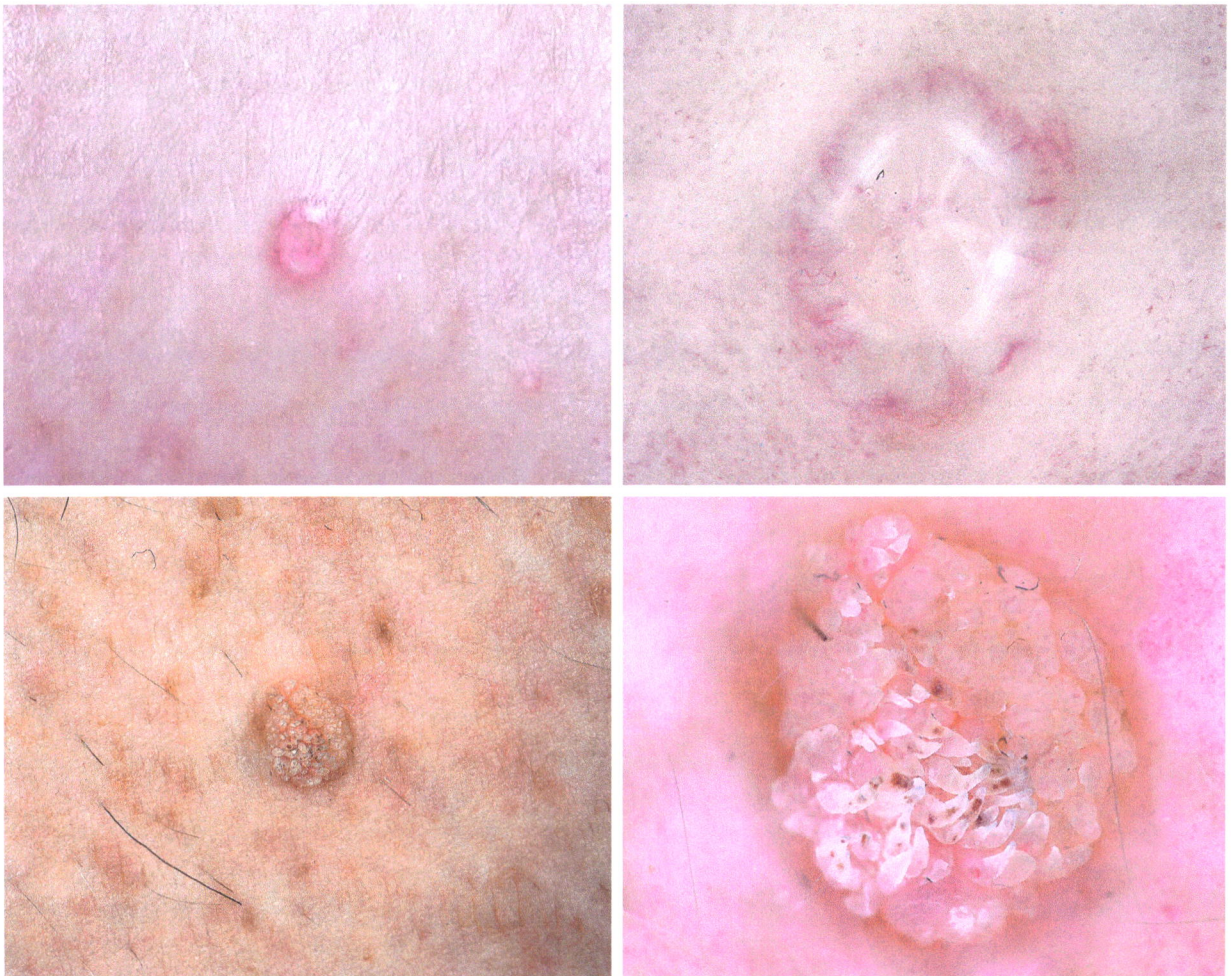

Figure 8.49: Viral warts.
*Clinical appearance **left**, dermatoscopy **right column**. **Top:** Molluscum contagiosum with yellow clods in the center and radial vessels that do not cross the center. **Bottom:** Viral wart with skin colored clods and centered vessels.*

areas. It is caused by the fungus *Hortaea werneckii*. Clinically this infection is easily confused with an acral nevus or a melanoma because it is seen as a more or less homogeneous, dirty brown or gray macule *(8.50)*. On dermatoscopy the differential diagnosis can be easily resolved because tinea nigra has no parallel lines but very thin brown or gray branched lines over the entire lesion (37).

Bacteria

Trichomycosis palmellina is probably the only bacterial infection whose diagnosis is facilitated even slightly by dermatoscopy. This disease is caused by *Coryne-bacterium tenuis* and is seen on dermatoscopy as a yellow, black or red structureless area that surrounds

the axillary hair (29). In most other bacterial infections one only finds unspecific hyperemia or pus.

Parasites

Scabies is a very common disease caused by the mite *Sarcoptes scabiei*. The mite lives in burrows in the stratum corneum and causes skin lesions and a sometimes intractable itch. To make the diagnosis without dermatoscopy the mite, which is barely visible with the unaided eye, has to be located microscopically in skin scrapings. However, the mite is easily demonstrated on dermatoscopy with no need for skin scrapings *(8.51)*. On dermatoscopy one sees a curved or serpentine line, which corresponds to the burrow *(8.52)*. At the end of the line the mite is seen as a small, dark triangle

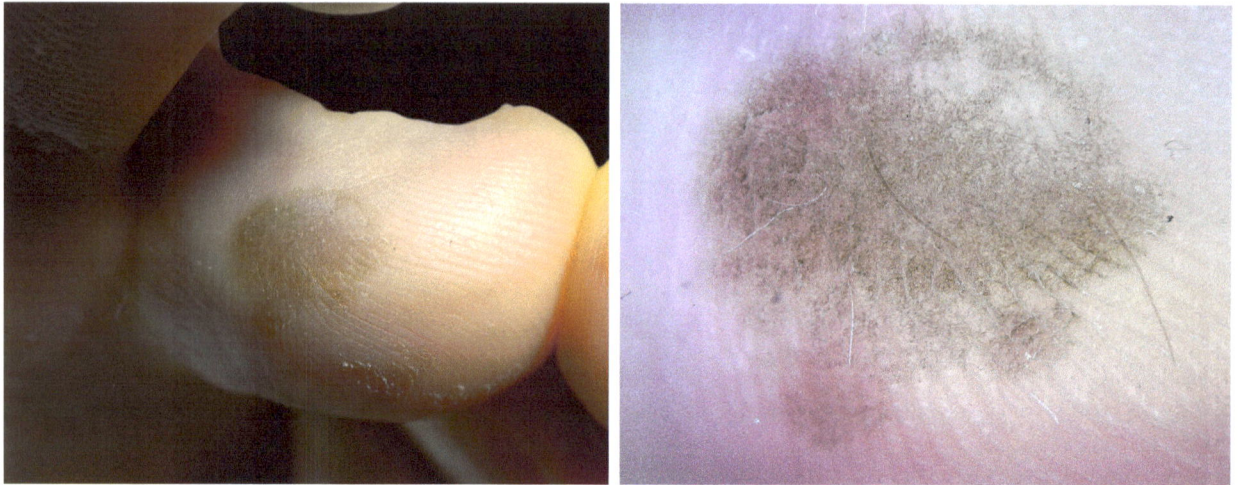

Figure 8.50: *Tinea nigra.*
The dermatoscopic appearance on the **right** *shows the typical thin branched gray lines of tinea nigra.*

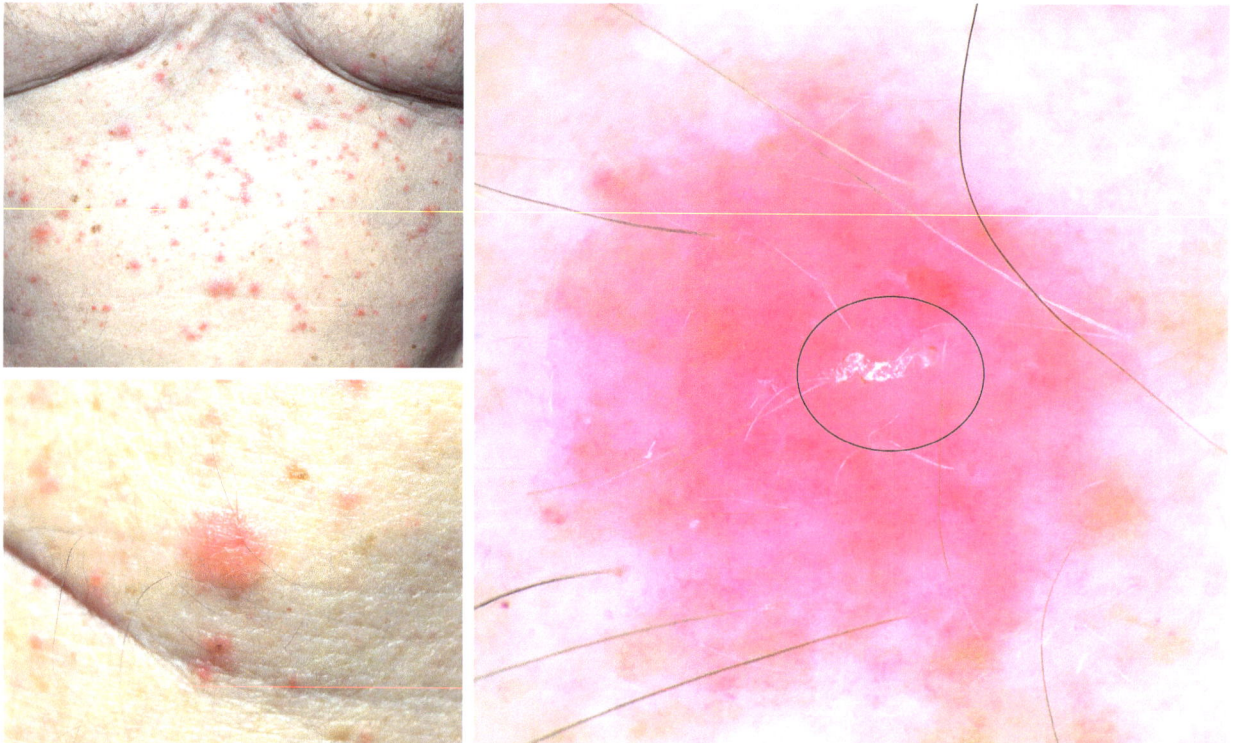

Figure 8.51: *Scabies diagnosed by dermatoscopy.*
The clinical overview **(top left)** *show a papular rash. On the clinical close-up* **(bottom left)** *one can see non-specific erythematous papules. The dermatoscopy* **(right)** *reveals the burrow and the scabies mite (circle).*

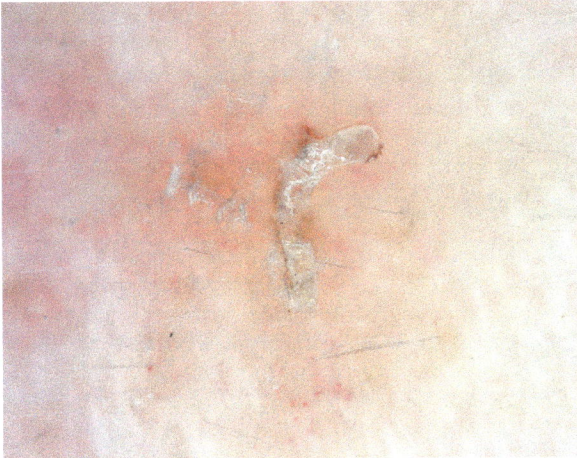

Figure 8.52: Scabies.
Diagnosis of scabies by dermatoscopy. On dermatoscopy one finds a thick curved line (the burrow). At the end of the line the mite is seen as a small, dark triangle (anterior portion of the parasite). Image courtesy of Iris Zalaudek and Giuseppe Argenziano.

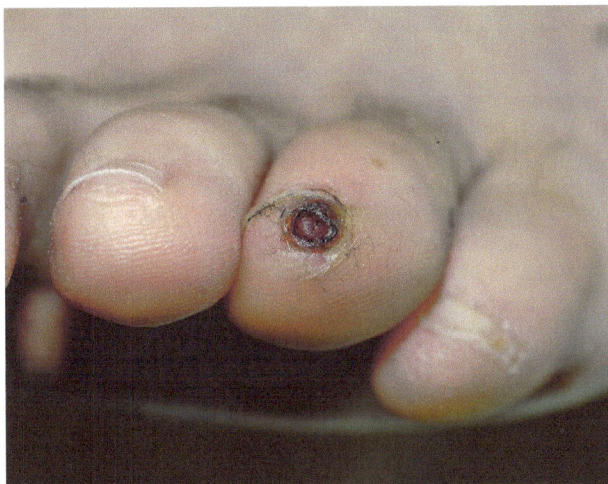
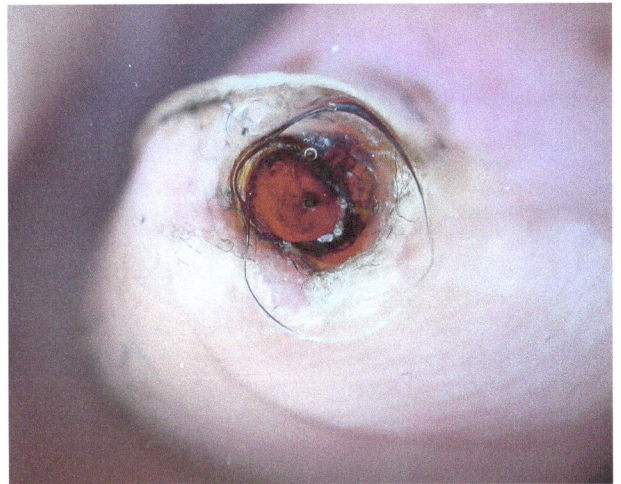

Figure 8.53: Dermatoscopy of tunga penetrans

(anterior portion of the parasite). This manifestation has been compared to a jet with a contrail. Occasionally mite excrement is seen as black dots within the thick curved line (38).

Lice (pediculosis capitis/phthiriasis pubis) can also be diagnosed in vivo with the dermatoscope. Nits may be distinguished from other structures such as dandruff. When the nit contains a nymph one sees brown oval clods on dermatoscopy. If they are empty (after the nymphs have hatched) there will be transparent clods with a flat end. These should be distinguished from debris of hair gel or dandruff, which will be seen as polygonal clods with white dots and lines (39).

A rather rare disease in high latitudes is caused by the sand flea *Tunga penetrans*. The main breeding areas are South-Central America, Africa or Asia. The sand flea bores its way through the epidermis, where it lays its eggs. The disease is manifested as dark papules that usually occur on acral locations. On dermatoscopy one finds a round, black or red structureless area with a central black clod or a dot (8.53). This feature correlates with the parasite's rump protruding out of the skin (40).

References

1   Braun RP, Baran R, Le Gal FA, Dalle S, Ronger S, Pandolfi R, et al. Diagnosis and management of nail pigmentations. J Am Acad Dermatol. 2007; 56; 835–847.

2   Thomas L, Dalle S. Dermoscopy provides useful information for the management of melanonychia striata. Dermatol Ther. 2007; 20; 3–10.

3   Jellinek N. Nail matrix biopsy of longitudinal melanonychia: diagnostic algorithm including the matrix shave biopsy. J Am Acad Dermatol. 2007; 56; 803–810.

4   Ronger S, Touzet S, Ligeron C, Balme B, Viallard AM, Barrut D, et al. Dermoscopic examination of nail pigmentation. Arch Dermatol. 2002; 138; 1327–1333.

5   Iorizzo M, Tosti A, Di Chiacchio N, Hirata SH, Misciali C, Michalany N, et al. Nail melanoma in children: differential diagnosis and management. Dermatol Surg. 2008; 34; 974–978.

6   Braun RP, Baran R, Saurat JH, Thomas L. Surgical Pearl: Dermoscopy of the free edge of the nail to determine the level of nail plate pigmentation and the location of its probable origin in the proximal or distal nail matrix. J Am Acad Dermatol. 2006; 55; 512–513.

7   Saida T, Koga H. Dermoscopic patterns of acral melanocytic nevi: their variations, changes, and significance. Arch Dermatol. 2007; 143; 1423–1426.

8   Miyazaki A, Saida T, Koga H, Oguchi S, Suzuki T, Tsuchida T. Anatomical and histopathological correlates of the dermoscopic patterns seen in melanocytic nevi on the sole: a retrospective study. J Am Acad Dermatol. 2005; 53; 230–236.

9   Malvehy J, Puig S. Dermoscopic patterns of benign volar melanocytic lesions in patients with atypical mole syndrome. Arch Dermatol. 2004; 140; 538–544.

10 Braun RP, Thomas L, Kolm I, French LE, Marghoob AA. The furrow ink test: a clue for the dermoscopic diagnosis of acral melanoma vs nevus. Arch Dermatol. 2008; 144; 1618–1620.

11 Saida T, Miyazaki A, Oguchi S, Ishihara Y, Yamazaki Y, Murase S, et al. Significance of dermoscopic patterns in detecting malignant melanoma on acral volar skin: results of a multicenter study in Japan. Arch Dermatol. 2004; 140; 1233–1238.

12 Ishihara Y, Saida T, Miyazaki A, Koga H, Taniguchi A, Tsuchida T, et al. Early acral melanoma in situ: correlation between the parallel ridge pattern on dermoscopy and microscopic features. Am J Dermatopathol. 2006; 28; 21–27.

13 Zalaudek I, Argenziano G, Soyer HP, Saurat JH, Braun RP. Dermoscopy of subcorneal hematoma. Dermatol Surg. 2004; 30; 1229–1232.

14 Sahin MT, Ozturkcan S, Ermertcan AT, Gunes AT. A comparison of dermoscopic features among lentigo senilis/initial seborrheic keratosis, seborrheic keratosis, lentigo maligna and lentigo maligna melanoma on the face. J Dermatol. 2004; 31; 884–889.

15 Stolz W, Schiffner R, Burgdorf WH. Dermatoscopy for facial pigmented skin lesions. Clin Dermatol. 2002; 20; 276–278.

16 Tschandl P, Rosendahl C, Kittler H. Dermatoscopy of flat pigmented facial lesions. J Eur Acad Dermatol Venereol. 2015; 29; 120–127.

17 de Carvalho N, Farnetani F, Ciardo S, Ruini C, Witkowski AM, Longo C, et al. Reflectance confocal microscopy correlates of dermoscopic patterns of facial lesions help to discriminate lentigo maligna from pigmented nonmelanocytic macules. Br J Dermatol. 2015; 173; 128–133.

18 Guitera P, Pellacani G, Crotty KA, Scolyer RA, Li LX, Bassoli S, et al. The impact of in vivo reflectance confocal microscopy on the diagnostic accuracy of lentigo maligna and equivocal pigmented and nonpigmented macules of the face. J Invest Dermatol. 2010; 130; 2080–2091.

19 Blum A, Simionescu O, Argenziano G, Braun R, Cabo H, Eichhorn A, et al. Dermoscopy of pigmented lesions of the mucosa and the mucocutaneous junction: results of a multicenter study by the International Dermoscopy Society (IDS). Arch Dermatol. 2011; 147; 1181–1187.

20 Ferrari A, Zalaudek I, Argenziano G, Buccini P, De Simone P, Silipo V, et al. Dermoscopy of pigmented lesions of the vulva: a retrospective morphological study. Dermatology. 2011; 222; 157–166.

21 Lin J, Koga H, Takata M, Saida T. Dermoscopy of pigmented lesions on mucocutaneous junction and mucous membrane. Br J Dermatol. 2009; 161; 1255–1261.

22 Blum A, Hofmann-Wellenhof R, Marghoob AA, Argenziano G, Cabo H, Carrera C, et al. Recurrent melanocytic nevi and melanomas in dermoscopy: results of a multicenter study of the International Dermoscopy Society. JAMA Dermatol. 2014; 150; 138–145.

23 Menzies SW, Kreusch J, Byth K, Pizzichetta MA, Marghoob A, Braun R, et al. Dermoscopic evaluation of amelanotic and hypomelanotic melanoma. Arch Dermatol. 2008; 144; 1120–1127.

24 Kittler H, Riedl E, Rosendahl C, Cameron A. Dermatoscopy of unpigmented lesions of the skin: a new classification of vessel morphology based on pattern analysis. Dermatopathol: Pract & Conc. 2008; 14.

25 Ferrara G, Zalaudek I, Cabo H, Soyer HP, Argenziano G. Collision of basal cell carcinoma with seborrhoeic keratosis: a dermoscopic aid to histopathology? Clin Exp Dermatol. 2005; 30; 586–587.

26 Zaballos P, Llambrich A, Puig S, Malvehy J. Dermoscopy is useful for the recognition of benign-malignant compound tumours. Br J Dermatol. 2005; 153; 653–656.

27 de Giorgi V, Massi D, Sestini S, Alfaioli B, Carelli G, Carli P. Cutaneous collision tumour (melanocytic naevus, basal cell carcinoma, seborrhoeic keratosis): a clinical, dermoscopic and pathological case report. Br J Dermatol. 2005; 152; 787–790.

28 Birnie AJ, Varma S. A dermatoscopically diagnosed collision tumour: malignant melanoma arising within a seborrhoeic keratosis. Clin Exp Dermatol. 2008; 33; 512–513.

29 Zalaudek I, Giacomel J, Cabo H, Di Stefani A, Ferrara G, Hofmann-Wellenhof R, et al. Entodermoscopy: a new tool for diagnosing skin infections and infestations. Dermatology. 2008; 216; 14–23.

30 Vazquez-Lopez F, Manjon-Haces JA, Maldonado-Seral C, Raya-Aguado C, Perez-Oliva N, Marghoob AA. Dermoscopic features of plaque psoriasis and lichen planus: new observations. Dermatology. 2003; 207; 151–156.

31 Pan Y, Chamberlain AJ, Bailey M, Chong AH, Haskett M, Kelly JW. Dermatoscopy aids in the diagnosis of the solitary red scaly patch or plaque-features distinguishing superficial basal cell carcinoma, intraepidermal carcinoma, and psoriasis. J Am Acad Dermatol. 2008; 59; 268–274.

32 Delfino M, Argenziano G, Nino M. Dermoscopy for the diagnosis of porokeratosis. J Eur Acad Dermatol Venereol. 2004; 18; 194–195.

33 Zalaudek I, Argenziano G. Dermoscopy subpatterns of inflammatory skin disorders. Arch Dermatol. 2006; 142; 808.

34 Morales A, Puig S, Malvehy J, Zaballos P. Dermoscopy of molluscum contagiosum. Arch Dermatol. 2005; 141; 1644.

35 Zaballos P, Ara M, Puig S, Malvehy J. Dermoscopy of molluscum contagiosum: a useful tool for clinical diagnosis in adulthood. J Eur Acad Dermatol Venereol. 2006; 20; 482–483.

36 Bae JM, Kang H, Kim HO, Park YM. Differential diagnosis of plantar wart from corn, callus and healed wart with the aid of dermoscopy. Br J Dermatol. 2009; 160; 220–222.

37 Smith SB, Beals SL, Elston DM, Meffert JJ. Dermoscopy in the diagnosis of tinea nigra plantaris. Cutis. 2001; 68; 377–380.

38 Argenziano G, Fabbrocini G, Delfino M. Epiluminescence microscopy. A new approach to in vivo detection of Sarcoptes scabiei. Arch Dermatol. 1997; 133; 751–753.

39 Di Stefani A, Hofmann-Wellenhof R, Zalaudek I. Dermoscopy for diagnosis and treatment monitoring of pediculosis capitis. J Am Acad Dermatol. 2006; 54; 909–911.

40 Bauer J, Forschner A, Garbe C, Rocken M. Dermoscopy of tungiasis. Arch Dermatol. 2004; 140; 761–763.

9 Digital Dermatoscopic Monitoring

Adding dermatoscopy to clinical examination allows earlier diagnosis of melanoma. However, in the earliest stages many melanomas lack the dermatoscopic criteria to allow diagnosis (1). Indeed, it seems likely that all melanomas go through a stage without any morphologic features to suggest the true diagnosis (2). *Figure 9.1* illustrates the appropriate technique of examination for each morphological stage and point in time of the developing melanoma. Melanomas which can be identified by the naked eye are usually larger than one centimeter in size and have usually been present for several years. As critics of dermatoscopy remark, in these advanced cases one does not require dermatoscopy at all. For smaller and earlier lesions however, naked eye examination does not perform so well, but the majority of these smaller melanomas are still easily diagnosed with the dermatoscope.

Moving further backward in the development of melanoma, i.e. shortly after it has emerged, we see many lesions which cannot be diagnosed by the naked eye or with the dermatoscope. There is one clue that is present in every malignancy, even when all others are lacking: change over time.

Digital dermatoscopic monitoring is comparison of serial dermatoscopic images to detect change over time, enabling the diagnosis of inconspicuous melanomas. Monitoring can also be used to reduce the number of biopsies of pigmented lesions with equivocal clues to malignancy. The disadvantage of this clue is that, unlike clues based on morphology, at least two sequential observations are needed. In other words, monitoring only works if a given lesion is imaged at an initial consultation, and the patient returns for subsequent examinations. In practical terms, it also requires sequential images of sufficient quality to detect change.

Monitoring is most useful for high risk individuals with a very large number of nevi. Over their lifetimes many of these patients are subjected to large numbers of biopsies. Sometimes this is unavoidable, but far too often it is an indiscriminate process, of no benefit to the patient. The monitoring strategies outlined below greatly reduce the number of biopsies needed, without increasing the risk of missing a melanoma.

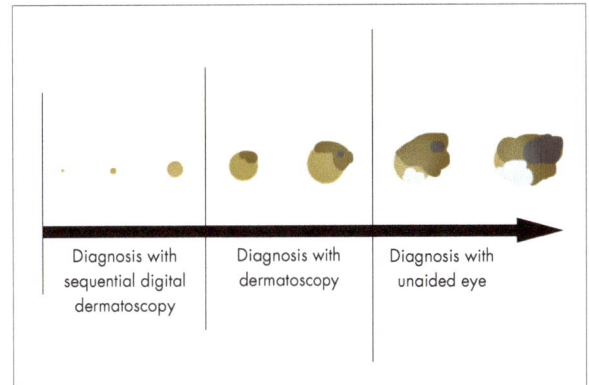

Figure 9.1: *Development of a melanoma over time. Initially melanomas are small and inconspicuous and lack any characteristic clues. It takes some time for melanomas to develop their typical clinical characteristics, such as asymmetry, variegate colors, and irregular borders. Different diagnostic methods are required at different stages in this development.*

An increasing number of so-called digital dermatoscopes are being offered on the market. The basic principle of digital dermatoscopes is simple: instead of the operator looking through the instrument to see the image, a hand-held dermatoscope is attached to a digital video camera. The camera is connected to a monitor that displays the dermatoscopic image in real time, and also to a computer to allow capture and storage of images from the camera *(9.2)*.

Dedicated software permits efficient administration of the saved images, which makes comparing images obtained at different points in time much easier. The image quality of these digital dermatoscopes has lagged behind that of images captured by attaching a camera to a conventional hand-held dermatoscope, but the development of high resolution digital imaging systems is seeing this gap narrowing.

A frequently underestimated advantage of digital dermatoscopy is patient participation in the examination. When using a conventional dermatoscope the patient cannot see the lesion being examined. During digital dermatoscopy the patient and the doctor can view the image on the monitor simultaneously. In the authors' experience, most patients appreciate this participation in the diagnostic process.

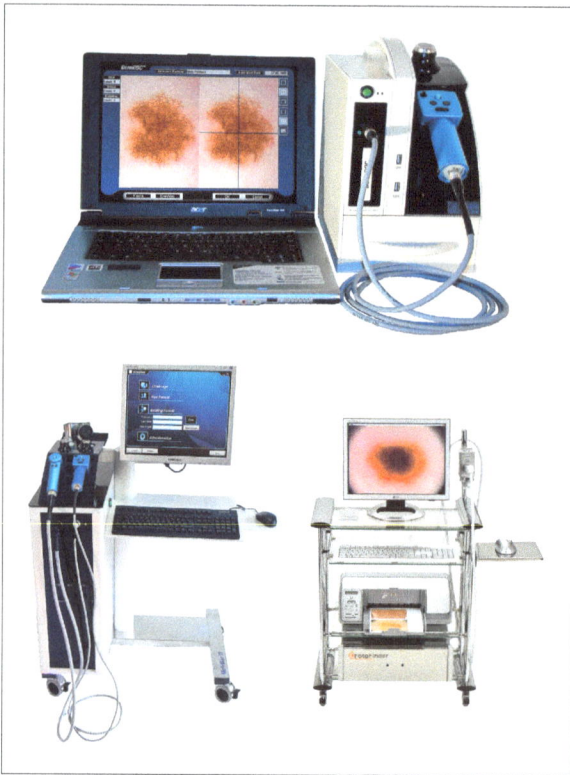

Figure 9.2: Digital Dermatoscopy Systems.
The main use of digital dermatoscopes is monitoring of pigment-ed lesions. These are three such systems. On the top and on the bottom left are two MoleMax systems (Derma Medical Systems, Vienna, Austria) on the bottom right is a Fotofinder (Fotofinder Systems GmbH, Bad Birnbach, Germany).

While monitoring is conceptually very simple, there are issues around which lesions should be monitored. As nevi also change over time, there are also issues regarding what changes indicate a diagnosis of melanoma.

9.1 Choice of lesions to monitor

While it is attractive to think that monitoring can detect nevi transforming into melanomas, a moment's reflection will show this is a very rare occurrence. Rather, monitoring is detecting actual melanomas, but earlier than is possible by observation of morphology alone. Most issues regarding monitoring are clarified if this fact is kept in mind; what one is monitoring is potentially already a melanoma.

A "back of the envelope" calculation shows malignant transformation in a nevus is a very rare event. If one assumes that populations with lighter skin phototypes have an average of 20 nevi per person and the incidence of melanoma in this group is 20 per 100,000 persons per year, then, one may anticipate 200 mel-

anomas per year in a population of 1 million. Given approximately 20% of melanomas arise in a pre-existing nevus, of these 200 melanomas, 40 would have arisen in a pre-existing nevus. As these 40 melanomas have arisen in a population with 20 million nevi, the annual risk of a single nevus undergoing malignant transformation is therefore 1:500,000. In other words, one would have to observe 500,000 nevi for a year in order to detect a single melanoma emerging in a pre-existing nevus, or one would have to prophylactically excise 500,000 nevi in order to prevent one melanoma per year. Even if the actual rate of transformation was 10 times this estimate, the basic argument remains valid as the observation or excision of even "only" 50,000 lesions to detect or prevent one melanoma annually is still absurd. The strategy of monitoring of nevi for malignant transformation is therefore only feasible if the clinician is able to identify lesions which are hundreds or even thousands of times more likely than the average nevus to undergo malignant transformation.

Unfortunately, the morphology of a nevus says nothing about its risk of malignant transformation *(9.3, 9.4)*. "Atypical" or "dysplastic" nevi are at no greater risk of turning into a melanoma. However, there is a risk that a lesion thought to be an "atypical" or "dysplastic" nevus may actually be a melanoma, but not recognized as such. That is, these terms are used when there is diagnostic uncertainty regarding the distinction between these lesions and melanoma. "Increasing" degrees of "dysplasia" or "atypia" actually represent increasing likelihood that the lesion being examined is not a nevus but actually a melanoma. Once this has been under-stood, the concept of the "dysplastic" or "atypical" nevus loses meaning.

Digital monitoring is of most utility for small and flat melanocytic lesions that demonstrate no obvious clues to melanoma, in a patient with multiple pigmented lesions. Lesions selected must be flat, to avoid the pos-sibility of monitoring a thick melanoma. There are several possible approaches. Firstly, lesions can be selected on the basis of criteria which are considered to suggest that the lesion has some likelihood of being an early melanoma. Monitoring is generally restrict-ed to one or a few lesions, with a shorter monitoring interval, usually 3 months. This method has been best put forward by Menzies (3). Lesions to be monitored are flat and nearly symmetrical, and have either a) no clues to malignancy but have changed according to the patient or b) a certain "architectural disorder" which falls short of clear-cut clues to malignancy. This method of monitoring is thus an alternative to excision when some residual uncertainty remains after an initial

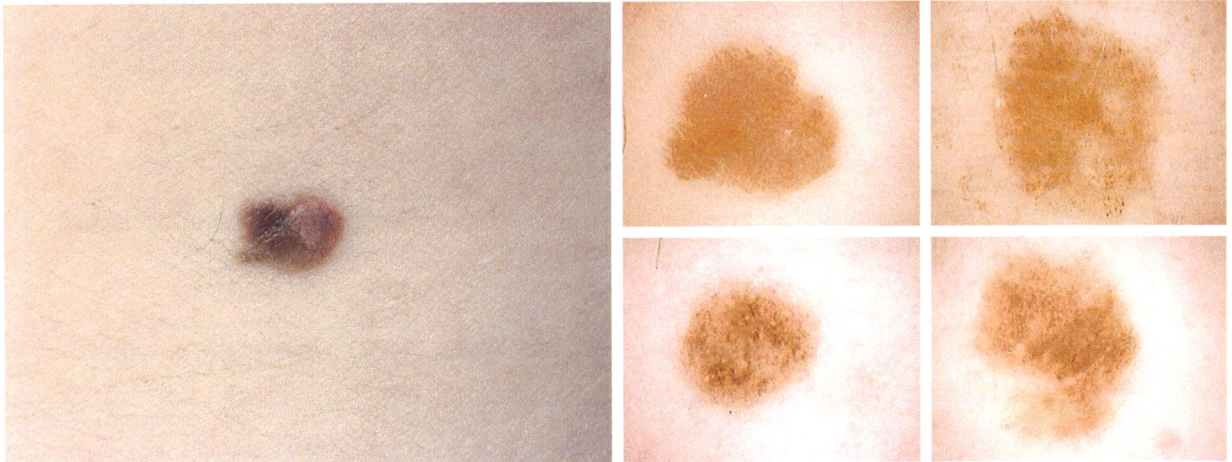

Figure 9.3: *The morphology of a nevus is not predictive of the risk that a melanoma will develop in this nevus.*
The clinical image on the **left** *shows a melanoma that developed in a pre-existing nevus. On the* **right** *one can see digital dermatoscopic images of four nevi of the same patient. Can you predict by morphology which nevus is the precursor lesion of the melanoma on the left? Answer see Figure 9.4.*

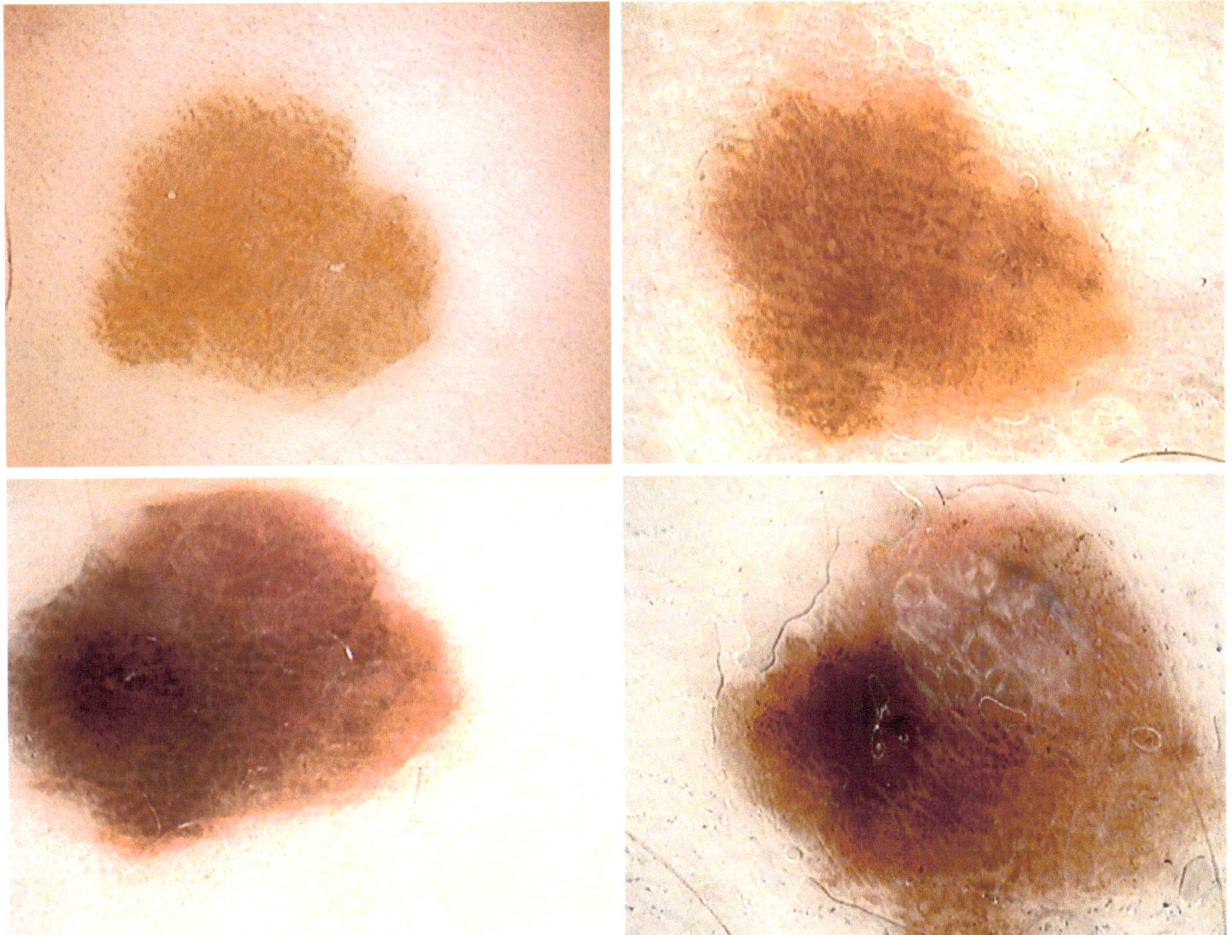

Figure 9.4: *The morphology of a nevus is not predictive of the risk that a melanoma will develop in this nevus.*
Sequence of images which demonstrates the development of the melanoma in one of the four nevi shown in Figure 9.3. By morphology it cannot be predicted which nevus will be the precursor lesion. The concept of the "dysplastic" or "atypical" nevus is flawed fundamentally because the morphology of a nevus is not predictive of its biological fate.

examination of lesions without clear clues to melanoma. A second type of monitoring may be used for high risk patients with multiple nevi *(9.5).* Lesions to be monitored are selected randomly, with as many lesions as possible documented at the initial examination and re-imaged at each consultation (4). There are no criteria for the selection of lesions because one wishes to identify melanomas that demonstrate no clues – at least on initial inspection. One therefore relies on chance and increases the likelihood of identifying a melanoma by documenting as many lesions as possible and confining the investigation to high-risk patients. The intervals between examinations are longer – typically six to twelve months. This type of monitoring is an alternative to indiscriminate excision of nevi in patients with multiple nevi.

A meta-analysis by Salerni et al. (5) shows the different outcomes of these two monitoring strategies *(Table 9.1).*

Short term monitoring is more efficient – one needs to monitor fewer lesions to detect one melanoma. Short term monitoring, however, will only increase the specificity by reducing the number of excisions. It sorts out false positives but does not find additional false negatives. To find additional false negatives one must include inconspicuous lesions (long term monitoring). Because inconspicuous lesions are monitored one needs to monitor a lot of lesions to detect one melanoma, more than 1000 in some settings. Long term monitoring, however, will increase specificity and sensitivity because it will detect melanomas that do not have any clues and cannot be diagnosed otherwise.

A third possible approach is to identify new or changed pigmented lesions by comparison of serial clinical total body photographs, and then subjecting these lesions to digital monitoring. Another study by Salerni et al showed this to be an effective strategy, detecting more

Table 9.1

Authors	Patients (n)	Lesions (n)	Follow-up interval (months)	Melanomas detected during follow-up (n)	In-situ melanomas (%)	Lesions excised (n)	Relative frequency of lesions excised (%)	Malignant/ benign ratio	Frequency of melanomas among excised lesions (%)
Kittler 2000, Austria (4)	202	1,862	3, 6, 12	8	62.5%	75	4	1: 8.4	10.7
Menzies 2001, Australia (3)	245	318	3	7	71.4%	53	16.6	1:6.5	13.2
Malvehy 2002, Spain (14)	290	3,170	3, 6	8	25%	42	1.3	1: 4.2	19
Schiffner 2003, Germany (15)	145	272	3, 6, 12	0	–	7	2.6	–	–
Robinson 2004, USA (16)	100	3,482	12	4	100%	193	5.5	1:47.3	2.1
Haenssle 2004, Germany (17)	212	2,939	3, 6, 12	17	52.9%	112	3.8	1:5.5	15.2
Bauer 2005, Germany (18)	196	2,015	3, 6, 12	2	100%	33	1.6	1:15.5	6.1
Haenssle 2006, Germany (19)	530	7,001	3, 6, 12	53	52.8%	637	9.1	1:12	8.3
Fuller 2007, USA (20)	297	5,945	6, 12	6	33.3%	324	5.4	1:53	1.9
Altamura 2008, Australia (21)	1,859	2,602	1.5, 3	81	67.9%	487	18.7	1:5	16.6
Argenziano 2008, Italy (10)	405	600	3, 6, 12	12	50%	54	9	1: 3.4	22.2
Haenssle 2010, Germany (22)	688	11,137	3, 6, 12	87	43.6%	1,219	10.9	1:8.5	10.4
Salerni 2011, Spain (6)	618	11,396	3, 6, 12	98	54%	1,152	10.1	1:10.7	8.5

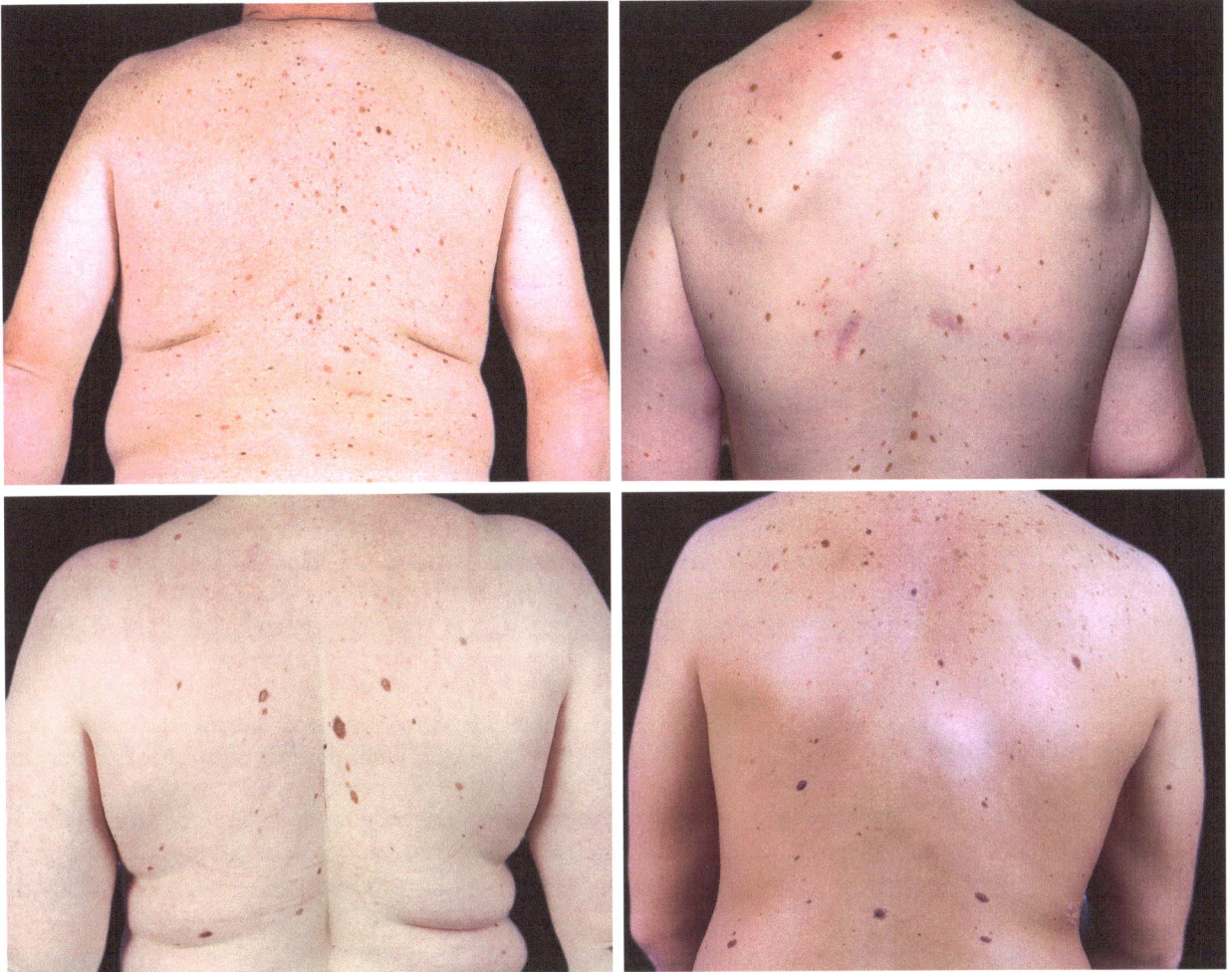

Figure 9.5: Patients with multiple nevi.
*Monitoring by digital dermatoscopy is especially suitable for patients with multiple nevi. It is an appropriate but time-consuming alternative to indiscriminate excision of nevi. The patients in the **lower row** have several large nevi; the majority of these are probably congenital. Digital monitoring of lesions of this size is unnecessary – if a lesion this large is a melanoma, it almost invariably has clear-cut clues to the diagnosis. Large, symmetrical and single-colored lesions can safely be diagnosed as nevi. If doubt remains after dermatoscopy, histopathology should be obtained at the initial examination. Monitoring should be reserved for small, flat lesions. The yield will still be small. Even in a high-risk population, one has to monitor 500 lesions in order to discover one melanoma. In an unselected population the yield will be much smaller. Therefore the benefit of this type of monitoring outside specialized pigmented lesion clinics is questionable.*

melanomas than by short-term monitoring, but requiring far fewer lesions to be monitored than random long-term monitoring. In practice, a combination of strategies seems to be most useful (6, 7).

Regardless of how one uses monitoring, knowing which lesions are unsafe to monitor is essential. By definition, monitoring is performed on potential melanomas. Monitoring must therefore be confined to lesions which, should melanoma be confirmed, will still have an excellent prognosis after the monitoring period. In practice this means flat and small melanocytic lesions, preferably with a reticular pattern on dermatoscopy. Even if such

a lesion is a melanoma, it will nearly always be slow growing at this stage of its growth. More than 50 % of melanomas discovered only by the use of monitoring are in situ melanomas, and nearly all the invasive melanomas are thinner than 1 mm, meaning that the risk of metastasis is either nil (in cases of in situ melanomas) or very low (in cases of thin invasive melanomas).

Nodular lesions that cannot be diagnosed as benign with absolute certainty must be excised at the initial consultation. If one monitors a nodule, one may be monitoring a rapidly growing nodular melanoma that could conceivably have already reached a Breslow thickness of several millimeters by the review. To a

Table 9.2

	Nevus	Melanoma
Change in size	No or symmetrical increase in size	Sometimes an asymmetrical increase in size
Change in color	No or lighter/darker brown or more/less erythema	Sometimes a new color
Changes in structure	No or non-essential changes in structure (the pre-existing structure becomes more prominent/less prominent) or pre-existing basic elements (e.g. clods or dots) are more/less numerous	Occasionally a new structure (includes clues to melanoma)

lesser extent this is true for larger (over 1 cm diameter) flat lesions as well.

When examining patients with multiple nevi, the question obviously arises as to how many lesions one should document. An unequivocal answer cannot be provided for this question. In clinical practice, the availability of time and personnel resources limits the number of dermatoscopic images one can obtain and record. For practical reasons it would be advisable to dispense with the documentation of melanocytic lesions that are smaller than 3 mm in diameter; otherwise one will have to record far too many images for each patient.

9.2 Interpretation of changes

The interpretation of changes seen in monitored lesions depends on the type of monitoring being performed, and the monitoring interval chosen. What is an appropriate interval between examinations? If the observation period is too short, even changes in melanomas will be difficult to notice.

For adults, reasonable monitoring intervals range between 3 and 12 months. Three months is a generally accepted period, over which most melanomas are expected to change (although this is too short an observation period for many lentiginous melanomas). Over longer observation periods, a significant number of benign nevi will change, and so criteria must be established for "acceptable" and "unacceptable" change. As many nevi change even in the short term in children, and melanomas are very rare, monitoring of pigmented lesions in pre-pubertal children is best avoided.

Short term monitoring (three months or less) is usually performed for lesions that, because of history or appearance, cannot be deemed benign with absolute certainty at the initial examination. For short-term monitoring, even small changes are regarded as significant, and all lesions showing changes (even to a "more benign" appearance) over 3 months or less should be submitted for histopathology.

Longer monitoring intervals – six months to one year – are mainly used for lesions with no features to suggest malignancy, typically in patients with multiple nevi.

When longer intervals are used, a distinction must be made between significant and insignificant changes. The latter are much more common. For instance, the transient stimulation of melanin production provoked by UV exposure may cause nevi to initially darken and then become lighter after a few weeks.

Distinctions are made on the basis of changes in size, color, and structure (9.6). Changes in size may be symmetrical (the shape of the lesion remains the same) or asymmetrical (the shape changes). The color of a lesion may change in that a pre-existing color (usually brown) may appear lighter or darker, or that a new color is seen. With regard to structure, an existing pattern (for instance reticular lines) may disappear, a new pattern may appear, or basic elements of a pattern such as dots or clods may be present in greater numbers or reduced numbers. A change in the number of brown clods is relatively common and is not relevant. However, any change in size, any new color, and any new structure should be regarded as a significant change.

Initially one tends to over-interpret changes, and in particular fail to realize that "changes" in lesions are often produced by variations in the imaging process, rather than changes in the lesion itself. Different exposure or color balance is common if the digital dermatoscope is not calibrated. Stretching of the skin during imaging distorts lesions, and rotation of the dermatoscope produces different lesion orientation. Of course, if the wrong lesion is imaged at the follow-up examination, "change" is inevitably produced. When patients have multiple nevi, this is not at all uncommon.

9.3 Growing nevus or melanoma?

An important criticism of digital monitoring is the fact that nevi also change. This is basically true, but nevi stop growing at some time whereas melanomas do not. Melanomas and nevi also grow in different ways — nevi tend to grow symmetrically, whereas melanomas grow asymmetrically, i.e. their shape changes (9.6, 9.8, Table 9.2). The rate of change for nevi varies, mainly depending on the type of nevus and the patient's age. Spitz or Reed nevi, for instance, grow faster than

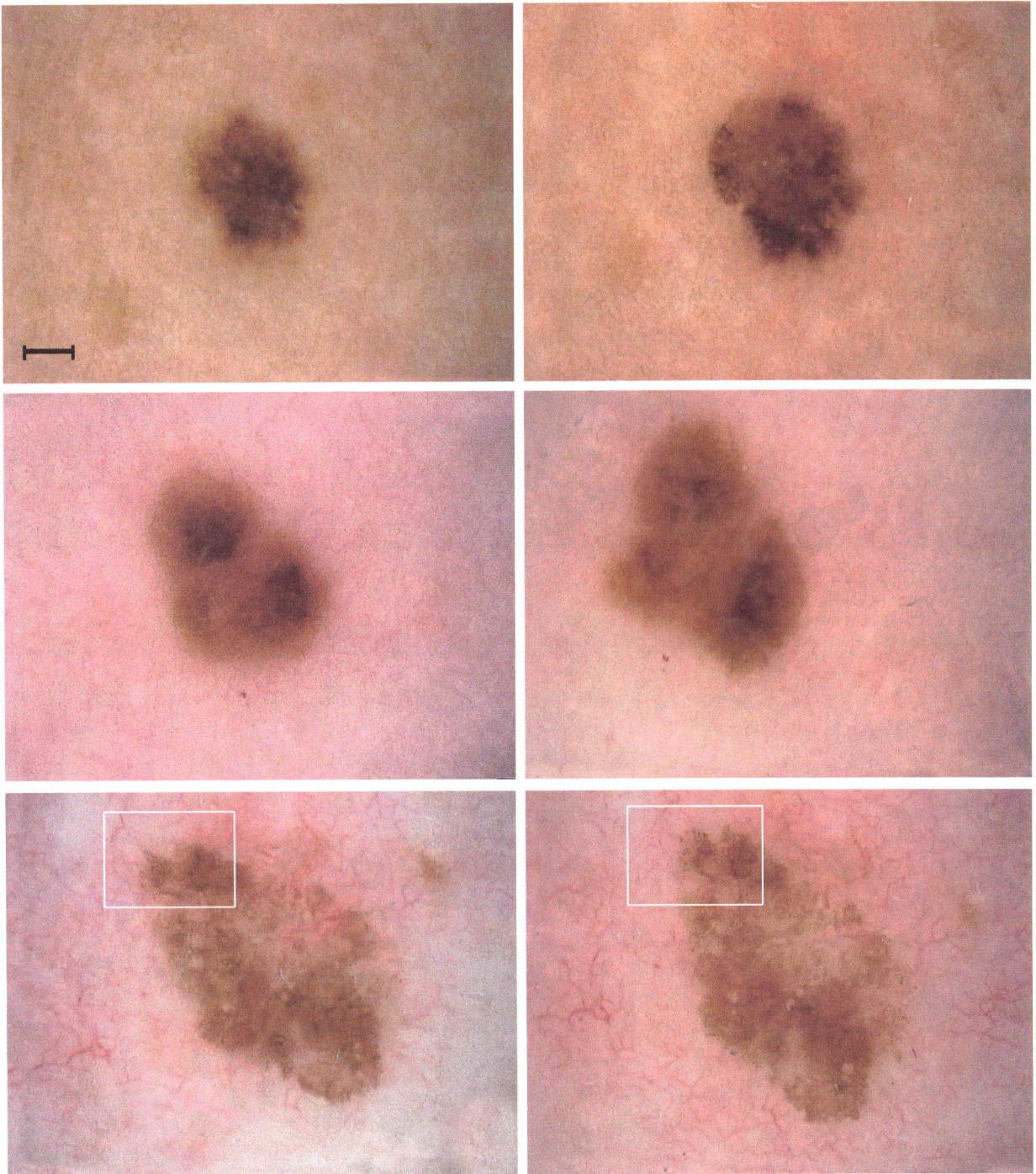

Figure 9.6: Digital dermatoscopic monitoring.
*The initial image is shown on the **left** and the corresponding follow-up image on the **right.** In all three cases the lesions were melanomas a few millimeters in size (the scale on the upper left image corresponds to 1 mm). **Top:** Monitoring interval 11 months, asymmetrical increase in size; in situ melanoma. **Middle:** Monitoring interval 10 months, melanoma (Breslow thickness < 1 mm). **Bottom:** Monitoring interval < 6 months, no change in size but new structures at the periphery (white rectangle); in situ melanoma.*

Clark nevi, and nevi in children generally grow faster than in adults.

There are 3 basic patterns of growth in nevi *(9.7)*. The most common growth pattern is the lentiginous pattern *(9.7, top)*. It occurs most often in flat, reticular lesions, which are usually Clark nevi. This growth pattern indicates slow growth. It is termed lentiginous growth pattern because histopathologically one sees mainly single melanoyctes at the dermo-epidermal junction. The second pattern is the nested growth pattern *(9.7, middle)*. It occurs in "superficial" or "superficial and deep" congenital nevi, Spitz nevi, and Clark nevi and is typified by a rim of clods or dots at the periphery of the nevus *(9.8)*. It is termed nested growth pattern because the clods correspond to nests of melanocytes in the epidermis. The third and fastest growth pattern is the fascicular growth pattern *(9.7 bottom)*, which is typified by radial lines or pseudopods dermatoscopically. It is typical for Reed nevi and for the initial phase of Spitz nevi. It is termed fascicular growth pattern because the radial lines and pseudopods correspond to fascicles of melanocytes at the dermo-epidermal junction.

Changes in color almost never occur in nevi *(9.9)*. The only exceptions – as mentioned earlier – are changes in the shade of brown induced by UV radiation. Melanomas, however, may develop a new color, especially during longer observation periods. Significant structural changes, i.e. the appearance of new patterns and particularly the clues to melanoma are, of course, mainly observed in melanomas *(9.6, 9.10)*. While 95 % of nevi do not change over one year, over longer intervals changes in nevi are commonly seen. For this reason,

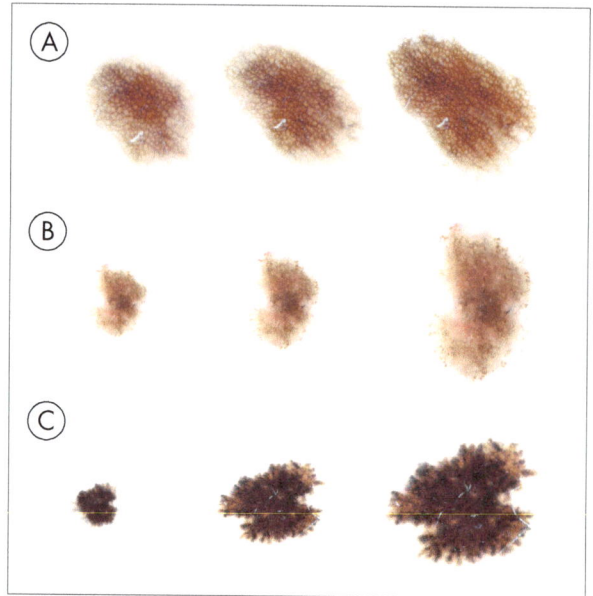

Figure 9.7: *Growth patterns of nevi.*
Top: *Lentiginous growth pattern.* **Middle:** *Nested growth pattern.* **Bottom:** *Fascicular growth pattern.*

monitoring over intervals longer than one year is not recommended.

The changes observed in melanomas also depend on the length of the monitoring period. Over intervals shorter than 3 months, even melanomas may not change appreciably. Melanoma in situ on the face, for example, may grow very slowly. In one study, while 93 % of all melanomas were detected by change over 3 months, only 75 % of facial lentigo maligna changed over this

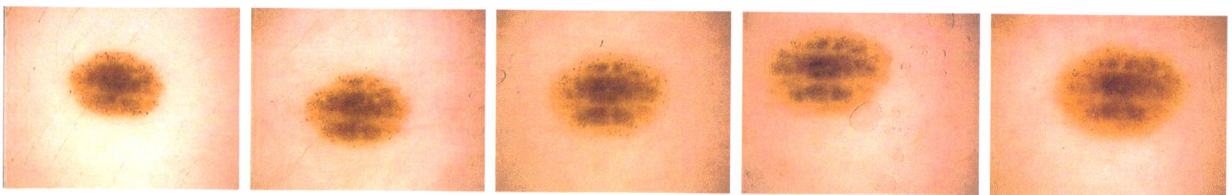

Figure 9.8: *Growing nevus.*
Growing nevus in a child, with a peripheral ring of brown clods or dots (nested growth pattern) – a typical characteristic of this phase of growth. Monitoring period: two years.

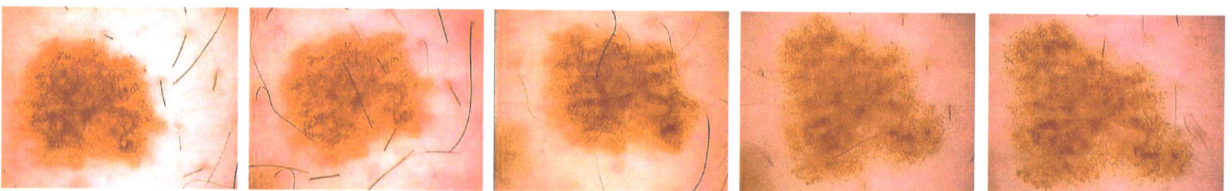

Figure 9.9: *Growing nevus.*
Growing nevus (adult patient) with a reticular pattern (lentiginous growth pattern). Note that there is a change in shape but not in structure or color. Monitoring period: three years.

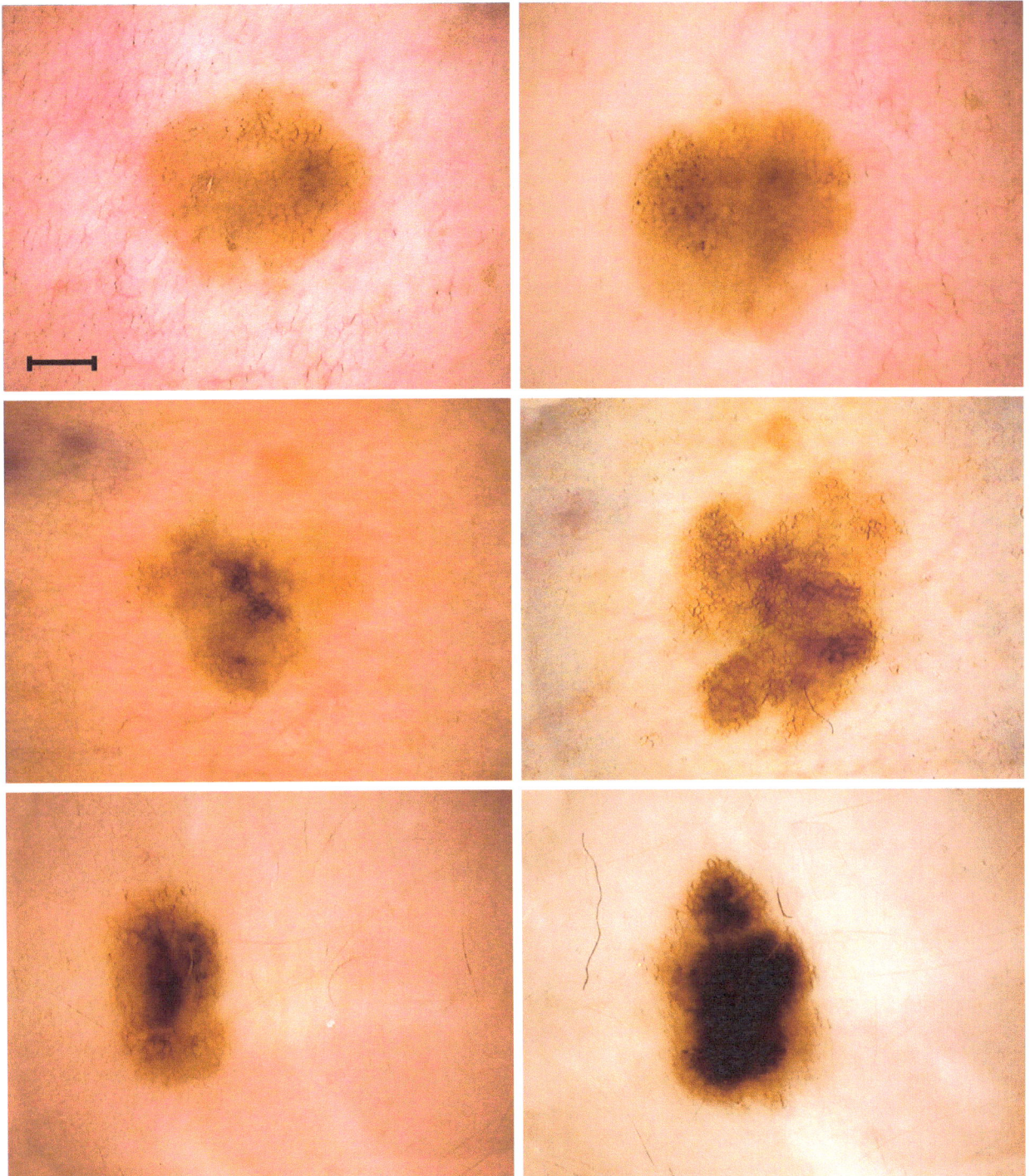

Figure 9.10: Monitoring by digital dermatoscopy.
*The initial appearance is shown on the **left** side and the corresponding follow-up image on the **right.** The monitoring interval in all three cases was between 4 and 8 months. The scale in the upper left image corresponds to 1 mm. **Top:** Asymmetrical increase in size (change of shape), structural change. Diagnosis: In situ melanoma. **Middle:** Asymmetrical increase in size (change in shape). Diagnosis: In situ melanoma. **Bottom:** Asymmetrical increase in size (change in shape). Diagnosis: In situ melanoma.*

time period. For these slowly growing melanomas, a monitoring period longer than 3 months is required` (8–10).

In adults the proportion of nevi that show significant changes in the course of a year is less than 5%. This remains true for patients with multiple nevi and patients with the so-called "dysplastic nevus syndrome". The number increases with longer observation periods and reduces with advancing age. As mentioned earlier, one finds a large number of growing nevi in children and adolescents.

Critics of digital monitoring assert that the procedure may document features which could have diagnosed a melanoma at the initial examination. The contention has been examined and refuted. In a study in which experienced dermatologists were shown the initial pictures of melanomas diagnosed by monitoring, but were not shown the follow-up sequences, the best dermatologists achieved a sensitivity of just 27% (11). Lacking the additional information about the change, it was impossible to identify these melanomas. Without explicitly saying so, these critics are arguing that melanomas should be allowed to grow until they demonstrate conventional clinical or dermatoscopic clues.

Although the majority of melanomas occur de novo, a melanoma may develop in a pre-existing nevus. A melanoma may develop in any nevus, but most often they arise in "superficial and deep" congenital nevi or in Clark nevi. However, this is very rarely the case from a prospective point of view, making it unlikely that one will document a melanoma developing in a pre-existing nevus – unless one observes tens of thousands of nevi per year. Figure 9.11 shows a melanoma that developed in a pre-existing Clark nevus.

9.4 Benefits and Risks

The availability of monitoring can change the clinician's threshold for biopsy of suspicious pigmented lesions, and this change in threshold is not without risk. At the initial examination one is more willing not to excise a borderline lesion when monitoring is available (11, 12). As a result the sensitivity of the initial examination, i.e. the number of excised melanomas, falls, whereas the specificity of the examination rises because the number of excised nevi also falls. At the follow-up examination, those melanomas that were not biopsied at the initial examination are identified by visible changes and excised. Thus, assessed across the two visits, the sensitivity of the investigation increases again, and the additional information about change increases the sensitivity to a greater extent than it would in the

case of two separate sequential examinations with no comparison of images. In other words, the increase in sensitivity at the follow-up examination outweighs the losses at the initial examination. The specificity of the follow-up examination is not significantly influenced by the use of monitoring, so the overall benefit remains.

It is this dependence on the subsequent examination that is the greatest weakness of sequential dermatoscopy. When the patient does not report for the follow-up examination, the loss in sensitivity at the initial examination is not counterbalanced by increased melanoma detection at the (missed) second visit. As a result the excision of some melanomas is delayed. In other words, the benefits of monitoring depend on the patient's compliance. Therefore, the use of sequential dermatoscopic monitoring should only be offered as an alternative to biopsy, after patients are appropriately informed about the procedure, and preferably provide written consent.

To summarize, the successful application of digital monitoring requires correct selection of lesions, an informed and motivated patient, and a fail-safe patient recall system. Provided these principles are strictly adhered to, monitoring is a safe and useful method of investigation that both improves the early detection of melanomas and reduces the number of excised nevi (13).

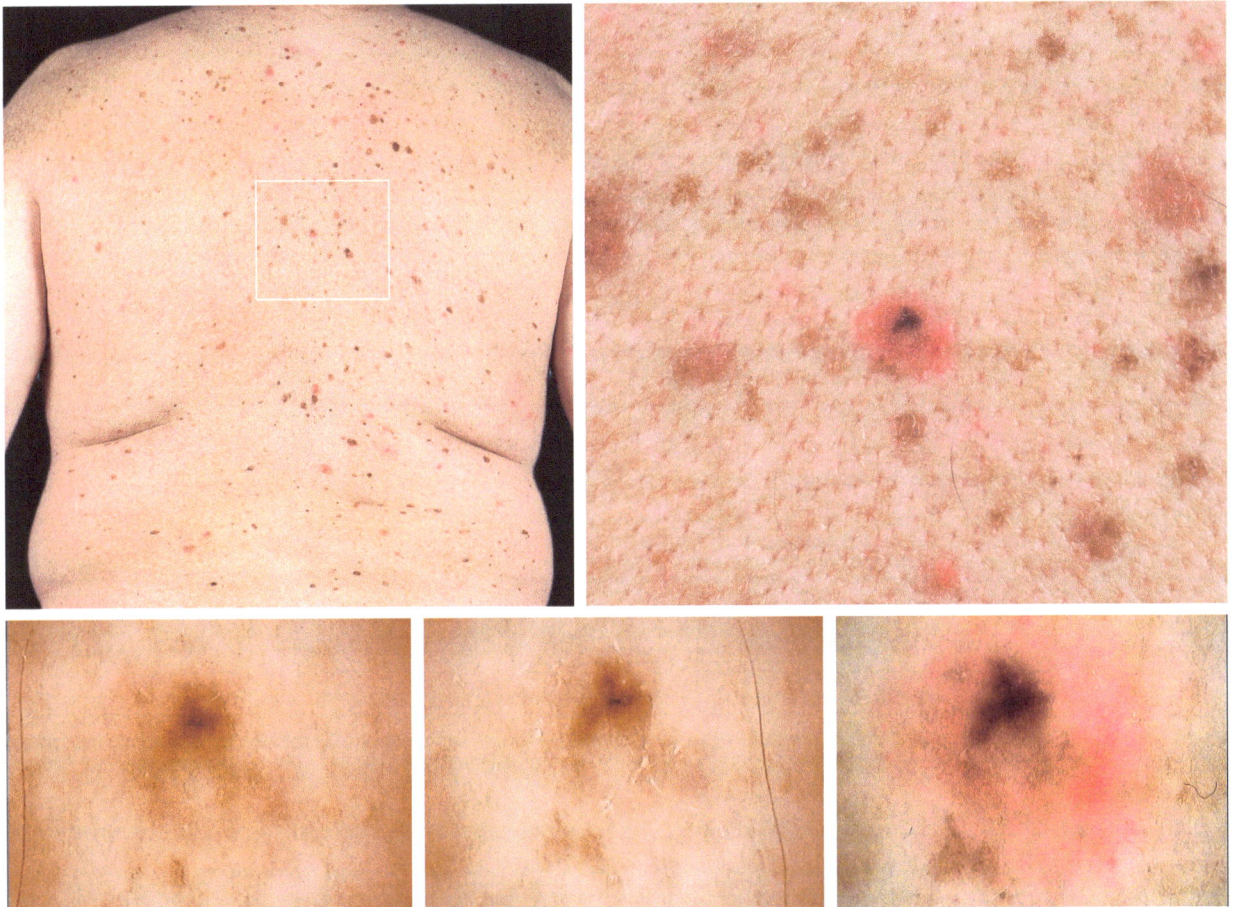

Figure 9.11: Development of a melanoma in a Clark nevus.
Top left: Clinical overview. **Top right:** Close-up of an asymmetrical reddened and unevenly pigmented plaque. **Bottom:** Digital dermatoscopic monitoring (initial picture on the **left,** first follow-up in the middle, second follow-up on the **right)** reveals no major change at the first follow-up examination. At the second monitoring examination one finds new structures (white lines and polymorphous vessels). Diagnosis: Melanoma in a pre-existing Clark nevus.

References

1 Skvara H, Teban L, Fiebiger M, Binder M, Kittler H. Limitations of dermoscopy in the recognition of melanoma. Arch Dermatol. 2005; 141(2): 155–160.
2 Kittler H, Guitera P, Riedl E, et al. Identification of clinically featureless incipient melanoma using sequential dermoscopy imaging. Arch Dermatol. 2006; 142(9): 1113–1119.
3 Menzies SW, Gutenev A, Avramidis M, Batrac A, McCarthy WH. Short-term digital surface microscopic monitoring of atypical or changing melanocytic lesions. Arch Dermatol. 2001; 137(12): 1583–1589.
4 Kittler H, Pehamberger H, Wolff K, Binder M. Follow-up of melanocytic skin lesions with digital epiluminescence microscopy: patterns of modifications observed in early melanoma, atypical nevi, and common nevi. J Am Acad Dermatol. 2000; 43(3): 467–476.
5 Salerni G, Teran T, Puig S, et al. Meta-analysis of digital dermoscopy follow-up of melanocytic skin lesions: a study on behalf of the International Dermoscopy Society. J Eur Acad Dermatol Venereol. 2013; 27(7): 805–814.
6 Salerni G, Carrera C, Lovatto L, et al. Benefits of total body photography and digital dermatoscopy ("two-step method of digital follow-up") in the early diagnosis of melanoma in patients at high risk for melanoma. J Am Acad Dermatol. 2012; 67(1): e17–27.
7 Salerni G, Carrera C, Lovatto L, et al. Characterization of 1152 lesions excised over 10 years using total-body photography and digital dermatoscopy in the surveillance of patients at high risk for melanoma. J Am Acad Dermatol. 2012; 67(5): 836–845.
8 Terushkin V, Dusza SW, Scope A, et al. Changes observed in slow-growing melanomas during long-term dermoscopic monitoring. Br J Dermatol. 2012; 166(6): 1213–1220.
9 Argenziano G, Kittler H, Ferrara G, et al. Slow-growing melanoma: a dermoscopy follow-up study. Br J Dermatol. 2010; 162(2): 267–273.
10 Argenziano G, Mordente I, Ferrara G, Sgambato A, Annese P, Zalaudek I. Dermoscopic monitoring of melanocytic skin lesions: clinical outcome and patient compliance vary according to follow-up protocols. Br J Dermatol. 2008; 159(2): 331–336.
11 Kittler H, Binder M. Follow-up of melanocytic skin lesions with digital dermoscopy: risks and benefits. Arch Dermatol. 2002; 138(10): 1379.
12 Kittler H. Use of digital dermoscopy to monitor melanocytic lesions: risks and benefits. J Drugs Dermatol. 2003; 2(3): 309–311.
13 Moloney FJ, Guitera P, Coates E, et al. Detection of primary melanoma in individuals at extreme high risk: a prospective 5-year follow-up study. JAMA Dermatol. 2014; 150(8): 819–827.
14 Malvehy J, Puig S. Follow-up of melanocytic skin lesions with digital total-body photography and digital dermoscopy: a two-step method. Clin Dermatol. 2002; 20(3): 297–304.
15 Schiffner R, Schiffner-Rohe J, Landthaler M, Stolz W. Long-term dermoscopic follow-up of melanocytic naevi: clinical outcome and patient compliance. Br J Dermatol. 2003; 149(1): 79–86.
16 Robinson JK, Nickoloff BJ. Digital epiluminescence microscopy monitoring of high-risk patients. Arch Dermatol. 2004; 140(1): 49–56.
17 Haenssle HA, Vente C, Bertsch HP, et al. Results of a surveillance programme for patients at high risk of malignant melanoma using digital and conventional dermoscopy. Eur J Cancer Prev. 2004; 13(2): 133–138.
18 Bauer J, Blum A, Strohhacker U, Garbe C. Surveillance of patients at high risk for cutaneous malignant melanoma using digital dermoscopy. Br J Dermatol. 2005; 152(1): 87–92.
19 Haenssle HA, Krueger U, Vente C, et al. Results from an observational trial: digital epiluminescence microscopy follow-up of atypical nevi increases the sensitivity and the chance of success of conventional dermoscopy in detecting melanoma. J Invest Dermatol. 2006; 126(5): 980–985.
20 Fuller SR, Bowen GM, Tanner B, Florell SR, Grossman D. Digital dermoscopic monitoring of atypical nevi in patients at risk for melanoma. Dermatol Surg. 2007; 33(10): 1198–1206; discussion 1205–1196.
21 Altamura D, Avramidis M, Menzies SW. Assessment of the optimal interval for and sensitivity of short-term sequential digital dermoscopy monitoring for the diagnosis of melanoma. Arch Dermatol. 2008; 144(4): 502–506.
22 Haenssle HA, Korpas B, Hansen-Hagge C, et al. Selection of patients for long-term surveillance with digital dermoscopy by assessment of melanoma risk factors. Arch Dermatol. 2010; 146(3): 257–264.

10 Cases

The following cases are best used to apply and test your knowledge of pattern analysis. Each right-hand page presents paired clinical and dermatoscopy images. Each left-hand page shows our description of each lesion using the method of pattern analysis, a dermatoscopic diagnosis or differential diagnosis derived from this description, and, where obtained, the histopathologic diagnosis.

In order to maximize the learning effect, we recommend you do not look at our descriptions or diagnoses until after you have attempted to describe the dermatoscopic image yourself using pattern analysis, and reached a reasoned diagnosis or differential diagnosis on the basis of this description. Alternatively, you may use the simplified algorithm "Chaos and Clues" described in chapter 5 to determine whether a lesion should be excised or not. Do not forget that the assessment of pattern and color is based on overall impression. Pattern and color indicate the direction in which one should proceed; differential diagnoses are resolved by the use of clues. The principle of pattern analysis is:

Pattern + Color + Clues = Diagnosis

Do not allow "at-a-glance" diagnoses to tempt you into making a short description or into not making a description at all. Part of the learning process is to proceed on the basis of pattern analysis even in cases of obvious diagnoses. Experience is needed to establish and perfect your own version of pattern analysis, and this includes banal lesions.

As in actual clinical practice, not all of these lesions permit an unequivocal diagnosis. In these cases you should weigh the clues and select the most likely diagnosis. Sometimes, even after careful consideration several equally likely diagnoses may remain. You should take the process of diagnosis as far as possible, but no further. If you are uncertain as to how to proceed from description to diagnosis, refer to chapter 5 and follow the algorithm. A standardized description that follows this principle, and with which you can compare your description is shown on the left-hand page opposite the images. Your description and the one given may

not always be exactly the same. In these cases you should ask yourself whether the differing descriptions have led to different diagnoses. As mentioned earlier, the algorithm is redundant so that for most lesions, most plausible descriptions lead to the same diagnosis. Most of the lesions shown here were excised, so conspicuous, equivocal and malignant lesions are over-represented. In order to restore some balance, we have also shown some lesions that were not excised because dermatoscopy could confidently confirm a benign diagnosis. It is still important to use pattern analysis for these lesions so that one gets a feeling for the full range of appearances of common and – if one may say so – banal lesions. A strong grounding in the appearance of common benign lesions is essential in becoming an expert, as variation from these benign patterns is in itself a clue to malignancy.

Like all morphological methods, pattern analysis occasionally leads to an incorrect diagnosis. We do however firmly believe that adherence to the principles of pattern analysis will lead more often to the correct diagnosis than any other method (including no method!). We have provided some examples of such incorrect diagnoses, and have attempted not to alter our descriptions of these lesions to better fit with the histological diagnosis. The algorithm is designed so the most common type of misdiagnosis is the false positive for melanoma, i.e. those cases in which dermatoscopy suggests the diagnosis of a melanoma while the histopathological investigation yields a benign condition. As overlooking a melanoma is a far more serious matter than excising a benign lesion, maximizing true positive findings for melanoma (sensitivity) must take priority over maximizing true positive findings for benign lesions (specificity).

Table 10.1					
	Pattern	Color	Clues	Dermatoscopic diagnosis	Histopathologic diagnosis
Top	More than one pattern (structureless, reticular, and clods), arranged asymmetrically (chaotic)	More than one color (light brown and dark brown)	Clue to melanoma: Thick reticular lines (between 9 and 11 o'clock)	Melanoma must be excluded	"Superficial and deep" congenital nevus
Middle	One pattern (reticular)	Eccentric hyperpigmentation	None	Clark nevus	Clark nevus
Bottom	More than one pattern (structureless, and branched lines), arranged asymmetrically (chaotic)	More than one color (brown and pink)	Clues to melanoma: Polymorphous vascular pattern, segmental radial lines	Melanoma	Melanoma

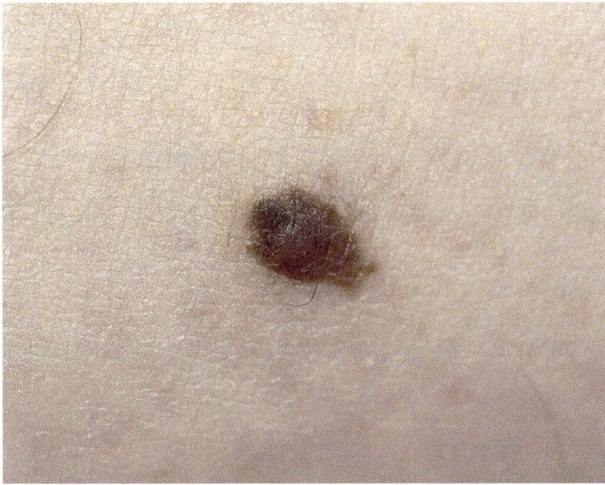
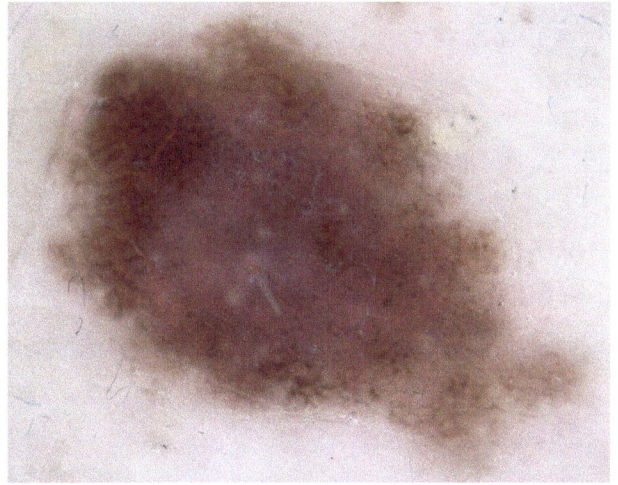
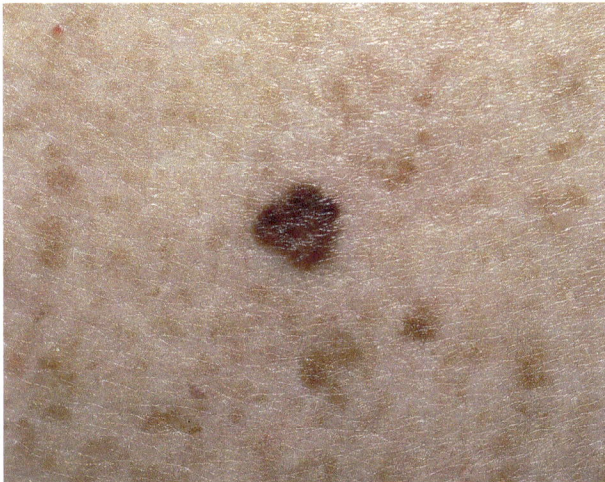
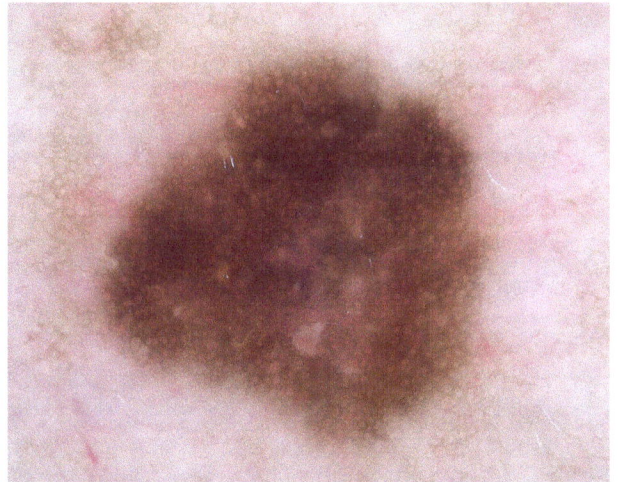
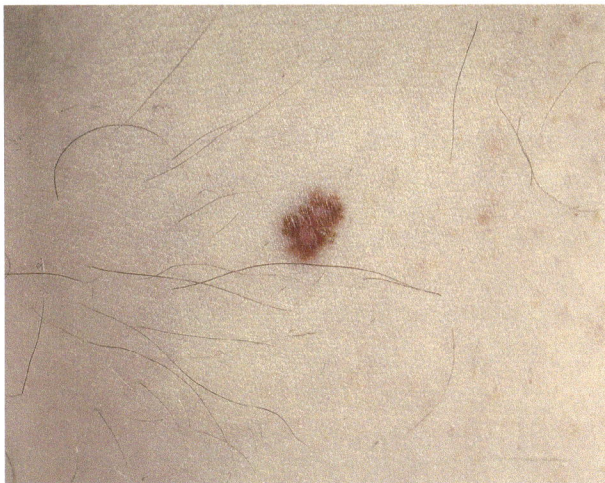
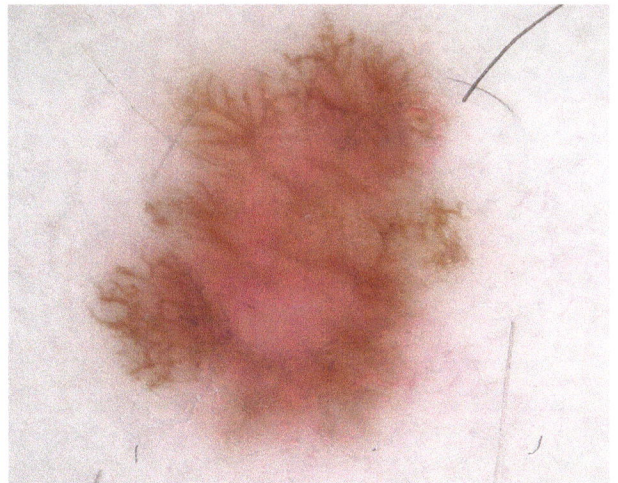

Table 10.2

	Pattern	Color	Clues	Dermatoscopic diagnosis	Histopathologic diagnosis
Top	One pattern (reticular)	Variegate	None	Clark nevus or "superficial" congenital nevus	Clark nevus
Middle	One pattern (reticular)	One color (light brown)	None	Clark nevus	Clark nevus
Bottom	One pattern (structureless)	More than one color (melanin)	Clues to melanoma: Gray lines and black dots at the periphery	Melanoma	Melanoma

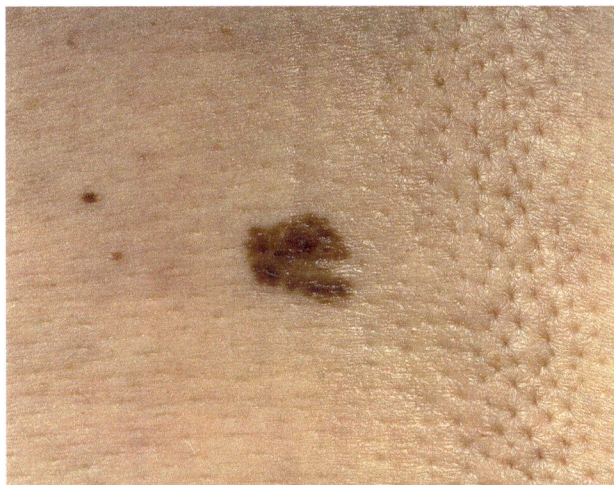
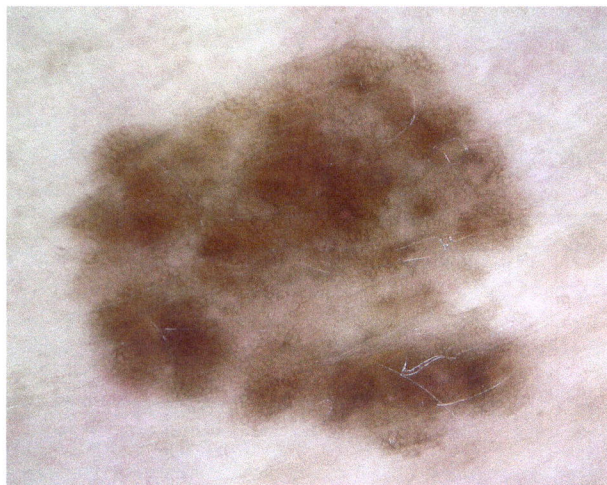
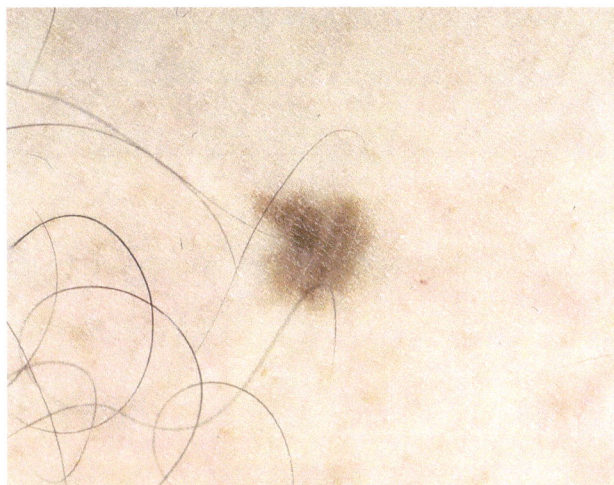
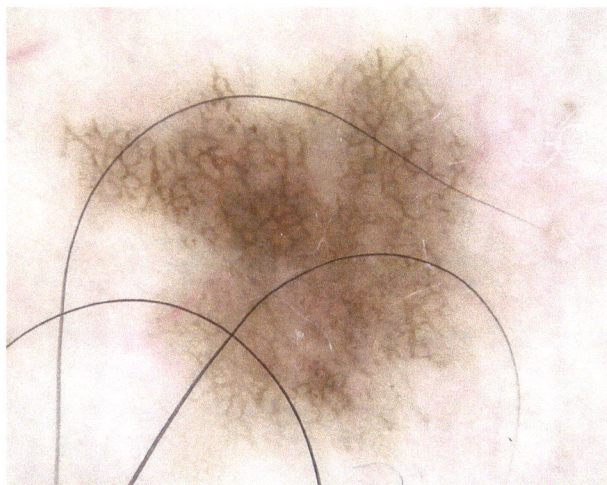
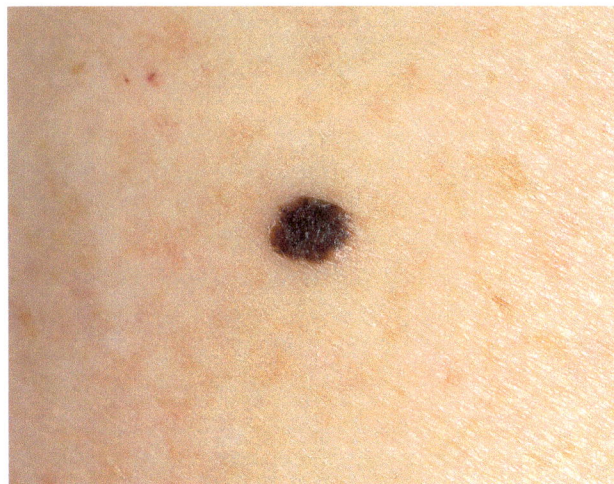
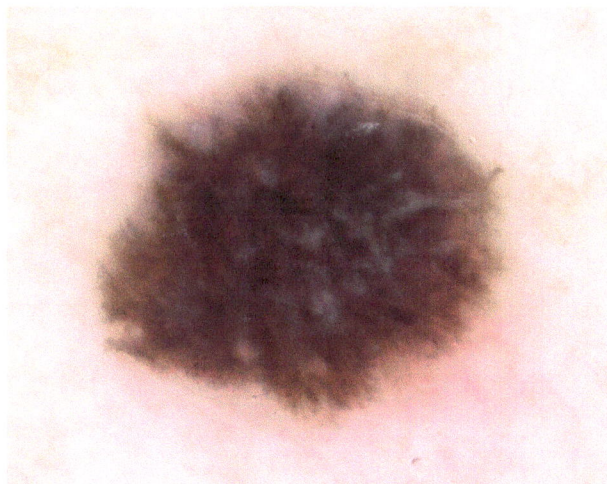

Table 10.3

	Pattern	Color	Clues	Dermatoscopic diagnosis	Histopathologic diagnosis
Top	More than one pattern (structureless in the center, clods in the periphery), no chaos	Dark-brown in the center, light brown in the periphery, no chaos	Maybe some segmental pseudopods but difficult to differentiate from clods	Most likely Spitz nevus (symmetry of pattern and color)	Spitz nevus
Middle	One pattern (clods)	Light brown and gray	Clue to melanoma: Gray clods	Unna nevus (the typical pattern of clods and the symmetry is more important than a single clue)	Unna nevus
Bottom	One pattern (clods)	Multiple colors arranged asymmetrically (chaos), melanin dominates	Clues to melanoma: Black dots and clods in the periphery, perpendicular white lines	Melanoma	Melanoma

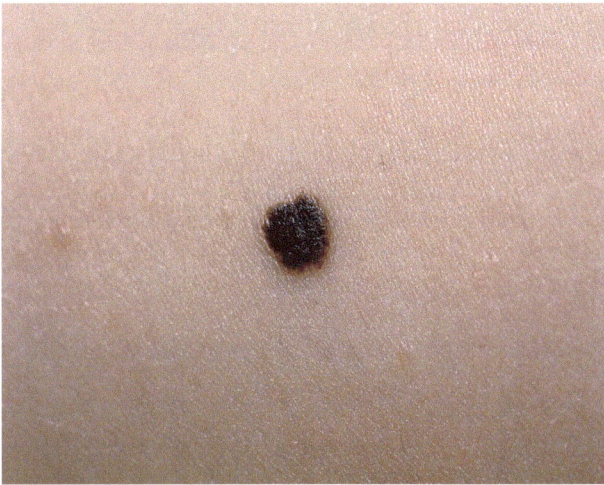
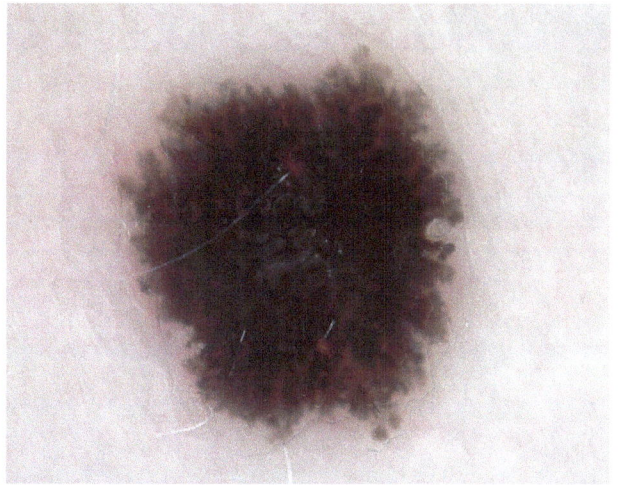
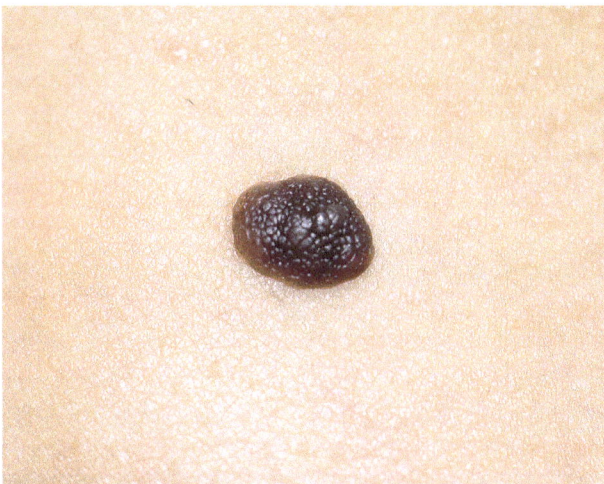
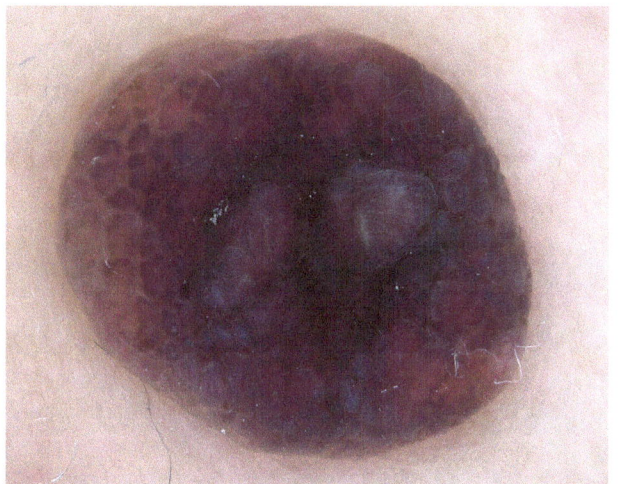
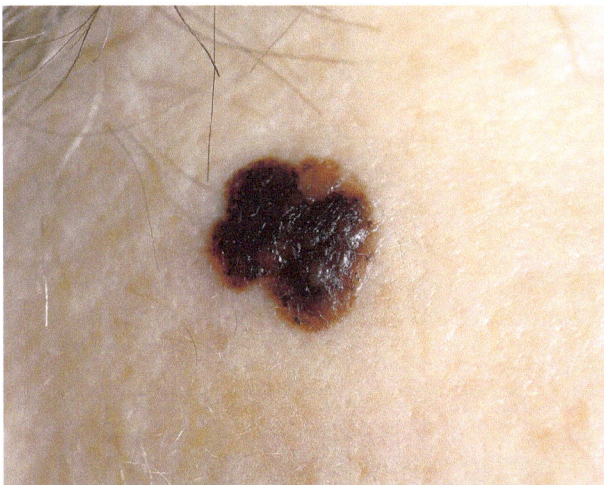
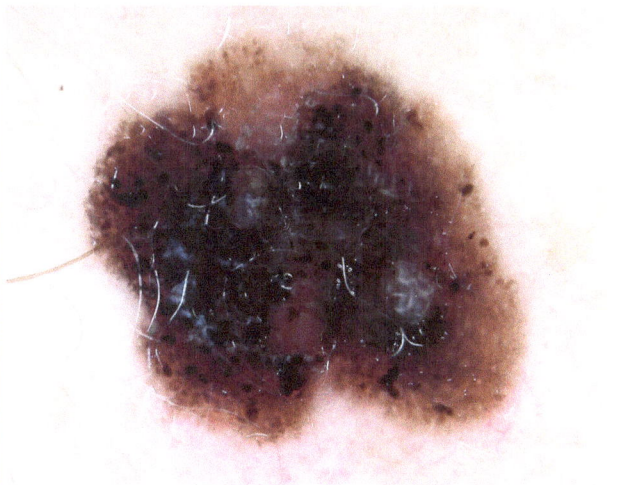

Table 10.4

	Pattern	Color	Clues	Dermatoscopic diagnosis	Histopathologic diagnosis
Top	More than one pattern (structureless and clods), arranged asymmetrically (chaotic)	More than one color (melanin dominates)	Clues to melanoma: Gray lines; structureless eccentric area	Melanoma	Melanoma
Middle	More than one pattern (reticular and dots), arranged asymmetrically (chaotic)	More than one color	Clues to melanoma: Black dots in the periphery, white lines	Melanoma	Melanoma
Bottom	One pattern (reticular)	Eccentric hyperpigmentation	None	Clark nevus	Clark nevus

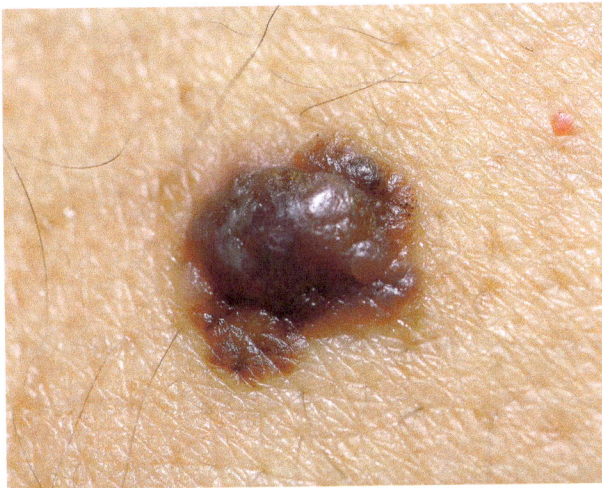
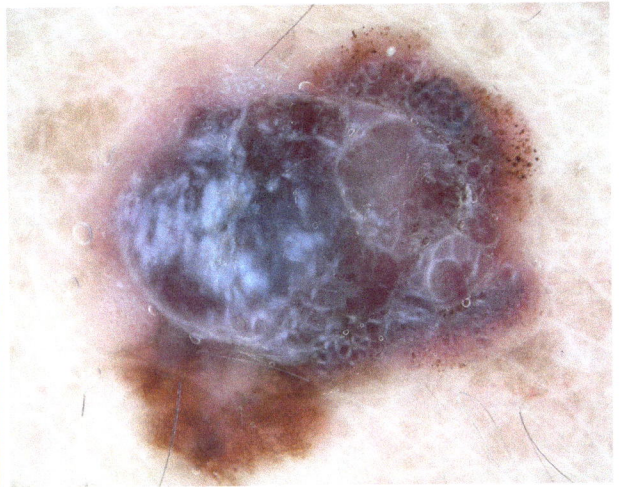
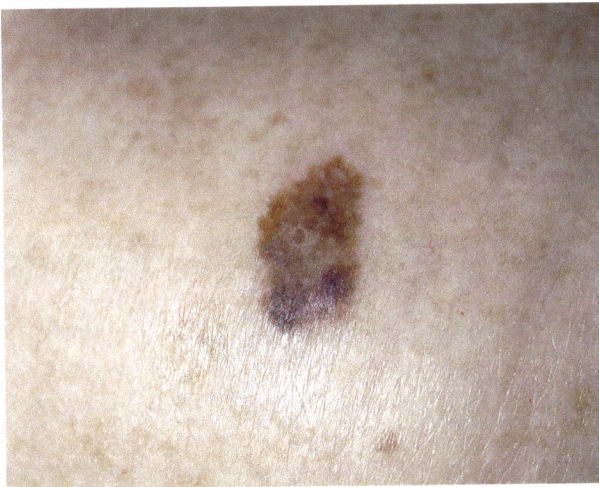
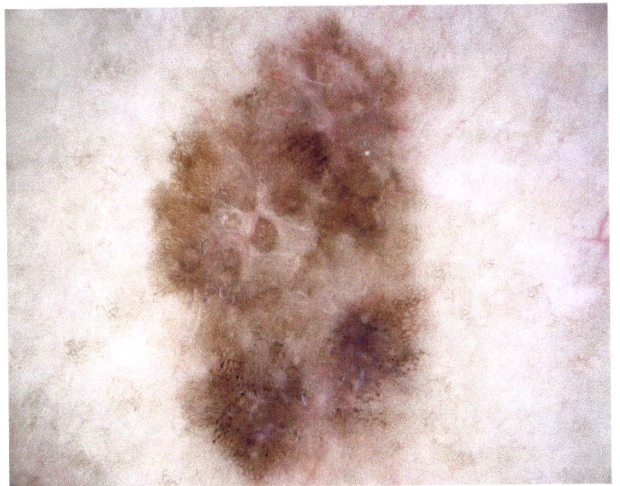
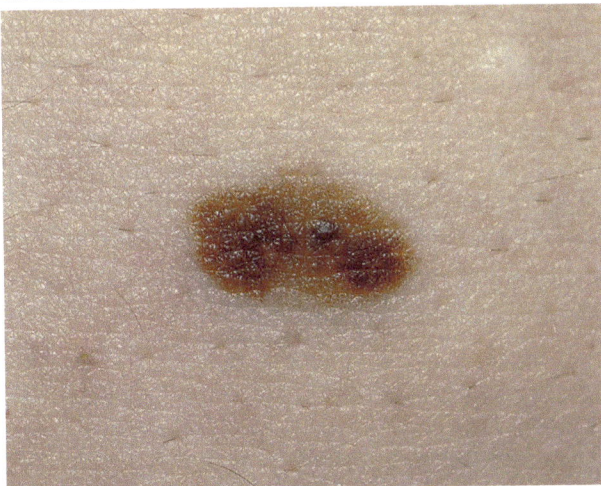
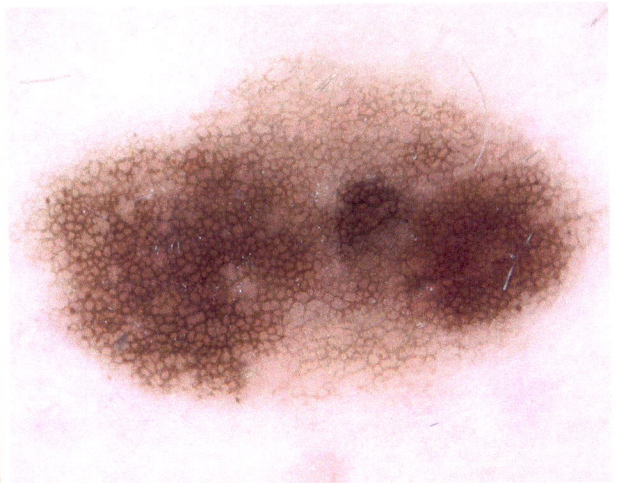

Table 10.5

	Pattern	Color	Clues	Dermatoscopic diagnosis	Histopathologic diagnosis
Top	One pattern (structureless). The single peripheral orange clod is an erosion due to trauma and has been ignored.	One color (blue) (By definition if there is one pattern and one color there is no chaos)	None	Blue nevus	Blue nevus
Middle	One pattern (reticular)	Central hyperpigmentation	None	Clark nevus	Clark nevus
Bottom	One pattern (reticular)	Variegate	None	Clark nevus or "superficial" congenital nevus	Clark nevus

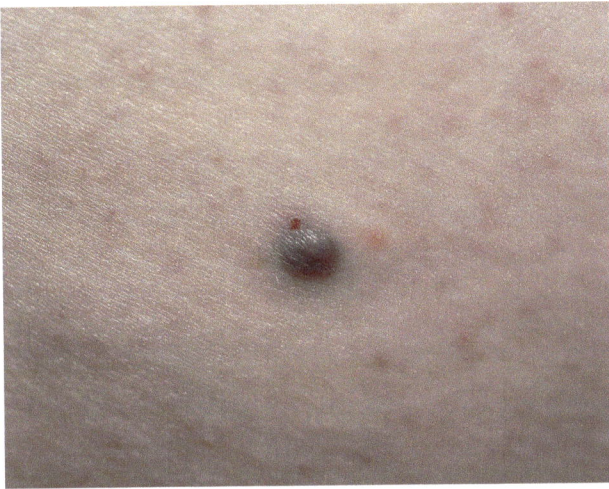
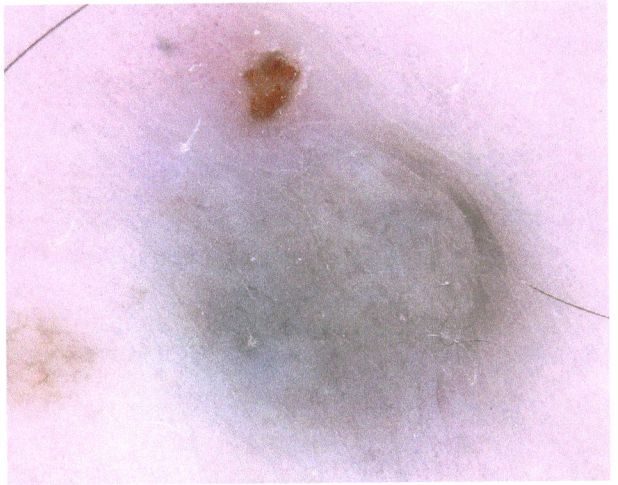
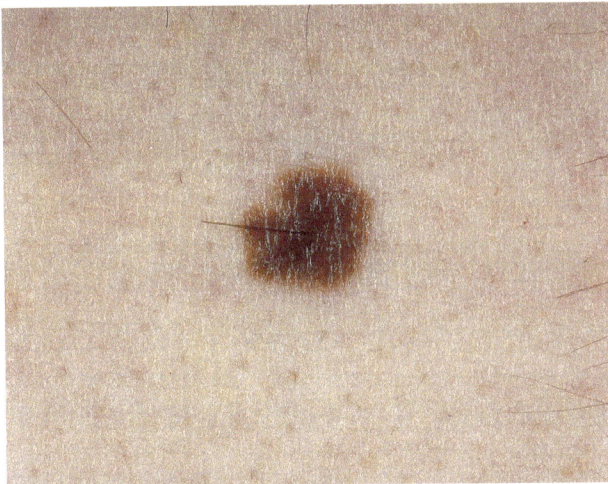
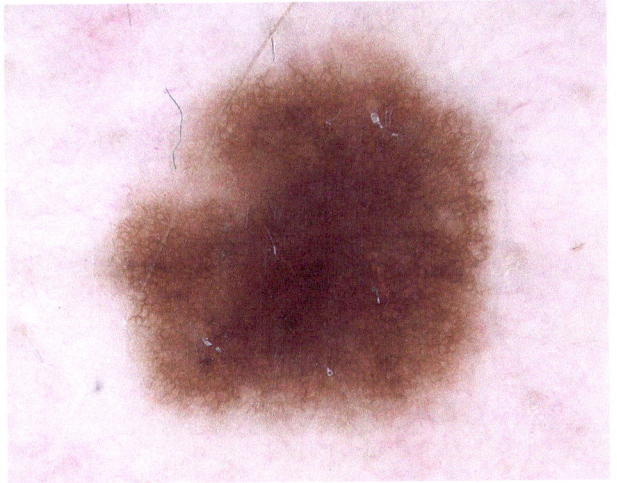
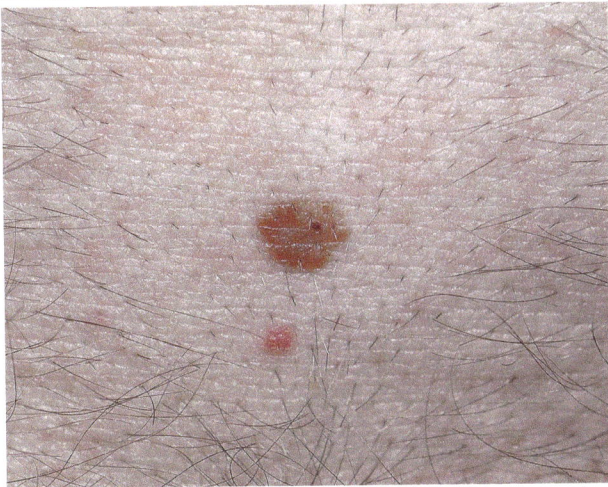
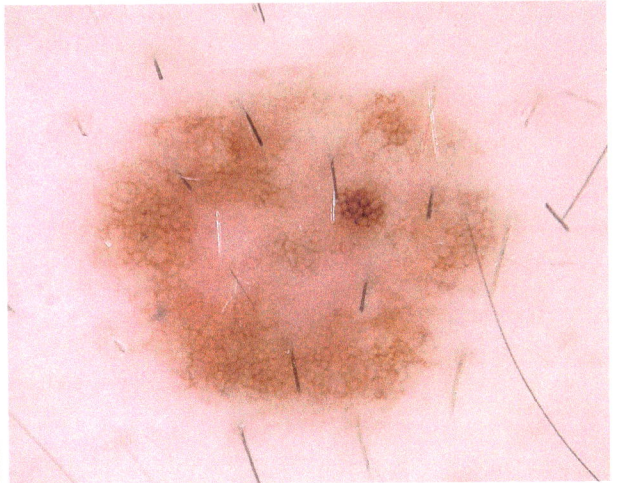

Table 10.6

	Pattern	Color	Clues	Dermatoscopic diagnosis	Histopathologic diagnosis
Top	More than one pattern (structureless in the center, reticular and dots in the periphery). The patterns are arranged symmetrically (no chaos).	More than one color, central hyperpigmentation	None	Clark nevus or "superficial" congenital nevus	Clark nevus
Middle	More than one pattern (reticular and dots), arranged asymmetrically (chaotic)	More than one color, eccentric hyperpigmentation	None. The dots in the periphery are brown and not black.	Clark nevus	Clark nevus
Bottom	One pattern (reticular)	One color (brown)	None	Clark nevus	Clark nevus

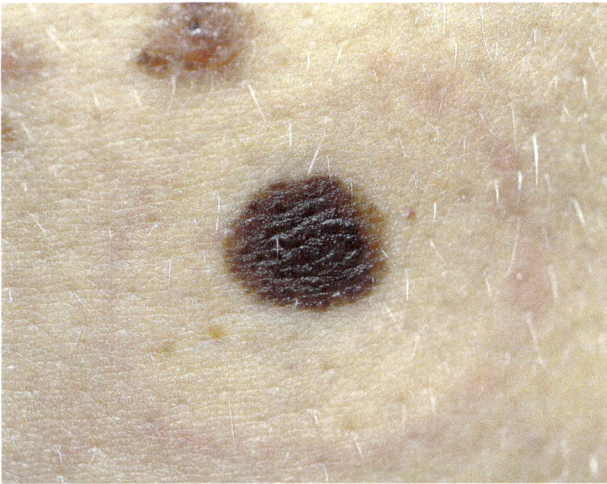
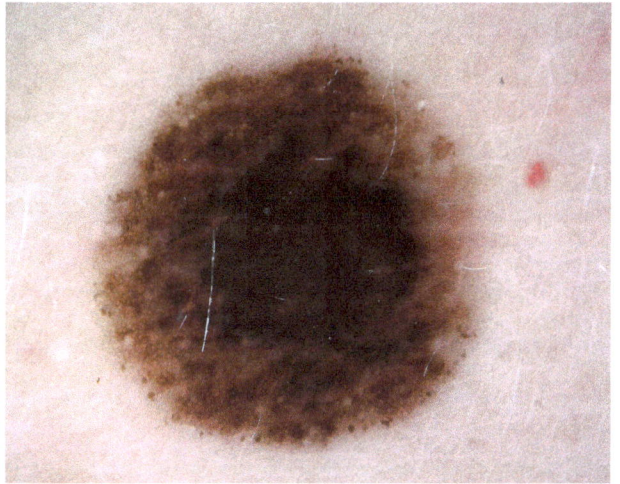
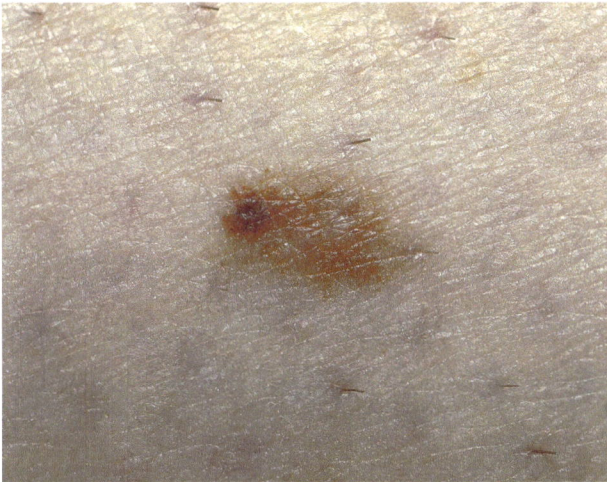
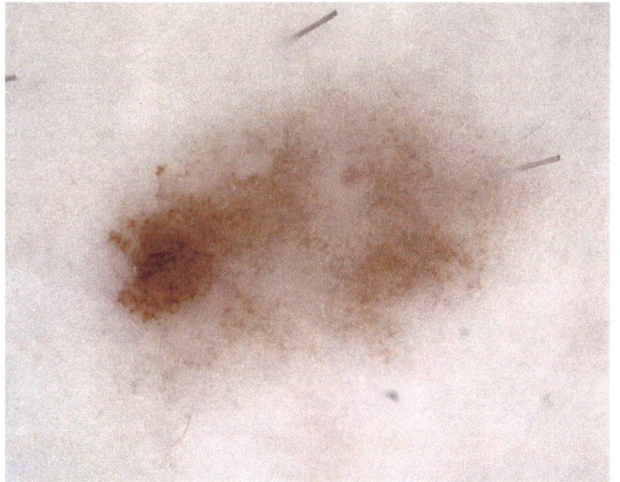
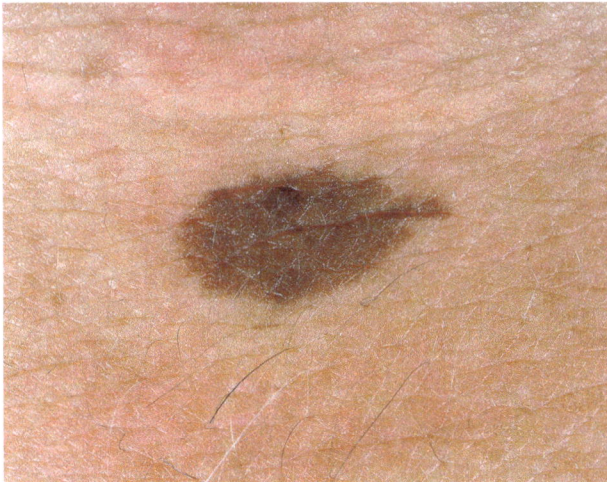
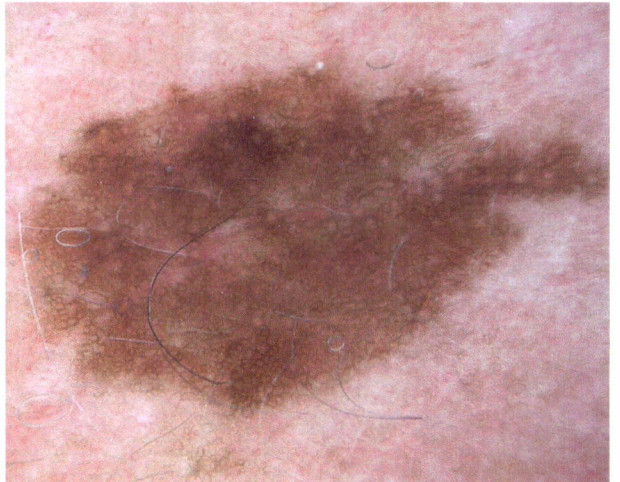

Table 10.7

	Pattern	Color	Clues	Dermatoscopic diagnosis	Histopathologic diagnosis
Top	More than one pattern (structureless in the center, reticular in the periphery). The patterns are arranged symmetrically (no chaos).	More than one color, white in the center	Thin reticular lines in the periphery and a white structureless center are a clue to dermatofibroma.	Dermatofibroma	Not excised
Middle	More than one pattern (clods and structureless), arranged asymmetrically (chaotic)	More than one color, eccentric hyperpigmentation	Clue to melanoma: Eccentric structureless area	Melanoma or melanoma in association with a nevus	Combined congenital nevus
Bottom	One pattern (circles)	Brown (not gray or black)	Clue to seborrheic keratosis: Some circles are "distorted", i.e. they appear oval or even polygonal (see also figure 7.4 for higher magnification)	Seborrheic keratosis or solar lentigo	Seborrheic keratosis

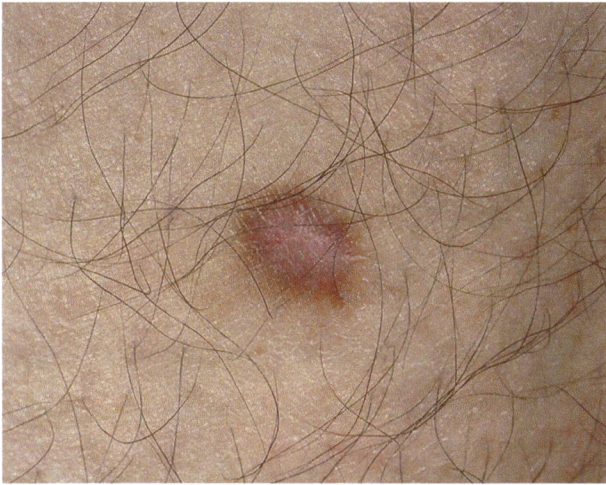
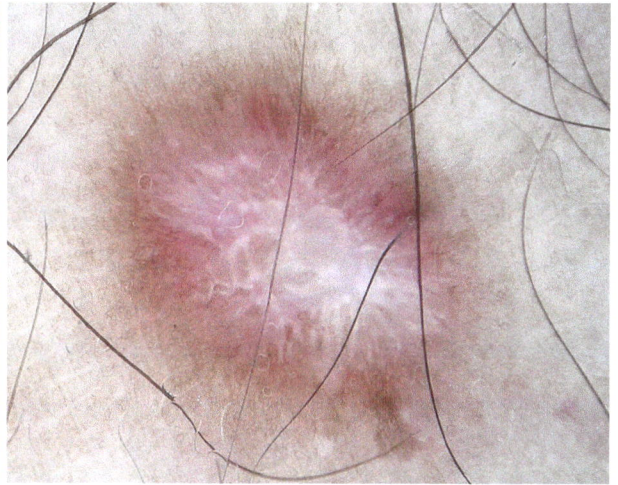
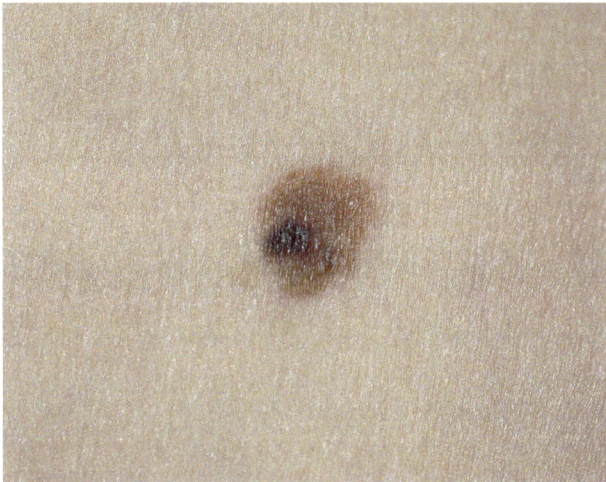
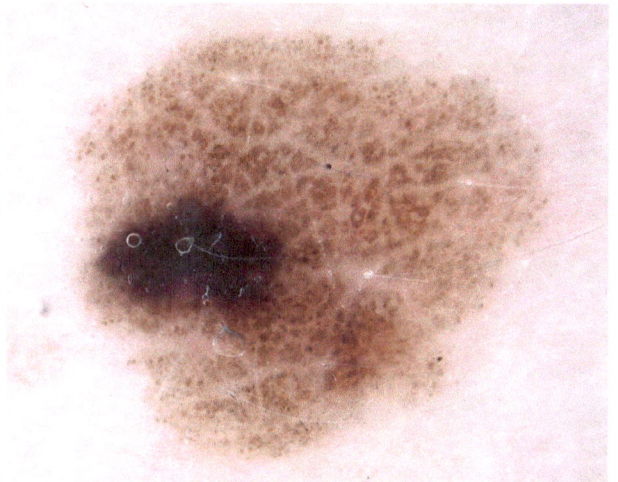
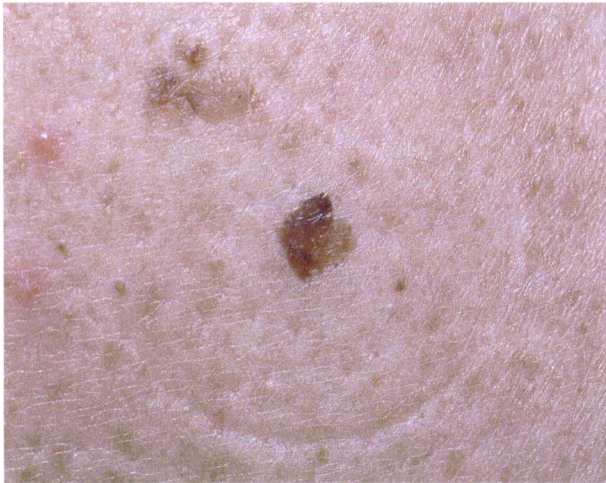
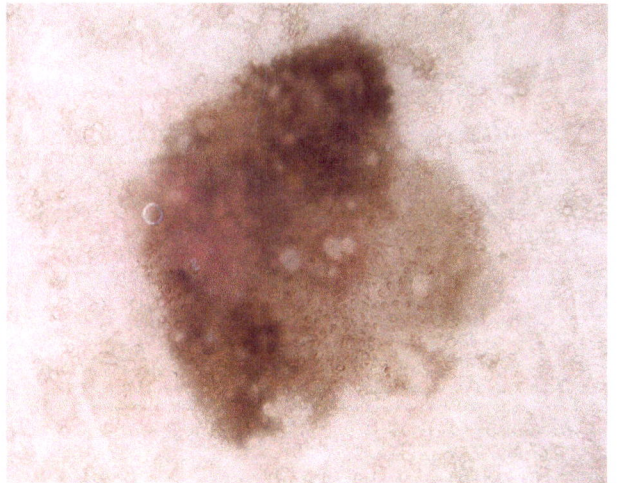

Table 10.8

	Pattern	Color	Clues	Dermatoscopic diagnosis	Histopathologic diagnosis
Top	More than one pattern (clods and curved lines). The few circles were not counted as a pattern. If the circles are regarded as an additional pattern the diagnosis would be the same.	Brown	Discrete circles and curved lines are clues to seborrheic keratosis	Seborrheic keratosis	Seborrheic keratosis
Middle	One pattern (reticular)	One color (brown)	None	Clark nevus	Not excised but no change during follow-up therefore Clark nevus
Bottom	One pattern (structureless)	More than one color, melanin (blue and gray), the colors are arranged asymmetrically (chaos)	Polymorphous vascular pattern, gray and blue structures	Melanoma (a basal cell carcinoma does not occur on acral skin)	Melanoma (invasion thickness > 1 mm)

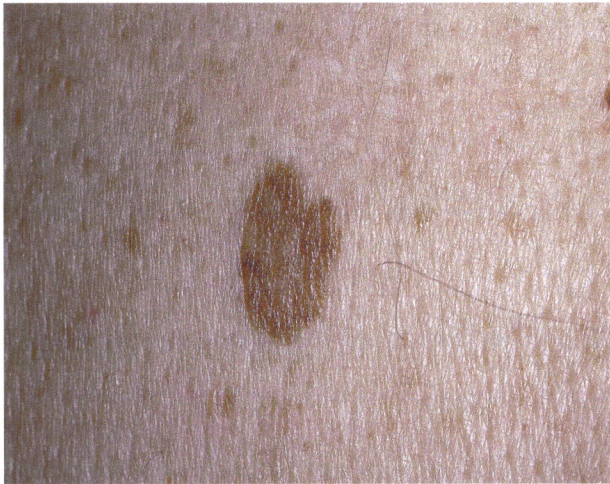
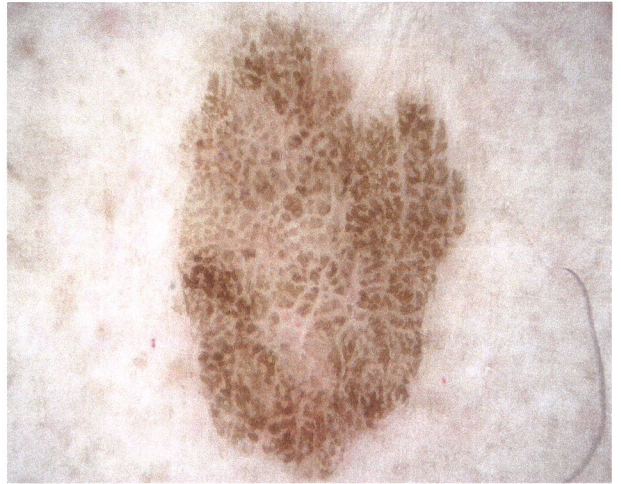
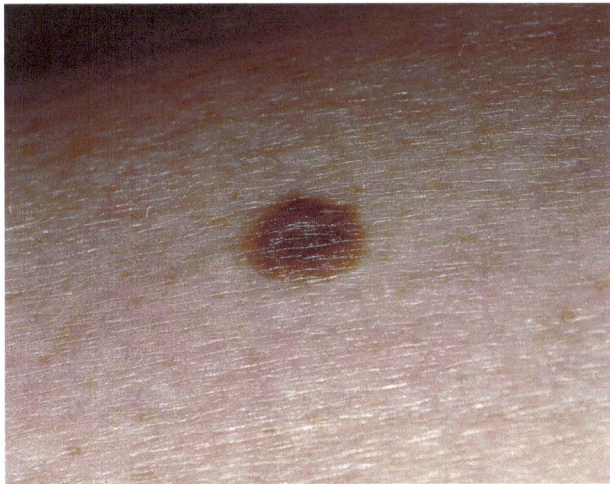
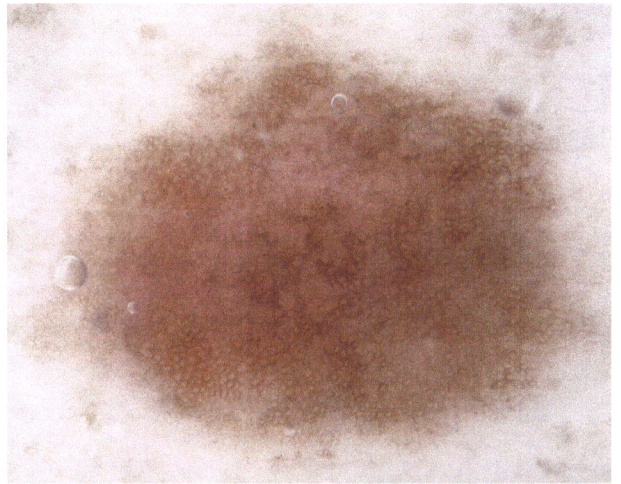
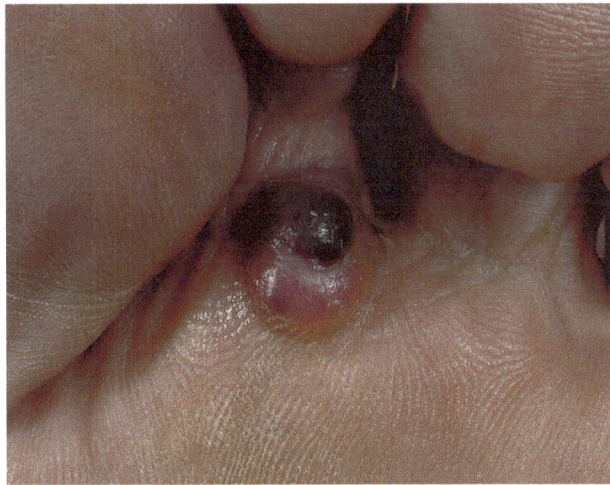
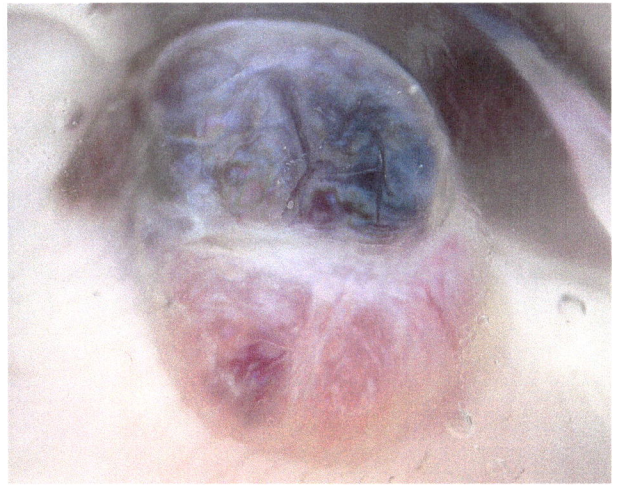

Table 10.9

	Pattern	Color	Clues	Dermatoscopic diagnosis	Histopathologic diagnosis
Top	One pattern (reticular)	One color (brown)	None	Clark nevus or "superficial" congenital nevus	Not excised but no change during follow-up
Middle	One pattern (reticular)	Variegate	Terminal hairs are a clue to a congenital nevus. No clue to melanoma.	"Superficial" or "superficial and deep" congenital nevus	"Superficial and deep" congenital nevus
Bottom	More than one pattern (clods and structureless)	Structureless = brown Clods = white	White clods are a clue to seborrheic keratosis	Seborrheic keratosis	Seborrheic keratosis

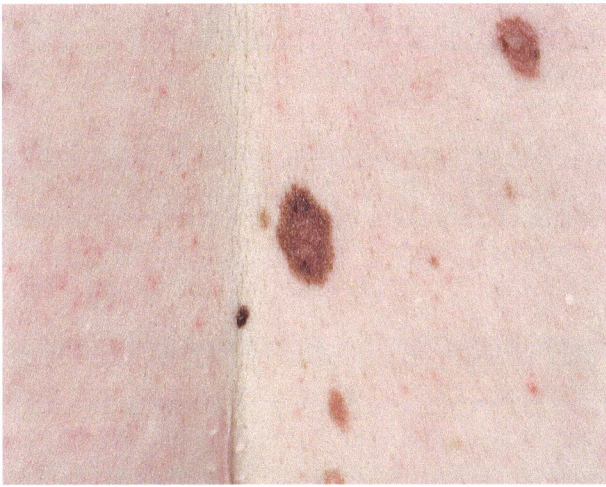
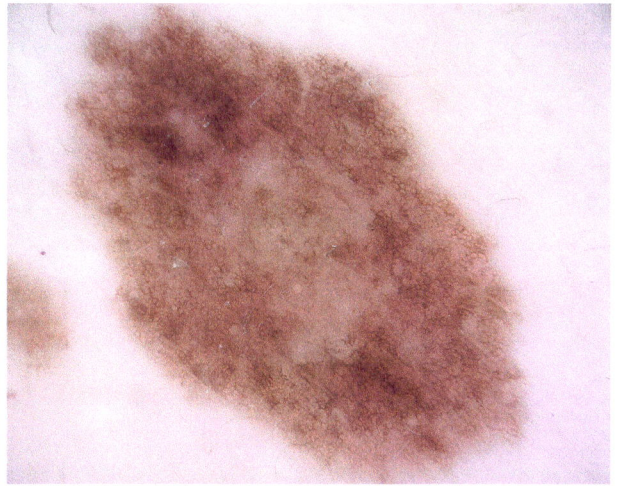
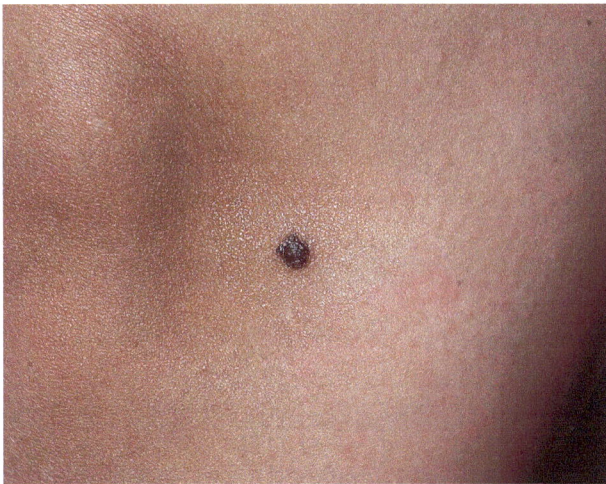
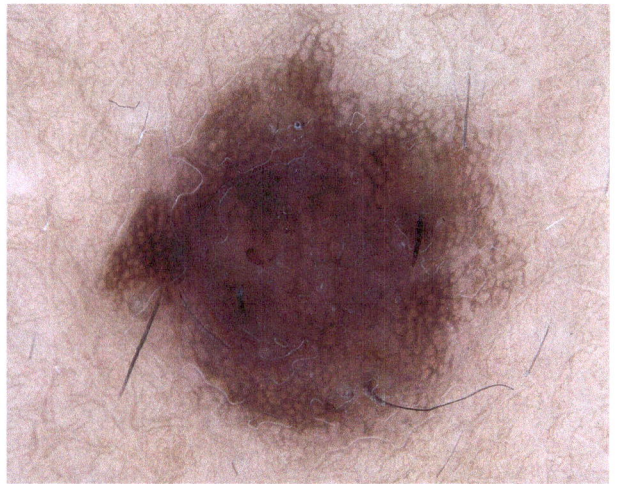
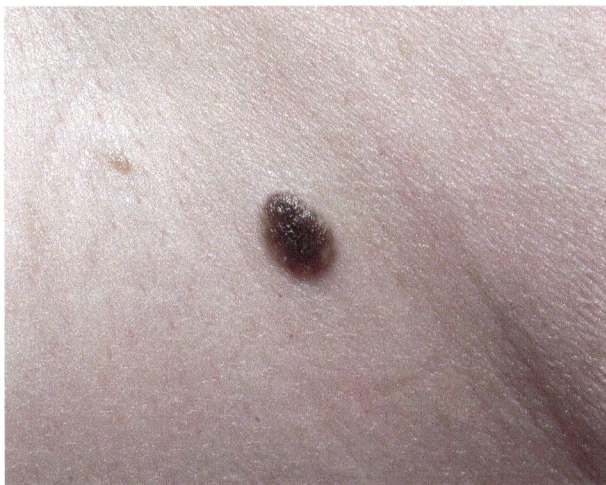
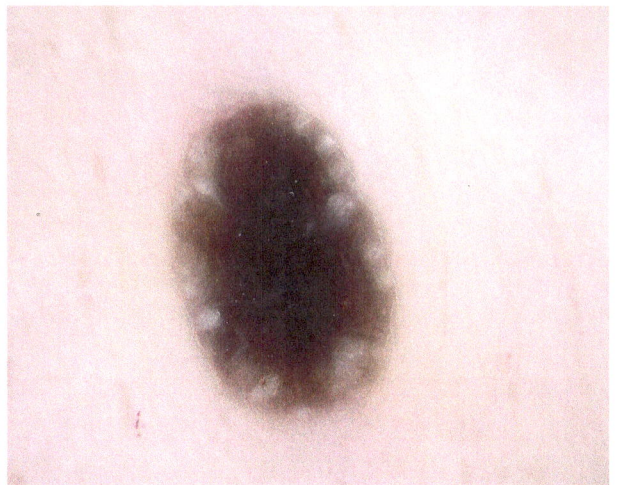

Table 10.10

	Pattern	Color	Clues	Dermatoscopic diagnosis	Histopathologic diagnosis
Top	More than one pattern (clods and structureless). The patterns are arranged asymmetrically (chaos).	Brown and black	Clues to melanoma: Pseudopods in the periphery, black clods in the periphery	Melanoma	Melanoma
Middle	One pattern (clods)	Brown and gray	Discrete orange and yellow clods and sharp circumscription point to a seborrheic keratosis	Seborrheic keratosis with unconventional criteria (gray clods are rarely found in a seborrheic keratosis)	Seborrheic keratosis, clonal type
Bottom	One pattern (large polygonal clods)	Skin colored and light brown	Curved vessels in the center of skin colored clods. Hyperkeratotic zone at 3 o'clock.	Unna nevus (in combination with a viral wart)	Unna nevus (in combination with a viral wart)

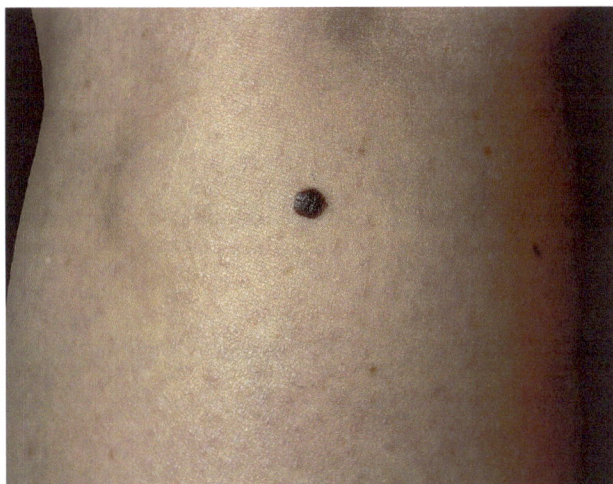
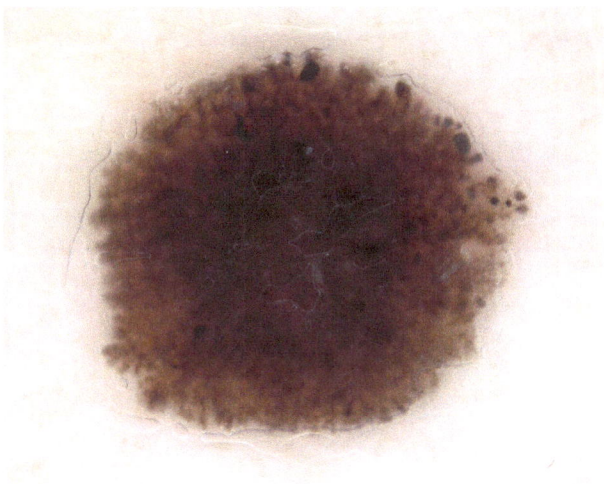
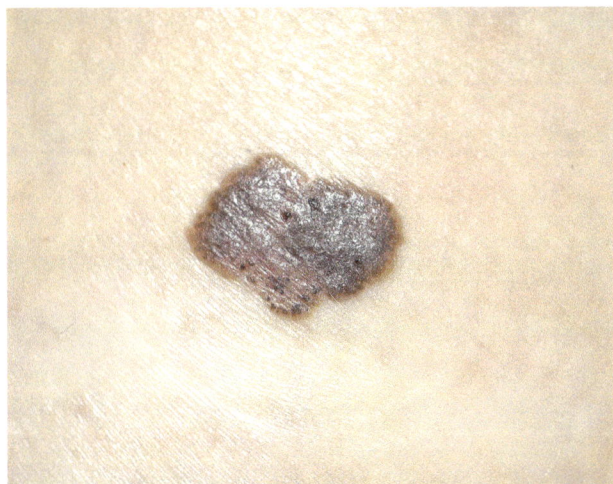
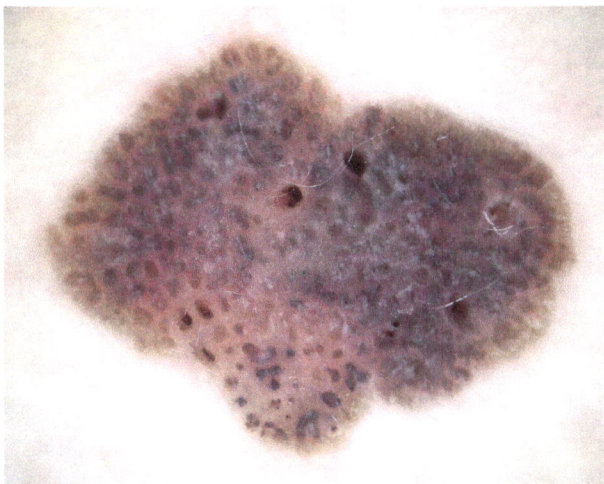
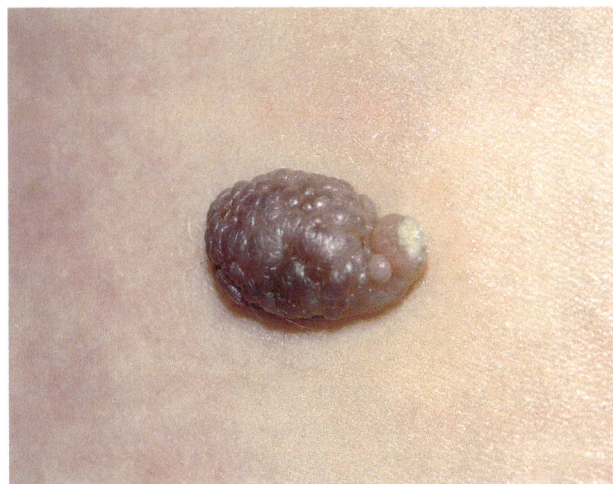
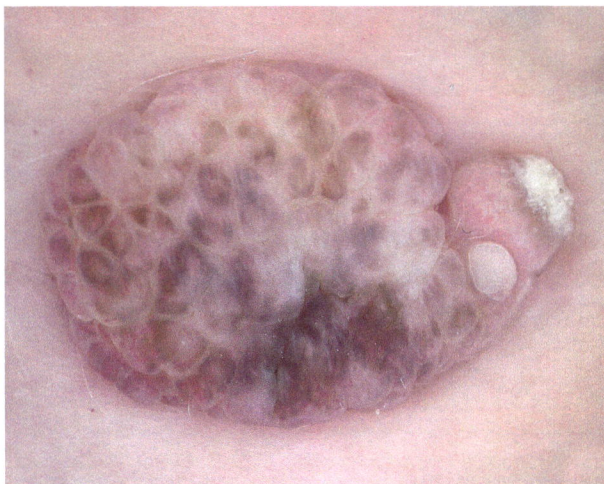

Table 10.11

	Pattern	Color	Clues	Dermatoscopic diagnosis	Histopathologic diagnosis
Top	One pattern (structureless)	More than one color including brown and gray (melanin), arranged asymmetrically (chaos)	Clues to basal cell carcinoma: serpentine vessels, some of which are branched	Basal cell carcinoma	Basal cell carcinoma
Middle	One pattern (clods)	Orange and white clods	Clues to seborrheic keratosis: White clods and orange clods, looped vessels	Seborrheic keratosis	Seborrheic keratosis
Bottom	One pattern (structureless)	Skin colored, light brown, blue (melanin) arranged symmetrically (no chaos)	None	Most likely combined congenital nevus	"Superficial and deep" congenital nevus

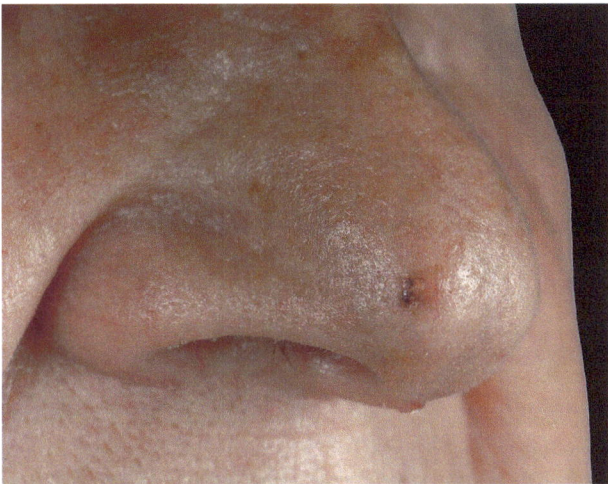

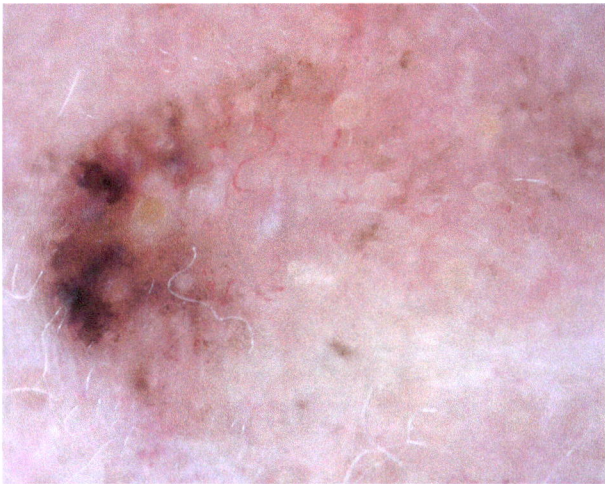

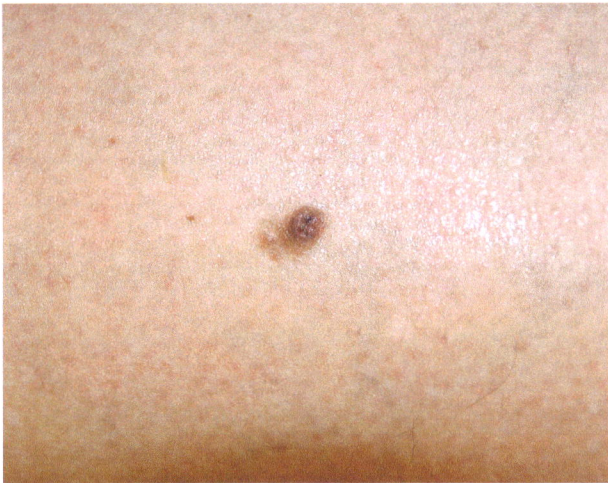

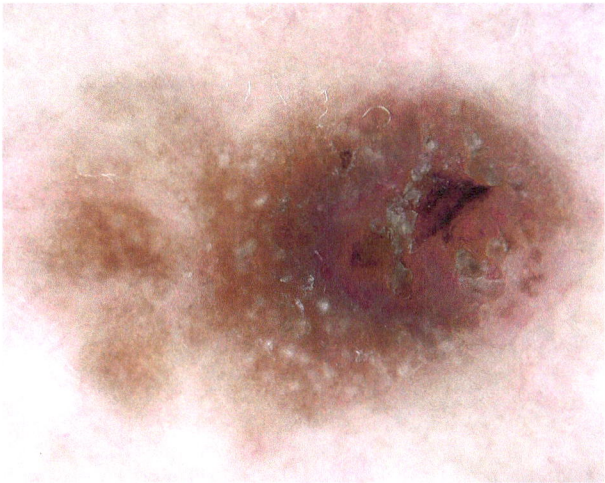

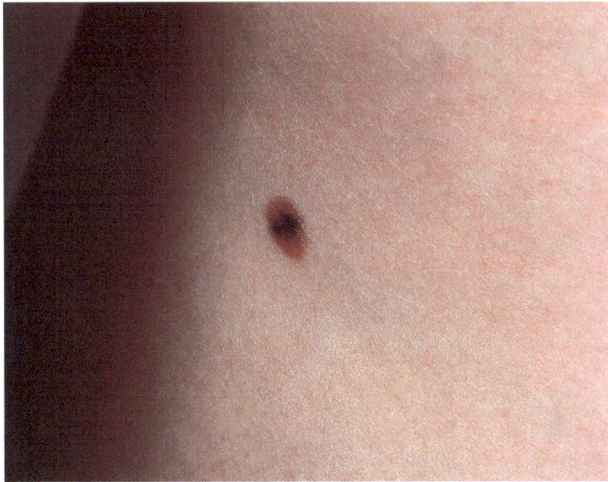

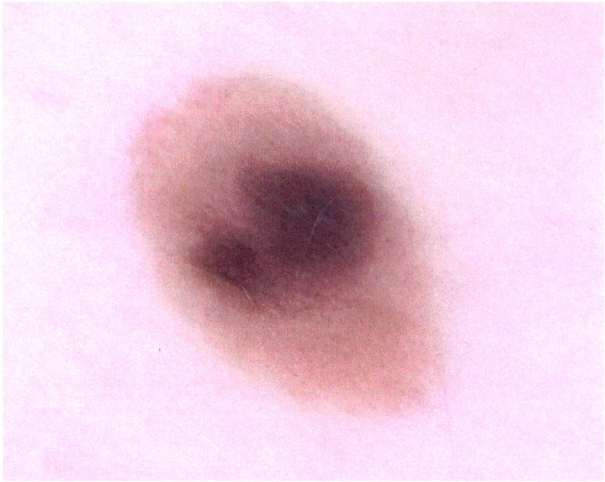

Table 10.12

	Pattern	Color	Clues	Dermatoscopic diagnosis	Histopathologic diagnosis
Top	One pattern (structureless)	More than one color including brown and gray, arranged asymmetrically (chaos)	Clues to seborrheic keratosis: discrete circles, sharp circumscription, blue structureless area, white clods	Seborrheic keratosis	Seborrheic keratosis
Middle	More than one pattern (reticular in the periphery, structureless in the center), arranged symmetrically	Central hyperpigmentation	Clues to melanoma: thick reticular lines	Clark nevus or, less likely, melanoma. The symmetry favors a Clark nevus but thick reticular lines are a clue to melanoma.	Melanoma in situ
Bottom	More than one pattern (clods and structureless), arranged asymmetrically (chaos)	Skin colored, light brown, gray (melanin)	Clues to basal cell carcinoma: Serpentine vessels, adherent fiber	Basal cell carcinoma	Basal cell carcinoma

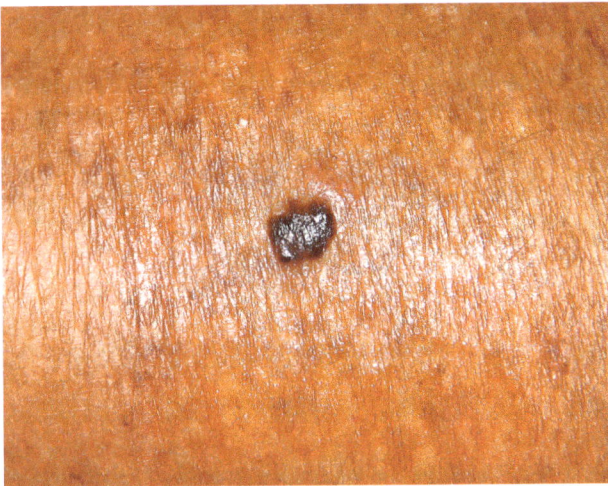
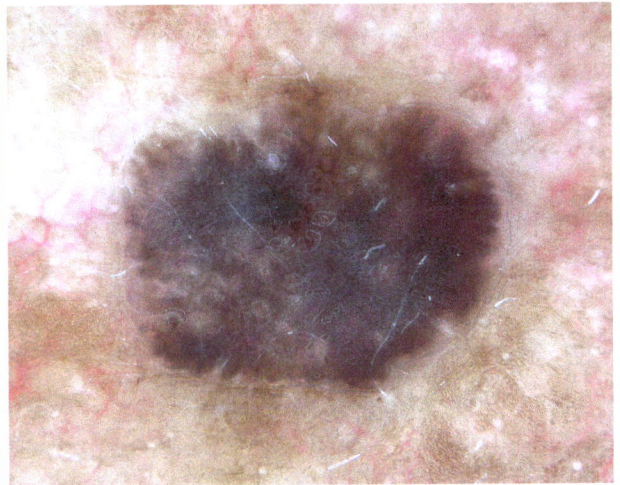
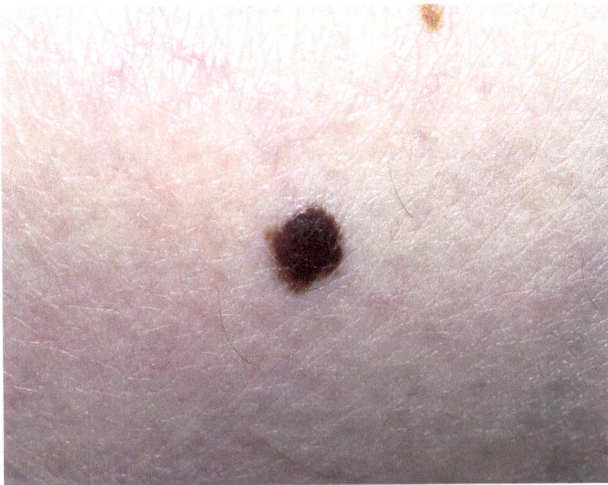

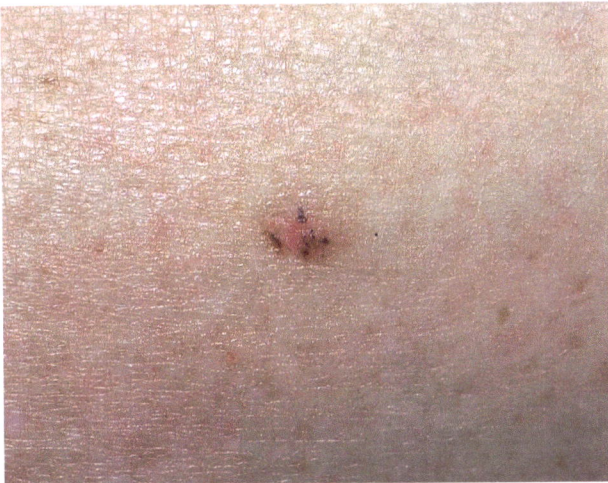
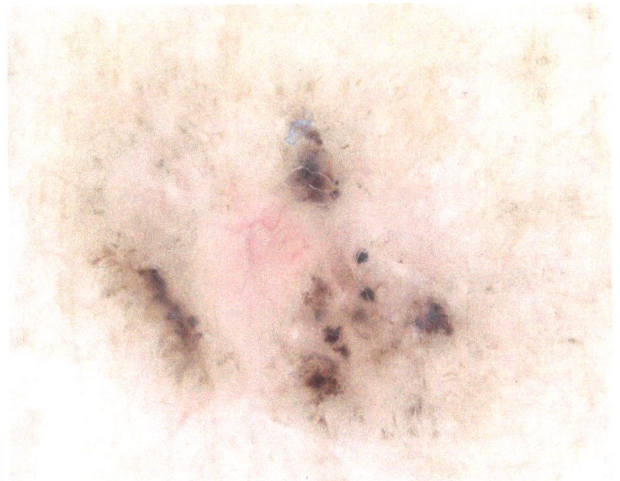

Table 10.13

	Pattern	Color	Clues	Dermatoscopic diagnosis	Histopathologic diagnosis
Top	More than one pattern (clods in the periphery, structureless in the center), arranged symmetrically (no chaos)	Brown in the periphery, gray in the center (no chaos)	None	Combined congenital nevus or "superficial and deep" congenital nevus	"Superficial and deep" congenital nevus
Middle	More than one pattern (circles and structureless), arranged asymmetrically (chaos)	Brown	None	Clark nevus or "superficial and deep" congenital nevus	Clark nevus
Bottom	More than one pattern (clods in the periphery, structureless in the center), arranged symmetrically (no chaos)	Brown	A peripheral rim of clods or dots is a clue to a growing nevus	Growing "superficial and deep" congenital nevus or Spitz nevus. In a growing Clark nevus one expects the reticular pattern in the center.	"Superficial and deep" congenital nevus

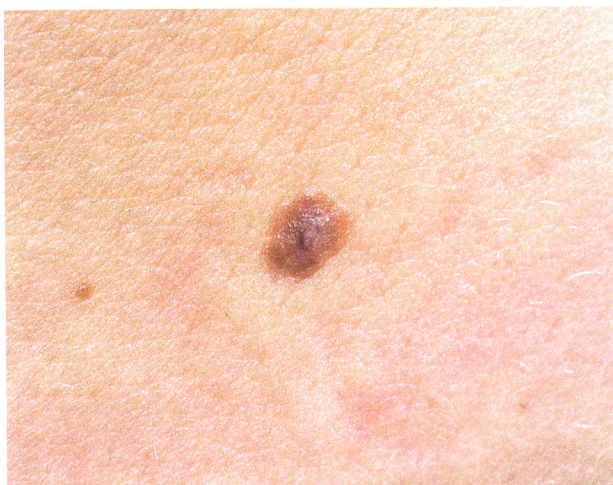
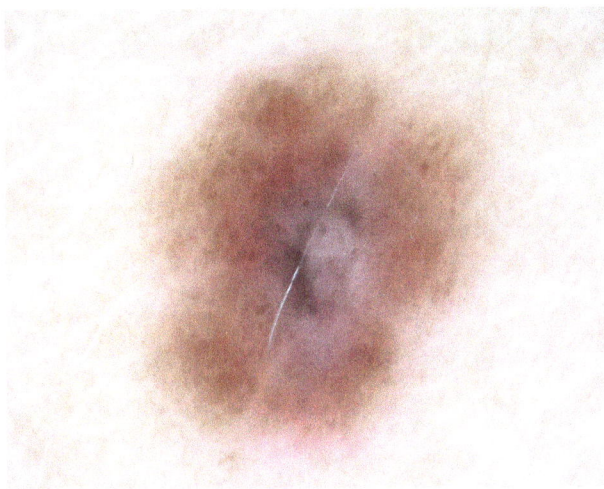
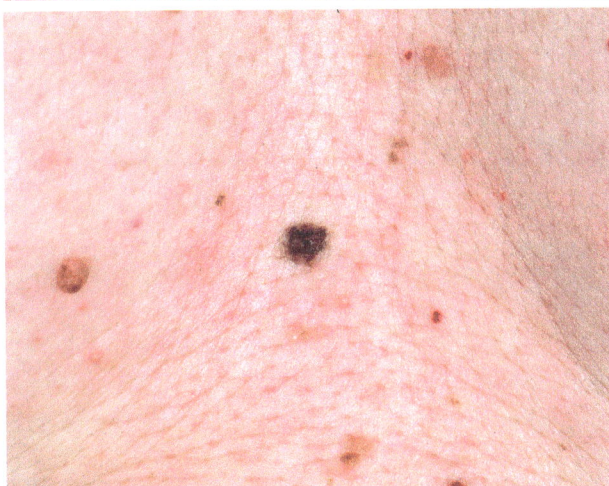
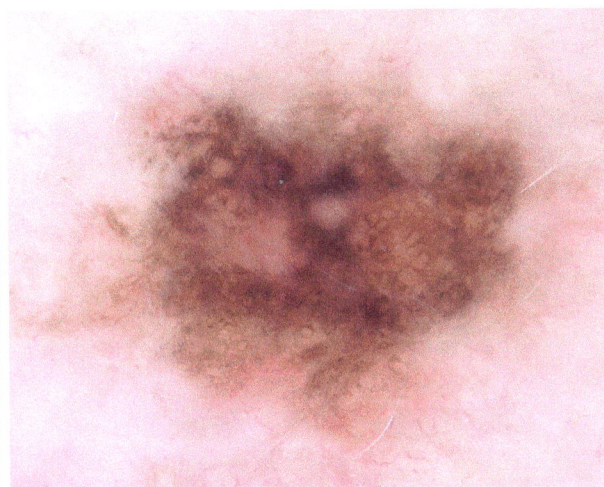
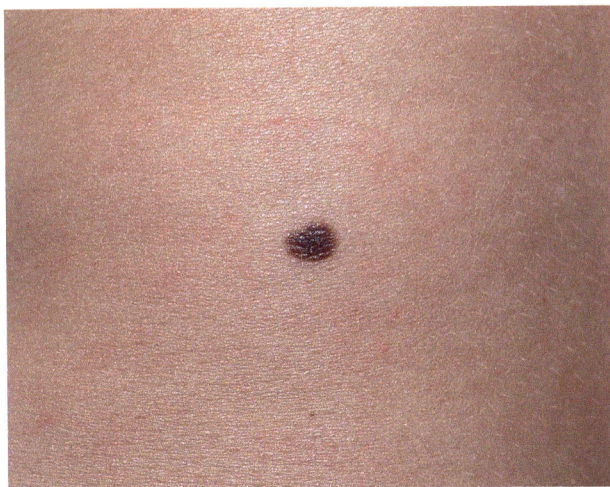
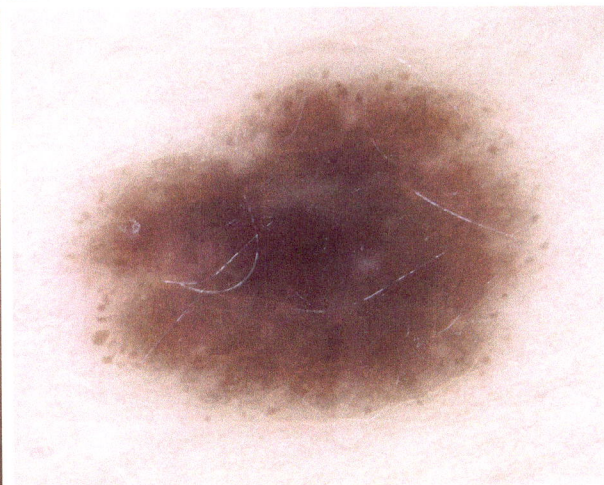

Table 10.14

	Pattern	Color	Clues	Dermatoscopic diagnosis	Histopathologic diagnosis
Top	One pattern (reticular)	Brown	None. Some brown dots in the periphery are not specific.	Clark nevus	Not excised
Middle	One pattern (structureless)	Skin colored, pink, and brown	Clues to melanoma: polymorphous vascular pattern, the presence of vessels as dots are in favor of melanoma and exclude other diagnoses such as basal cell carcinoma	Melanoma	Melanoma in a pre-existing Clark nevus
Bottom	More than one pattern (clods in the periphery, structureless in the center), arranged symmetrically (no chaos)	Brown	A peripheral rim of clods or dots is a clue to a growing nevus	Growing "superficial and deep" congenital nevus or Spitz nevus. In a growing Clark nevus one expects the reticular pattern in the center.	"Superficial and deep" congenital nevus

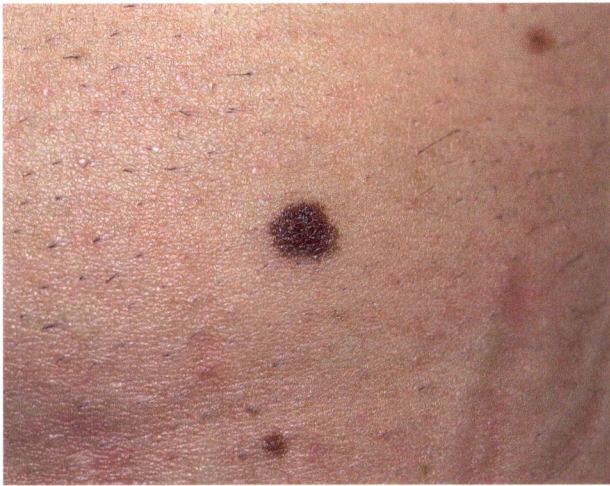
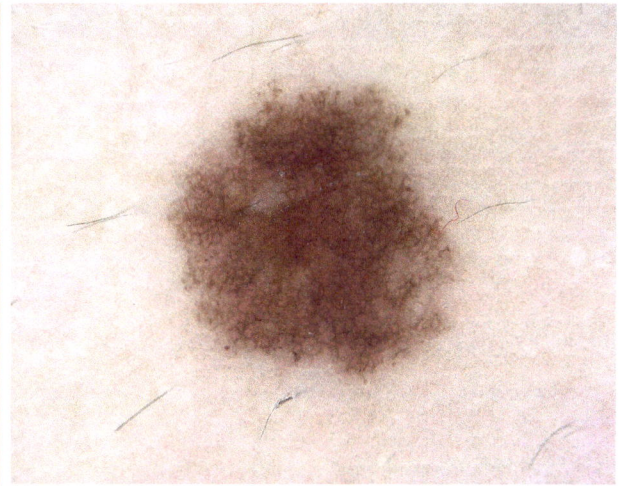
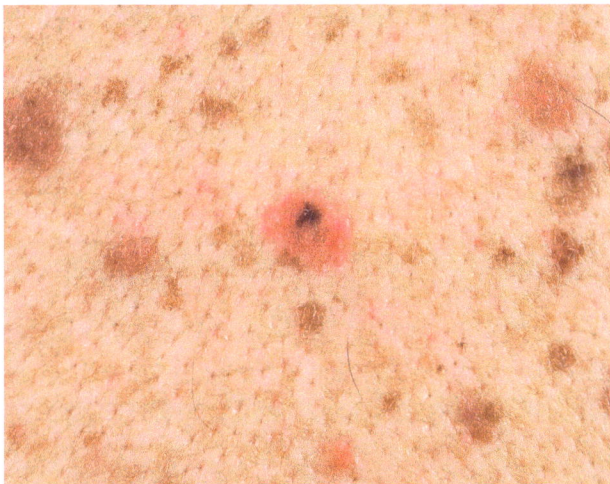
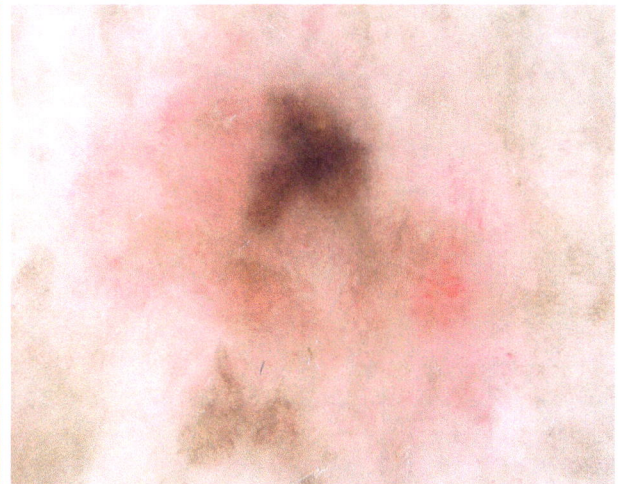
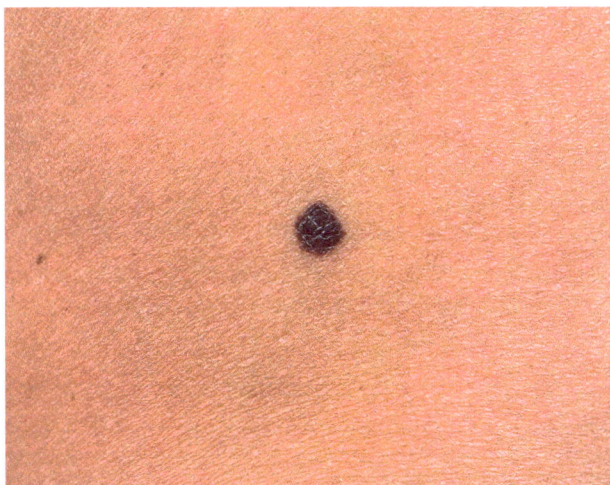
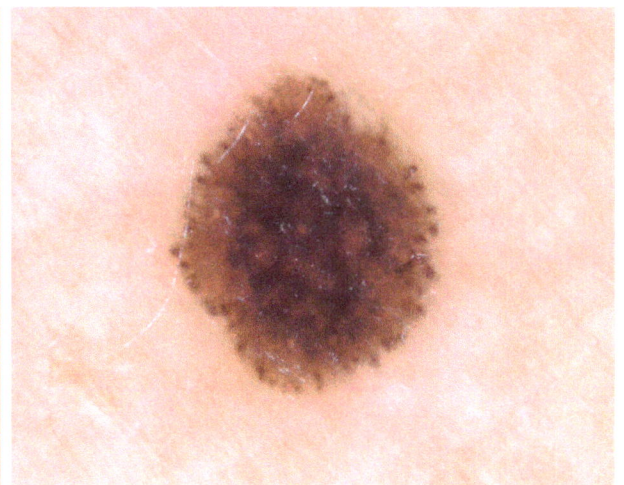

Table 10.15

	Pattern	Color	Clues	Dermatoscopic diagnosis	Histopathologic diagnosis
Top	More than one pattern (clods in the periphery, structureless in the center), arranged symmetrically (no chaos)	Brown	A peripheral rim of clods or dots is a clue to a growing nevus	Growing "superficial and deep" congenital nevus or Spitz nevus. In a growing Clark nevus one expects the reticular pattern in the center.	Not excised
Middle	One pattern (structureless)	Black in the center, brown at the periphery	None	Clark nevus or Reed nevus	Clark nevus
Bottom	More than one pattern (radial lines in the periphery, structureless in the center), arranged asymmetrically (chaos)	Central hyperpigmentation	Clue to melanoma: Segmental radial lines	Melanoma	Clark nevus

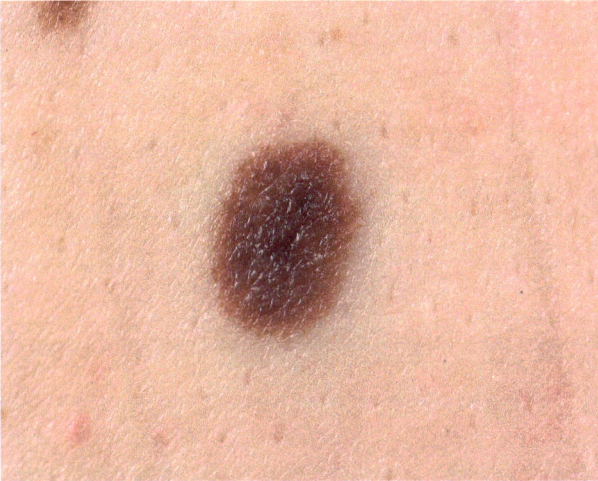
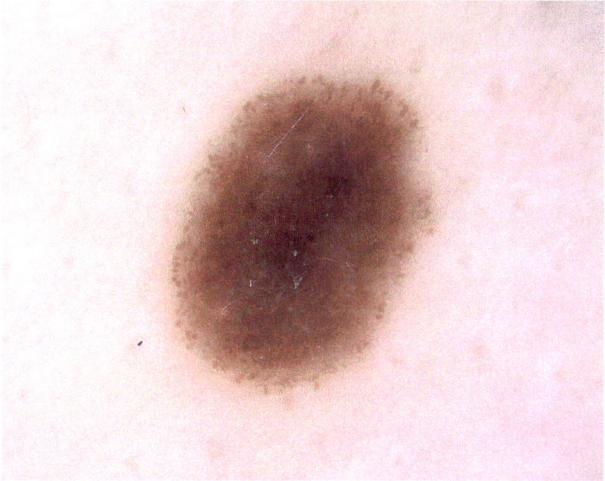
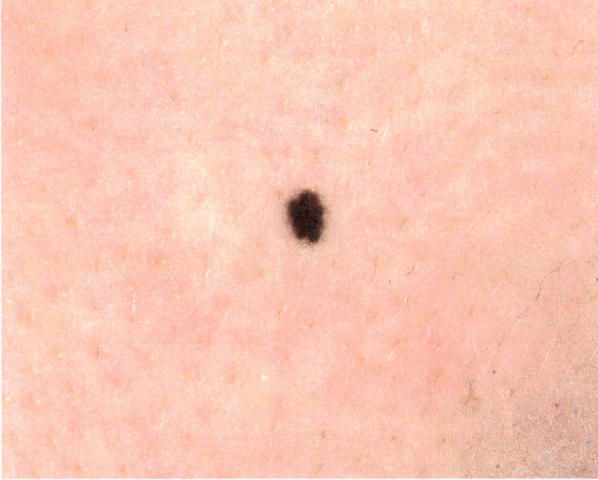
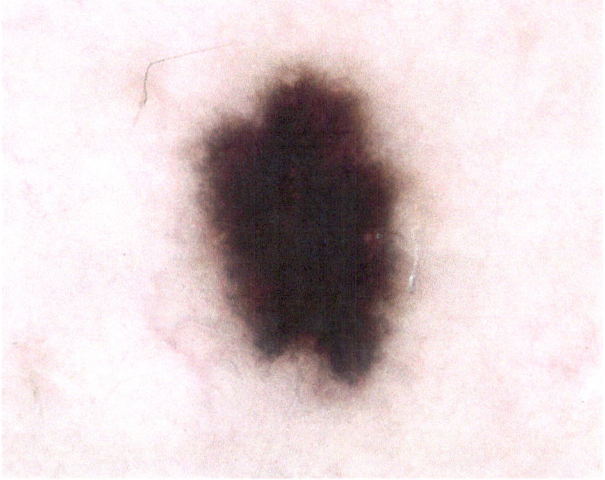
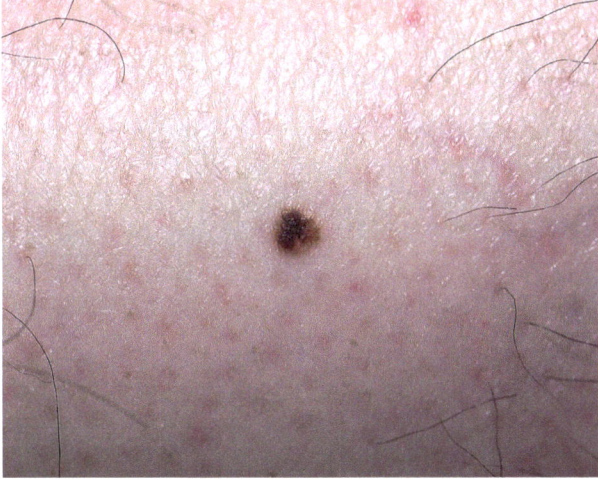
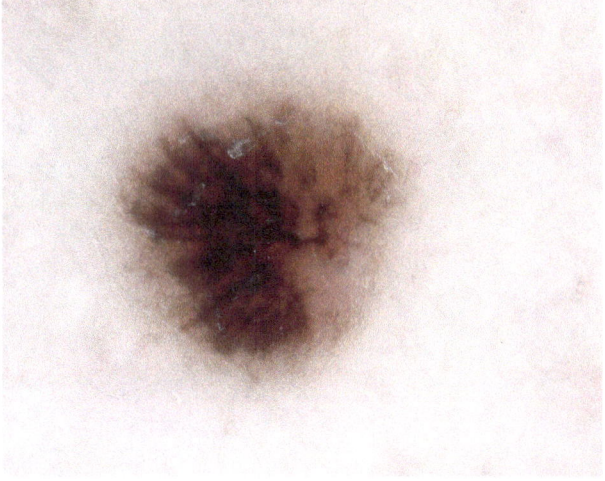

Table 10.16

	Pattern	Color	Clues	Dermatoscopic diagnosis	Histopathologic diagnosis
Top	More than one pattern (dots and structureless) arranged asymmetrically (chaos)	Brown, gray, and skin colored	Serpentine vessels are a clue to basal cell carcinoma, one or two blue clods (too few to form a pattern) support this diagnosis	Basal cell carcinoma	Basal cell carcinoma
Middle	More than one pattern (clods, dots, structureless) arranged asymmetrically	Clods are mostly black and dots are gray	Clues to seborrheic keratosis: White and yellow clods, looped vessels, sharp demarcation	Seborrheic keratosis in regression (lichen planus-like keratosis)	Seborrheic keratosis
Bottom	One pattern (reticular)	Eccentric hyperpigmentation	Clues to melanoma: thick reticular lines	Melanoma	Clark nevus

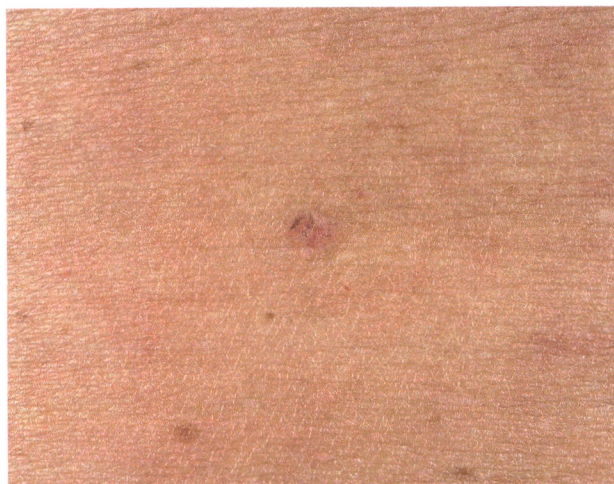
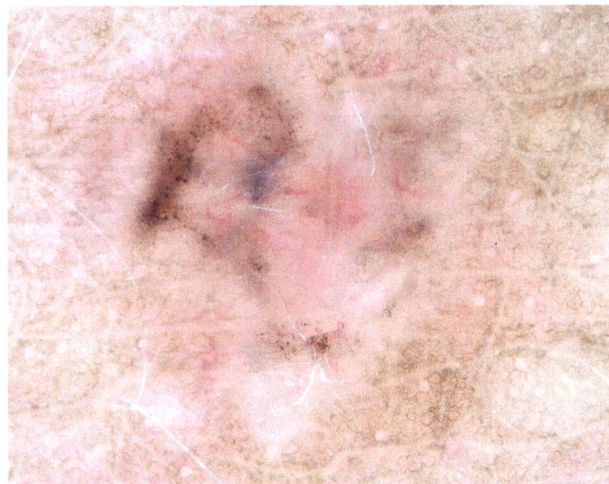

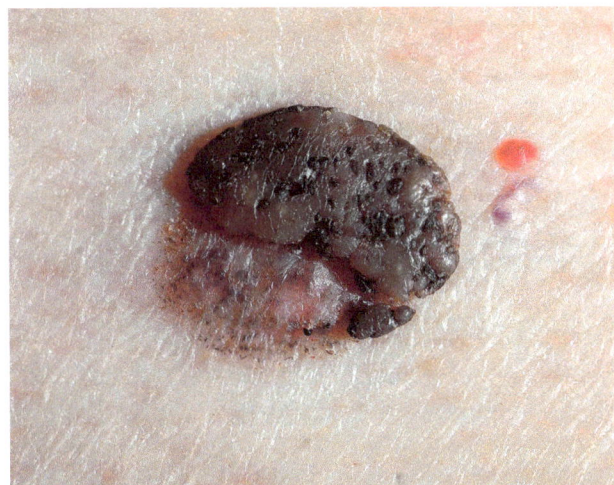
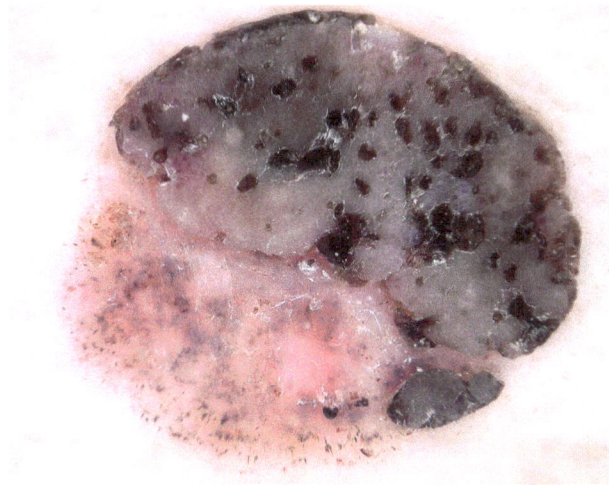

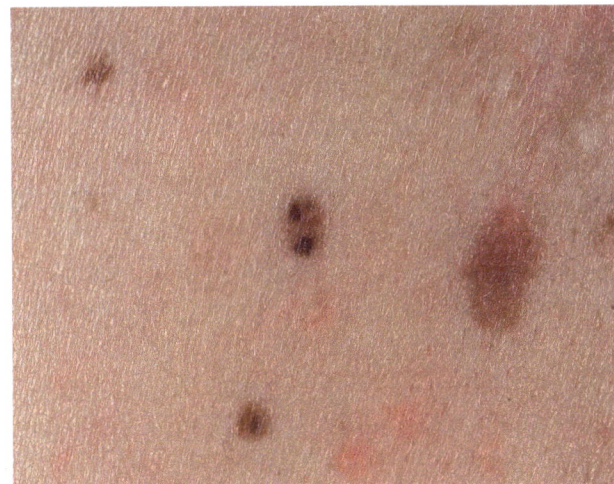
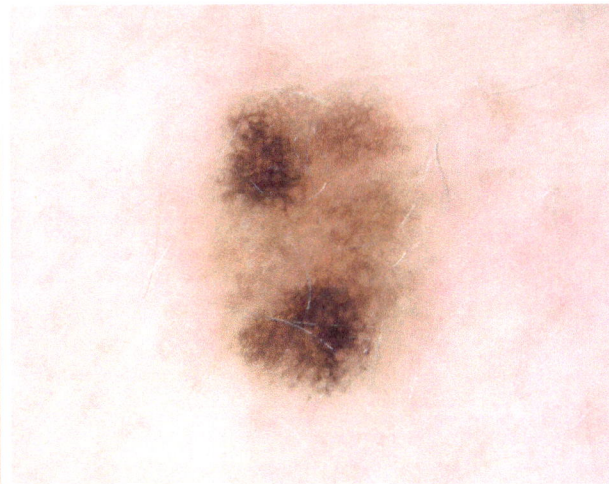

Table 10.17

	Pattern	Color	Clues	Dermatoscopic diagnosis	Histopathologic diagnosis
Top	One pattern (dots). If one prefers structureless it would lead to the same diagnosis.	Gray (dots) and red	Clues to melanoma: Gray dots and white lines	Melanoma	Melanoma
Middle	One pattern (clods)	Clods are grey, yellow and white	Clues to seborrheic keratosis: Yellow and white clods	Seborrheic keratosis	Seborrheic keratosis
Bottom	One pattern (reticular)	Eccentric hyperpigmentation	None	Clark nevus, "superficial" congenital nevus, or "superficial and deep" congenital nevus	Clark nevus

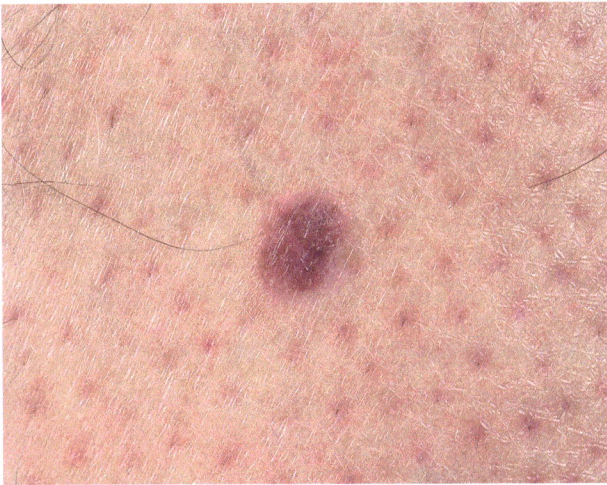

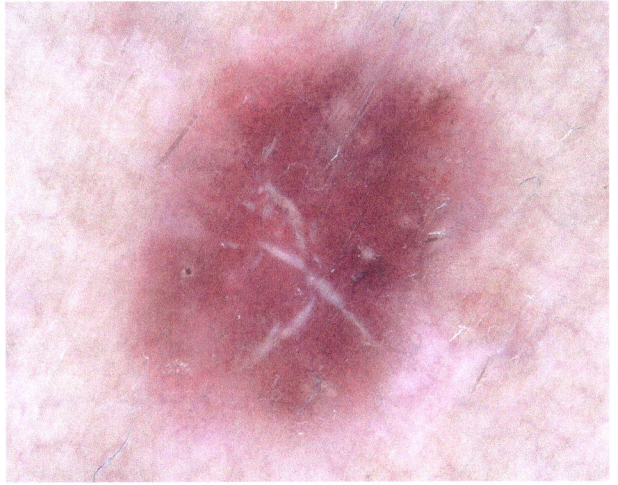

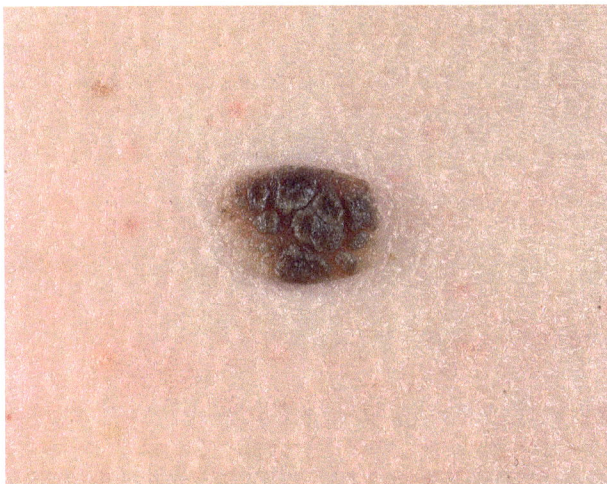

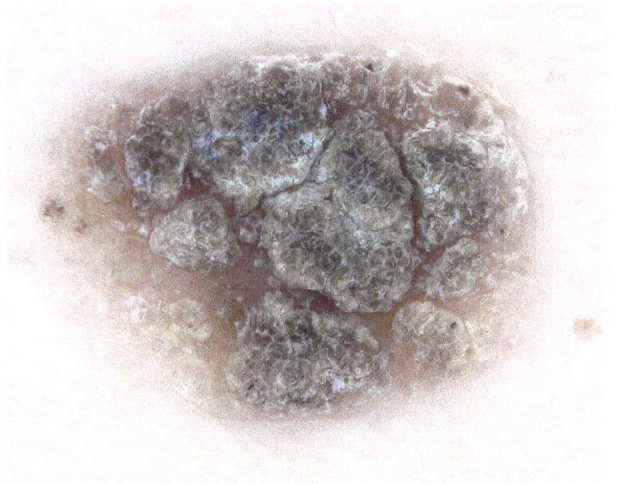

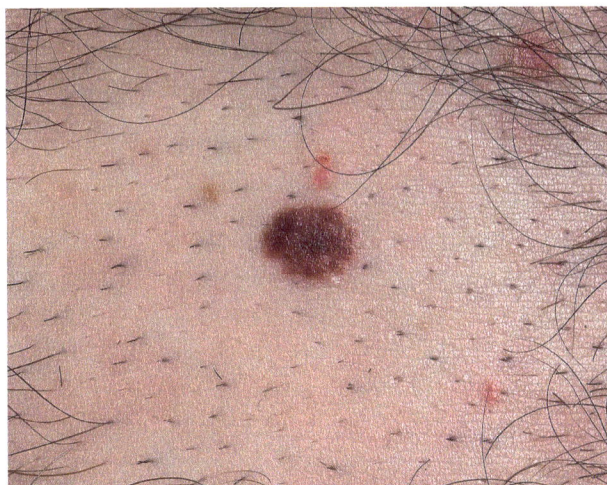

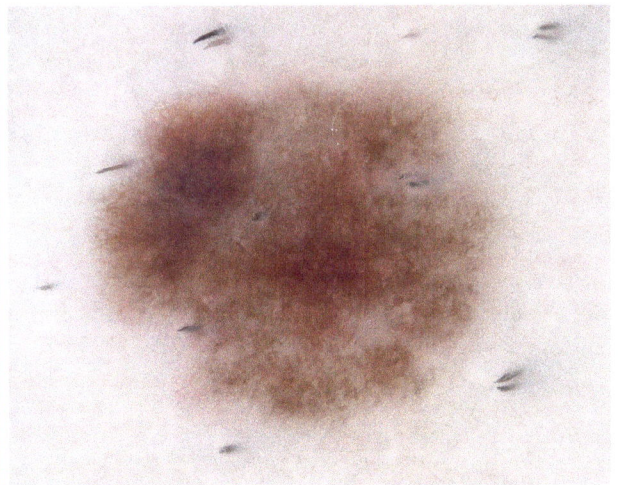

Table 10.18

	Pattern	Color	Clues	Dermatoscopic diagnosis	Histopathologic diagnosis
Top	More than one pattern (reticular and clods). If one prefers only reticular it would lead to the same differential diagnosis.	Eccentric hyperpigmentation	None	Clark nevus, "superficial" congenital nevus, or "superficial and deep" congenital nevus	Clark nevus
Middle	One pattern (reticular)	Eccentric hyperpigmentation	None	Clark nevus	Clark nevus
Bottom	One pattern (reticular)	Central hyperpigmentation	None	Clark nevus	Not excised

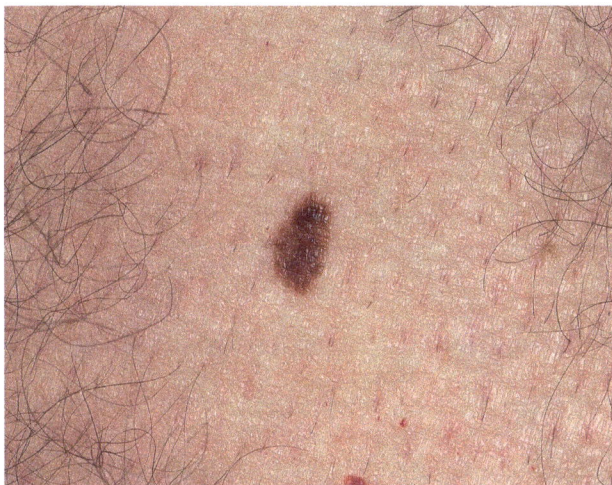
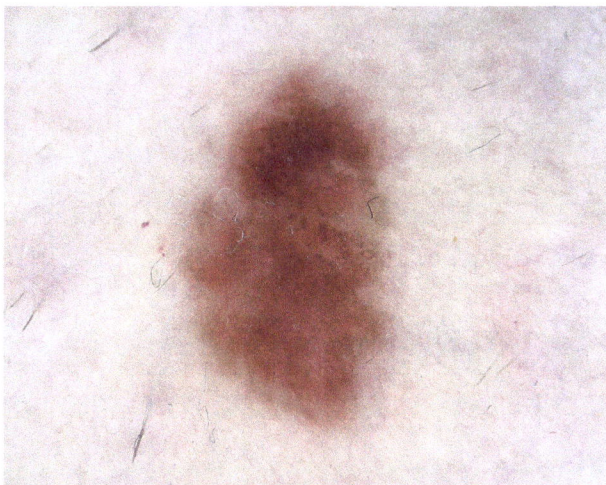
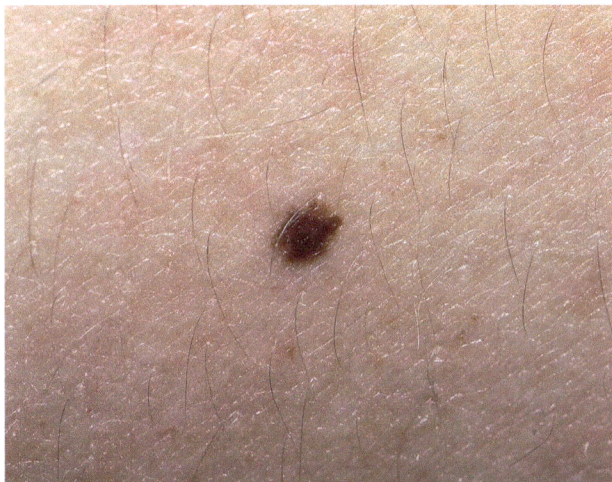
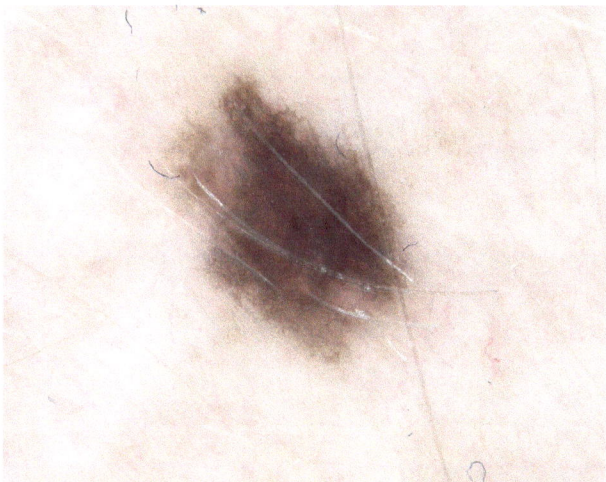
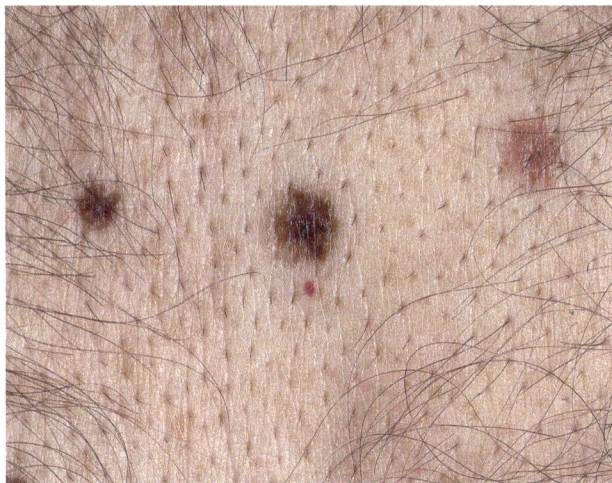
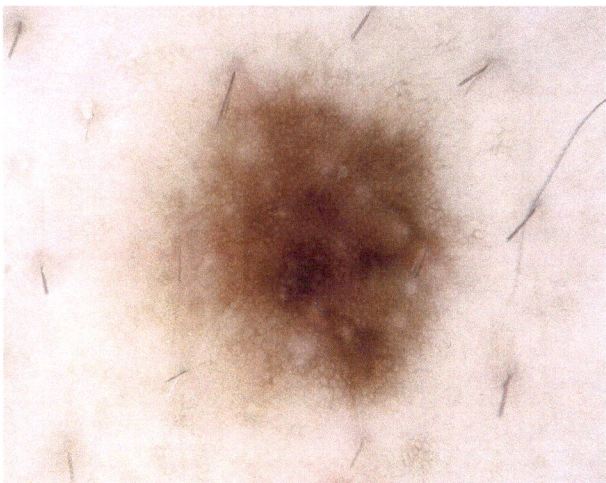

Table 10.19

	Pattern	Color	Clues	Dermatoscopic diagnosis	Histopathologic diagnosis
Top	More than one pattern (reticular in the periphery, structureless in the center), arranged symmetrically	Central hypopigmentation	Clues to melanoma: Gray dots	"Superficial and deep" congenital nevus. Symmetry of pattern and color takes precedence over a single clue (gray dots).	"Superficial and deep" congenital nevus
Middle	One pattern (reticular)	Central hyperpigmentation	Clue to melanoma: Thick reticular lines	As a general principle symmetry of pattern and color takes precedence over a single clue. Therefore the most likely diagnosis is Clark nevus. However, a melanoma in situ cannot be excluded with certainty.	Clark nevus
Bottom	More than one pattern (reticular in the periphery, clods in the center), arranged symmetrically. Note that the two eccentric clods are too insignificant to disturb the overall symmetry.	Central hyperpigmentation	Clue to melanoma: Gray clods	As a general principle symmetry of pattern and color takes precedence over a single clue. Therefore the most likely diagnosis is Clark nevus. However, a melanoma in situ cannot be excluded with certainty.	Clark nevus

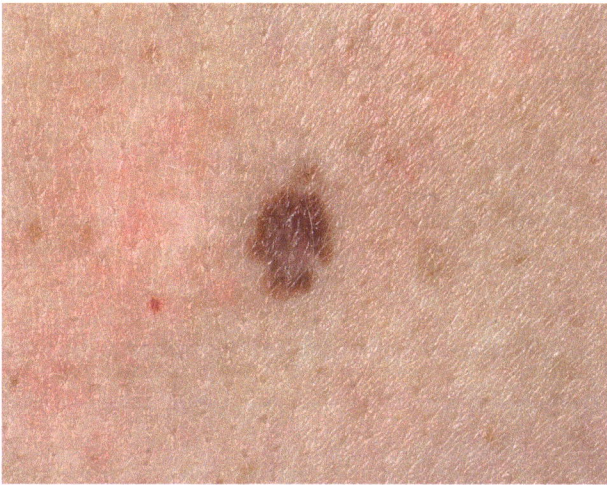
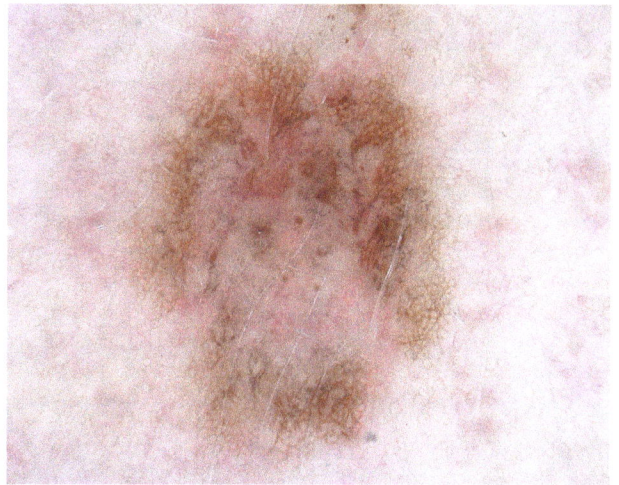
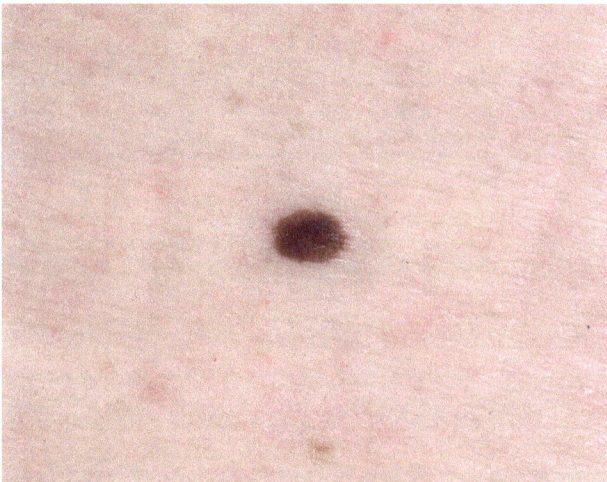
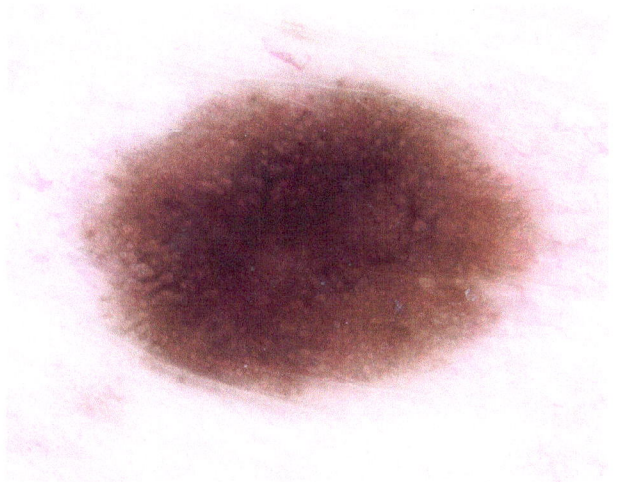
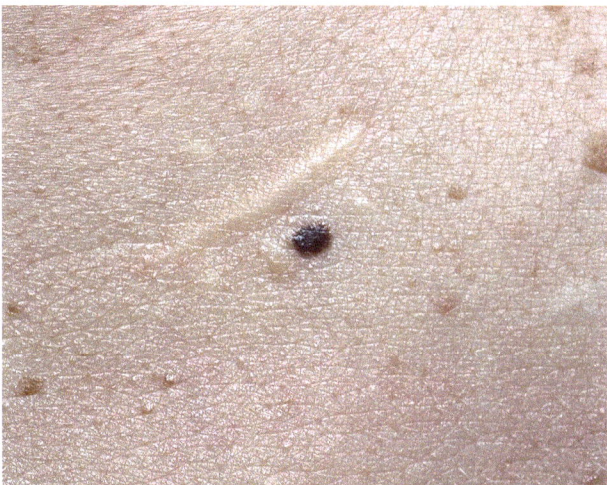
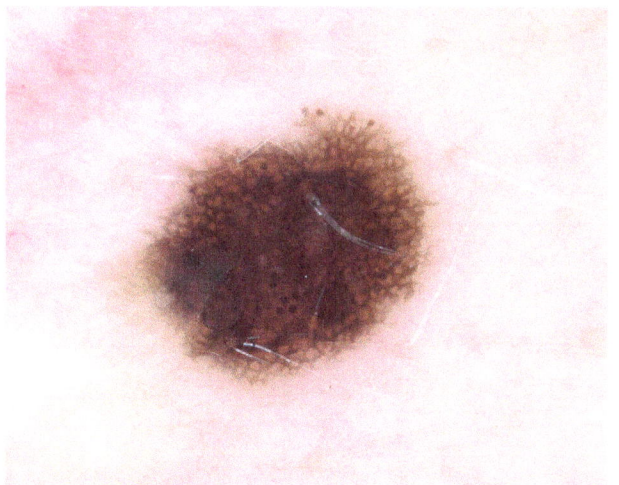

Table 10.20

	Pattern	Color	Clues	Dermatoscopic diagnosis	Histopathologic diagnosis
Top	More than one pattern (clods and structureless)	Brown, orange, yellow, white	Clues to seborrheic keratosis: White and yellow clods, looped vessels	Seborrheic keratosis	Seborrheic keratosis
Middle	More than one pattern (dots and structureless), arranged asymmetrically (chaos)	Brown and skin-colored, central hypopigmentation	Clue to melanoma: None, the brown dots at the periphery are not specific	Most likely "superficial and deep" congenital nevus	"Superficial and deep" congenital nevus
Bottom	More than one pattern (reticular and structureless), arranged asymmetrically (chaos)	More than one color	Clues to melanoma: Gray clods and white lines	Melanoma	Melanoma

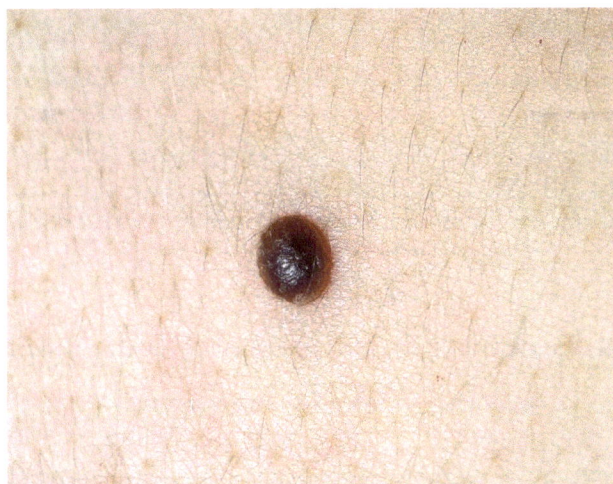
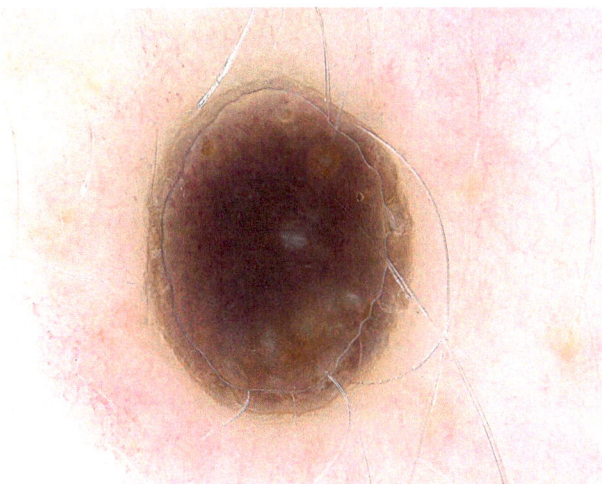
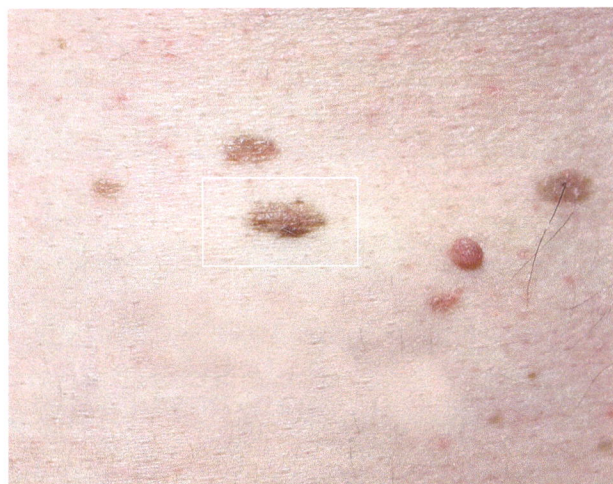

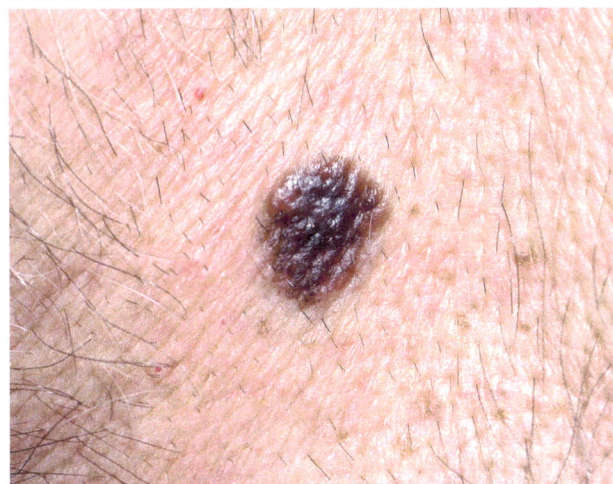
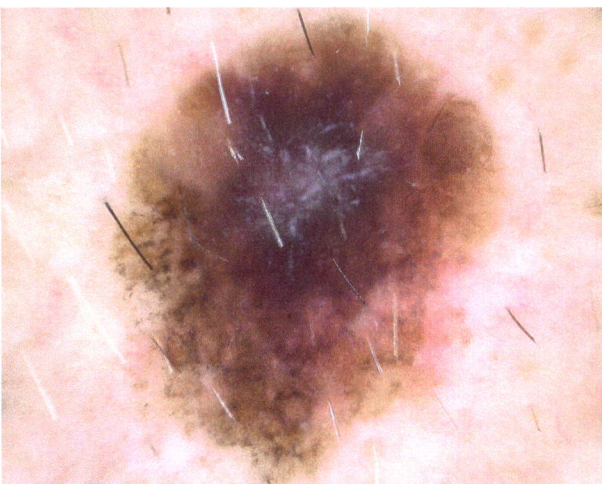

Table 10.21

	Pattern	Color	Clues	Dermatoscopic diagnosis	Histopathologic diagnosis
Top	More than one pattern (thick curved lines and clods)	Brown	Clues to seborrheic keratosis: Discrete circles and thick curved lines	Seborrheic keratosis	Seborrheic keratosis
Middle	One pattern (structureless)	Blue and brown (arranged symmetrically)	None	Blue nevus. The discrete brown pigmentation in the periphery is unusual but in keeping with the diagnosis of a blue nevus.	Blue nevus
Bottom	One pattern (angulated lines)	Gray and brown	Clues to melanoma: Gray dots	Most likely melanoma in situ. Pigmented actinic keratosis or lichen planus-like keratosis (solar lentigo with regression) are less likely but not impossible.	Melanoma in situ (lentigo maligna)

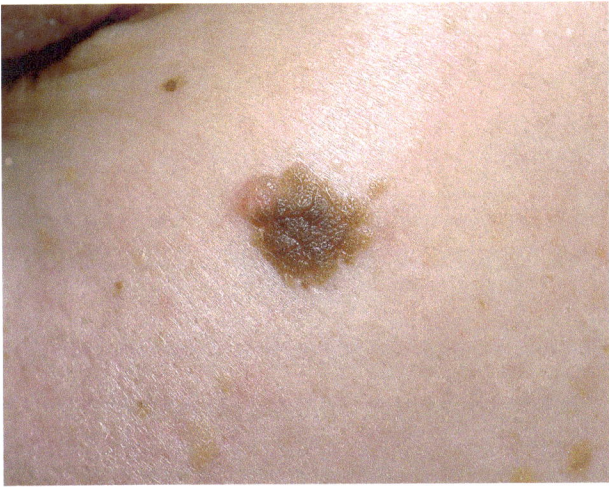
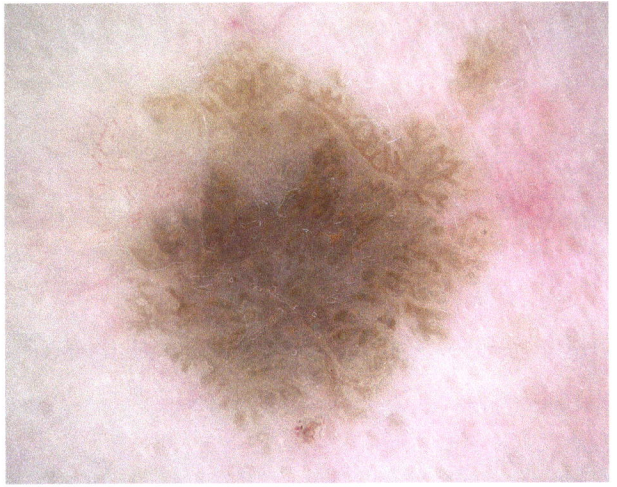
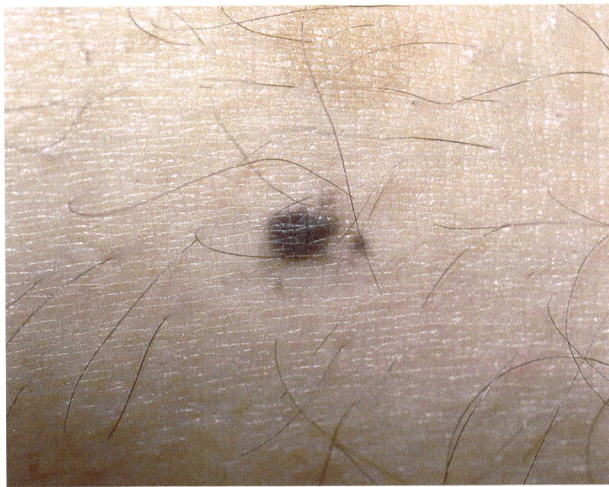
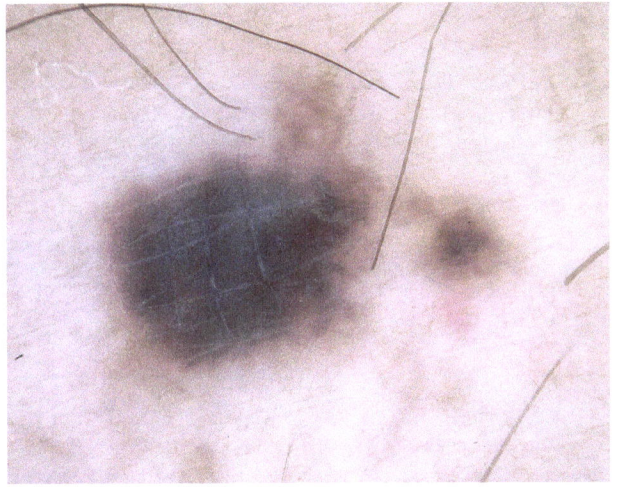
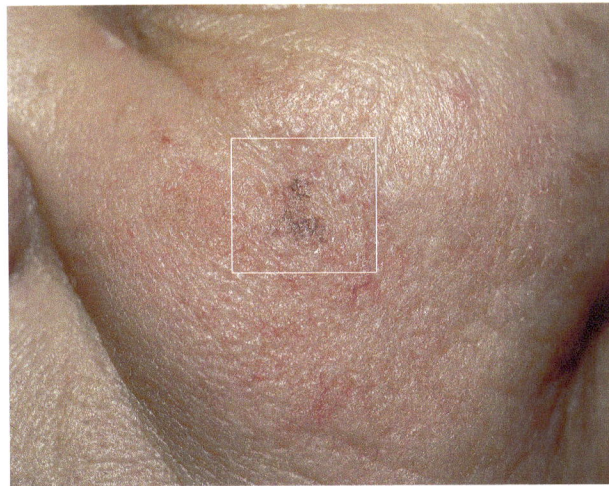
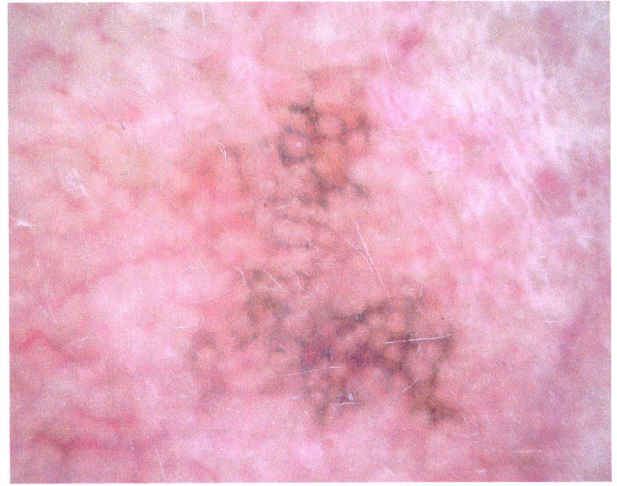

Table 10.22

	Pattern	Color	Clues	Dermatoscopic diagnosis	Histopathologic diagnosis
Top	One pattern (reticular)	Brown	None	Clark nevus	Not excised
Middle	More than one pattern (reticular in the periphery, structureless in the center), arranged symmetrically	Brown	None	Clark nevus, "superficial" congenital nevus, or "superficial and deep" congenital nevus	Not excised
Bottom	One pattern (structureless)	Brown	Terminal hairs are a clue to a congenital nevus	"Superficial and deep" congenital nevus	Not excised

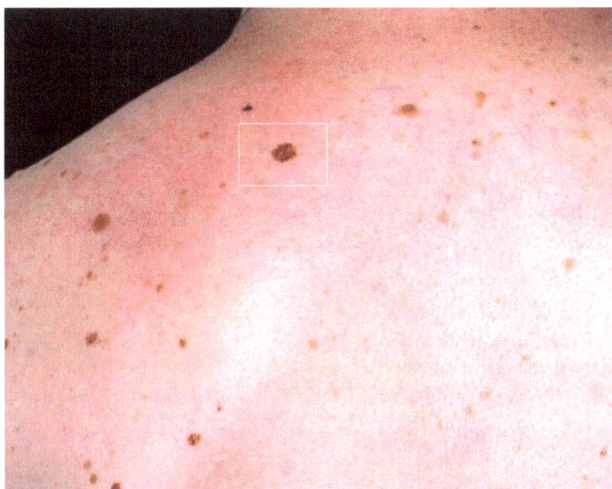
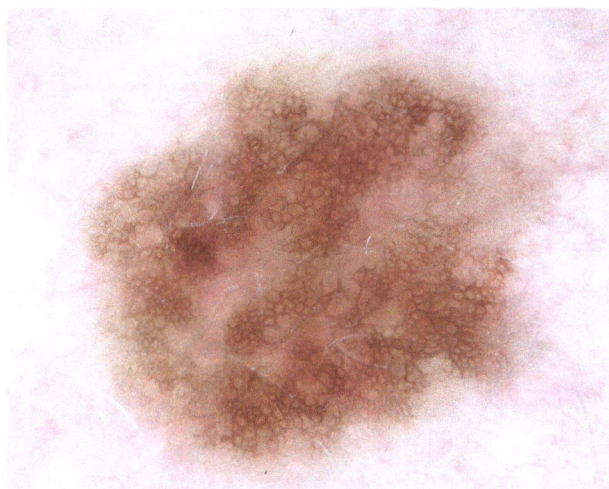
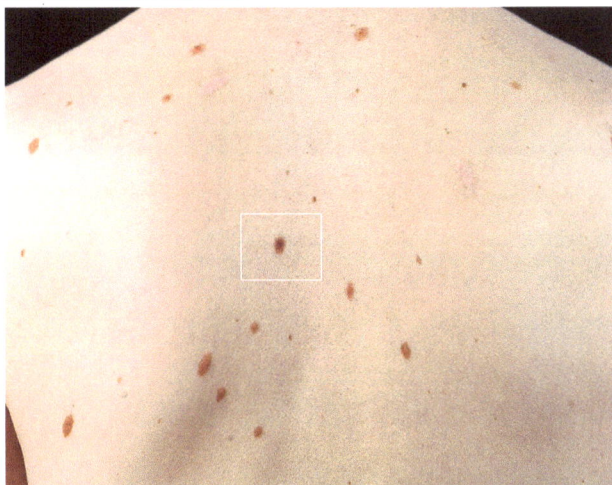
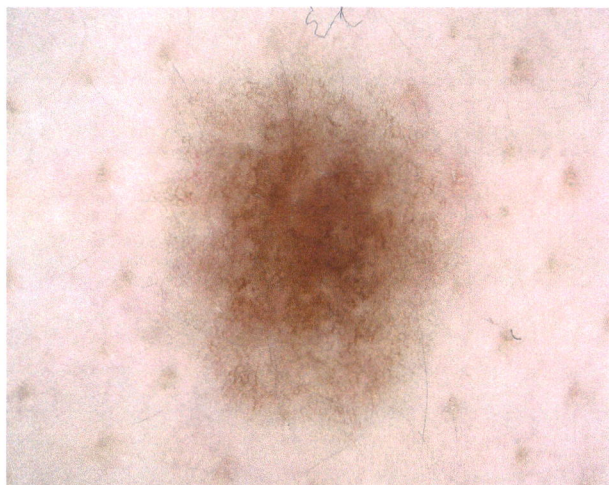
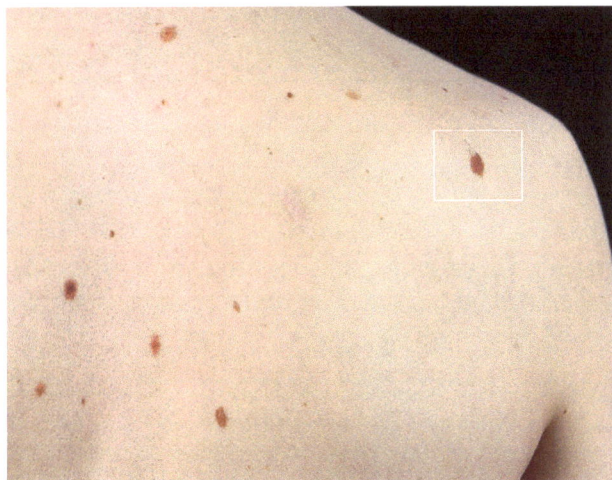
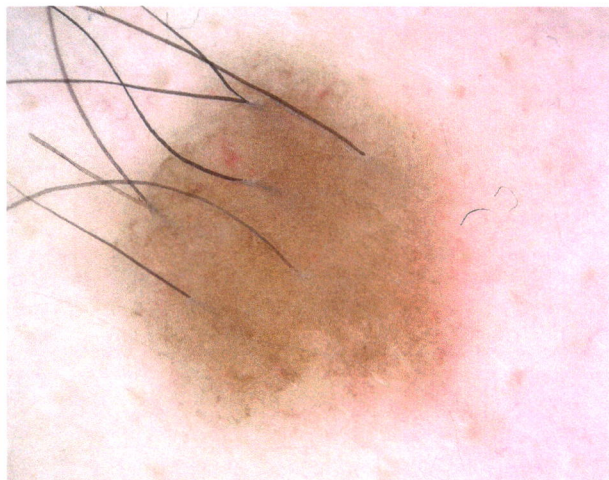

Table 10.23

	Pattern	Color	Clues	Dermatoscopic diagnosis	Histopathologic diagnosis
Top	One pattern (clods)	Yellow, orange, brown, and white	Yellow, orange, and white clods are a clues to seborrheic keratosis	Seborrheic keratosis	Seborrheic keratosis
Middle	More than one pattern (clods in the periphery, structureless in the center), arranged symmetrically	Central hyperpigmentation (dark brown)	Clods in the periphery are a clue to a growing nevus	Growing Clark nevus or Spitz nevus	Clark nevus
Bottom	One pattern (reticular)	Eccentric hyperpigmentation	Clue to melanoma: Thick reticular lines	Melanoma	"Superficial" congenital nevus

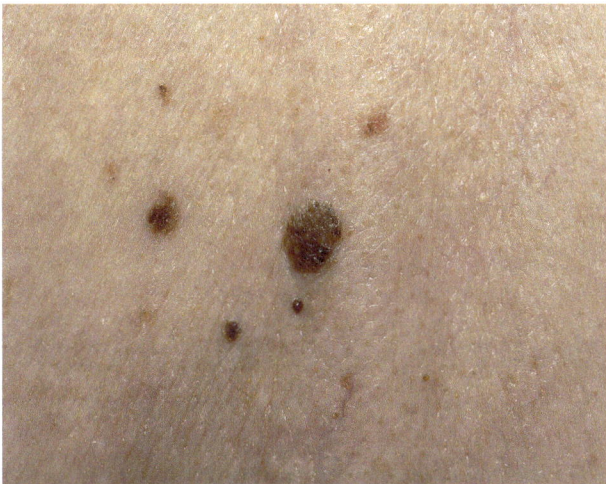
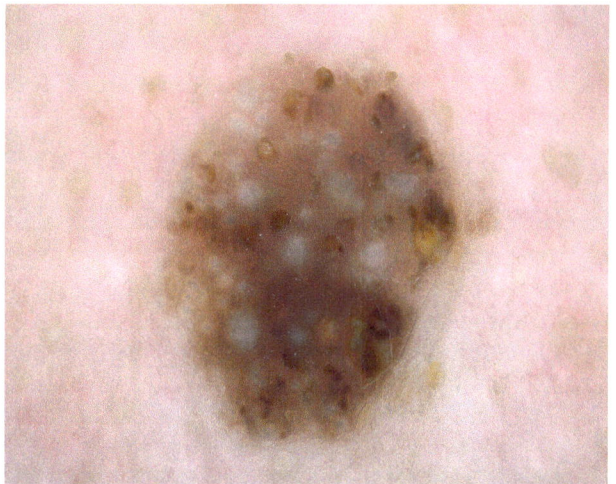
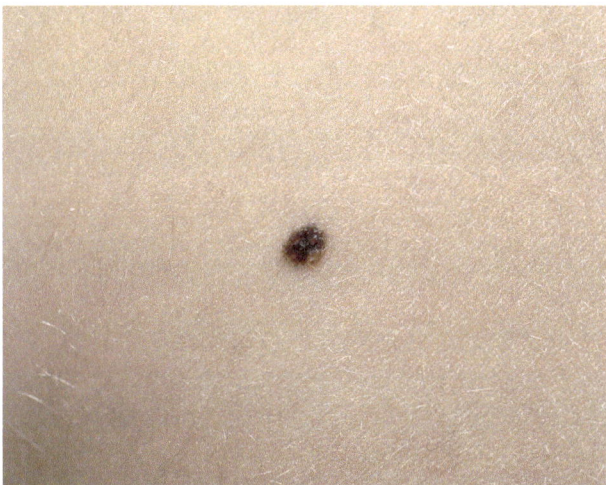
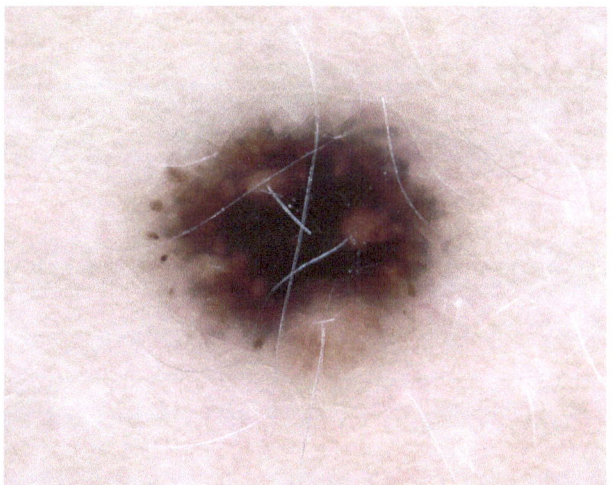
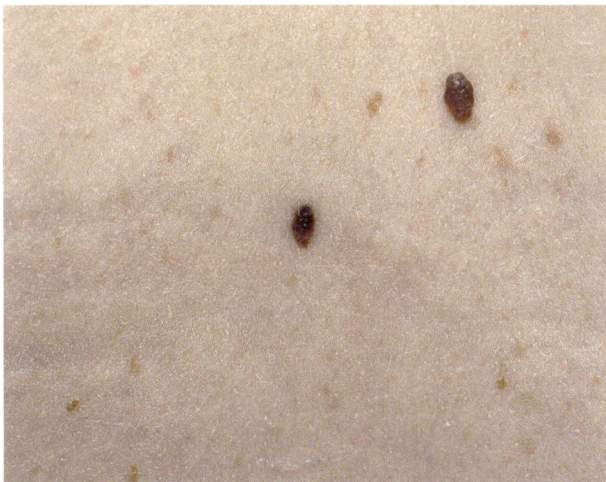
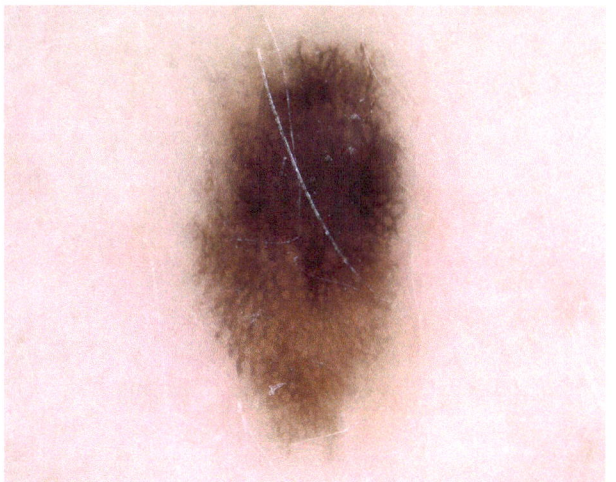

Table 10.24

	Pattern	Color	Clues	Dermatoscopic diagnosis	Histopathologic diagnosis
Top	Non-pigmented lesion, nodule	Pink	Serpentine vessels, branched	Most likely basal cell carcinoma but any neoplasm that grows underneath the superficial vascular plexus may have serpentine branched vessels on dermatoscopy	Basal cell carcinoma
Middle	One pattern (curved lines)	Brown	Curved lines and a well-demarcated scalloped border are clues to solar lentigo	Solar lentigo	Not excised
Bottom	More than one pattern (dots and structureless) arranged asymmetrically (chaos). The alternative interpretation of one pattern (structureless) would lead to the same diagnosis.	Gray (dots) and orange and pink	Clue to basal cell carcinoma: Gray clods, orange structureless zone (ulceration), and serpentine vessels	Basal cell carcinoma	Basal cell carcinoma

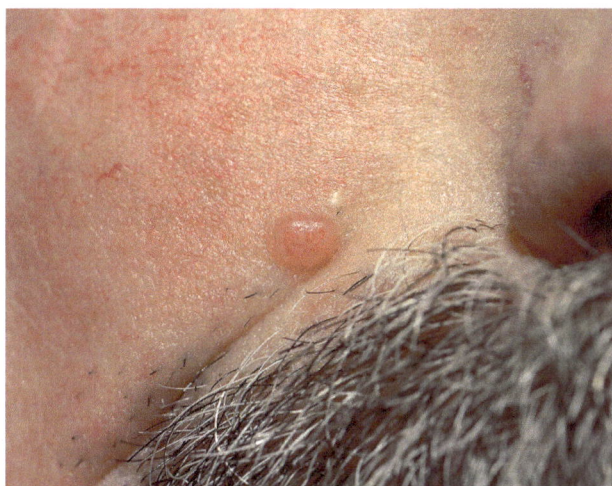
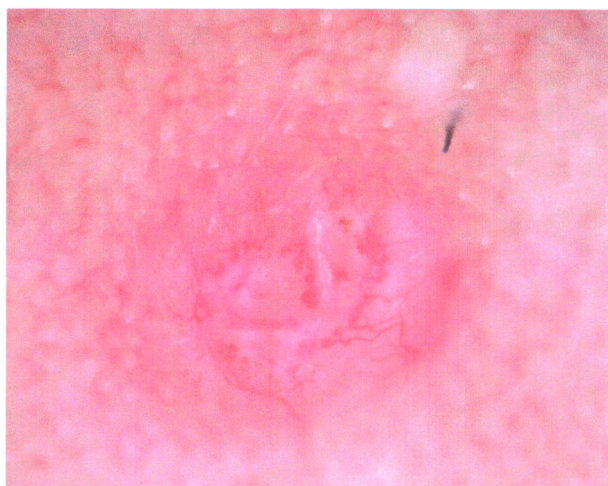
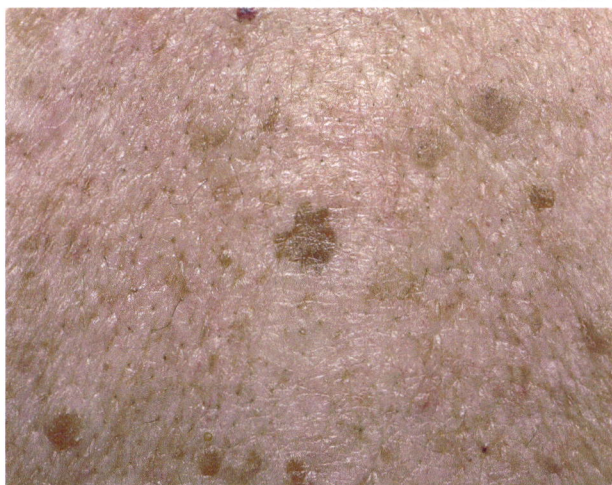
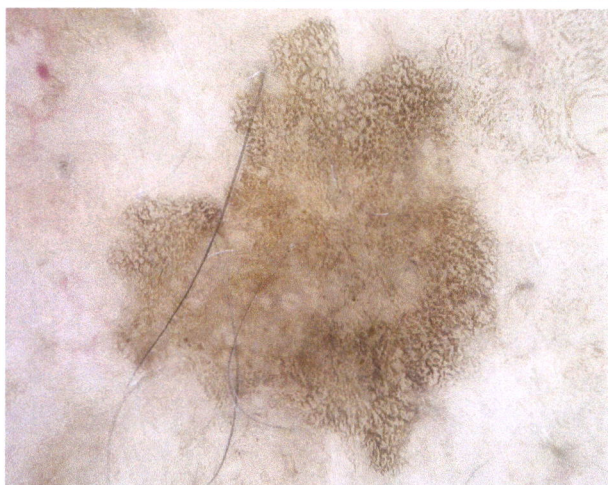
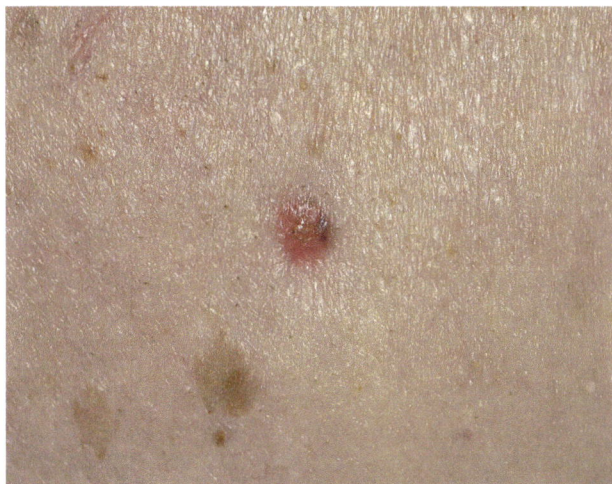
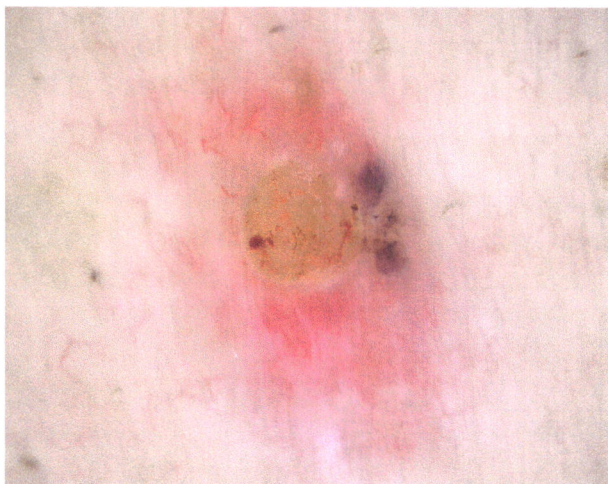

Table 10.25

	Pattern	Color	Clues	Dermatoscopic diagnosis	Histopathologic diagnosis
Top	Non-pigmented lesion, nodule	Pink	White lines (clue to malignancy), serpentine vessels, branched	Most likely basal cell carcinoma but any neoplasm that grows underneath the superficial vascular plexus may have serpentine branched vessels on dermatoscopy	Metastasis of a malignant peripheral nerve sheath tumor
Middle	More than one pattern (reticular in the periphery, structureless in the center)	Central hypopigmentation	A structureless white center in the context of reticular lines in the periphery is a clue to dermatofibroma	Dermatofibroma	Not excised
Bottom	More than one pattern (reticular, clods, structureless) arranged asymmetrically (chaos)	More than one color (brown, gray, skin)	Clue to melanoma: Gray clods	Melanoma	Melanoma

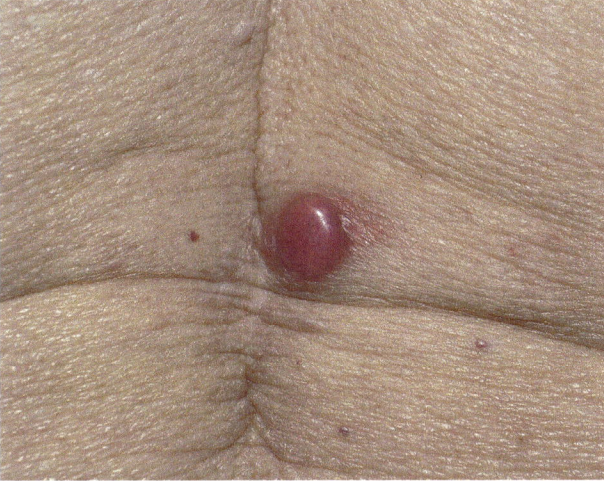
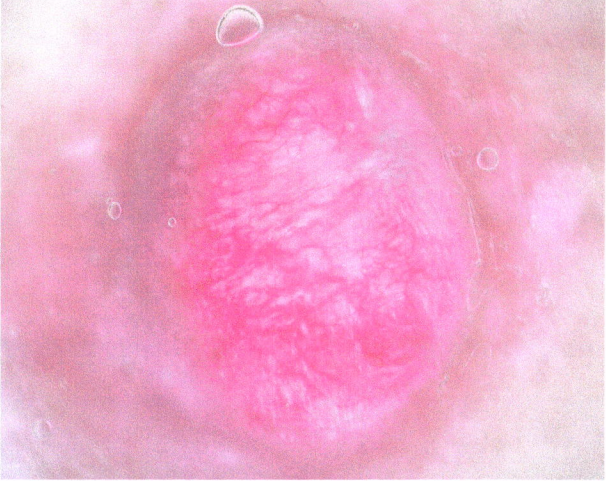
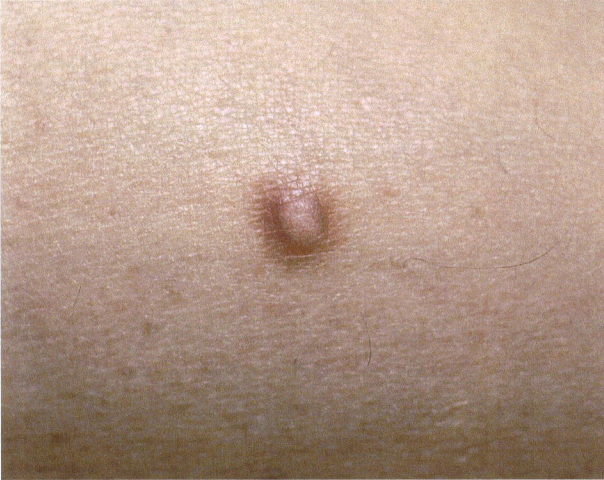
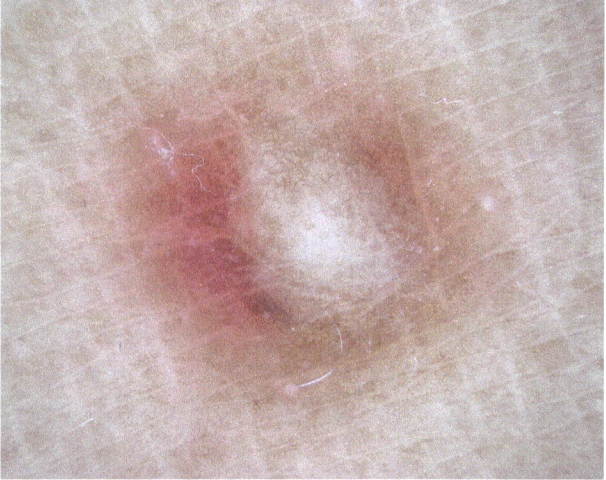
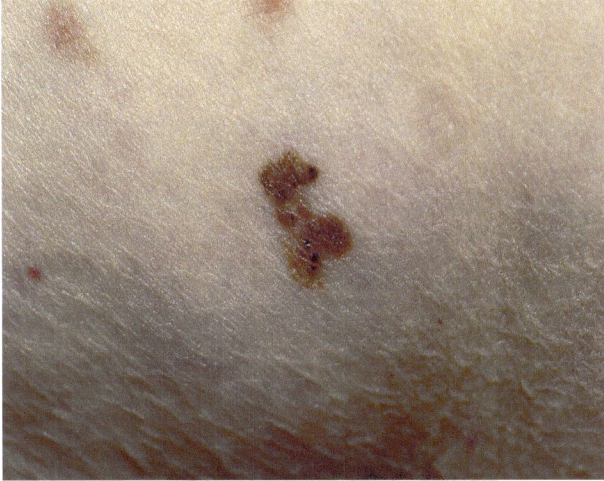
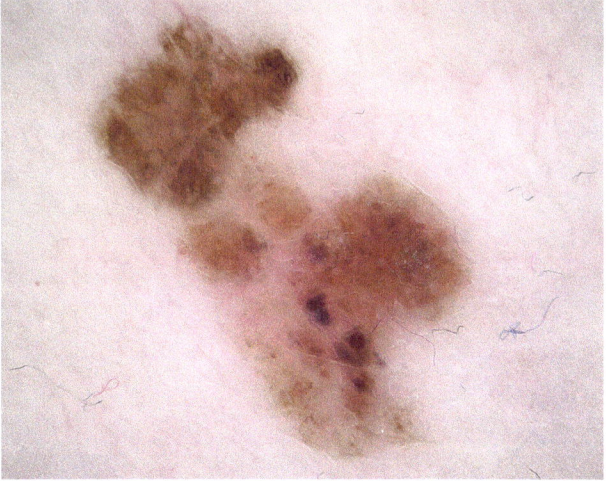

Table 10.26

	Pattern	Color	Clues	Dermatoscopic diagnosis	Histopathologic diagnosis
Top	More than one pattern (reticular in the periphery, structureless in the center) arranged symmetrically	Brown	Terminal hairs are clues to a congenital nevus	"Superficial and deep" congenital nevus	Not excised
Middle	More than one pattern (reticular in the periphery, structureless in the center) arranged symmetrically	Central hypopigmentation	None	"Superficial and deep" congenital nevus	Not excised
Bottom	More than one pattern (reticular in the periphery, structureless in the center) arranged symmetrically	Brown	Terminal hairs are clues to a congenital nevus	"Superficial and deep" congenital nevus	Not excised

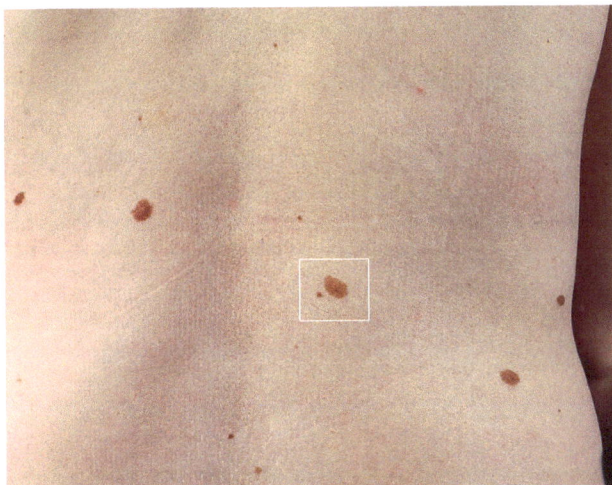
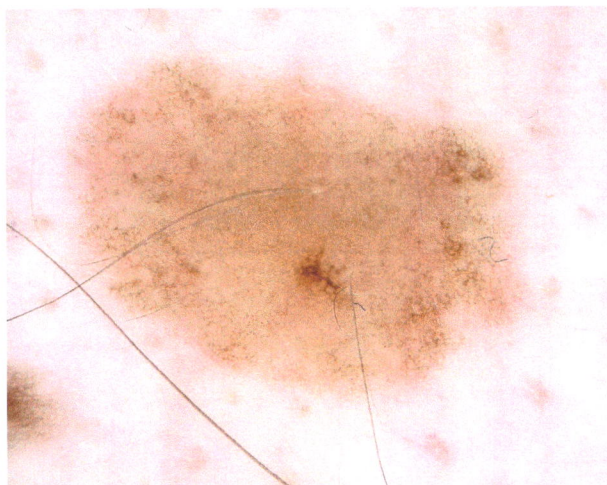
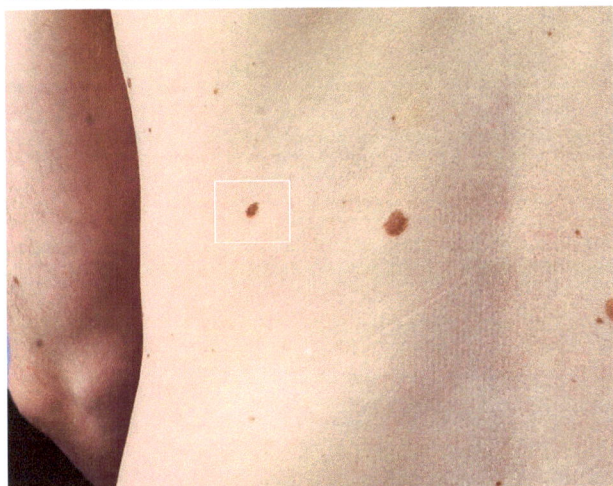
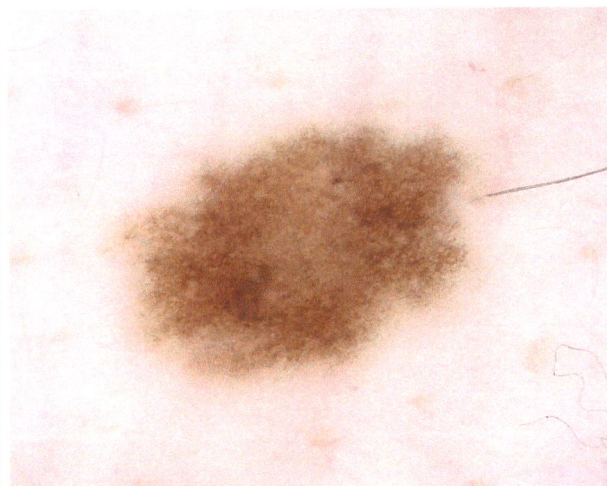
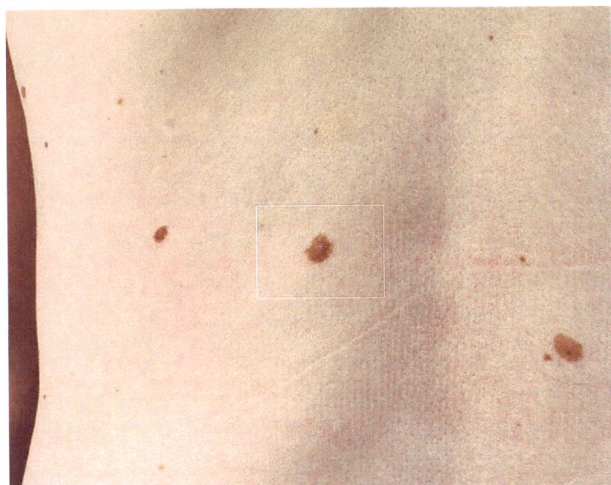
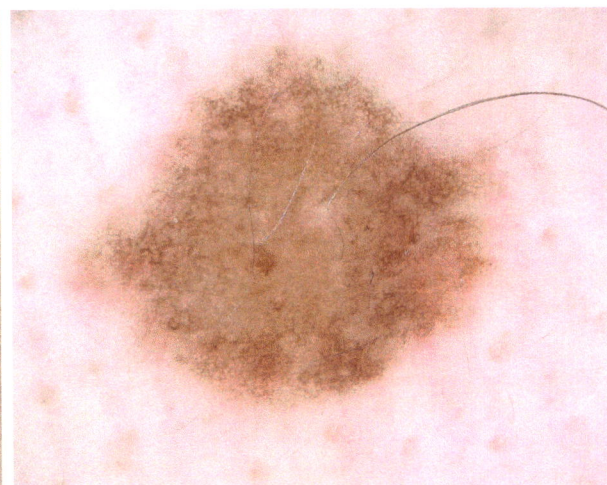

Table 10.27

	Pattern	Color	Clues	Dermatoscopic diagnosis	Histopathologic diagnosis
Top	More than one pattern (reticular and dots) arranged asymmetrically (chaos)	Brown and gray	Clues to melanoma: Gray dots, peripheral black dots	Melanoma	Melanoma
Middle	One pattern (clods)	Brown	None	"Superficial and deep" congenital nevus	"Superficial and deep" congenital nevus
Bottom	More than one pattern (clods, dots, structureless) arranged asymmetrically (chaos)	Brown, orange, gray, and white	White and orange clods are clues to a seborrheic keratosis. Gray clods are clues to basal cell carcinoma. However, the sharp circumscription and coiled vessels favor the diagnosis of seborrheic keratosis over basal cell carcinoma.	Most likely seborrheic keratosis	Seborrheic keratosis

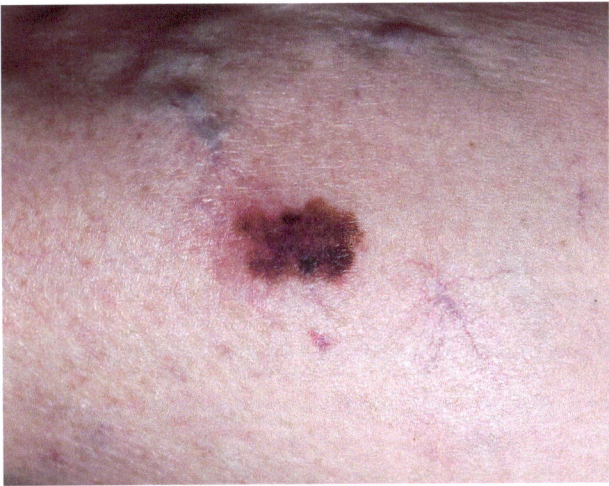
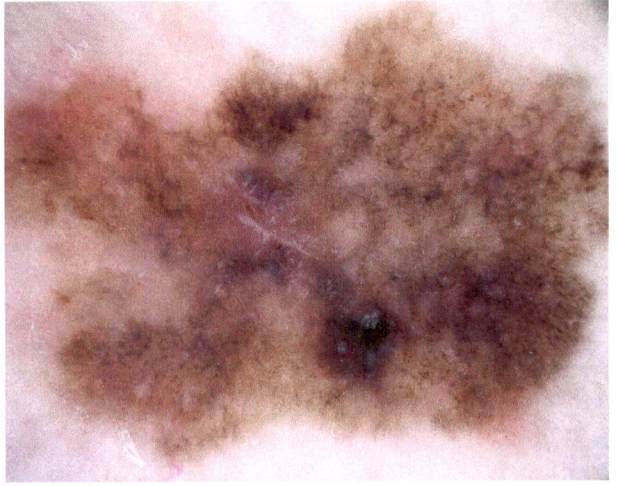
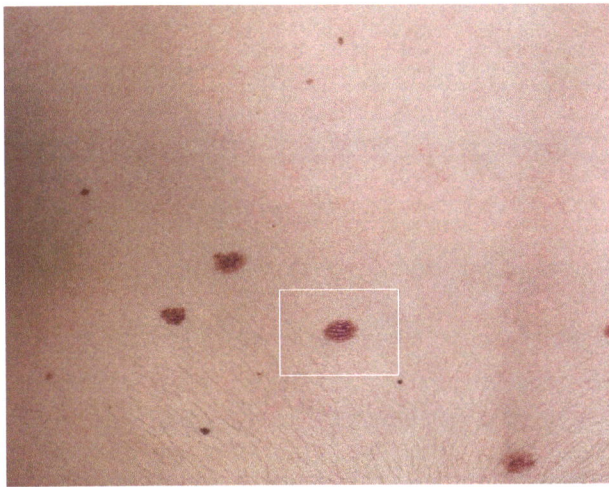
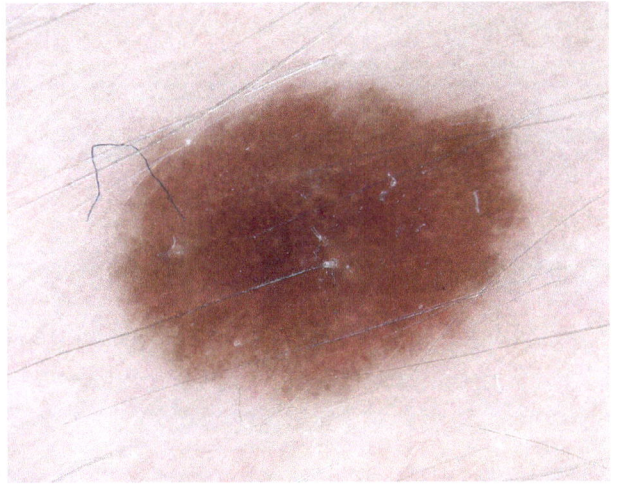
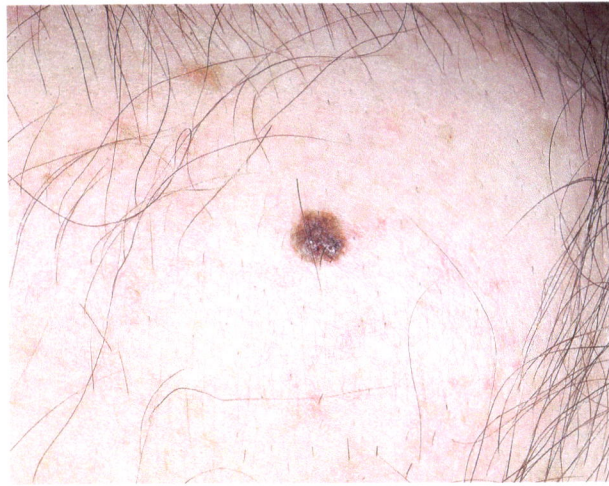
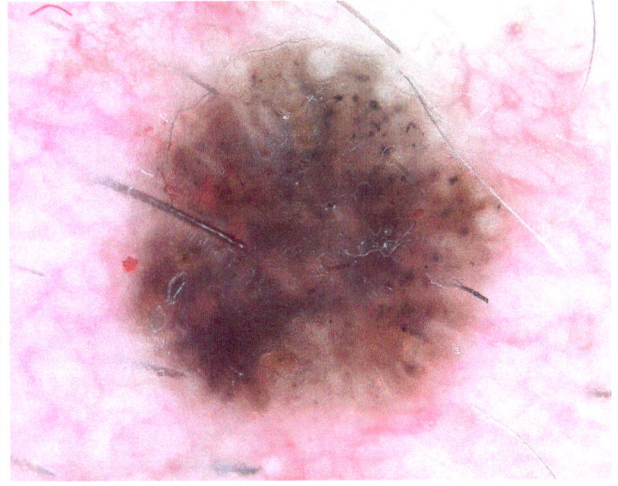

Table 10.28

	Pattern	Color	Clues	Dermatoscopic diagnosis	Histopathologic diagnosis
Top	More than one pattern (clods and structureless) arranged asymmetrically (chaos)	Clods are blue and gray	Clues to basal cell carcinoma: Blue and gray clods; serpentine, branched vessels	Basal cell carcinoma	Basal cell carcinoma
Middle	One pattern (large polygonal clods)	Brown	None	Unna nevus (a congenital nevus of one type)	Not excised
Bottom	More than one pattern (clods, and structureless) arranged asymmetrically (chaos)	More than one color (melanin dominant)	Clues to melanoma: White lines and gray clods	Melanoma	Melanoma

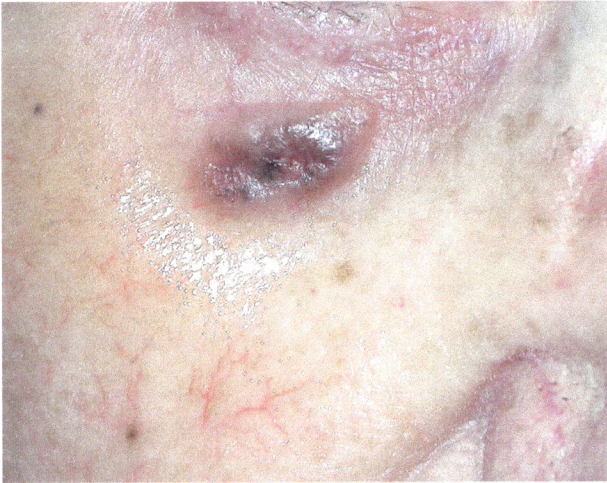
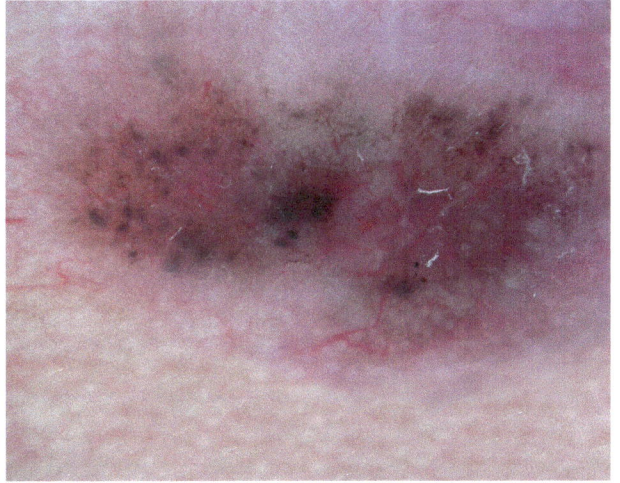
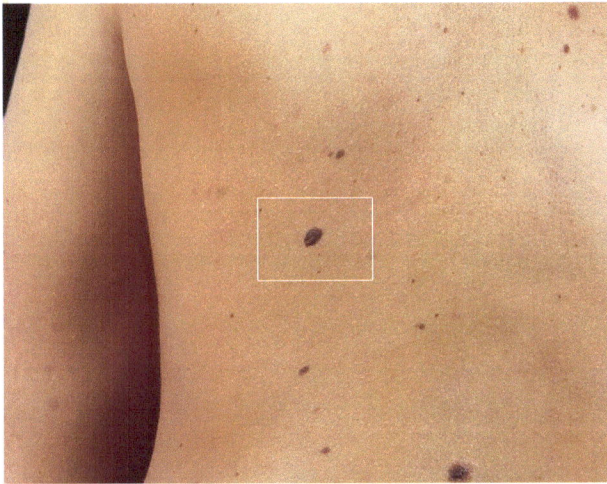
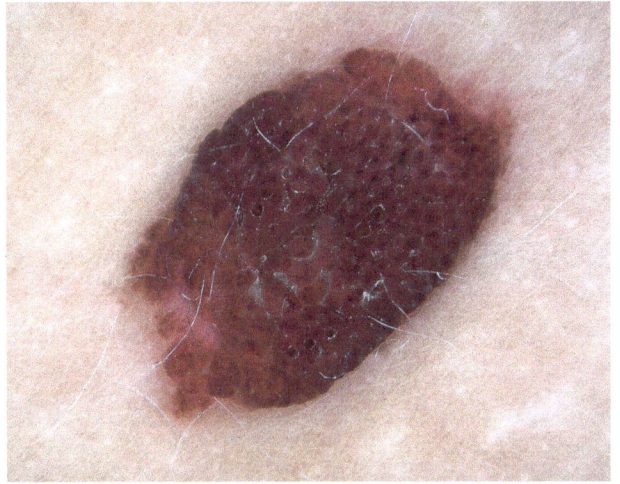
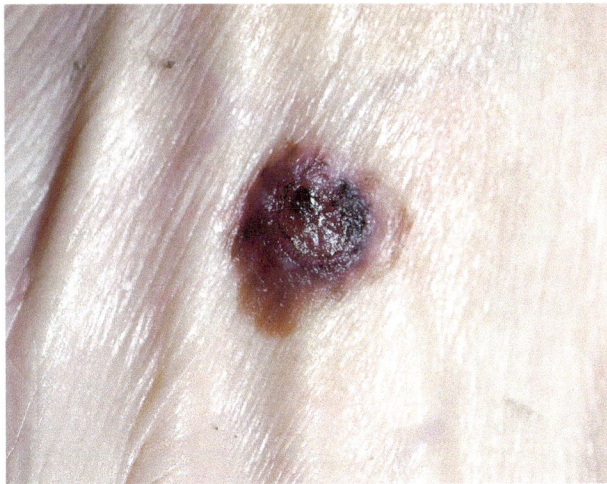
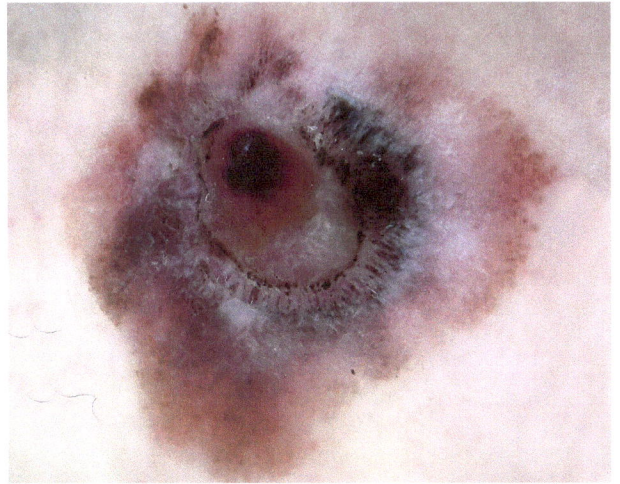

Table 10.29

	Pattern	Color	Clues	Dermatoscopic diagnosis	Histopathologic diagnosis
Top	More than one pattern (clods and structureless) arranged asymmetrically (chaos)	Black, gray and brown (melanin dominates)	Some seborrheic keratosis are so heavily pigmented that the clods appear black or dark brown and not yellow, orange, or white	Seborrheic keratosis	Seborrheic keratosis
Middle	One pattern (large polygonal clods)	Brown and skin-colored	Large polygonal, skin-colored or light brown clods are clues to a mainly intradermal congenital nevus (Unna nevus)	Unna nevus (a congenital nevus of one type)	Unna nevus
Bottom	More than one pattern (clods, and structureless) arranged asymmetrically (chaos)	More than color (melanin dominant)	Clues to melanoma: Gray clods, white lines, pseudopods, eccentric structureless area	Melanoma	Melanoma

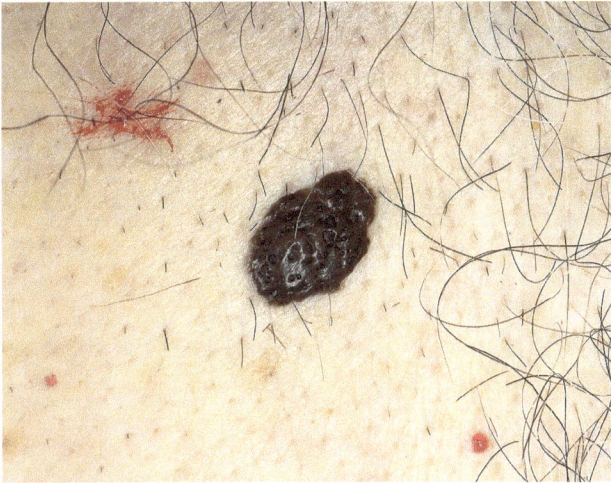
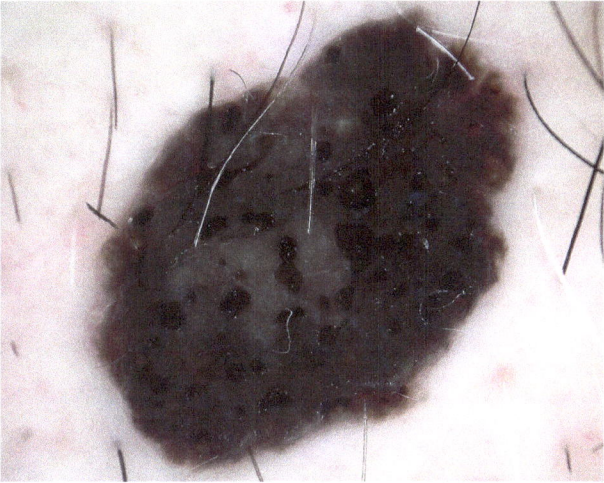
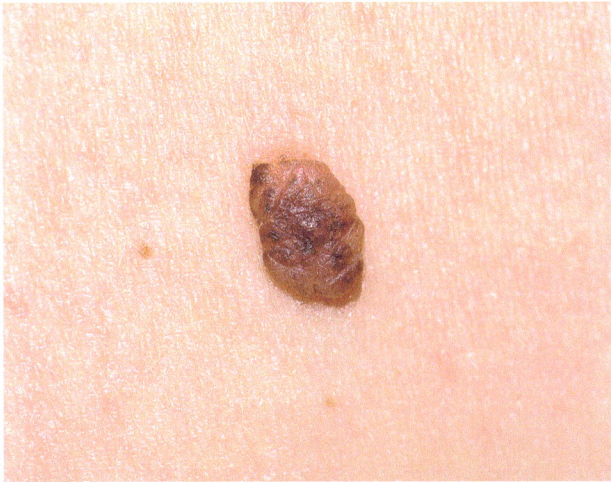
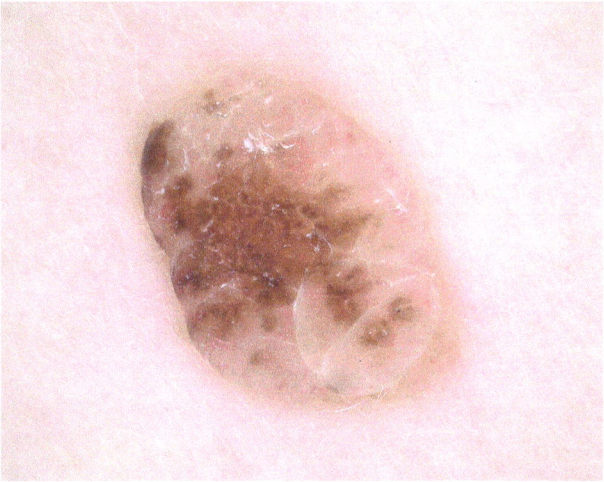
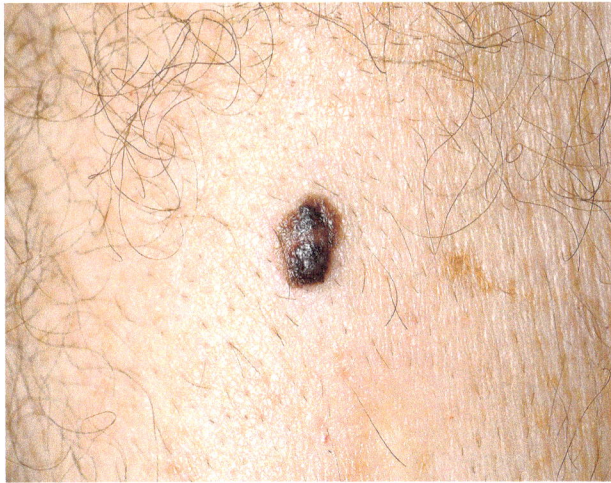
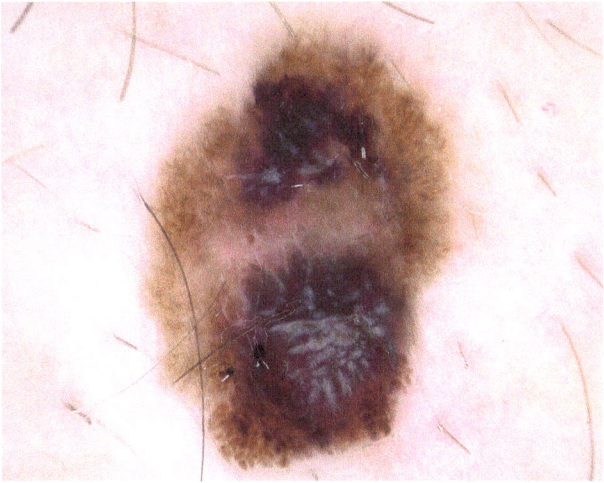

Table 10.30

	Pattern	Color	Clues	Dermatoscopic diagnosis	Histopathologic diagnosis
Top	One pattern (clods). The clods are arranged in the furrows but this does not make them parallel lines.	Brown	None	"Superficial and deep" congenital nevus	"Superficial and deep" congenital nevus
Middle	More than one pattern (clods, and structureless) arranged asymmetrically (chaos)	Clods are gray and brown	Clues to malignancy: Gray clods and white lines. The small zone of ulceration (small red clod) favors basal cell carcinoma.	Basal cell carcinoma	Basal cell carcinoma
Bottom	More than one pattern (clods and structureless) arranged asymmetrically (chaos)	More than one color (melanin dominant)	Clues to melanoma: Black dots in the periphery, segmental radial lines, eccentric, structureless area	Melanoma	Melanoma

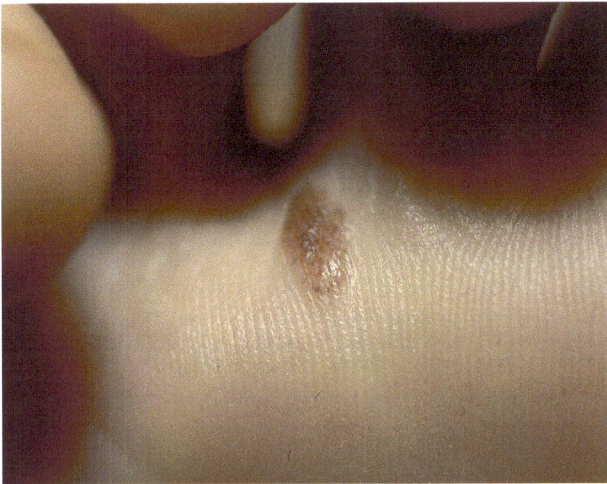

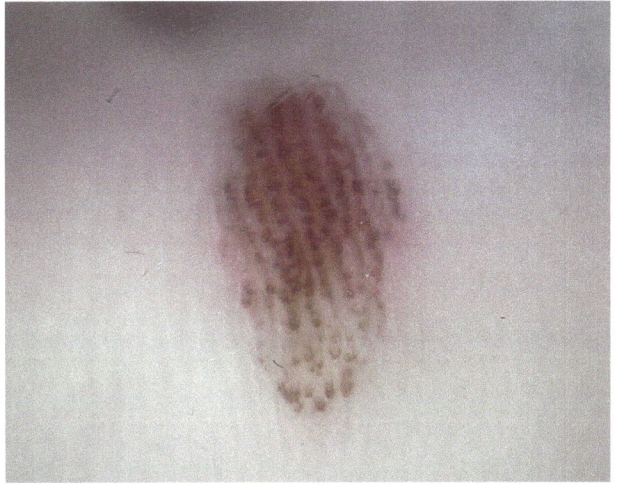

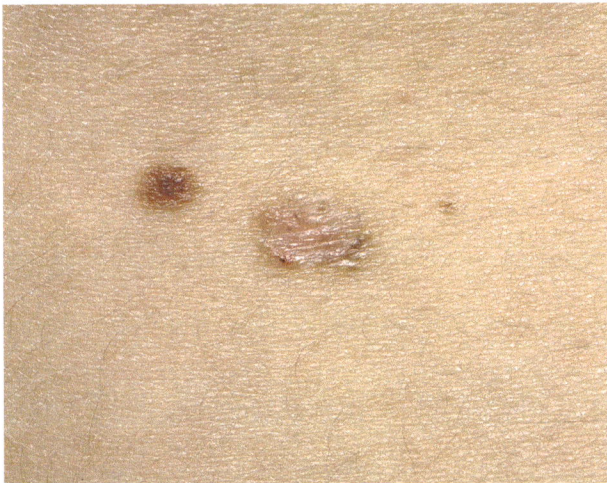

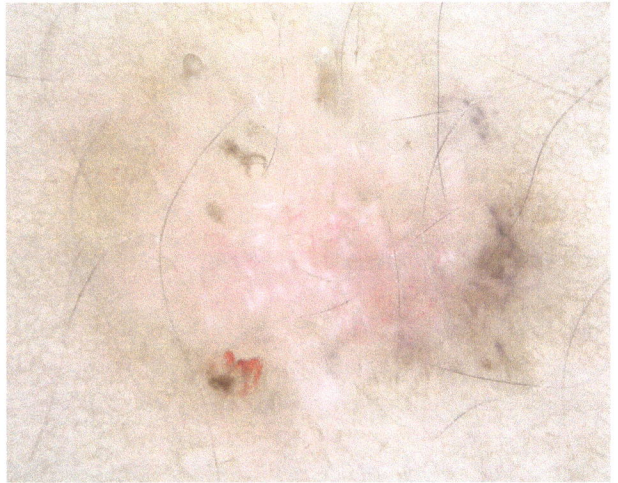

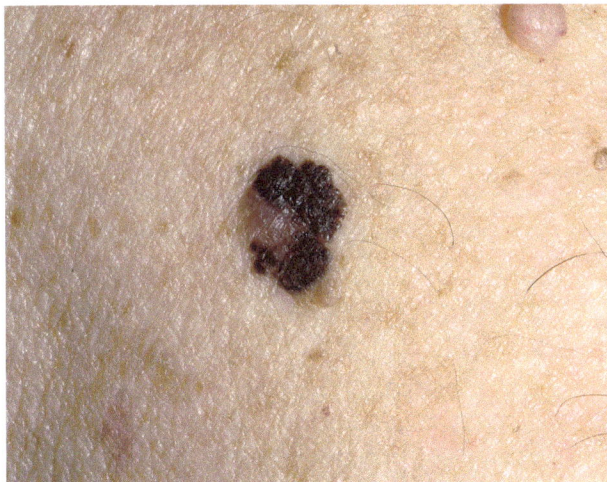

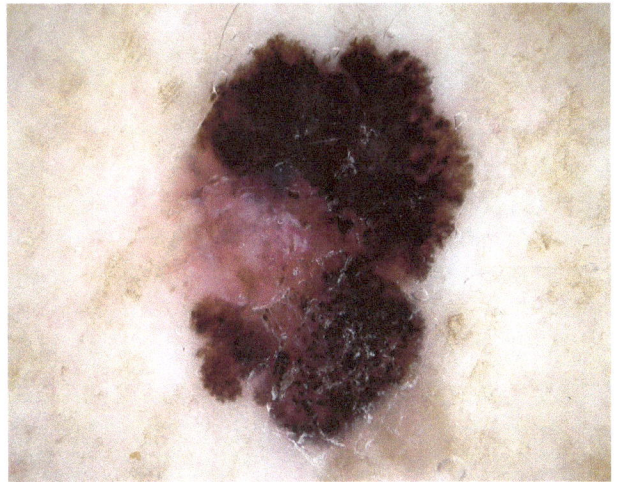

Table 10.31

	Pattern	Color	Clues	Dermatoscopic diagnosis	Histopathologic diagnosis
Top	One pattern (reticular)	Brown	None	Clark nevus	Clark nevus
Middle	One pattern (parallel lines on the ridges)	Brown	Parallel lines on the ridges are found in acral melanoma, hemorrhage, and exogenous pigmentation	Acral melanoma, hemorrhage, or exogenous pigmentation	Intracorneal hemorrhage
Bottom	One pattern (parallel lines on the ridges)	Brown	Parallel lines on the ridges are found in acral melanoma, hemorrhage, and exogenous pigmentation	Acral melanoma, hemorrhage, or exogenous pigmentation	Intracorneal hemorrhage

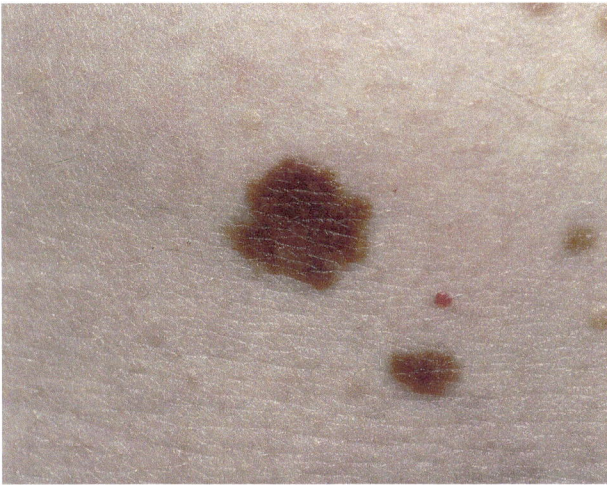
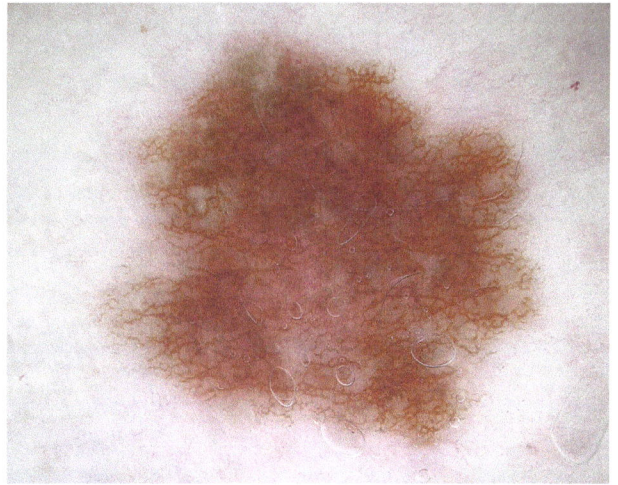
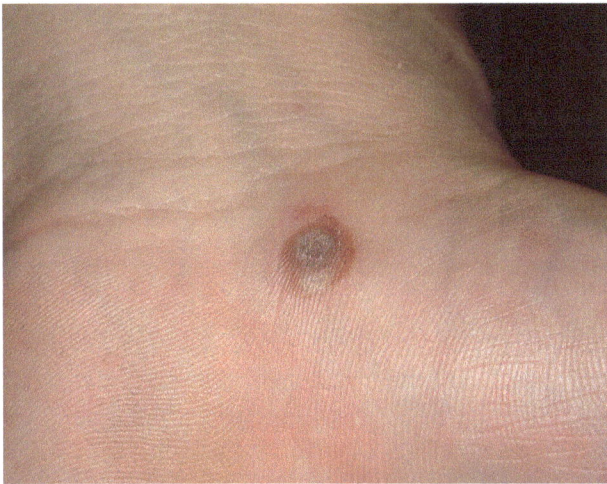
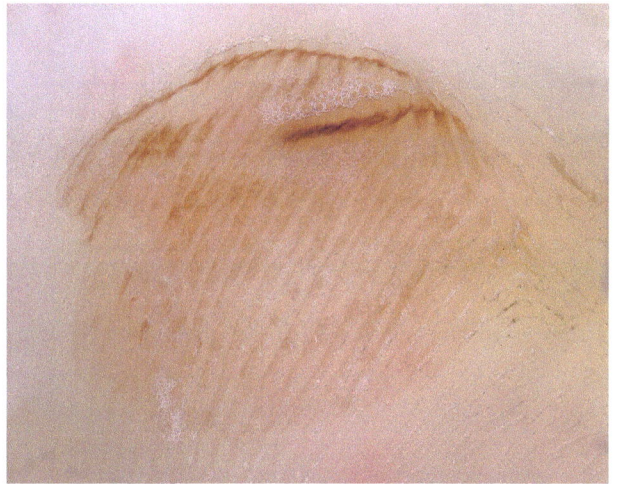
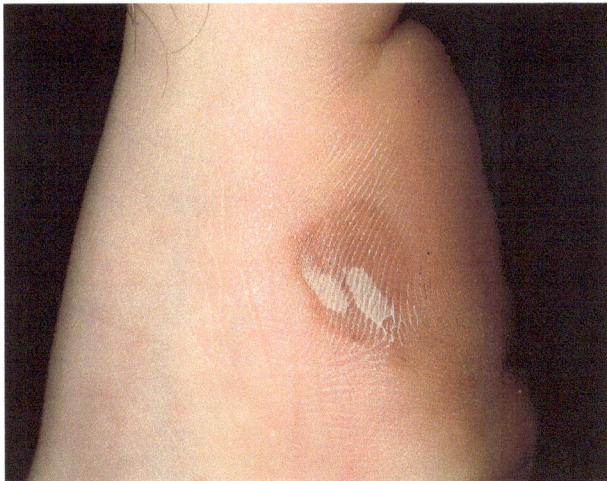
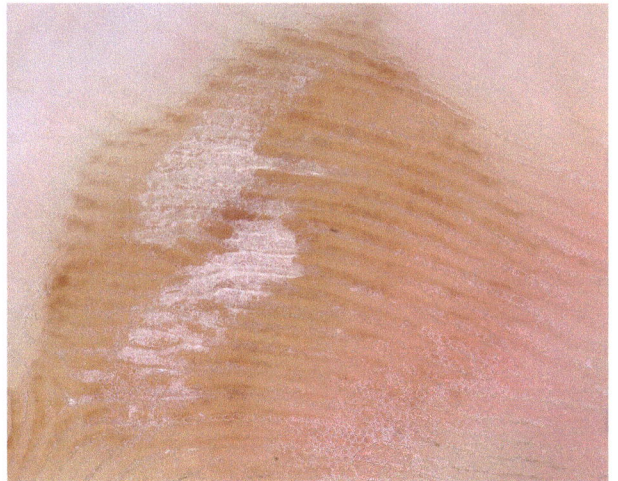

11 Dermatoscopic-dermatopathologic correlation

Knowledge of histopathology and correlation with the dermatoscopic findings increases understanding of dermatoscopy (1–6). It permits a significant level of interpretation of dermatoscopic patterns and clues even when a specific diagnosis cannot be reached. To a degree, it is also possible to predict histopathology from the findings on dermatoscopy. An example is the interpretation of reticular lines, which may have six different histopathological correlates *(11.1).* The most common cause of reticular lines is hyperpigmentation of basal keratinocytes. While melanin is produced in melanocytes it is often transferred to keratinocytes in the form of melanosomes. Thus an increase in the number of melanocytes is not necessary to produce reticular lines. Hyperpigmentation of basal keratinocytes is seen as reticular lines on dermatoscopy because in the rete ridges several keratinocytes filled with melanin are superimposed on each other while just a thin layer of pigmented keratinocytes is found on the tips of the dermal papillae *(11.1A).* The hypopigmented intervening spaces correlate with the dermal papilla lying below it. Quite often a capillary is centered in the papilla, which is seen on dermatoscopy as a dot vessel as in a hypopigmented space. The hyperpigmented lines correspond to the rete ridges. It should be noted that dermal papillae shrink to a greater extent than epithelial rete ridges during histopathologic processing.

Keeping these anatomical features in mind, the base of the rete ridges should also be hypopigmented because

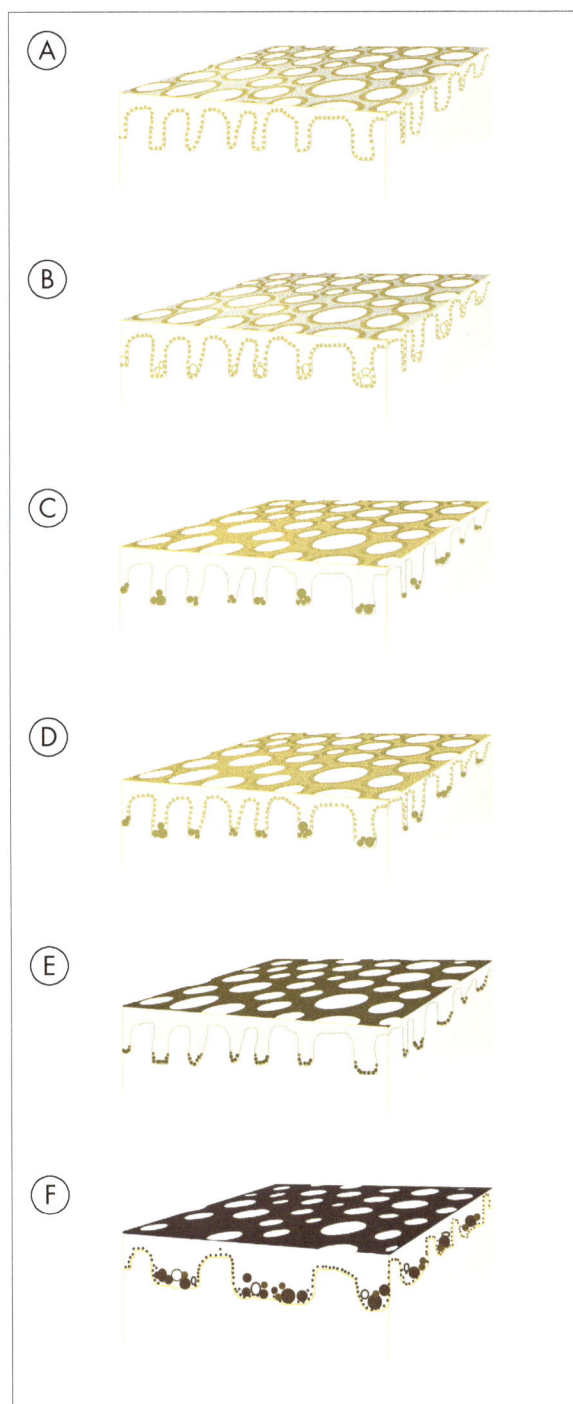

Figure 11.1: Correlation of dermatoscopy and histopathology – reticular lines.
A: Hyperpigmentation of basal keratinocytes, no increase in melanocytes, B: Hyperpigmentation of basal keratinocytes with an increased number of melanocytes which are arranged in nests. In this case the melanocytes are unpigmented and therefore invisible on dermatoscopy, C: Proliferation of pigmented melanocytes at the base of rete ridges. The melanocytes are spread out like a carpet and coat the base of the rete ridges. Viewed from above with dermatoscopy this appears as reticular lines (network). Viewed in cross-section on histopathology the melanocytes appear to be arranged as single cells or in small nests. D: Mixture of A and C, E: Hyperpigmentation of basal keratinocytes, but only at the base of rete ridges, F: The rete ridges are broadened and filled with pigmented melanocytes. This appears as thick reticular lines on dermatoscopy.

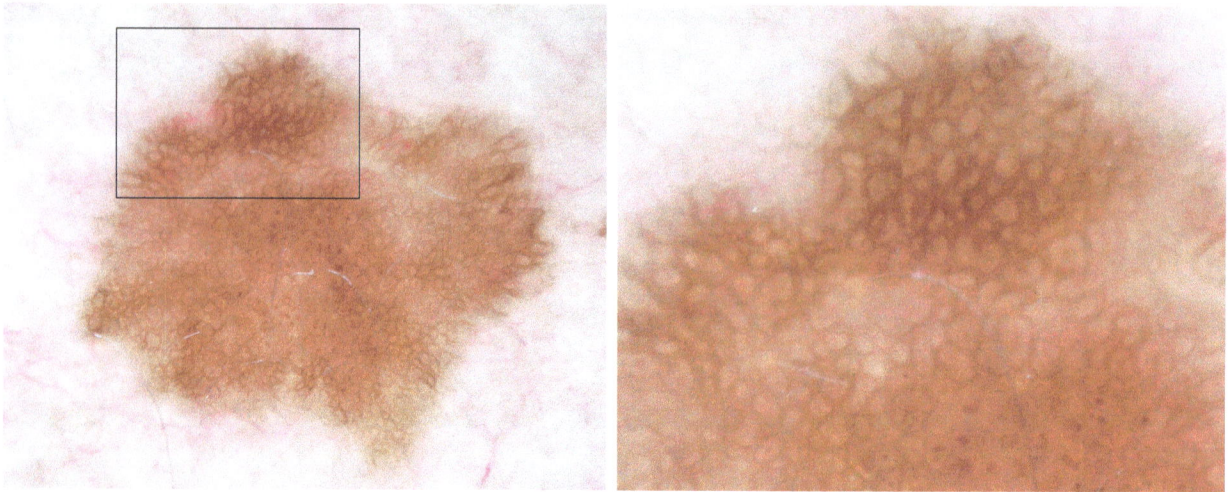

Figure 11.2: Reticular double lines.
With magnification one sees that the reticular lines in this Clark nevus have a hypopigmented zone in their center. This zone corresponds to the base of the rete ridges.

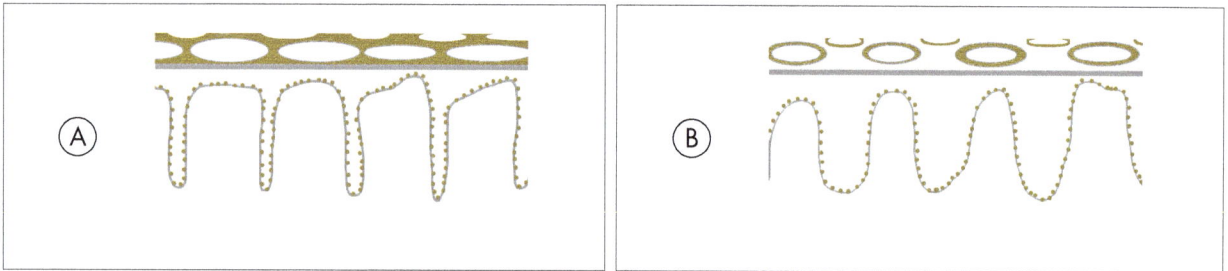

Figure 11.3: Relationship between reticular lines and circles.
When the rete ridges are narrow compared to the dermal papillae, hyperpigmentation of basal keratinocytes is seen as a reticular pattern **(A)**. When the papillae are broad one sees circles instead of reticular lines **(B)**. On the face, circles are produced by a different mechanism, pigmentation surrounding the infundibular openings.

one finds just a thin layer of melanin at this site as well, and occasionally one does actually see double lines *(11.2)*.

However, compared to the dermal papilla this zone is quite narrow and therefore usually creates the impression of a single line. Very broad rete ridges create a pattern of circles rather than reticular lines *(11.3)*.

For this reason, a pattern of closely adjacent circles in lesions on the trunk or limbs should be interpreted identically to a pattern of reticular lines.

As a proliferation of melanocytes is not necessary to produce reticular lines, it is not surprising that some non-melanocytic lesions have reticular lines on dermatoscopy. Typical examples are solar lentigines, flat seborrheic keratoses and dermatofibromas.

Therefore it is impossible to establish, on the basis of reticular lines, whether a lesion is melanocytic or non-melanocytic *(11.4)*.

In melanocytic lesions the melanocytes are increased in number and at least partly arranged in nests. When a nevus is situated in the epidermis the nests are mainly at the base of the rete ridges. However, if the melanocytes that constitute the nests are not filled with melanin they are invisible on dermatoscopy. Even so, a reticular pattern may still be seen, due entirely to hyperpigmentation of basal keratinocytes *(11.1B)*. Nests of pigmented melanocytes are seen as brown dots or small brown clods. However, pigmented melanocytes at the base of rete ridges may not be arranged in nests, but may be spread out as a confluent proliferation of single cells. To use an analogy: dermal papillae extend vertically like mountain tops while the rete ridges form the intervening valleys. The valleys (base of rete ridges) are coated with a confluent proliferation of melanocytes that, when viewed from above, appear as reticular lines. However, on histological (cross-) sections the

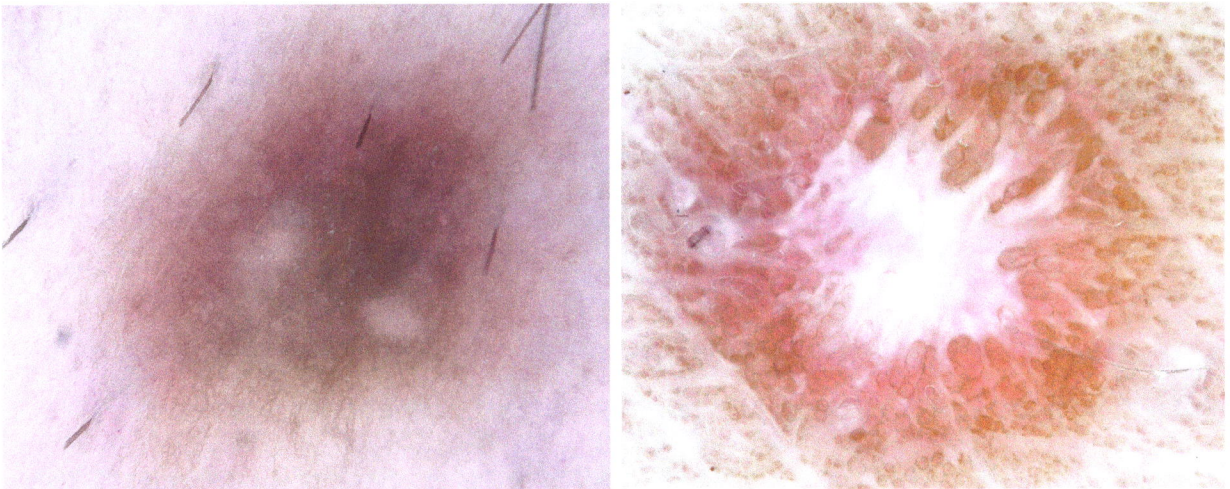

Figure 11.4: *Reticular lines and circles in dermatofibromas.*
*The dermatofibroma on the left shows reticular lines while the dermatofibroma on the right reveals circles on dermatoscopy. The histopathological correlate in both cases is hyperpigmentation of basal keratinocytes, but differing width of rete ridges produces different dermatoscopic patterns – narrow rete ridges produce reticular lines (**left**) and widened rete ridges (in this case due to acanthosis) produce circles (**right**).*

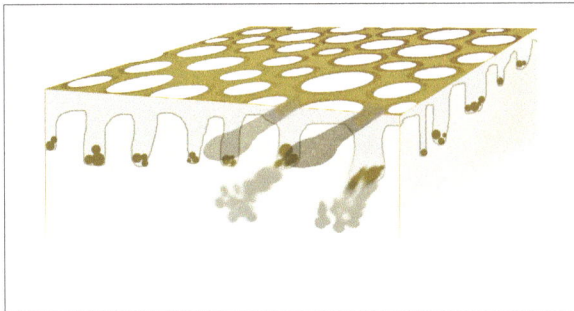

Figure 11.5: *Pseudopods.*
Pseudopods are epidermal aggregates of melanocytes (fascicles) that proliferate along the base of rete ridges. They constitute the front of a rapidly growing neoplasia and therefore spread outward from the body of the lesion. When the pseudopods occupy the entire periphery of the lesion in a symmetrical arrangement the pattern is benign, but when the pseudopods occur in only some segments the lesion is usually malignant (melanoma). Pseudopods are only identifiable on histological sections when cut lengthwise. On crosswise sections, they look like nests.

proliferation of melanocytes at the base of rete ridges look like small nests, although the melanocytes are spread out in a single layer *(11.1C)*. For the same reason, in "ink-spot" lentigo (which is marked by very strongly hyperpigmented keratinocytes at the base of rete ridges) one finds reticular lines *(11.1E)* although the melanocytes are not increased in number. When rete ridges are broadened by melanocytes filled with melanin pigment, this produces thick reticular lines and not thin ones *(11.1F)*. For this reason thick reticular lines are a dermatoscopic clue to melanoma. Pseudopods

and peripheral radial lines, on the other hand, are cohesive aggregates (fascicles) of melanocytes which are joined by bridging as a radial proliferation at the base of rete ridges *(11.5)*. White reticular lines correspond to fibrosis of the papillary dermis in conjunction with nests of pigmented melanocytes in the rete ridges. The specific histopathologic correlates of angulated lines is unclear.

Brown clods are produced by nests of melanin-filled melanocytes in the epidermis, whereas blue or gray clods are produced by nests of melanin-filled melanocytes in the dermis *(11.6)*.

Melanocytes or nests of melanocytes that are not filled with melanin are invisible on dermatoscopy. Black or dark brown dots are aggregates of melanin in melanocytes either as single cells or small nests, close to the stratum corneum *(11.6)*. Similar aggregates of melanin deeper in the epidermis produce lighter brown dots. Melanin pigment in the dermis, when located in melanophages, produces gray or blue dots *(11.6)*. The special anatomy of acral skin explains the dermatoscopic patterns of parallel lines on the ridges and furrows, as well as that of lines crossing ridges and furrows. In histological sections cut across the papillary lines, two types of rete ridges alternate on acral skin. In the middle there is a broad rete ridge located exactly below the epidermal ridge. This rete ridge is flanked by two rete ridges located below the furrows. The duct (acrosyringium) of the eccrine sweat glands extends from the middle rete ridge to the surface of the skin, emerging on the epidermal ridge. Proliferation

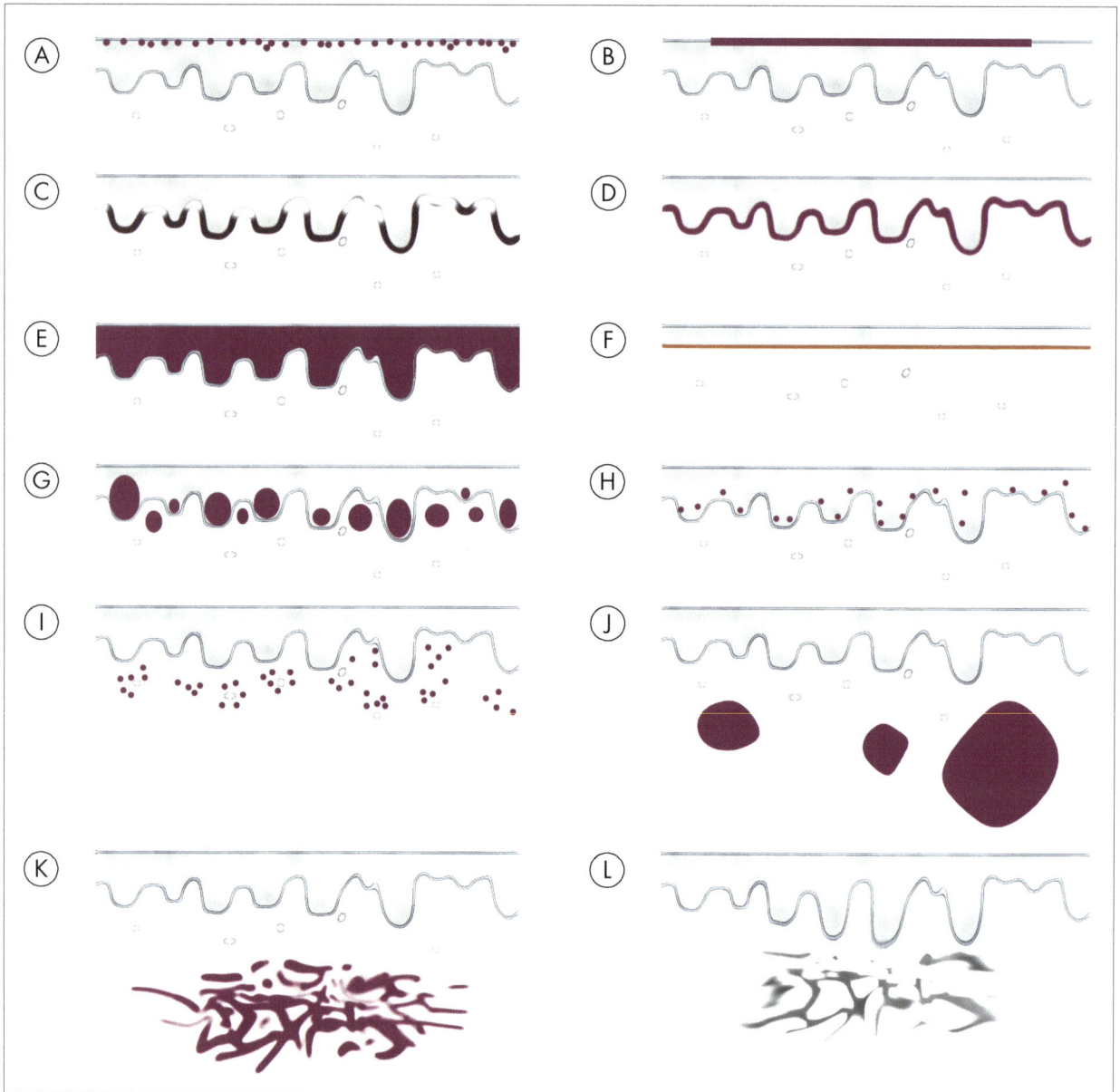

Figure 11.6: Histopathologic correlates of common dermatoscopic patterns.
A: black dots, **B:** black structureless, **C:** reticular; type ink-spot lentigo, **D:** reticular; type solar lentigo and junctional nevus, **E:** brown structureless; type seborrheic keratosis, **F:** brown structureless with loss of rete ridges, **G:** brown clods, **H:** brown dots, **I:** gray dots, **J:** gray and blue clods, **K:** blue structureless, **L:** white structureless.

of melanocytes within the flanking rete ridges causes pigmentation of the epidermal furrows while proliferation of melanocytes in the broader middle rete ridges causes pigmentation of the epidermal ridge *(11.7)*. The ridges are usually broader than the furrows, and the eccrine duct openings are seen as a row of white dots along the middle of the ridge.

In histological cross-sections cut across ridges and furrows, a contiguous proliferation of melanocytes may look like nests. However, when one looks at the dermatoscopy, pigmentation on the ridges or in the furrows is nearly always seen as lines and not as dots or clods arranged as lines, suggesting that the melanocytes are indeed arranged as a contiguous strand.

The pigmentation above the rete ridges continues up to the relatively thick stratum corneum. At weightbearing sites, like the ball of the big toe or heel, these pigment columns above the rete ridges in the stratum corneum may be forced obliquely by pressure, resulting in a crossing pattern composed of short parallel lines. The crossing pattern usually arises from the furrow pattern.

On the face of elderly persons the rete ridges are absent, leading to a flattened epidermis. With no rete ridges, melanin in the basal layers of the epidermis is seen on dermatoscopy not as reticular lines but as a brown structureless area.

A special feature of facial skin is the numerous hair follicles. These funnel-shaped follicular openings (infundibula) appear round from above and dominate the dermatoscopic appearance of pigmented lesions on the face. When these unpigmented openings are surrounded by brown or gray pigmentation (melanin in the epithelium), a pattern of circles is seen. One may also see this pigmentation as brown, gray or black dots arranged as circles around the unpigmented follicular openings.

The histopathologic correlate of structureless areas is different for different colors *(11.6)*. Black structureless areas indicate a collection of melanin in the stratum corneum. Brown structureless areas are produced by melanin in the basal epidermal layers, but only when the rete ridges are absent and the epidermis is flattened. In the presence of rete ridges, basal hyperpigmentation due to melanin is seen as a reticular pattern. Blue and gray structureless areas arise due to melanin aggregates in the dermis. A notable exception is the acanthotic seborrheic keratosis, in which a large increase in thickness of the epidermis (acanthosis) and hyperkeratosis may make epidermal melanin appear gray or even blue. White structureless areas usually correspond to dermal fibrosis.

In summary, a basic knowledge of the microanatomy of the skin is essential for the interpretation of dermatoscopic appearances, and a profound understanding of dermatoscopy only comes with a good understanding of dermatopathology.

Whenever possible dermatoscopic findings should be correlated with histopathology; this is best achieved by viewing the histopathological section oneself with a microscope. For clinicians who do not read their own histopathology slides, communication of dermatoscopic findings to the pathologist is very worthwhile. We have presented a few pigmented lesions with their clinical, dermatoscopic and histopathological correlates as an

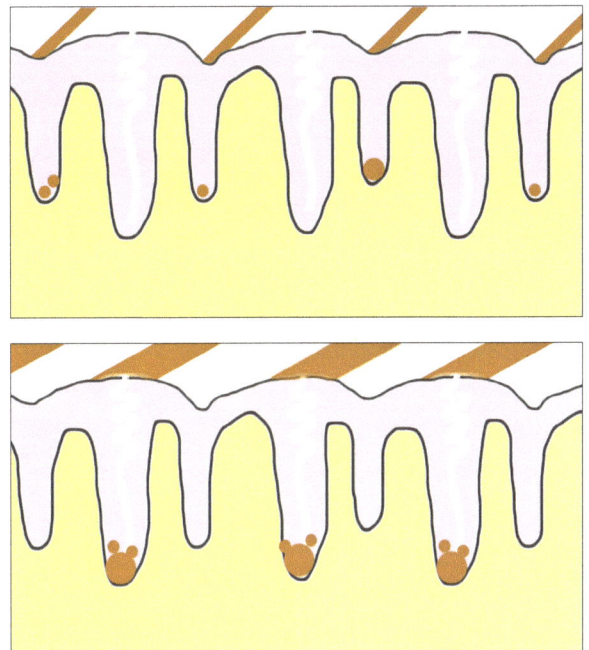

*Figure 11.7: Schematic diagram of the microanatomy of melanocytic lesions on acral skin. **Above:** Furrow pattern. **Below:** Ridge pattern.*

introduction to the field. Further cases may be seen at the Internet sites recommended in the supplement.

References

1. Yadav S, Vossaert KA, Kopf AW et al. Histopathologic correlates of structures seen on dermoscopy (epiluminescence microscopy). Am J Dermatopathol. 1993 Aug; 15(4): 297–305.
2. Soyer HP, Kenet RO, Wolf IH et al. Clinicopathological correlation of pigmented skin lesions using dermoscopy. Eur J Dermatol. 2000 Jan–Feb; 10(1): 22–8.
3. Massi D, De Giorgi V, Soyer HP. Histopathologic correlates of dermoscopic criteria. Dermatol Clin. 2001 Apr; 19(2): 259–68, vii.
4. Ferrara G, Argenziano G, Soyer HP et al. Dermoscopicpathologic correlation: an atlas of 15 cases. Clin Dermatol. 2002 May–Jun; 20(3): 228–35.
5. Ferrara G, Argenyi Z, Argenziano G et al. The influence of clinical information in the histopathologic diagnosis of melanocytic skin neoplasms. PLoS One. 2009; 4(4): e5375.
6. Ferrara G, Argenziano G, Giorgio CM, et al. Dermoscopicpathologic correlation: apropos of six equivocal cases. Semin Cutan Med Surg. 2009 Sep; 28(3): 157–64.

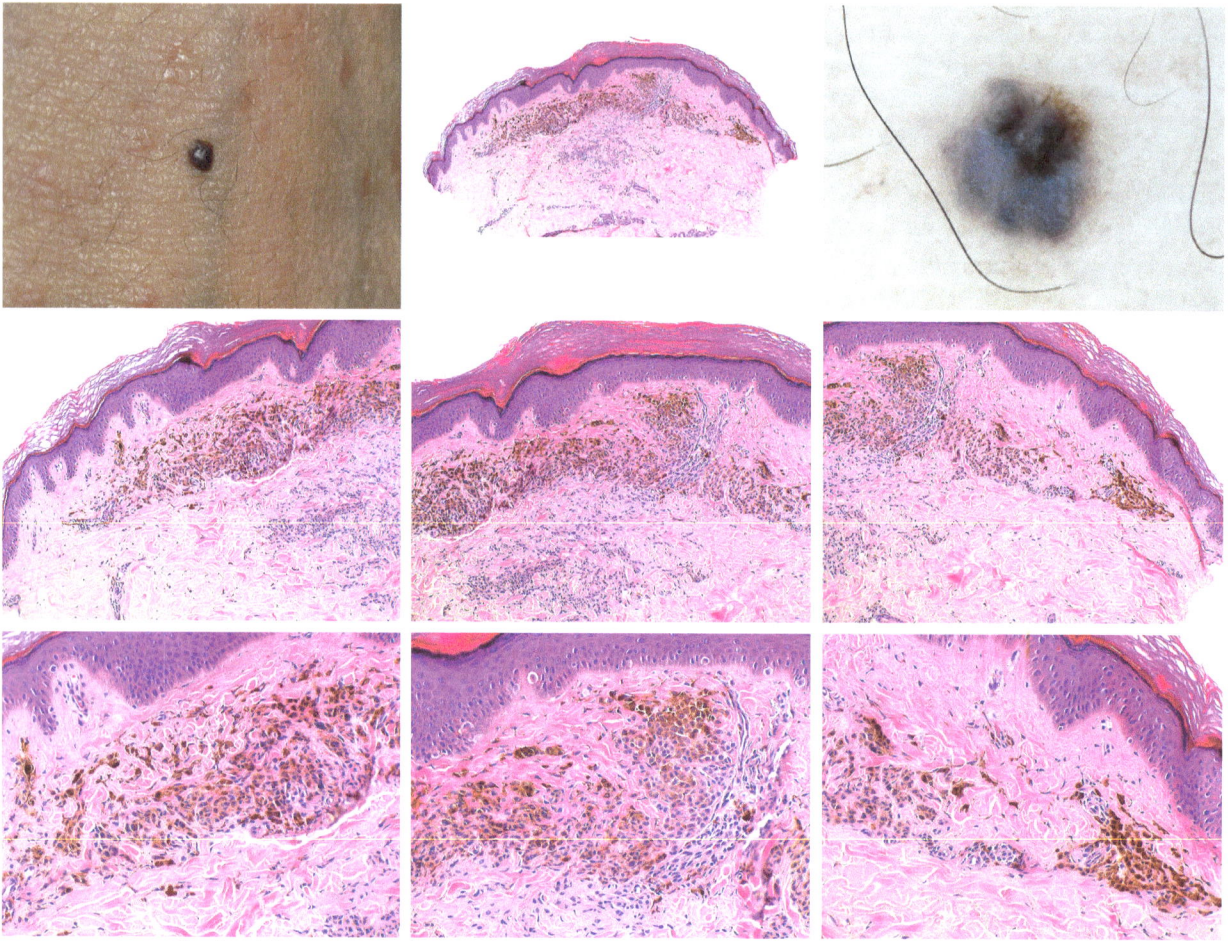

Figure 11.8: "Superficial and deep" congenital nevus.
The clinical and the dermatoscopic image are suggestive of a blue nevus. On dermatoscopy the pattern is structureless blue. The micrographs reveal that the blue structureless area corresponds to a collection of pigmented melanocytes in the dermis, the majority of which are located in the papillary dermis. The melanocytes in the reticular dermis are not pigmented. This example demonstrates that color on dermatoscopy depends not only on the location but also on the density and the distribution of melanin. If melanin in the papillary dermis is situated in macrophages and not in melanocytes one sees gray dots or clods and not a blue structureless area. If melanin in the papillary dermis is sparse and not dense it appears as gray and not as blue structureless area. It is also instructive to see that not all blue lesions are blue nevi. Dermatopathologists call a nevus "blue nevus" if melanocytes in the dermis are dendritic and associated closely with delicate fibrillary bundles of collagen, which is not the case here. The overall architecture and the morphology of melanocytes are that of a "superficial and deep" congenital nevus.

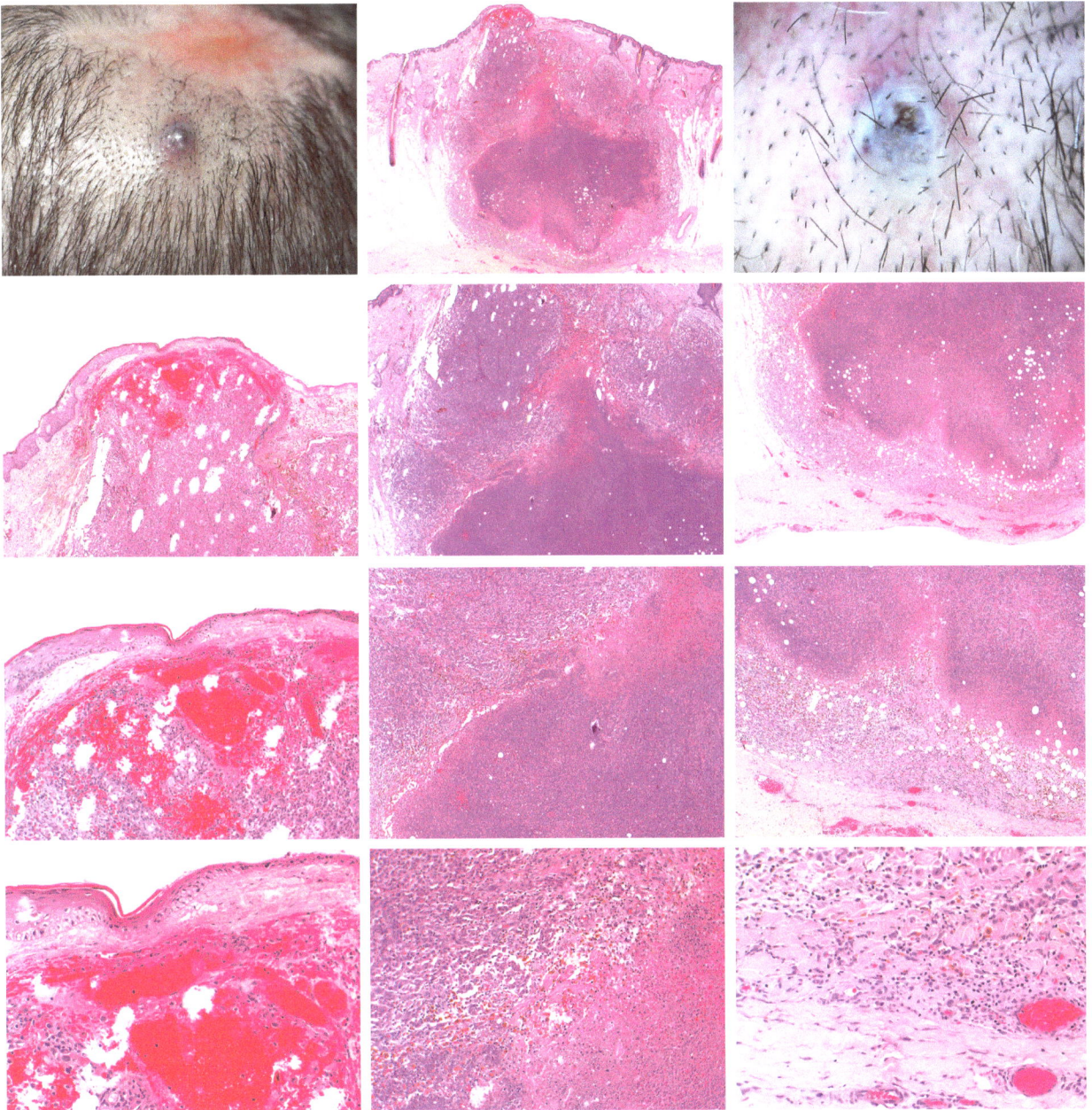

Figure 11.9: Melanoma metastasis.

On dermatoscopy one can see a pigmented lesion with a structureless pattern and blue color similar to the lesion shown in figure 11.8. In the center there is a small black and orange structureless zone which corresponds to a zone of erosion histopathologically (black corresponds to congealed blood and orange to dried serum). Underneath the erosion one can see a nodular proliferation of neoplastic, partly pigmented, melanocytes in the dermis and in the subcutaneous fat. This proliferation of melanocytes appears structureless blue on dermatoscopy. The pleomorphic melanocytes, numerous mitoses, the arrangement of neoplastic melanocytes in the dermis and the lack of an epidermal component make this a melanoma metastasis. This example demonstrates why dermatoscopy cannot replace dermatopathologic examination. Dermatoscopy cannot differentiate between a blue nevus, a melanoma or a melanoma metastasis.

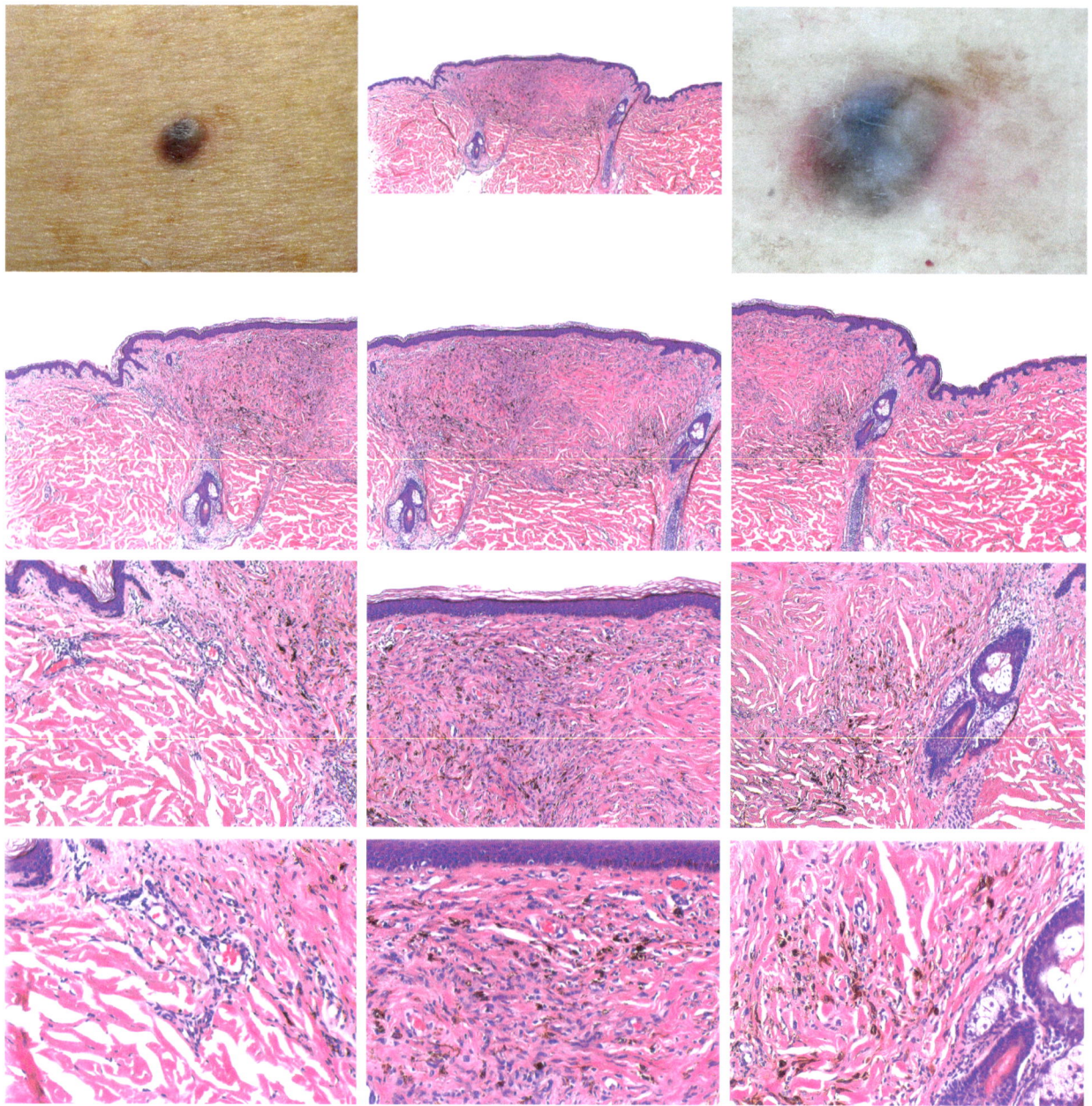

Figure 11.10: *Blue nevus.*
The dermatoscopy of this lesion is identical with the lesion in figure 11.8. One finds a blue structureless area, which corresponds to melanin in the dermis. In contrast to the "superficial and deep" congenital nevus in figure 11.8 one can see a dermal proliferation of deeply pigmented melanocytes with prominent dendrites. Ackerman believed that which has been designated "blue nevus" is really several very different kinds of melanocytic nevi that he named eponymously, such as for Tièche (so-called common blue nevus), Allen (so-called cellular blue nevus), and Masson (so-called blue-neuronevus). The distinctive congenital nevus pictured here is the one described first by Tièche in collaboration with Jadassohn.

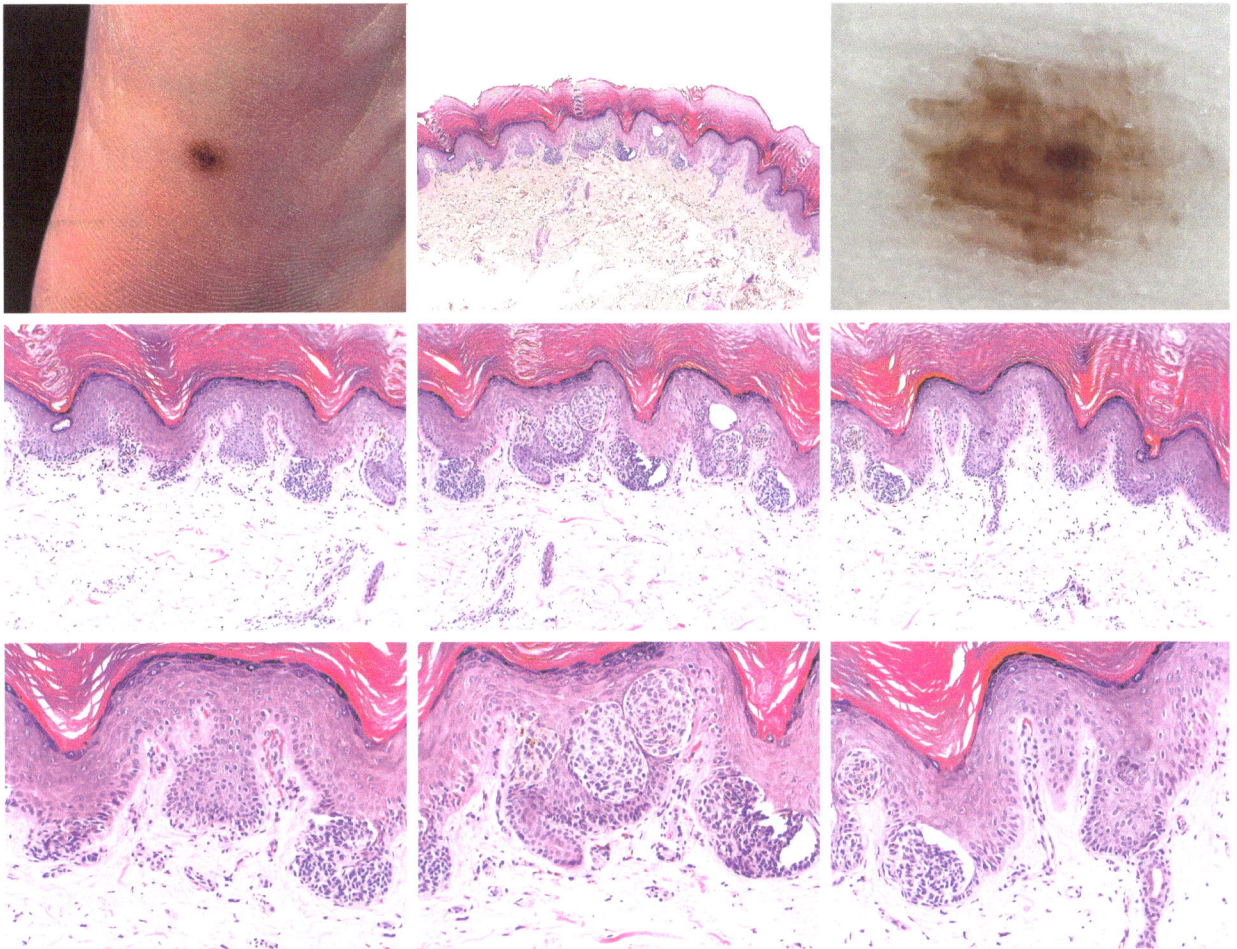

Figure 11.11: *"Superficial" congenital nevus.*
The dermatoscopic image of this nevus reveals a pattern of clods. Histopathologically the clods correspond to large nests of melanocytes in the epidermis. It can be seen that clods are located on the ridges and in the furrows. Accordingly the nests of melanocytes can be found in all rete ridges. This is a "superficial" congenital nevus and not a classic acral nevus, because in the latter the epidermal nests are smaller and located preferentially in the rete ridges underneath the furrows. The pattern of clods is typical for congenital nevi, irrespective of the anatomic site. The terminology of acral nevi is confusing. In general almost all types of nevi may be found on acral skin but some types prefer other locations. Clark nevi for example practically never appear on acral skin and only rarely on the face.

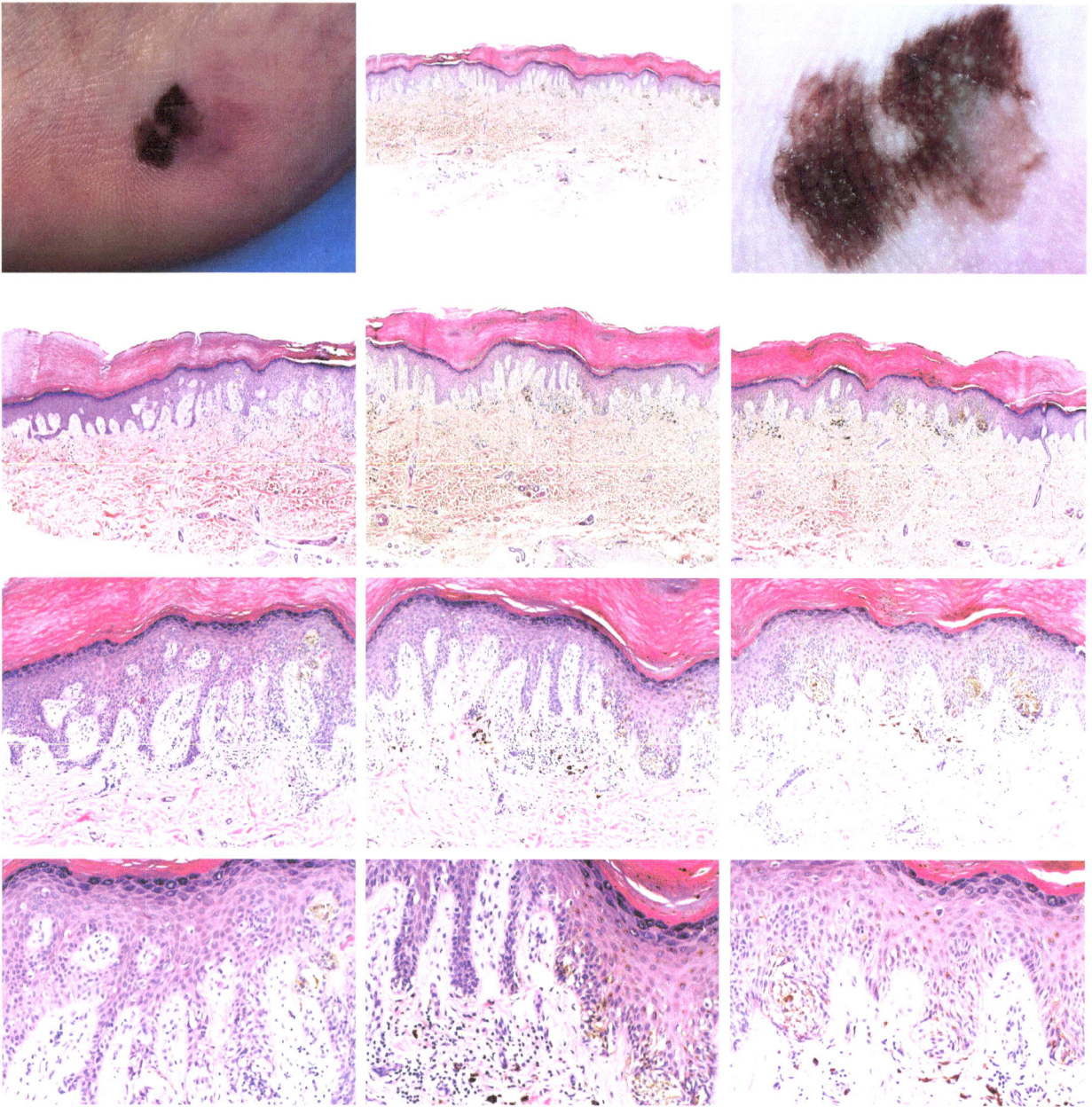

Figure 11.12: Melanoma, acral.

Dermatoscopy of this melanoma on acral skin reveals chaos. One can see several patterns and colors arranged asymmetrically. There are dots, lines (on the ridges but also in the furrows), and a structureless area; the colors are brown, gray and black. Neoplastic melanocytes in the epidermis are arranged as nests, strands and as single cells. The lack of clods on dermatoscopy suggests that the appearance of nests has actually been created by crosswise sectioning of strands. The black dots seen on dermatoscopy correspond to small collections of melanin in the stratum corneum.

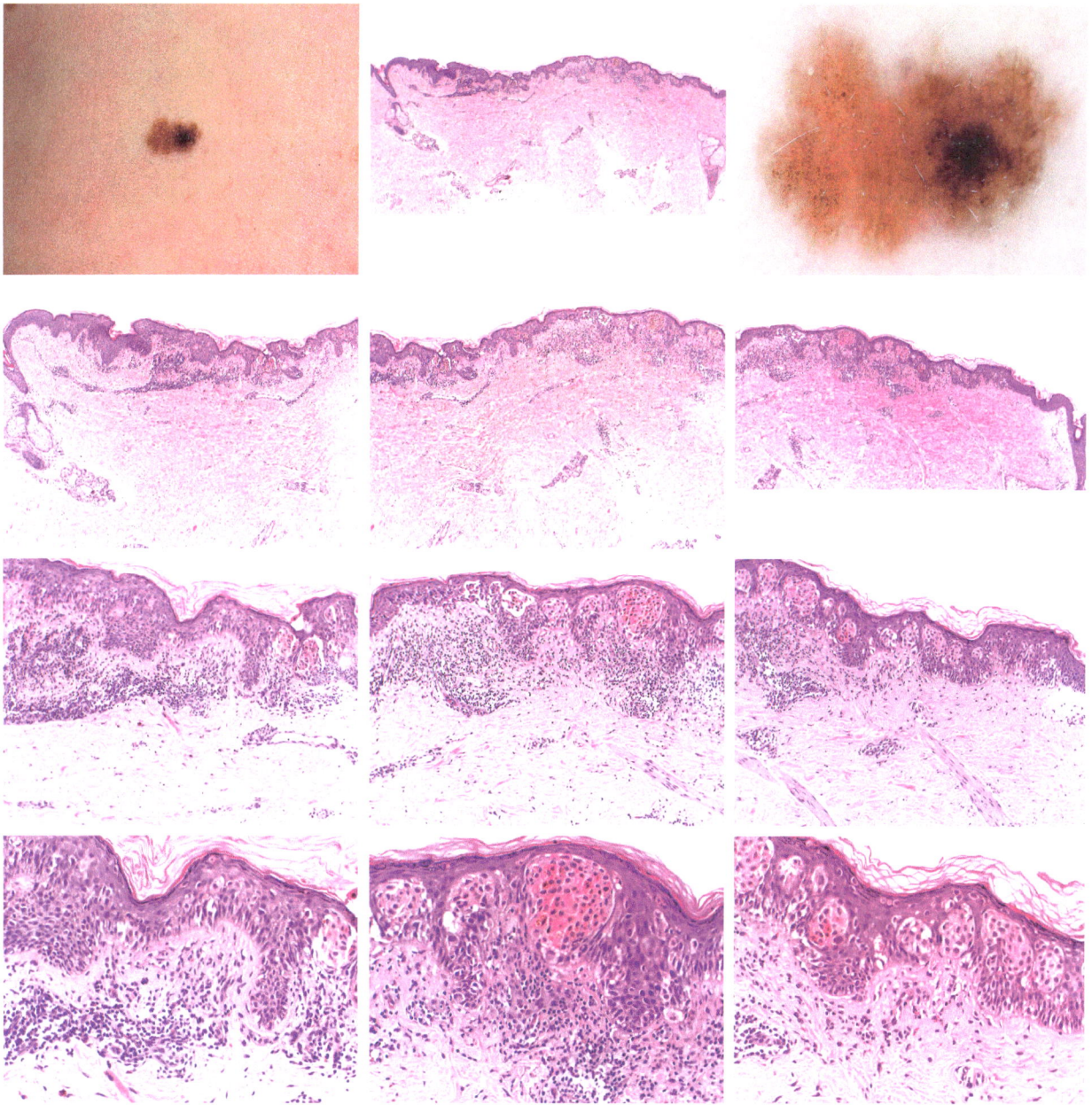

Figure 11.13: *Melanoma in situ.*
On the clinical image one can see asymmetry of color but the striking structural asymmetry (asymmetry of pattern) is only revealed by dermatoscopy. On one side there is a pattern of reticular lines and a structureless brown area, on the other side one can see clods that vary in size and shape. The brown clods on dermatoscopy correspond to large nests of neoplastic melanocytes in the epidermis. The melanocytes are replete with melanin.

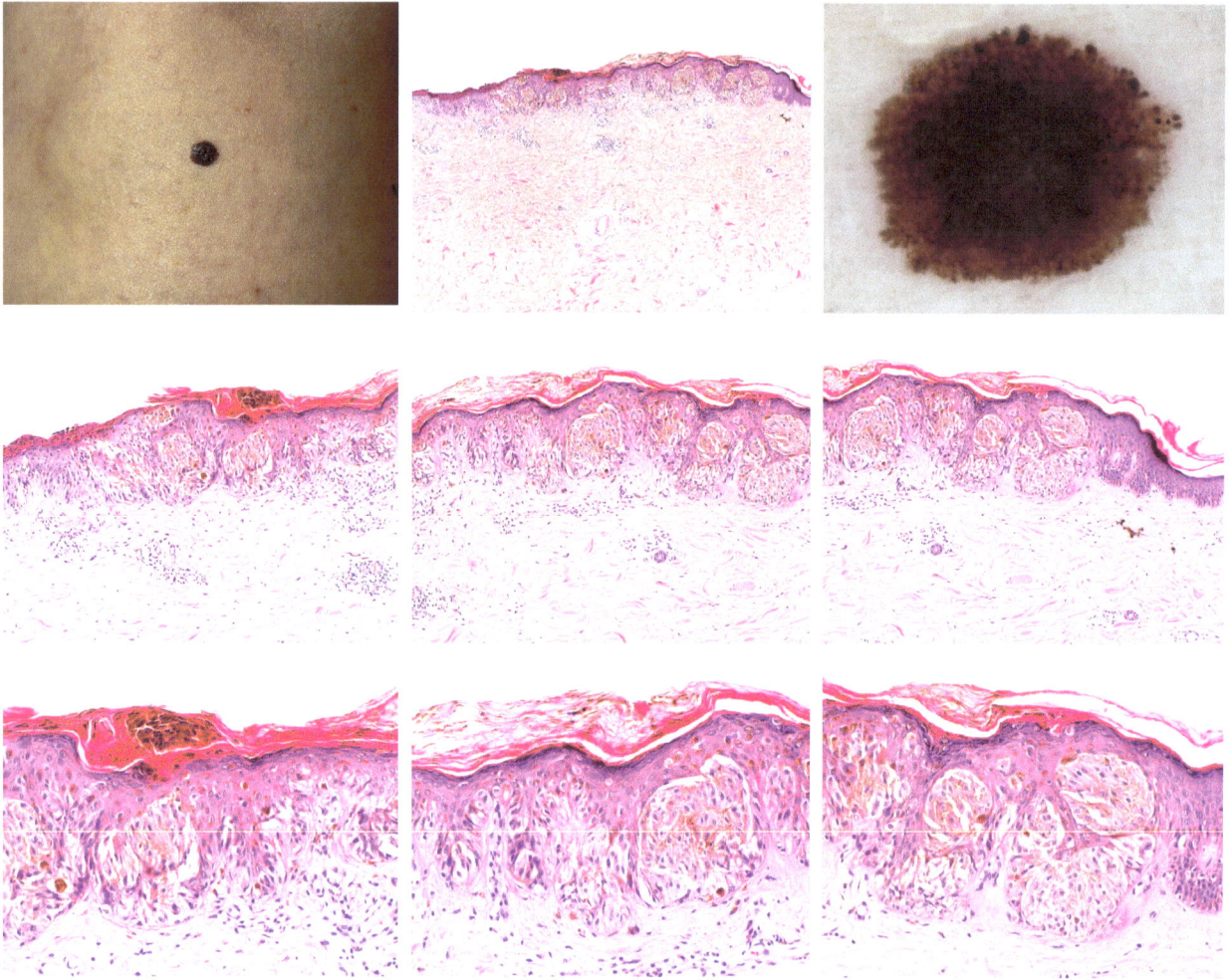

Figure 11.14: *Melanoma in situ.*
This heavily pigmented lesion is reminiscent of a Reed nevus clinically. On dermatoscopy one sees a dark brown and black structureless area in the center and clods and pseudopods in the periphery. Histopathologically the clods correspond to epidermal nests of pleomorphic melanocytes. The clods and the nests vary in size and shape. The pseudopods correspond to melanocytes arranged in fascicles that are not visible on the micrographs. If the fascicles are cut crosswise and not tangentially they look like nests histopathologically. In the center there is a dense accumulation of melanin in the stratum corneum which corresponds to the black structureless zone seen on dermatoscopy. One of the black clods at the periphery can be identified on the micrographs as a collection of melanin in the stratum corneum.

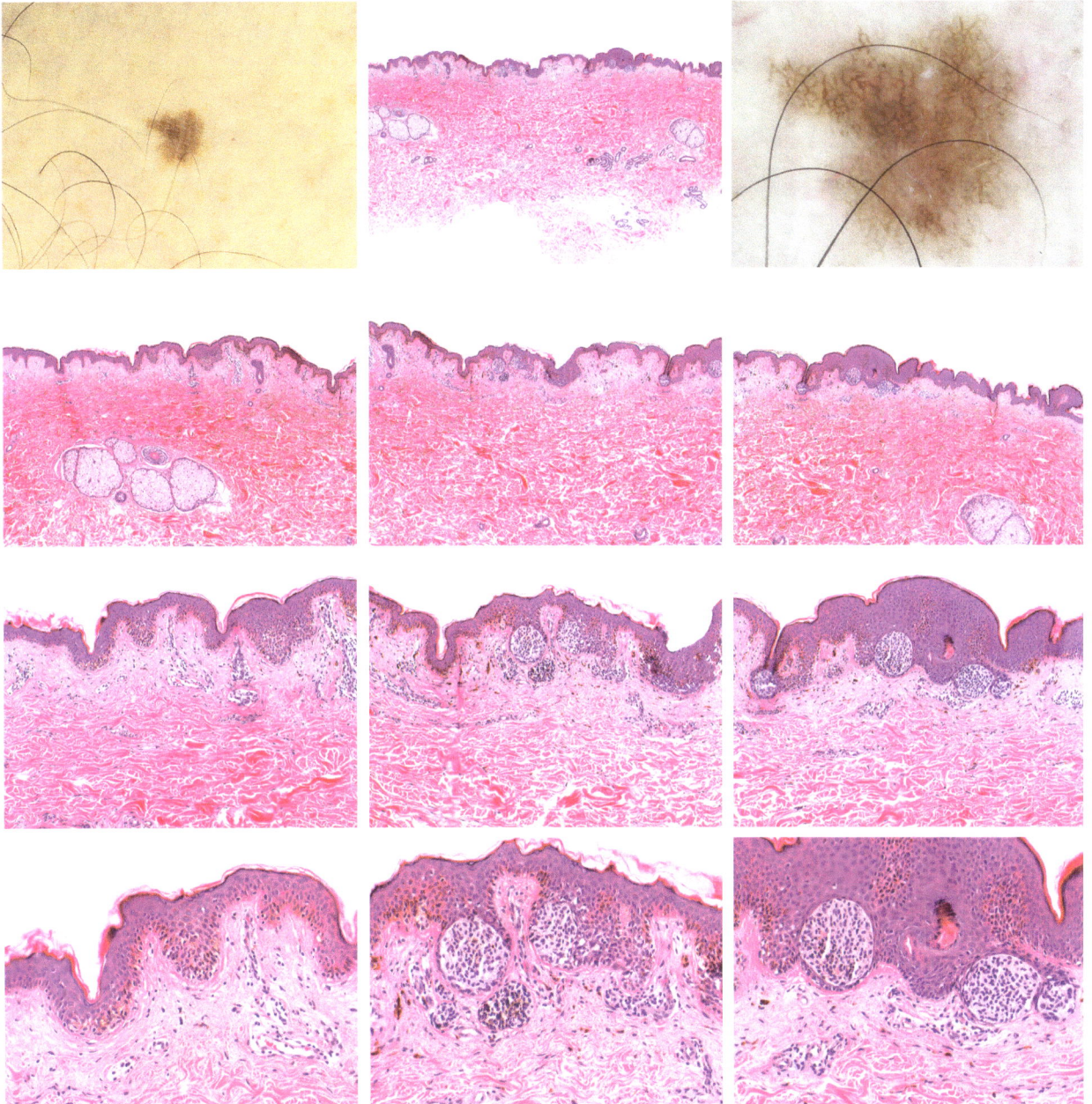

Figure 11.15: *Clark nevus.*
The only pattern visible on dermatoscopy is reticular lines. There are a few brown dots but they are too sparse to form a pattern. Histopathologically the reticular lines correspond to hyperpigmented basal keratinocytes. The small epidermal nests are composed of pigmented and non-pigmented melanocytes that are small and monomorphous. Only those nests that house pigmented melanocytes are visible as brown dots on dermatoscopy. The nests that are situated in the rete ridges are located on the reticular lines dermatoscopically. Dots or clods that are located between the lines are situated in the dermal papilla and indicate that the lesion involves the dermis. Small nests of melanocytes positioned entirely at the dermo-epidermal junction (or in the papillary dermis in the center of the lesion), are typical of Clark nevus.

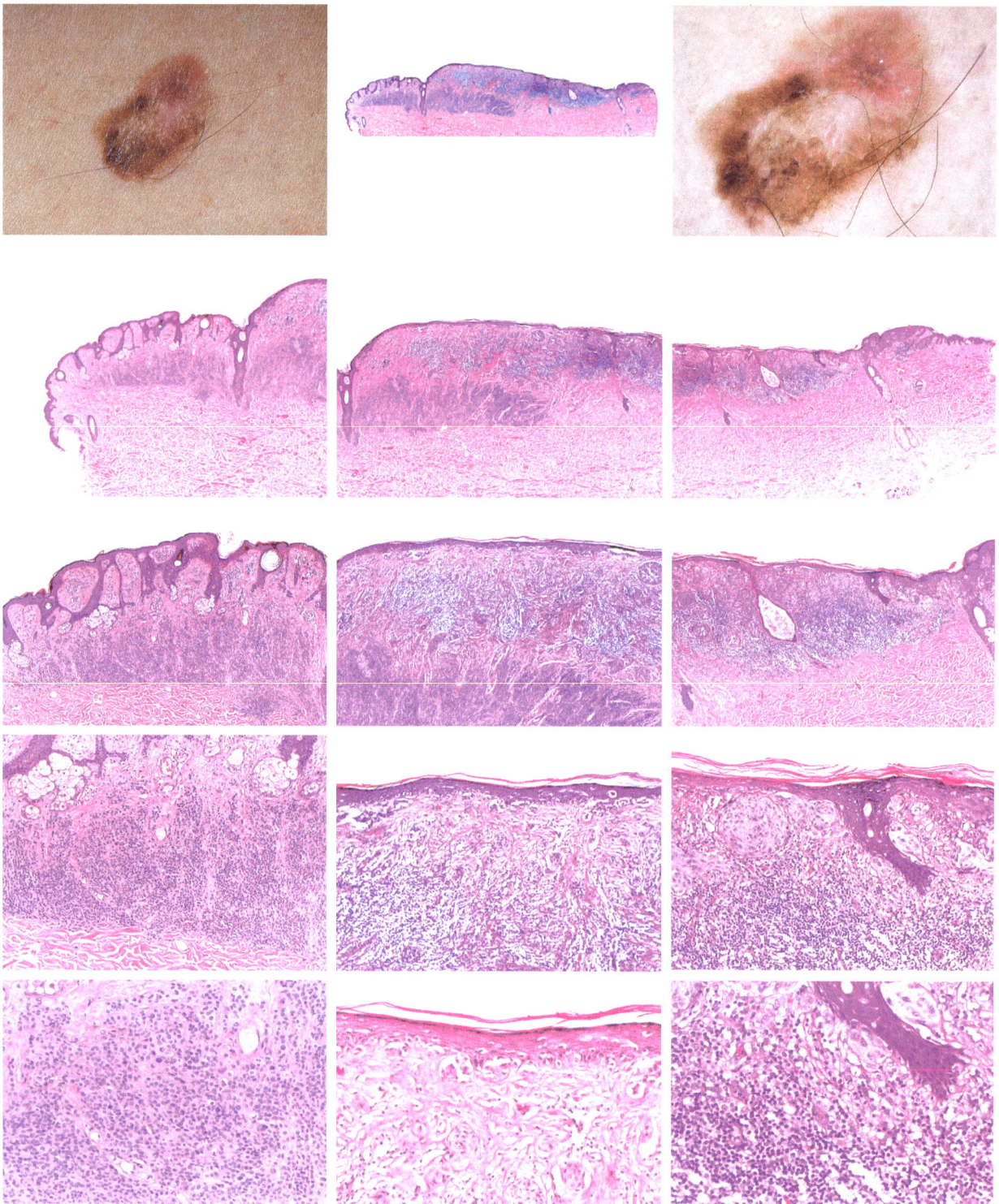

Figure 11.16: *Melanoma in association with a "superficial and deep" congenital nevus.*
Most melanomas, i.e. about 80–85% of them in "Caucasians", develop de novo. When, however, melanoma develops in a pre-existing nevus, that nevus is likely to be congenital, usually one "superficial and deep" and not a Clark nevus. Clinically this lesion is multicolored and asymmetric. One can see an increased number of terminal hairs. On dermatoscopy the lesion is chaotic with white reticular lines as a clue to melanoma. At scanning power magnification, two completely different architectural patterns are evident, namely, that of a "superficial and deep" congenital nevus on the left and a melanoma on the right. The patterns contrast sharply, the congenital nevus being present in abundance in the upper part of the reticular dermis, thereby qualifying it as "superficial and deep", with no nests at the dermoepidermal junction. The melanoma is housed mostly in the epidermis, but also in the papillary dermis, and shows a dense infiltrate of lymphocytes. The reticular lines correspond to pigmented keratinocytes in the epidermis, especially the basal layer. White reticular lines correspond to fibroplasia of the papillary dermis beneath an epidermis that displays distinct rete ridges. The white lines are thick because the dermal papillae are broad.

Supplement

Recommended websites for continuous education

www.derm101.com
Comprehensive online library of resources for the diagnosis and treatment of skin diseases. One of the resources is dedicated to dermatoscopy. Five new cases every month with clinical-derma-toscopic-dermatopathologic correlation. High quality images.

Dermatoscopy on Facebook
Great cases, great members, easy to use (if you like Facebook).
www.facebook.com/groups/dermatoscopy

www.dermoscopyatlas.com
Comprehensive online atlas

www.dermoscopy.org
Dermatoscopy from a different point of view. Good image quality.

www.dermoscopy-ids.org
Official website of the International Society of Dermoscopy (IDS). High quality images. Discussion group.

Skin Cancer College Australasia
For access to the Skin Cancer College Australasia Skin Cancer Blog international registered medical practitioners can email info@skincancercollege.org to request guest access.

dermoscopic.blogspot.com
Comprehensive collection of dermatoscopic images

Other sites
www.dermoscopyconsult.com
dermnetnz.org/doctors/dermoscopy-course
www.dermatology.org.uk/dermoscopy-courses.html
www.dermnet.com/dermoscopy-videos
www.dermoscopy.co.uk

Master of science in dermatoscopy
www.medunigraz.at/dermoscopy

Master of Medicine (Skin Cancer) Program
The University of Queensland, Australia
www.skincancermasters.com
or email cliffrosendahl@bigpond.com

"One of the symptoms of an approaching nervous breakdown is the belief that one's work is terribly important."
Bertrand Russell

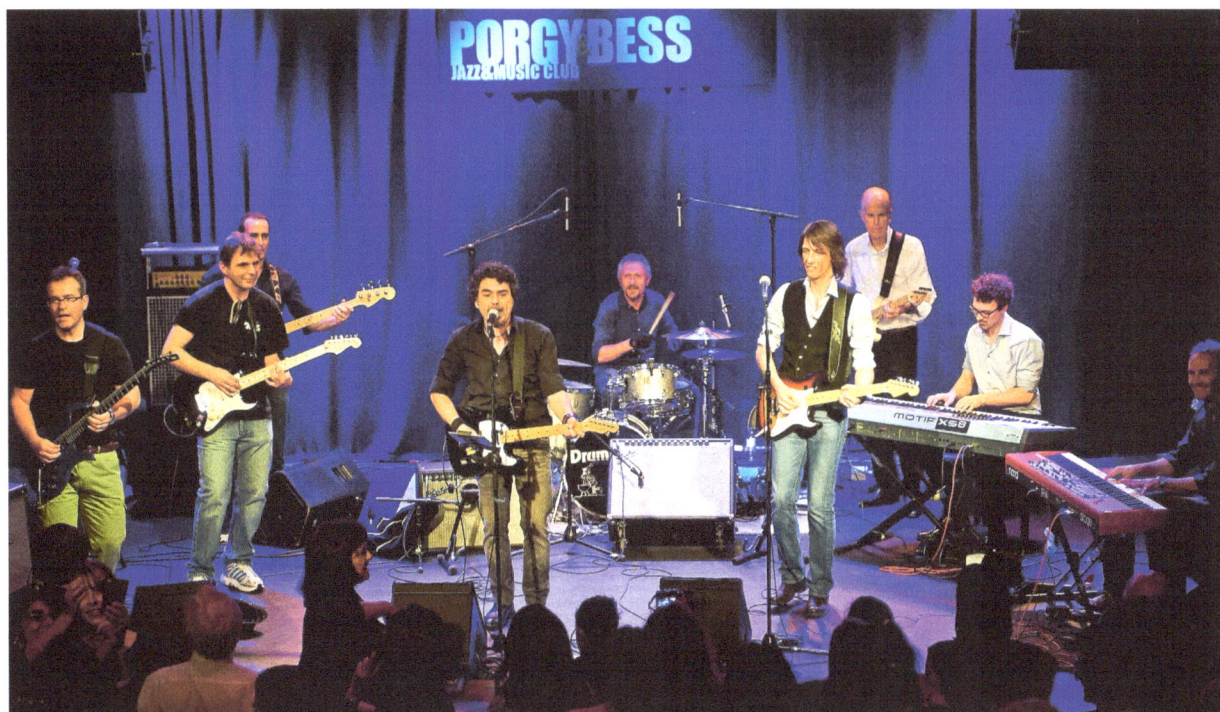

"Los globulos marrones" with Harald Kittler (guitar), Philipp Tschandl (keyboard), Giuseppe Argenziano (drums), Luc Thomas (guitar), Peter Bourne (guitar) live in Vienna, Austria during the World Congress of Dermatoscopy 2015.

Index

3-point checklist 17
4-dot clod 210
7-point check-list (Argenziano) 17
   "atypical" Spitz nevus 35

A

ABCD rule (Stolz) 17
accessory nipple 285
Ackerman nevus 31
acral lesion 260
acral nevus 28
actinic keratosis 50, 215
adherent fiber 235f
adnexal neoplasm 50
age spots 49
amelanotic melanoma 229
angiokeratoma 42ff
angulated lines 55, 125f, 242
annular-granular pattern 126
apocrine cysts 51
atypical fibroxanthoma 230
atypical nevus 37
atypical pigment network 127
atypical Spitz nevus 35

B

bacteria 291
Bannayan-Riley-Ruvalcaba syndrome 49
BAPomas 40
basal cell carcinoma 50, 89, 215
biopsy of the nail matrix 257
black heel 45
blotch 127, 140
blue nevus 29, 106
blue veil 128
blue-gray ovoid nests 128
blue-white veil 128
Bowen's disease 50, 93, 215
brain-like pattern 129
branched lines 55
branched streaks 129
broadened pigment network 129

C

calcinosis cutis 210, 221
Carney complex 49
CASH algorithm 17
central white patch 129
cerebriform pattern 129
chaos 191f
chaos and clues 18, 190
cherry angioma (tardive angioma) 42
chrysalids 130
chrysalis 130
circles 55
Clark nevus 29f, 97
clear cell acanthoma 221, 223
cliché 243ff
clods 55
clues 66f, 193ff
clues to malignancy 192f
cobblestone pattern 130
combined congenital nevus 32f, 104
combined nevus 33
comedo-like openings 130
compound nevus 39
congenital nevus 31f
crown vessels 132
crypts 132
crystalline 130
curved lines 55
cutaneous amyloidosis 290
cutaneous Lupus erythematosus 287f

D

dermal nevus 35, 39, 228
dermatofibroma 51, 81
dermatoscopy of nail pigmentation 253
digital dermatoscopic monitoring 297ff
digital mucoid (myxoid) cyst 225
dots 55
double reticular lines 238
dysplastic nevus 37

E

eccrine poroma	221, 224, 232
exogenous pigmentation	266

F

fat fingers	132
fibrillar pattern	132
fibropithelioma of Pinkus	231
fingerprinting	132
fissures and ridges	133
folliculitis	207, 209
four dots in a square (four-dot clod)	238
four-dot clod	210
freckle	49
fungal infection of the nail plate	259
fungi	290f
furuncle	207

G

genital lentiginosis	47, 280
genital lentigo	89
globules (globuli)	133
granulomatous inflammation	210
Grover's disease	286, 290
gyri	129

H

hemangioma	42, 74f
hemoglobin	64
hemorrhage	45
high-grade dysplastic nevus	37
homogeneous pattern	133
Hortaea werneckii	51
Hutchinson's sign	255
hypermelanotic nevus	40

I

ink-spot lentigo	47f, 81
intracorneal hemorrhage	77
intraepidermal carcinoma	50
inverse (negative) pigment network	134
irregular peripheral extensions	136
irregular pigment network	127

J

junctional nevus	39

K

Kaposi sarcoma	43f, 284
Kaposi's disease (Kaposi sarcoma)	44f
keratin	204
keratinocyte cancer	50
keratoacanthoma	224, 226

L

labial lentigo	89, 279
large cell anaplastic T-cell lymphoma	232
lattice-like pattern	134
Laugier-Hunziker syndrome	47, 49
leaf-like structure	135
leishmaniasis	210, 221
lentigines (melanotic macules)	280
lentiginosis of the lip	47
lentigo	45
lentigo solaris	49
LEOPARD syndrome	47, 49
lichen planus	215, 286, 288f
lichen planus-like keratosis	50, 81, 278
liver spots	49
Lupus erythematosus	215, 286
lymphangioma	210

M

malignant peripheral nerve sheath tumor	230
maple leaf-like areas	135
melanin	62
melanocytoma	40
melanoma	42, 113
melanoma of the nail plate	255
melanotic macule	45, 81
MELTUMP	35
Menzies' method	17
Merkel cell carcinoma	221, 227
metastases of melanoma	121
metastasis	221
Meyerson nevus	40
micro-Hutchinson's sign	255
Miescher nevus	35, 113
milia-like cysts	135
milky red areas	136
Molluscum contagiosum	221, 286, 290
monomorphous	215
moth-eaten border	136
mucosal lentiginosis	280
mucosal lesions	280
mucosal melanoma	280
myiasis	207

N

nails	253f.
nevus araneus ("spider nevus")	42, 44
nevus flammeus ("port-wine stain")	44
nevus sebaceous	211
nevus spilus	35
non-pigmented (amelanotic) lesions	203
nummular dermatitis	215

P

parallel lines	55
parasites	291
pattern analysis	16, 18
pediculosis	286
penile lentiginosis	279
peppering	136
peripheral streaks	136
periungual pigmented Bowen's disease	267
Peutz-Jeghers syndrome	47, 49
picker's nodule	221
pigment network	136f
pigmented actinic keratosis	89, 278
pigmented purpura	51
pilomatrixoma	207, 210, 221
pityriasis rosea	215, 286
polygons	125f, 242
porokeratosis	215, 286, 288
prurigo	221
pseudo-Hutchinson sign	256
Pseudomonas aeruginosa	259
pseudo-network	137, 269
pseudopods	55
psoriasis	215, 286, 287
PUVA lentigines	47f
pyogenic granuloma	42, 76, 207

R

radial lines	55
radial streaming	137
rainbow pattern	138
recurrent melanocytic lesions	280
recurrent nevus	35, 106
red lacunes	138
Reed nevus	35, 106
reticular depigmentation	134, 138
reticular lines	53
rhomboids	126, 139
rosettes	139, 238

S

sarcoidal rosacea	286
sarcoidosis	286
scabies	286, 291
scale	203
scar-like depigmentation	139
sebaceous gland hyperplasia	207, 209, 221
seborrheic keratosis	49, 80
shiny white lines	130
shiny white streaks	130, 140
solar lentigines with regression	278
solar lentigo	77
solitary angiokeratoma	76
spider nevus (nevus araneus)	42, 215
Spitz nevus	35, 106
spoke-wheel areas	140
spongiotic dermatitis	215, 286
squamous cell carcinoma	50, 89
starburst pattern	141
stasis purpura	51
strands	140
strawberry pattern	141
string of pearls	142
structureless pattern	55
subungual bleeding	258
sulci	129
superficial and deep congenital nevus	31, 97
superficial congenital nevus	31, 97
surface scale	203
Sutton nevus (Halo nevus)	35

T

tardive angioma (cherry angioma)	42
targetoid dots	142
targetoid vessels	142
tattoo	51, 284
telangiectasia macularis perstans	215
Tinea nigra	51, 286, 290, 292
trichoblastoma	50
trichoepithelioma	224
Trichomycosis palmellina	286, 291
tungiasis	286

U

ulceration	203
Unna nevus	35, 113, 228

V

Verruca genitalis 286
Verruca palmaris 286
Verruca plana 286
Verruca vulgaris 286
vessels 70ff
viral warts 221, 290
vulvar melanoma 279

W

white circles 208, 242
white clues 205
white lines 241
white scale 215
Wiesner nevus 40

X

xanthelasma 210
xanthogranuloma 210f

Z

zig-zag pattern 126, 142
Zitelli nevus 31f

www.ingramcontent.com/pod-product-compliance
Lightning Source LLC
Chambersburg PA
CBHW050800220326
41598CB00006B/82